WITHDRAWN

MACROPHAGES AND LYMPHOCYTES

Nature, Functions, and Interaction

PART A

ADVANCES IN EXPERIMENTAL MEDICINE AND BIOLOGY

Editorial Board:

NATHAN BACK, *State University of New York at Buffalo*

N. R. DI LUZIO, *Tulane University School of Medicine*

EPHRAIM KATCHALSKI-KATZIR, *The Weizmann Institute of Science*

DAVID KRITCHEVSKY, *Wistar Institute*

ABEL LAJTHA, *New York State Research Institute for Neurochemistry and Drug Addiction*

RODOLFO PAOLETTI, *University of Milan*

Recent Volumes in this Series

Volume 117
STEROID HORMONE RECEPTOR SYSTEMS
Edited by Wendell W. Leavitt and James H. Clark

Volume 118
CELL SUBSTRATES: Their Use in the Production of Vaccines and Other Biologicals
Edited by John C. Petricciani, Hope E. Hopps, and Paul J. Chapple

Volume 119
TREATMENT OF EARLY DIABETES
Edited by Rafael A. Camerini-Davalos and Bernard Hanover

Volume 120A
KININS – II: Biochemistry, Pathophysiology, and Clinical Aspects
Edited by Setsuro Fujii, Hiroshi Moriya, and Tomoji Suzuki

Volume 120B
KININS – II: Systemic Proteases and Cellular Function
Edited by Setsuro Fujii, Hiroshi Moriya, and Tomoji Suzuki

Volume 121A
MACROPHAGES AND LYMPHOCYTES: Nature, Functions, and Interaction, Part A
Edited by Mario R. Escobar and Herman Friedman

Volume 121B
MACROPHAGES AND LYMPHOCYTES: Nature, Functions, and Interaction, Part B
Edited by Mario R. Escobar and Herman Friedman

Volume 122A
PURINE METABOLISM IN MAN – III: Clinical and Theoretical Aspects
Edited by Aurelio Rapado, C. H. M. M. de Bruyn, and R. W. E. Watts

Volume 122B
PURINE METABOLISM IN MAN – III: Biochemical, Immunological, and Cancer Research
Edited by Aurelio Rapado, C. H. M. M. de Bruyn, and R. W. E. Watts

Volume 123
GABA – Biochemistry and CNS Functions
Edited by Paul Mandel and Francis V. DeFeudis

Volume 124
THE ENDOCRINE PANCREAS AND JUVENILE DIABETES
Edited by David M. Klachko, Ralph R. Anderson, Thomas W. Burns, and Harold V. Werner

MACROPHAGES AND LYMPHOCYTES

Nature, Functions, and Interaction

PART A

Edited by

Mario R. Escobar

Medical College of Virginia
Richmond, Virginia

and

Herman Friedman

University of South Florida
Tampa, Florida

WITHDRAWN

PLENUM PRESS • NEW YORK AND LONDON

Library of Congress Cataloging in Publication Data

Reticuloendothelial Society.
Macrophages and lymphocytes, nature, functions, and interaction.

(Advances in experimental medicine and biology; v. 121)
"Proceedings of the eighth international congress of the Reticuloendothelial Society, held in Jerusalem, Israel, June 18–23, 1978."
Includes index.
1. Macrophages – Congresses. 2. Lymphocytes – Congresses. 3. Reticulo-endothelial system – Congresses. 4. Immune response – Congresses. I. Escobar, Mario R. II. Friedman, Herman, 1931- III. Title. IV. Series.
QR185.8.M3R47 1979 599'.02'9 79-9566
ISBN 0-306-40285-8 (Part A)

Proceedings of the Eight International Congress of the Reticuloendothelial Society, held in Jerusalem, Israel, June 18–23, 1978, of which this is part one.

© 1980 Plenum Press, New York
A Division of Plenum Publishing Corporation
227 West 17th Street, New York, N.Y. 10011

All rights reserved

No part of this book may be reproduced, stored in a retrieval system, or transmitted, in any form or by any means, electronic, mechanical, photocopying, microfilming, recording, or otherwise, without written permission from the publisher

Printed in the United States of America

599.029
R438m
v.1

PROCEEDINGS OF THE

VIII INTERNATIONAL CONGRESS OF THE RETICULOENDOTHELIAL SOCIETY

Jerusalem, Israel   *June 18-23, 1978*

ORGANIZING AND PROGRAM COMMITTEE: M. Schlesinger, M. M. Sigel, H. Friedman and M. R. Escobar

ISRAELI HOST COMMITTEE: M. Schlesinger, M. Feldman, R. Gallily, C. Greenblatt, D. Pluznik and J. Yoffey

LIAISON MEMBERS: S. M. Reichard, W. Th. Daems, M. Kojima, M. G. Hanna, J. Harris and M. La Via

INTERNATIONAL REPRESENTATIVES: J. Babnik, L. A. Chedid, V. Esmann, K. Flemming, P. Garzon, J. Gras Riera, P. J. Jacques, D. Nelson, G. Nitulescu, F. Rossi, B. E. Schildt, O. Stendahl, A. E. Stuart, M. Timar and I. Toro

This meeting is dedicated
to the memory of
NEWTON B. EVERETT
May 12, 1916
May 23, 1979

34557

Preface

The Reticuloendothelial (RE) Society, which is concerned with advancement of knowledge concerning the many diverse functions of RE cells, organizes national and international meetings and publishes a scientific journal. The VIII International Congress of the RE Society was held in Jerusalem, Israel, June 18-23, 1978. The Congress had as its scientific objective a wide range of subjects concerning the RE System, especially as related to macrophage function and interaction with lymphocytes. Emphasis of the Congress was placed on the nature and function of macrophages and other cells of the RE System with reference to immune responses, anti-infectious activity, tumor immunity, autoimmunity, and transplant rejection. The secretion of soluble factors by macrophages and lymphocytes and the mode of action of these factors on other cells was stressed. During the Congress some discussion was entertained concerning the controversy as to what constitutes the "RE System" per se. Some investigators feel that the phagocytic activity of macrophages is the most important aspect of the RE System playing also a major role in many parameters of immunity. Mononuclear phagocytes include tissue macrophages as well as circulating monocytes and their precursors. Although phagocytosis is a major functional activity of these cells, it is only one of several activities. The important role of mononuclear phagocytes and other mononuclear cells in immune responsiveness, - including humoral and cell mediated immunity, specific and nonspecific resistance to microorganisms and tumor cells, as well as homeostatic activities in general - has become the focus of attention of many investigators and served as a focal point for the exchange of scientific information during the Congress.

The Congress was immediately preceded by the 6th International Conference on Germinal Centers and Lymphatic Tissues in Immune Reactions being held in Kiel, Germany, June 11-16, 1978. The RES Congress was followed by the 12th International Leukocyte Culture Conference being held in Beersheba, Israel June 25-30, 1978. An attempt was made by the Organizing and Program Committees for the 3 conventions to interrelate the scientific topics planned for presentation. Thus, the RES Congress dealt mainly with macrophage nature and functions whereas the Leukocyte Culture Conference devoted much attention to the role and activities of lymphocytes. The RES Congress was divided into symposia, contributed papers, and workshop sessions. Five symposia were held during each morning on the following topics: I. Regulatory Functions of the RE System, II. Enzymatic Activities of Macrophages, III. Role of Macrophages in Tumor Activity, IV. Environmental Factors Influencing the RES, and V. Interactions of Macrophages and Lymphocytes in the Immune Response.

Each afternoon was devoted to several simultaneous scientific sessions with short papers presented on subjects of current interest to the RE System. Although workshops devoted to particularly important areas of the RE System were useful and well-attended, their publication is not included in these volumes because of the priority given to the large number of formal papers selected for their high quality and relevance.

These volumes constitute the published records of the proceedings of the Congress, including only the symposia and selected proffered papers. However, the written contributions are not arranged exactly as presented at the Congress but rather they are interspersed according to the central theme of each of the four sections for each volume. The first volume deals with the enzymatic and metabolic activities of RE cells, the immunopharmacology and regulatory functions of the RE System, as well as with environmental factors influencing the latter. The second volume includes papers concerned with immunity and infection, interaction of cells in the RE System and immunomodulation in cancer.

M. R. Escobar

H. Friedman

Acknowledgments

The editors are indebted to Drs. N. R. Di Luzio, K. B. P. Flemming, C. Greenblatt, M. G. Hanna, T. Mekori-Felsteiner, Q. N. Myrvik, D. Nachtigal, D. H. Pluznik, J. J. Oppenheim, M. Quastel, F. Rossi, J. B. Solomon, K. Stern and N. Trainin who chaired the Symposia. Many thanks to Drs. P. Abramoff, J. Battisto, T. K. Eisenstein, T. N. Harris, P. J. Jacques, A. M., Kaplan, M. Kojima, F. J. Lejeune, T. J. Linna, Q. N. Myrvik, S. J. Normann, P. Patriarca, J. Pitt, S. M. Reichard, B. V. Siegel, R. N. Taub, G. Wertheim and E. F. Wheelock who chaired the Short Paper Sessions. Gratitude is expressed to Drs. N. R. Di Luzio, T. K. Eisenstein, A. Ghaffar, C. Greenblatt, H. W. Holy, P. J. Jacques, H. Koren, P. Patriarca, W. Regelson, M. M. Sigel and others for their valuable assistance in preparing the workshops. This Congress could not have succeeded without the financial support of Accurate Chemical and Scientific Corporation; Battelle Memorial Institute; Dako of Denmark; Merck and Company; Nyegaard of Norway; Ortho Pharmaceutical Company; Owens-Illinois; The Upjohn Company; USV Pharmaceutical Company; and especially, the generous donation from the Fogharty International Center of the National Institutes of Health (USA). Recognition is extended to M. A. Dearing, I. Friedman and L. Sylte who shared in the monumental task of typing all the manuscripts; to the staff of Plenum Publishing Corporation for their expert assistance; and, to Mr. R. J. Burk, Jr. and his staff, from the Central Office of the Reticuloendothelial Society, for their advice and encouragement.

Contents of Part A

Contents of Part B.. xix

Introduction.. xxvii

SECTION 1
ENZYMATIC AND METABOLIC ACTIVITIES OF THE
RETICULOENDOTHELIAL SYSTEM

FOREWORD.. 2

Association of Some Metabolic Activities of
Leukocytes with the Immune Response.......................... 3

R. R. Strauss

Role of the RES in Lead Salt Sensitization to
Endotoxin Shock... 21

J. P. Filkins

A Metabolic Comparison Between Human Blood
Monocytes and Neutrophils....................................... 29

D. Roos, M. Reiss, A. J. M. Balm, A. M. Palache,
P. H. Cambier and J. S. Van Der Stijl-Neijenhuis

The Regulation of Macrophage Activities: Role of the
Energy-Dependent Intracellular Ca^{2+} Buffering Systems....... 37

D. Romeo, C. Schneider, R. Gennaro and C. Mottola

O_2^- and H_2O_2 Production During the Respiratory Burst in Alveolar Macrophages 53

F. Rossi, G. Zabucchi, P. Dri, P. Bellavite and G. Berton

Biochemical and Biological Properties of Leukocyte Intracellular Inhibitors of Proteinases 75

M. Kopitar, T. Giraldi, P. Locnikar and V. Turk

Immunological Studies of Intracellular Leukocyte Proteinase Inhibitor by Granular Extract and Cathepsin D 85

J. Babnik, M. Kopitar and V. Turk

A Comparative Study of the Biochemical Properties of Myeloperoxidase and Eosinophil Peroxidase 91

R. Cramer, B. Bisiacchi, G. de Nicola and P. Patriarca

Glucocorticoid Protection of Hepatic Phagocytosis in Hypoxia 101

M. J. Galvin and A. M. Lefer

Evidence that Phagocytosing Chicken Polymorphonuclear Leukocytes Generate Hydrogen Peroxide and Superoxide Anion 111

P. Dri, P. Bellavite, R. Cramer, B. Bisiacchi, F. Cian and P. Patriarca

The Role of Leukocyte Extracts and Myeloperoxidase in the Lysis of Staphylococci and the Inhibition of Bacteriolysis by Anionic Polyelectrolytes and by Inflammatory Exudates 123

I. Ginsburg, N. Neeman, M. Lahav and M. N. Sela

Biological and Biochemical Characteristics of the Tetrapeptide Tuftsin, Thr-Lsy-Pro-Arg....................... 131

V. A. Najjar

Angiotensin Converting Enzyme: Induction in Rabbit Alveolar Macrophages and Human Monocytes in Culture......... 149

E. Silverstein, J. Friedland and C. Setton

Effect of Proteinases on EA (IgG)-Binding Receptors of Rat Macrophages... 157

G. Boltz-Nitulescu and O. Forster

Endotoxin-Induced SAA Elevation in the Mouse - Lack of A Role For Complement or Acid Proteases............ 167

Y. Levo, P. D. Gorevic, P. Chatpar, E. C. Franklin and B. Frangione

Differential Effect of Polycations on Uptake and Desulphation of Heparin................................ 175

I. Fabian, I. Bleiberg and M. Aronson

The Purification of Plasma Membranes from Guinea Pig Peritoneal Macrophages.................................. 183

G. Chauvet, A. Anteunis and R. Robineaux

Cytological Characteristics of Bone Marrow Reticular Cells, Tissue Macrophages and Monocytic Cell Line.. 195

M. Kojima and T. Sato

Leukocyte Enzyme Assays by Flow Cytophotometry............. 211

L. S. Kaplow

SECTION 2
IMMUNOPHARMACOLOGY OF THE RETICULOENDOTHELIAL SYSTEM

FOREWORD.. 224

Alterations of Rat Liver Lysosomes After Treatment With Particulate β 1-3 Glucan From *Saccharomyces cerevisiae*.................................... 225

P. Jacques and F. Lambert

Suppressor Cell Induction and Reticuloendothelial Cell Activation Produced in the Mouse By β 1-3 Glucan....... 235

F. J. LeJeune, A. Vercammen-Grandjean, P. Mendes da Costa, D. Bron and V. Defleur

Therapeutic Effect of Intravenously Administered Yeast Glucan, in Mice Locally Infected by *Mycobacterium leprae*.................................... 245

J. Delville and P. J. Jacques

Comparative Biological and Antitoxoplasmic Effects of Particulate and Water-Soluble Polysaccharides *In Vitro*.................................... 255

B. T. Nguyen and S. Stadtsbaeder

Glucan Induced Inhibition of Tumor Growth and Enhancement of Survival in a Variety of Transplantable and Spontaneous Murine Tumor Models........................ 269

N. Di Luzio, R. B. McNamee, D. L. Williams, K. M. Gilbert and M. A. Spanjers

Glucan Induced Modification of Experimental *Staphylococcus aureus* Infection in Normal, Leukemic and Immunosuppressed Mice......................... 291

D. L. Williams and N. Di Luzio

Particulate β 1-3 Glucan and Causal Prophylaxis of Mouse Malaria (Plasmodium berghei) 307

J. Gillet, P. J. Jacques and F. Herman

Restoration of Depressed Antibody Responses of Leukemic Splenocytes Treated with LPS-Induced Factors....... 315

R. C. Butler, H. Friedman and A. Nowotny

Functional Similarity and Diversity in Peritoneal Macrophage Populations Induced In Vivo by Various Stimuli 323

R. Goldman, Z. Bar-Shavit and A. Raz

Activation of Pleural Macrophages by Intrapleural Application of Corynebacterium parvum 333

I. Bašić, B. Rodé, A. Kaštelan and L. Milas

Modulation of T Cells and Macrophages by Cholera Toxin Treatment In Vivo and In Vitro 343

H. Friedman and S. Lyons

In Vivo Activation of Murine Peritoneal Macrophages by Nocardia Water Soluble Mitogen (NWSM) 351

I. Löwy, D. Juy, C. Bona and L. Chedid

Suppression of Immunological Responsiveness in Aged Mice and Its Relationship with Coenzyme Q Deficiency 361

E. G. Bliznakov

Quercetin, A Regulator of Polymorphonuclear Leukocyte (PMNL) Functions 371

C. Schneider, G. Berton, S. Spisani, S. Traniello and D. Romeo

The Effect of Cyclophosphamide on A Secondary Ocular Immune Response in Rabbits 381

J. M. Hall and J. F. Pribnow

SECTION 3
REGULATORY FUNCTIONS OF THE RETICULOENDOTHELIAL SYSTEM

FOREWORD 390

RES Function and Glucose Homeostasis 391

J. P. Filkins

Role of RES and Leukocytic Endogenous Mediator in Iron, Zinc and Copper Metabolism 403

R. F. Kampschmidt

Function of Macrophage Prostaglandins in the Process of Phagocytosis 413

E. Razin, U. Zor and A. Globerson

The Mononuclear Phagocyte System and Hemopoiesis 419

M. Rachmilewitz, B. Rachmilewitz, M. Chaouat, H. Zlotnik and M. Schlesinger

Macrophages as Regulators of Granulopoiesis 433

R. N. Apte, E. Heller, C. F. Hertogs and D. H. Pluznik

Regulation of Antigen Binding to T Cells: The Role of Products of Adherent Cells, and the H-2 Restriction of the Antigen Bound 451

P. Lonai, J. Puri, M. Zeicher and L. Steinman

Alveolar Macrophage - Induced Suppression of the Immune Response 459

H. B. Herscowitz, R. E. Conrad and K. J. Pennline

Suppression of Antibody Forming Cells by Rat Spleen Macrophages 485

S. M. Reichard

SECTION 4
ENVIRONMENTAL FACTORS INFLUENCING THE RETICULOENDOTHELIAL SYSTEM AND IMMUNE RESPONSES

FOREWORD 498

Environmental Chemical-Induced Modification of Cell-Mediated Immune Responses 499

J. B. Silkworth and L. D. Loose

The Immunodepressive Effect of Phenol Derivatives 523

M. F. La Via, L. D. Loose, D. S. La Via and M. S. Silberman

Alveolar Macrophage - Splenic Lymphocyte Interactions Following Chronic Asbestos Inhalation in the Rat 539

E. Kagan and K. Miller

Tobacco Smoke and the Pulmonary Alveolar Macrophage 555

D. B. Drath, P. Davies, M. L. Karnovsky and G. L. Huber

Effects of Pesticides on the Reticuloendothelial System 569

W. S. Ceglowski, C. D. Ercegrovich and N. S. Pearson

Substances from Marine Organisms Influencing Tumor Growth and Immune Responses.................................. 577

M. M. Sigel, W. Lichter, A. Ghaffar, L. L. Wellham and A. J. Weinheimer

Effects of UV Radiation on the Immune System: Consequences for UV Carcinogenesis.......................... 589

M. L. Kripke

In Vitro and *In Vivo* Parameters of Humoral and Cellular Immunity in an Animal Model for Protein-Calorie Malnutrition............................ 599

M. A. Taylor, B. A. Israel, M. R. Escobar and D. Berlinerman

Participants 607

Index 617

Contents of Part B

Contents of Part A.. xix

Introduction.. xxvii

SECTION 1
THE RETICULOENDOTHELIAL SYSTEM AND IMMUNE
RESPONSES IN INFECTION

FOREWORD.. 2

Genetic Modification of Macrophage Functions in Relation to Antibody Responsiveness and Resistance to Infection.. 3

C. Stiffel, D. Mouton, Y. Bouthillier and G. Biozzi

The Chemotactic, Phagocytic, and Microbial Killing Abilities of Primate Polymorphonuclear Leukocytes (PML).. 13

J. W. Eichberg, S. S. Kalter, W. T. Kniker, R. W. Steel and R. L. Heberling

Protective Effect of PSK, A Protein-Bound Polysaccharide Preparation Against Candidiasis in Tumor Bearing Mice.. 21

A. Uetsuka, S. Satoh and Y. Ohno

Phagocytosis of Candida Albicans by Polymorphonuclear Leukocytes from Normal and Diabetic Subjects................ 33

R. A. Jackson, C. S. Bryan and B. A. Weeks

Relationship Between Protective Immunity, Mitogenicity, and B Cell Activation by Salmonella Vaccines.................................... 39

T. K. Eisenstein, C. R. Angerman, S. O'Donnell, S. Specter and H. Friedman

Effects of Bacterial Products on Granulopoiesis............ 51

R. Urbaschek

Interaction of Murine T-Cell Surface Antigens with *Mycoplasma hyorhinis*.................................. 65

K. S. Wise, P. B. Asa and R. T. Acton

Alveolar Macrophage Dysfunction Associated With Viral Pneumonitis.................................... 81

G. J. Jakab, G. A. Warr and P. L. Sannes

B and T Lymphocyte Activation by Murine Leukemia Virus Infection.................................. 91

M. Bendinelli and H. Friedman

Abolition of Lymphocyte Blastogenesis by Oncornaviral Components.................................... 99

A. Hellman, A. K. Fowler, D. R. Twardzik, O. S. Weislow and C. D. Reed

Distinguishable Biological Effects of Murine Leukemia and Sarcoma Viruses in Long Term Bone Marrow Culture.. 111

J. S. Greenberger, P. B. Davisson and P. J. Gans

SECTION 2
NATURE, ACTIVATION AND INTERACTIONS OF THE RETICULOENDOTHELIAL SYSTEM

FOREWORD.. 126

Lymphocytes and Macrophages in the
Lymphomyeloid Complex.................................... 127

J. M. Yoffey

Ultrastructural Studies on Bronchial-Associated
Lymphoid Tissue (BALT) and Lymphoepithelium in
Pulmonary Cell-Mediated Reactions in the Rabbit............ 145

Q. N. Myrvik, P. Racz, and K. T. Racz

Ultrastructural and Cytochemical Studies of Mouse
Natural Killer (NK) Cells................................. 155

R. Kiessling, J. C. Roder and P. Biberfeld

Macrophage-Lymphocyte Interaction and Genetic
Control of Immune Responsiveness........................... 165

J. W. Thomas, J. Schroer, K. Yokomuro, J. T. Blake
and A. S. Rosenthal

Enhancement of Spreading, Phagocytosis and Chemotaxis
by Macrophage Stimulating Protein (MSP).................... 181

E. J. Leonard and A. H. Skeel

BCG-Activated Macrophages: Comparison as Effectors
in Direct Tumor-Cell Cytotoxicity and Antibody
Dependent Cell-Mediated Cytotoxicity....................... 195

D. O. Adams and H. S. Koren

Activation of Macrophages Assessed by _In Vivo_
and _In Vitro_ Tests.. 203

J. M. Rhodes and J. Bennedsen

A Novel Biological Function of Macrophages Associated With Antigen Discrimination Properties 211

R. M. Gorczynski

Macrophage-Like Properties of Human Hyalocytes 223

G. Boltz-Nitulescu, G. Grabner and O. Forster

Correlation of B Cell Acquisition of Differentiation Antigens with Capacity to Interact with Allogeneic Effect Factor (AEF) 229

J. R. Battisto, J. H. Finke and B. Yen

Partial Immunochemical Characterization of a Human B-Lymphocyte Differentiation Antigen (BDA-1) 239

E. W. Ades, P. A. Dougherty and C. M. Balch

The Effect of Xenoantisera on T-Lymphocyte Functions in the Absence of Complement 247

R. Rabinowitz, R. Laskov and M. Schlesinger

Effect of Immune Sera Upon Enhanced *In Vitro* Antibody Responses 261

S. J. Frank, S. Specter, A. Nowotny and H. Friedman

Growth of Human T-Cells Following *In Vitro* Allograft Sensitization 269

J. L. Strausser and A. Rosenberg

SECTION 3
IMMUNOPATHOLOGY OF THE RETICULOENDOTHELIAL SYSTEM

FOREWORD 275

Immunosuppression as a Homeostatic Mechanism in Disease and Aging.................................... 277

H. R. Strausser and M. M. Rosenstein

Suppressor Monocytes in Human Disease: A Review............ 283

G. P. Schechter, L. M. Wahl and J. J. Oppenheim

Suppressor Cell Defect in Psoriasis.......................... 299

D. N. Sauder, P. L. Bailin and R. S. Krakauer

Stimulation of the Reticuloendothelial System and Autoimmunity...................................... 307

J. I. Morton and B. V. Siegel

Mitigation of Experimental Allergic Encephalomyelitis by Cathepsin D Inhibition.................................. 317

D. H. Boehme and N. Marks

Localization and Clearance of Passively Administered Immune Complexes and Aggregated Protein, in the Choroid Plexus of Mice...................... 325

P. M. Ford

Cardiac Specific Antigen and Antibody in Immunopathogenesis of Cardiac Disease...................... 335

K. Chang, H. Friedman and H. Goldberg

Phagocyte Functions in Familial Mediterranean Fever......... 341

M. Bar-Eli, M. Levy, M. Ehrenfeld, M. Eliakim and R. Gallily

SECTION 4
THE RETICULOENDOTHELIAL SYSTEM AND IMMUNOMODULATION IN CANCER

FOREWORD 351

Macrophages in Tumor Immunity 353

M. G. Hanna, Jr.

Macrophages as Regulators of Immune Responses Against Tumors 361

R. B. Herberman, H. T. Holden, J. Y. Djeu, T. R. Jerrells, L. Varesio, A. Tagliabue, S. L. White, J. R. Oehler and J. H. Dean

Macrophage Activation for Tumor Cytotoxicity: Mechanisms of Macrophage Activation by Lymphokines 381

M. S. Meltzer, L. P. Ruco and E. J. Leonard

The Treatment of Established Micrometastases with Syngeneic Macrophages 399

I. J. Fidler, W. E. Fogler, Z. Barnes and K. Fisher

Influence of Tumor Burden, Tumor Removal, Immune Stimulation, Plasmapheresis on Monocyte Mobilization in Cancer Patients 411

R. Samak, L. Israel and R. Edelstein

Protection from Malignancy by Nonimmune Lymphoid Cells 425

T. J. Linna and K. M. Lam

Modulation of the Tumoricidal Function of Activated Macrophages by Bacterial Endotoxin and Mammalian Macrophage Activation Factor(s).................. 433

J. B. Hibbs, J. B. Weinberg and H. A. Chapman

Studies on the Endotoxin Induced Tumor Resistance........... 455

A. Nowotny and R. C. Butler

A Macrophage Chemotaxis Inhibitor Produced by Neoplasms: Characterization of Its Biological Activity.. 471

R. Synderman and M. C. Pike

Enhancement of Tumor Growth by Peritoneal Macrophages of Normal and Tumor-Bearing Mice................ 485

A. Gabizon and N. Trainin

Macrophage Involvement in Leukemia Virus-Induced Tumorigenesis.. 493

M. Bendinelli, D. Matteucci, A. Toniolo and H. Friedman

Functional Heterogeneity and T Cell-Dependent Activation of Macrophages from Murine Sarcoma Virus (MSV)-Induced Tumors................................ 509

H. T. Holden, L. Varesio, T. Taniyama and P. Puccetti

Involvement of Peritoneal Macrophages in Cellular Responses to Mastocytoma in Resistant and Susceptible Mice.. 521

P. Farber, S. Specter and H. Friedman

Syngeneic Anti-Tumor Globulin: Suppression of Mouse Plasmacytoma by the IgG2 Fraction.................... 531

T. N. Harris and S. Harris

Mechanism of Resistance of Mice to Syngeneic Methylcholanthrene Induced Fibrosarcomas.................... 541

D. S. Nelson, M. Nelson and K. E. Hopper

Opsonization of Antitumor Reactive Lymphocytes in SJL/J Mice Bearing Spontaneous or Transplanted Reticulum Cell Sarcomas (RCS).............................. 553

I. V. Hutchinson, J. Roman and B. Bonavida

Anti Inflammatory Consequences of Transplanted Tumors....... 563

S. J. Normann, E. Sorkin and M. Schardt

Participants.. 575

Index... 585

Introduction

In this volume sections are included dealing with enzymatic and metabolic activities, immunopharmacology and regulatory functions of the Reticuloendothelial (RE) System. Environmental factors influencing the RE System and immunity are also discussed. It is difficult to separate topics dealing with enzymatic activities related to phagocytosis from those concerning antibody formation or cellular immunity. Thus, these papers are included in the same section. Immunopharmacology has become a major area of interest throughout the world. The relationship of pharmacological reactions to the functional activity of RE cells is an important topic. Thus, in the section dealing with immunopharmacology various agents which influence or modify resistance to bacteria, tumors and virus infections as well as those factors influencing the activity of macrophages and lymphocytes are discussed. Among these factors are those derived from bacteria and other infectious agents. The regulatory functions of the RE System are described in the third section. Included are discussions of hemopoiesis, granulopoiesis, glucose homeostasis, metabolism of iron, zinc and copper, etc. Environmental factors influencing the RE System and immune responses are also treated in detail. Recent studies from a large number of laboratories have implicated environmental contaminants as important modifiers of immune responsiveness, both _in vivo_ and _in vitro_. Cellular immunity and antibody formation can be depressed after exposure to a wide variety of chemicals including phenols. Asbestos, recently in the limelight because of its carcinogenic activity, was discussed in terms of its effects on macrophages. Furthermore, tobacco smoke, now considered an important cause of lung cancer, has been shown to influence pulmonary alveolar macrophage activity. Pesticides can also influence macrophage activity and immunity. Thus, all in all, it is quite apparent that many factors previously taken "for granted" as inert and necessary components of the environment, especially in an industrialized civilization, may have detrimental effects on selected cell populations of the RE System.

Part I
Enzymatic and Metabolic Activities of the Reticuloendothelial System

Biochemical aspects of the Reticuloendothelial (RE) System have been studied for many decades. It is quite apparent that functional activity of the RE System, including macrophages, is intimately dependent upon enzymatic activities, alterations in metabolism, etc. In this section a number of papers dealing with metabolic activities of monocytes, neutrophils and lymphoid cells is presented. The role of the RE System in endotoxin shock, the regulation of macrophage activity by energy dependent intracellular calcium as well as the biochemical properties of macrophages and leukocytes in the myeloperoxidase system, etc. are discussed in detail. The influence of agents such as bacteria, immunostimulatory substances, proteinases, endotoxin, etc., on biochemical aspects of macrophage function and activity is described in a number of papers. It is evident that much new work is underway in many laboratories concerning metabolic activities of leukocytes and macrophages in regard to immune responses and other reactions.

ASSOCIATION OF SOME METABOLIC ACTIVITIES OF LEUKOCYTES WITH THE IMMUNE RESPONSE

R. R. STRAUSS

Albert Einstein Medical Center, Northern Division

Philadelphia, Pennsylvania (USA)

Phagocytosis is a physiological function of many different mammalian cell types. These phagocytic cells remove dead cells, tissue, and foreign substances from the body by engulfment and digestion of these materials. Some phagocytic cells, notably the neutrophils, monocytes and macrophages, also serve as primary factors in the host-defense mechanism by engulfing, killing and digesting pathogenic microorganisms. Macrophages have also been implicated in the killing of tumor cells and the humoral immune response. Stimulation of a number of biochemical and metabolic parameters has been associated with phagocytosis. These include increased glucose utilization, $1^{14}C$-glucose oxidation, $6^{14}C$-glucose oxidation, oxygen consumption, NADPH oxidase activity, peroxidase activity, superoxide anion production, H_2O_2 production and chemoluminescence. These biochemical and metabolic activities of phagocytes and their relationship to particle engulfment and intracellular microbicidal activity have been reviewed in detail by Karnovsky (11) and others (23). This report will be concerned with the association of some metabolic activities of mouse macrophages and the immune response. It seems as if some of the metabolic activities that have been related to phagocytosis and killing of microorganisms by macrophage and neutorphils may also be associated with cellular and humoral immunity.

MATERIALS AND METHODS

Experimental animals. Male Balb/c mice were used in these studies. The animals were purchased from Cumberland View Farms (Clinton, Tennessee) and were maintained in the central animal facility at our institution. The mice weighed approximately

20 g at the start of each experiment. They were housed in plastic cages in groups of 6-10 and fed Purina mouse chown and water *ad libitum*.

Immunogens. Sheep erythrocyte (SRBC) suspensions were purchased from Flow Laboratories (Rockville, Maryland). They were washed and resuspended to 2% (v/v) in saline prior to use as immunogens.

Immunization. Mice were immunized by either the intraperitoneal (i. p.) or intravenous (i. v.) route with 0.5 ml of a 2% suspension of SRBC. *In vitro* immunization of spleen cell cultures in Marbrook chambers (11) was with SRBC at a ratio of 1 erythrocyte to 10 spleen cells. Cultures were maintained in RPM-1640 + 10% fetal calf serum (FCS) in a humidified atmosphere of 5% CO_2 in air. Enumeration of *in vitro* plaque forming cells (PFC) from immunized mice was done 4 days after immunization. PFC determination of Marbrook chamber cultures was done 5 days after *in vitro* immunization.

Detection of antibody forming cells. The hemolytic assay for antibody PFC in agar gel was performed essentially as described by Jerne and Nordin (10) for detecting direct IgM PFC to SRBC. Indirect IgG PFC were determined by addition of a previously determined appropriate dilution of goat antimouse IgG serum purchased from Microbiological Associates (Bethesda, Maryland) to the plates. The number of indirect PFC was then ascertained mathematically.

Preparation of lymphoid cells. Mice were killed by cervical dislocation and their spleens aseptically removed at autopsy. Dispersed spleen cell suspensions, relatively freed of erythrocytes by a brief (30 sec) period of osmotic shock, were prepared as previously described (24).

^{3}H-thymidine incorporation studies. Phytohemagglutinin P (PHA-P) and *Escherichia coli* endotoxin (LPS) both purchased from Difco Laboratories (Detroit, Michigan) were dissolved or suspended in sterile distilled water prior to dilution in sterile RPMI-1640 containing 10% FCS. The mitogen were added to cell cultures (16 x 125 mm screw cap tubes) containing 1 x 10^6 mouse spleen cells. The total volume per culture was 1.0 ml. Cultures were incubated 24 hr at 37 C in a humidified atmosphere containing 5% CO_2 in air. At this time 1 μCi of ^{3}H-thymidine (sp. Act. 6.7 Ci/m), New England Nuclear Corp. (Boston, Massachusetts) was added to each culture. Incorporation of ^{3}H-thymidine into acid insoluble products was determined as described in a previous report (25).

Enzyme assays. Homogenates of spleen cell suspensions were prepared from cells suspended in 0.25 M sucrose. Cells were homogenized for 2 min at 3800 rpm in an ice bath with a Potter-Elvevh-

TABLE I

Effect of Intraperitoneal Injection of 2-Deoxyglucose on Hemolytic PFC Response by Balb/c Mice to Sheep Erythrocytes[a]

Dose	Spleen Wt. (mg)	PFC/Spleen	PFC/10^6 Cells
None	192.3 ± 13.5	107611 ± 27903	272.0 ± 54
	169.1 ± 9.5	43683 ± 2992	132.0 ± 4.6
	161.2 ± 19.2	27153 ± 12656	112.7 ± 55.4
	114.7 ± 22.1	8565 ± 4174	42.3 ± 7.3

[a]Values are expressed as the mean ± S. E. of mean for 3 experiments. There were 3-4 mice/group in each experiment.

jem tissue homogenizer with a teflon-tipped motor driven pestle. Homogenates were fractionated by centriguation in a refrigerated Sorvall RC-2 centrifuge. Acid phosphatase and peroxidase activities were determined by previously described procedures (25, 26). All chemicals used in these procedures were purchased from commercial sources and were of reagent grade.

RESULTS

Intraperitoneal injection of the glycolytic antagonist 2-deoxyglucose (DOG) immediately after injection of sheep erythrocyte (SRBC) antigen by the same route resulted in a marked suppression in hemolytic plaque forming cells (PFC) by the Jerne procedure. The data shown in Table I reveal that doses of DOG as low as 1 mg/mouse were inhibitory to the PFC response. Spleen and thymus weights (thymus weight not shown) were not changed by 1 and 2 mg/mouse doses. Both organs were markedly decreased in weight when 4 mg/mouse were administered. The apparent toxic effect of the highest dose of DOG led us to examine the effect of this compound on the *in vitro* immune response of mouse spleen cells to the same antigen. The results presented in Table II show that DOG is much more effective as a suppressive agent in the *in vitro* system. Quantities as low as 5 μg/culture (0.5 μg/ml) resulted in marked suppression of the PFC response. This was statistically significant ($p < 0.01$) by Student's t test. The optimal time of addition of DOG for *in vitro* immunosuppression appears to be between 2 and 3 hr after addition of the SRBC antigen. These data are shown in Table III. There is little or no suppression of the PFC response if DOG is added 48 or 72 hr after addition of antigen (data not

TABLE II

Effect of Dose of 2-Deoxyglucose in *In vitro* PFC Response of Mouse Spleen Cells to Sheep Erythrocytes[a]

Additions	PFC/10^6 Cells	% Change
None	448 ± 34	-
1 μg/culture	509 ± 214	+ 13.6
5 μg/culture	108 ± 5	- 75.9
10 μg/culture	70 ± 15	- 84.4
20 μg/culture	60 ± 21	- 86.6
50 μg/culture	46 ± 27	- 89.7

[a]Values are expressed as the mean ± SEM of 3 cultures

TABLE III

Effect of Time of Addition of 2-Deoxyglucose on *In vitro* PFC Response to Sheep Erythrocytes

Dexoyglucose	Time of Addition[a]	PFC/10^6 Cells	% Change
-	-	1250	-
+	0	643	- 49
+	+ 1 hr	659	- 47
+	+ 2 hr	669	- 46
+	+ 3 hr	973	- 22
+	+ 5 hr	871	- 30
+	+24 hr	1067	- 15

[a]10 μg/culture of 2-deoxyglucose was added when indicated

shown). Since DOG is a known antagonist of glycolytic activity (5), the effect of excess glucose on *in vitro* immunosuppression in this compound was examined. The results presented in Table IV show that the addition of glucose does not change the inhibitory effect of the deoxy compound. If anything, there appears to be an enhancement of the effect in the presence of 20 μg of glucose.

TABLE IV

Effect of Glucose Addition on
In vitro PFC Inhibition by 2-Deoxyglucose[a]

Glucose	2-Deoxyglucose	PFC/10^6 Cells	% Change
-	-	2368	-
-	10 μg	1531	- 47
5 μg	10 μg	1423	- 50
10 μg	10 μg	1355	- 53
20 μg	10 μg	1199	- 58

[a]2-Deoxyglucose and glucose added to cultures as the same time as the SRBC antigen

TABLE V

Effect of H_2O_2 and the 20,000 x g Pellet
Fraction of Mouse Spleen on *In vitro* PFC Production[a]

Additions	PFC/Culture	PFC/10^6 Cells
None	1573 ± 48	990 ± 71
1 m M H_2O_2	840 ± 69	527 ± 56
H_2O_2 + pellet fraction	907 ± 308	744 ± 261
Pellet fraction	5213 ± 716	3546 ± 131

[a]Values are expressed as mean ± SEM of 4 cultures

Hydrogen peroxide (H_2O_2) is a toxic endproduct of glucose metabolism. It has been reported that H_2O_2 inhibits the production of immunoglobulins by cultured lymphoid cells (6). The effect of H_2O_2 on the *in vitro* PFC response of mouse spleen cells is shown in Table V. These data show that H_2O_2 also inhibits the PFC re-

TABLE VI

Effect of Immunization of Mice with Sheep Erythrocytes on Spleen Cell Peroxidase Activity

Day After Immunization[a]	Peroxidase Activity (guaiacol units)[b]		
	Per 10^8 Cells	Per Gm Spleen	Per Spleen
0	0.126 ± 0.015	2.520 ± 0.300	0.252 ± 0.028
1	0.138 ± 0.018	2.760 ± 0.358	0.328 ± 0.043
2	0.207 ± 0.022[c]	4.140 ± 0.442[c]	0.513 ± 0.055[c]
3	0.163 ± 0.020	3.260 ± 0.398	0.499 ± 0.061
4	0.114 ± 0.014	2.283 ± 0.441	0.299 ± 0.058
6	0.144 ± 0.014	2.884 ± 0.280	0.363 ± 0.035
7	0.121 ± 0.021	2.421 ± 0.420	0.315 ± 0.055

[a]Groups of mice immunized with 4 x 10^8 sheep erythrocytes on day indicated before assay for splenic peroxidase activity
[b]Average responses as mean value ± S. E. for spleens of 5-10 animals each in 2-4 separate experiments
[c]Statistically different from unimmunized controls ($p < 0.02$ by Student's t test

TABLE VII

Splenoperoxidase Activity of Mice Injected with Heterologous and Syngeneic Erythrocytes or Serum

Antigen Injected[a]	Peroxidase Activity Per 10^8 Cells[b]
None (controls)	0.091 ± 0.008
Rabbit RBCs (2.0%)	0.188 ± 0.016[c]
Rabbit serum (0.5 ml)	0.286 ± 0.119[c]
Mouse RBCs (2.0%)	0.111 ± 0.007
Mouse serum (0.5 ml)	0.107 ± 0.032

[a]Groups of mice injected i. p. with indicated antigen 2 days before assay for splenic peroxidase activity
[b]Average values ± S. E. for spleens of 3 mice/group
[c]Statistically different from unimmunized control value ($p < 0.01$)

sponse. Addition of the 20,000 x g pellet fraction of spleen cell suspensions (adjusted to 0.01 quaiacol units of peroxidase activity) along with the peroxide did not overcome this inhibition. The pellet fraction alone, however, has a markedly stimulatory effect on the PFC response.

The unexpected observation that the peroxidase containing fraction of mouse spleen cell stimulated the in vitro PFC response led to a study of peroxidase activity in spleen cell suspensions from immunized and control mice. The data in Table VI show that this activity is significantly ($p < 0.02$) increased 2 days after immunization with SRBC. As shown in Fig. 1, the increased peroxidase activity preceded the peak PFC response by 2 days and the splenomegaly by 1 day. Peroxidase activity was back to normal levels at the time of peak antibody production. Additional evidence linking the increased splenoperoxidase (SPO) activity to the immune response is provided by the data presented in Table VII. These results show that SPO activity is increased in homogenates of spleen cell suspensions obtained from mice immunized 2 days earlier with either rabbit serum or erythrocytes. Homogenates from animals injected with syngeneic mouse erythrocytes or serum exhibited no significant changes in SPO activity. In order to

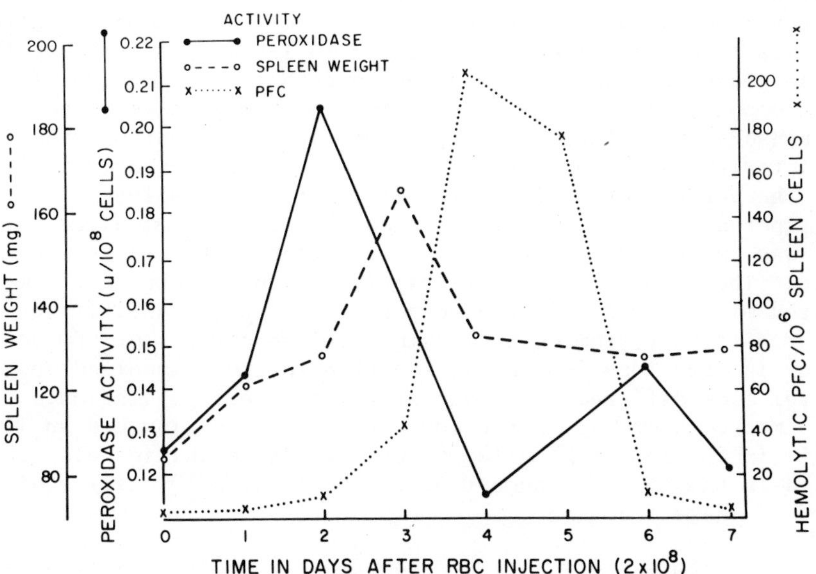

Fig. 1. Changes in peroxidase activity, spleen weight and hemolytic PFC response in spleens of mice after immunization with SRBC. Each point represents the average value of spleens from 5 to 8 mice on the day indicated after i. p. injection of 0.5 ml of 2% sheep erythrocytes. Peroxidase activity expressed as guaiacol units per 10^8 spleen cells.

TABLE VIII

Peroxidase Activity of Adherent and Non-adherent Spleen Cells from Immunized and Control Mice

Spleen Cell Preparation	Mouse Group[a]		
	Immunized[b]	Controls	→ P Values
Adherent	0.218 ± 0.027	0.125 ± 0.017	0.05
Non-Adherent	0.129 ± 0.22	0.092 ± 0.011	0.02
P Value ↓	< 0.05	< 0.1	

[a]Average peroxidase activity for 7 preparations each for 2 separate experiments; activity expressed as guaiacol units per 10^8 spleen cells

[b]Immunized mice injected 2 days earlier i. p. with 0.5 ml of a 2% suspension of sheep erythrocytes

ascertain the cell type involved in this reaction, SPO activity of adherent and nonadherent spleen cells from immunized and control mice was examined. The results shown in Table VIII indicate that the increased SPO activity was most marked in the adherent (macrophage population). Assay of fractions of homogenates of adherent and nonadherent spleen cells from immunized and control mice for SPO activity was done next. These results are presented in Table IX. The percent of SPO activity in the 600 x g pellet and 20,000 x g supernatant fractions of adherent cells from immunized animals was increased over those same fractions obtained from controls. The 20,000 x g pellet fraction of homogenates from immunized mice showed a decreased percentage of SPO activity when compared to that from control animals. The percent of SPO activity in fractions from nonadherent cells from immunized and control mice differed from that of the adherent population. There was a marked decrease in the 600 x g pellet fraction and an increase in the 1500 x g pellet fraction. These changes also occurred in the absolute number of guaiacol units/10^8 cell equivalents of these fractions.

Since SPO activity is largely associated with the lysosomal fraction of both adherent and nonadherent spleen cells (see Table IX), it was decided to determine the effect of an inhibitor of lysosomal enzyme activities on the immune response. Trypan blue was the compound chosen for these experiments. The data shown in Table X indicate that i. p. injection of 1.0 mg of trypan blue at

TABLE IX

Subcellular Distribution of Peroxidase Activity in Adherent and Non-adherent Spleen Cells from Immunized and Control Mice

	Percent Splenic Peroxidase Activity for[a]:							
	Immunized Mice[b]				Control Mice[a]			
	Adherent		Non-Adherent		Adherent		Non-Adherent	
	Units	Percent[c]	Units	Percent[c]	Units	Percent	Units	Percent
Total homogenate	0.171[a]	-	0.147	-	0.128	-	0.096	-
600 x g pellet	0.048	20.25	0.012	9.13	0.024	16.33	0.018	18.82
1,500 x g pellet	0.050	21.32	0.041	30.80	0.034	22.78	0.020	20.97
20,000 x g pellet	0.099	42.00	0.060	45.25	0.071	48.30	0.043	45.70
20,000 x g supernate	0.039	16.43	0.020	14.82	0.019	12.59	0.014	14.51

[a]Average peroxidase activity as percentage of total guaiacol units/10^8 cells for 2 assays with 3 pooled spleens in each sample; adherent _vs_ non-adherent cells prepared by glass separation procedures

[b]Mice injected 2 days earlier i. p. with 0.5 ml 2% sheep erythrocytes

TABLE X

Effect of Intraperitoneal Injection of Trypan Blue on the Immune Response to Sheep Erythrocytes by BALB/c Mice

Dose	Spleen Weight (mg)[a]	PFC/10^6 Cells	PFC/Spleen
0.5 mg	169.7 ± 10.2	248.5 ± 23.2	73448 ± 17398
1.0 mg	165.2 ± 12.2	87.3 ± 8.1[b]	27510 ± 6789[b]
2.0 mg	84.2 ± 7.5[b]	91.8 ± 8.9[b]	16192 ± 4160[b]
Control	187.8 ± 10.3	268.6 ± 18.1	01979 ± 11463

[a]All numbers represent the mean ± S. E. of mean of 5 mice/group
[b]Significantly different from control value ($p < 0.05$ by Student's t test

the time of immunization with SRBC is sufficient for significant inhibition of the PFC response. This dose of dye did not significantly change the spleen weights of the animals involved while the 2 mg/mouse dose was associated with a marked drop in spleen weight, as well as the PFC response. The effect of time of i. p. injection of trypan blue relative to immunization witn SRBC on the hemolytic PFC response is shown in Table XI. These data indicate that the time for maximal inhibition occurs within 6 hr after immunization. It was also determined that inhibition did not occur if the dye was injected 48 hr prior to or 48, 72 or 96 hr after the immunogen. The data presented in Table XII are indicative of a suppressive effect of trypan blue on immunologic memory. These results show that if the dye and immunogen are administered on day 0 and the SRBC are given again on day 10 without dye that there is an inhibition of both the direct (IgM) and indirect (IgG) hemolytic PFC response.

In order to rule out the possible *in vivo* stress effects of the dye, studies on the *in vitro* immune response were done next. The results presents in Table XIII show that trypan blue is immunosuppressive in this system with a dose as low as 0.32 mg/culture. There was no apparent effect of the dye on the viability of the lymphoid cells employed in these experiments. Preincubation of either adherent or nonadherent spleen cells for 6 hr before addition of the SRBC to the cultures indicated that both cell types are sensitive to the action of the dye. This occurred even if the cells were washed before antigen was added.

TABLE XI

Effect of Time in Hours of Trypan Blue Injection on the Hemolytic PFC Response by BALB/c Mice

Time[a]	Spleen Wt. (mg)	PFC/Spleen	PFC/10^6 Cells
- 24 hr	169 ± 14	41,180 ± 6,560[b]	194 ± 19[b]
0 hr	175 ± 18	39,060 ± 8,227	198 ± 26
+ 1 hr	179 ± 19	43,253 ± 6,826	194 ± 29
+ 2 hr	179 ± 16	33,057 ± 8,737	181 ± 54
+ 6 hr	168 ± 20	31,764 ± 10,781	180 ± 50
+ 24 hr	185 ± 11	51,674 ± 7,970	222 ± 21
Control[c]	171 ± 6	110,780 ± 12,198	489 ± 72

[a]Time of i. p. injection of 1.0 mg (0.5 ml) of trypan blue relative to immunization with 2% SRBC (0.5 ml) by the same route

[b]All data are presented as the mean ± S. E. of mean for 3 separate experiments (3-4 mice/group)

[c]Untreated, immunized control mice

TABLE XII

Effect of *In vivo* Administration of Trypan Blue on Direct and Indirect Hemolytic Plaque Formation[a]

Day 0		Day 10		PFC/Spleen	
SRBC	Trypan Blue	SRBC	Trypan Blue	Direct	Indirect
-	-	+	-	131,650	3,350
-	-	+	+	29,237	N.D.
-	+	+	-	119,720	N.D.
+	-	-	-	1,750	16,890
+	+	-	-	4,260	15,270
+	-	+	-	77,635	203,815
+	+	+	-	17,875	64,900

[a]All assays done on day 14. Results are average for 2 mice for each set of conditions (please see text for complete details)

TABLE XIII

Effect of Trypan Blue on *In vitro* PFC Response to Sheep Erythrocytes by BALB/c Mouse Spleen Cells[a]

Trypan Blue/ Culture	Viable Cells $\times 10^6$/Culture	PFC/10^6 Spleen Cells	P
0	0.95 ± 0.04	1497 ± 207	-
2.5 mg	0.66[b]	26	-
1.25 mg	0.92 ± 0.10	689 ± 48	<0.01
0.63 mg	0.91 ± 0.05	818 ± 31	<0.05
0.32 mg	0.92 ± 0.08	730 ± 108	<0.05
0.16 mg	0.98 ± 0.16	1150 ± 133	N.S.

[a]All values are expressed as the mean ± S. E. of mean for 5 cultures. Statistical evaluation was by Student's t test
[b]Average for 2 cultures

The *in vitro* mitogenic response of lymphoid cells has been considered to be a model for cellular immunity. Thus the effect of trypan blue on PHA and endotoxin mediated mitogenic response of mouse spleen cells was studied. The data presented in Table XIV show that trypan blue is inhibitory to PHA mediated stimulation of the incorporation of ^{3}H-thymidine into acid insoluble products. The dose required to inhibit this T cell response was 0.5 mg per culture which was the same as that required for suppression of the *in vitro* hemolytic PFC response. In order to determine the specificity of trypan blue associated inhibition of the mitogenic responses the dye was tested in the B cell mediated stimulation by bacterial endotoxin (LPS). The results shown in Table XV indicate that this dye is also inhibitory to LPS mediated mitogenesis. The minimal effective level of dye required is 0.5 mg/culture; the same amount previously found to inhibit the T cell and *in vitro* PFC response. Maximal inhibition occurred if the dye was added within 18 hr after the mitogen. The data presented in Table XVI indicate that trypan blue inhibits the mitogenic response only when both adherent and nonadherent cells are present in the cultures. This is an indication that the macrophage is the sensitive cell.

TABLE XIV

Effect of Trypan Blue on Phytohemagglutinin Stimulation of ^{3}H-thymidine Uptake by Mouse Spleen Cells[a]

Additions	DPM/10^6 Spleen Cells
None	7630 ± 485
PHA	22033 ± 2388
PHA + Trypan Blue 0.5 mg	9622 ± 821
PHA + Trypan Blue 0.05 mg	18756 ± 515
Trypan Blue 0.5 mg	8766 ± 737

[a]All values are expressed as the mean ± S. E. of mean (see text for complete details)

TABLE XV

Dose-Response Effect of Trypan Blue on *Escherichia coli*

LPS	Trypan Blue	CPM/Culture
-	-	6575
-	0.5 mg	6353
+	-	39260
+	0.05 mg	37537
+	0.25 mg	33288
+	0.50 mg	19120
+	1.00 mg	20868

DISCUSSION

This report has been concerned with the possible relationship between some enzymes of carbohydrate metabolism and by lysosomes with cellular and humoral immunity. Data have been presented that show that 2-deoxyglucose, a competitive inhibitor of phosphohexoseisomerase (5), can inhibit both *in vivo* and *in vitro* the hemolytic PFC response of mouse splenocytes to SRBC. This compound has previously been shown to be inhibitory to PHA mediated mitogenesis (19), phagocytosis by polymorphonuclear leukocytes (PMN) (4) and macrophages (15). Inhibition of mouse macrophage phagocytosis occurred only when opsonized erythrocytes were the particles involved. Engulfment of polystyrene latex particles was not

TABLE XVI

Effect of Trypan Blue on LPS Mediated Mitogenesis by Adherent, Non-Adherent and Unseparated Mouse Spleen Cells

Cell Preparation	Mitogenic Index[a]	
	Alone	+ Trypan Blue (0.5 mg)
Adherent	1.67	1.19
Non-adherent	2.31	2.63
Unseparated	2.21	1.11

[a] $\frac{\text{Cells + LPS}}{\text{Cells - LPS}}$

effected by DOG. The compound was inhibitory only to Fc receptor mediated phagocytosis by these cells. Phagocytosis of latex or albumin coated oil droplets by PMN leukocytes was also inhibited by DOG. This inhibition was overcome by the addition of glucose or pryuvate unless the DOG was removed from the culture medium. We have found that DOG suppresses the *in vitro* PFC response to SRBC. This suppression was not reversed by addition of glucose to the culture medium. These results appear to be similar to those of Boxer *et al.* obtained with PMN leukocytes. It has been proposed that DOG alters F_c or C_3 dependent areas of the PMN membrane thus inhibiting engulfment (4, 15). The glucose antagonist could also have an effect on the cellular ATP pool which in turn could alter the interactions of contractile proteins that have been associated with PMN phagocytosis (22). Either or both of these mechanisms could be involved with the DOG associated immunosuppression reported herein.

The *in vitro* immunosuppression noted in the presence of H_2O_2 is also of interest. This metabolite is produced by reactions catalyzed by several different enzymes. These include glucose oxidase, xanthine oxidase, and NAD(P)H oxidases. The latter reduced pryidine nucleotide oxidases have been reported to be involved in phagocytosis (11, 18). H_2O_2 is broken down in reactions catalyzed by catalase, myeloperoxidase or glutathione peroxidase. It has been shown that the H_2O_2 associated inhibition of microtubule assembly and function in leukocytes is really due to gluthathione disulfide (GSSG) that is produced by the glutathione peroxidase mediated reaction (17). Leukocyte microtubules have been reported to be involved in movement of membrane receptors (16), chemotaxis (2) and intracellular movement of lysosomes (28). One could therefore speculate that the H_2O_2 associated immunosuppression involves the production of GSSG with resulting inhibition of microtubule assembly and/or function. An effect on the movement of membrane receptors could inhibit phagocytosis and the mechanism for immunosuppression would be similar to that previously postulated for DOG. If the effect were on lysosomal degranulation, the mechanism could involve peroxidase or some other lysosomal enzymes.

The redistribution and increase in splenoperoxidase activity observed in spleen cell homogenates from immunized mice may also be related to a function of cytoplasmic microtubules. The activity of this enzyme is confined mainly to the lysosomal fraction of the cell (26) and as previously noted microtubules have been implicated in lysosomal degranulation (28). Since H_2O_2 is immunosuppressive in vitro, the peroxidase may simply function to control the level of metabolic peroxidases in the cell. This, however, does not rule out the possibility that other lysosomal enzymes have a role in the immune response.

The immunosuppression that was observed both in vivo and in vitro in the presence of trypan blue provides additional evidence for the involvement of lysosomal enzumes in immunity. This dye has been reported to be inhibitory to the activity of a number of lysosomal enzymes from rat liver (3). We have also found trypan blue to be inhibitory to the activity of acid phosphatase and peroxidase from murine spleen cells (27). In addition to suppression of the PFC response by spleen cells, we (27) and others (13) have reported that this dye also inhibits the response of these cells to several mitogens, such as PHA, Con A and LPS. The mitogenic response of lymphoid cells has often been used as an in vitro model for the immune response.

The relationship between cellular metabolism and the immune response that has been presented in this report tends to confirm the data of several earlier investigators. The glycolytic antagonist 2 deoxyglucose has been shown to inhibit the mitogenic response of lymphocytes (19). We have repeated this effect (data not presented) and also found this compound to be inhibitory to both in vivo and in vitro immune responses. Other have reported that the mitogenic response of lymphocytes is accompanied by an increased flow of glucose through the hexose monophosphate shunt (20). These investigators also speculated upon an increase in H_2O_2 production by the stimulated cells. It has been previously reported that mouse spleen cell contained NADPH oxidase activity and did produce H_2O_2 (24). In another report it was found that H_2O_2 was able to suppress immunoglobulin production by lymphoid cells in culture (6). We have found that H_2O_2 inhibits the in vitro hemolytic PFC response and that splenoperoxidase activity is increased by antigenic stimulation. There have been many reports implying a role for lysosomal enzyme activities other than peroxidase in the immune response. Leukocytes from immunized animals have been reported to have an increase in lysosomal nuclease activity (1) APTase (7) and other hydrolases (21). It has also been reported that human lymphocytes exhibit an increase in hydrolase rich granules after PHA stimulation of acid hydrolases from the 20,000 z pellet fraction to the supernatant fraction of human lymphocyte (9).

It would appear from the data presented in this report and that of previous investigators that there is an association between cellular metabolism and the immune response. One could speculate from our data that H_2O_2 produced from intermediary metabolism interacts with lysosomal peroxidase as a control mechanism for this response. The role(s) of other enzymes and metabolic pathways that have been found to be affected by antigenic stimulation would require additional studies before one could even postulate a possible mechanism. Such studies could prove to be valuable to researchers and clinicians who are interested in immunological disorders associated with a variety of conditions.

ACKNOWLEDGEMENTS

The author thanks Ms. Leoney Mills, Mr. Navin Patel, Mr. Chandu Patel and Mr. Matthew McConeghy for technical assistance and Ms. Marlene Banks for typing of this manuscript.

REFERENCES

1. Atwal, O. S. Experimentia 23 (1967) 185.
2. Bandmann, U., Rydgren, L. and Norberg, B. Exptl. Cell Res. 88 (1974) 63.
3. Beck, F., Lloyd, J. and Griffiths, A. Science (1967) 157.
4. Boxer, L. A., Baehner, R. L. and Davis, J. J. Cell. Physiol. 91 (1977) 89.
5. Brown, J. Metabolism 11 (1962) 1098.
6. Cohen, H. J. Experientia 29 (1973) 1285.
7. Friedman, H. and Kately, J. R. Proc. Soc. Exp. Biol. Med. 147 (1974) 460.
8. Hirschhorn, Rochelle, Brittinger, et al. In: Proceedings of the 3rd annual leukocyte culture conference (Ed. W. O. Rieke) N. Y., 639.
9. Hirschhorn, R., Brittinger, G., Hirschhorn, K. and Weissman, G. J. Cell. Biol. 37 (1968) 412.
10. Jerne, N. K. and Nordin, A. A. Science 140 (1963) 405.
11. Karnovsky, M. L. Seminars Hemat. 5 (1968) 156.
12. Karnovsky, M. L., Drath, D. and Lazdins, J. Plenum Press, New York, 121 (1976).
13. Kripke, M. L., Norbury, K. C., Gruyo, E. and Hibbs, J. B., Jr.

Infect. Immun. 17 (1977) 121.
14. Marbrook, J. Lancet II (1967) 1279.
15. Michl, J., Ohlbaum, D. J. and Silverstein, S. C. J. Exptl. Med. 144 (1976) 1461.
16. Oliver, J. M., Albertini, D. F. and Berlin, R. D. J. Cell Biol. 71 (1976) 921.
17. Oliver, J. M., Berlin, R, D., Baehner, R. L. and Boxer, L. K. Brit. J. Haematol. 37 (1977) 311.
18. Patriarca, P., Dri, P., Kakinuma, K. and Rossi, P. Mol. Cell. Biochem. 12 (1976) 137.
19. Polgar, P. R., Foster, J. M. and Cooperband, S. R. Exptl. Cell Res. 49 (1968) 231.
20. Sagone, A. L., Jr., LoBuglio, A. F. and Balcerzak, S. P. Cell. Immunol. 14 (1974) 443.
21. Shults, F. S. and Woodward, J. M. Canad. J. Microbiol. 13 (1967) 795.
22. Stossel, T. P. and Pollard, T. D. J. Biol. Chem. 248 (1973) 8288.
23. Stossel, T. P., N. E. J. Med. 290 (1974) 717.
24. Strauss, R. R., Paul, B. B., Jacobs, A. A. and Sbarra, A. J. Infect. Immun. 5 (1972) 114.
25. Strauss, R. R., Jacobs, A. A., Paul, B. B. and Sbarra, A. J. RES 11 (1972) 277.
26. Strauss, R. R., Friedman, H., Mills, L. and Zayon, G. Infect. Immun. 15 (1977) 197.
27. Strauss, R. R., Patel, N. and Patel, P. J. Reticuloendothel. Soc. 22 (1977) 533.
28. Zurier, R. B., Weissmann, G., Hoffstein, S., Kammerman, S. and Tai, H. H. J. Clin. Invest. 53 (1974) 297.

ROLE OF THE RES IN LEAD SALT SENSITIZATION TO ENDOTOXIN SHOCK

J. P. FILKINS

Stritch School of Medicine
Loyola University of Chicago
Chicago, Illinois (USA)

Lead salts when administered to experimental animals in doses which by themselves are quite innocuous render the lead-treated subject markedly sensitive to lethal endotoxicosis as well as other forms of shock (2, 9, 11). A role for the RES in lead-sensitization to endotoxin shock was suggested by the ability of lead acetate to depress the intravascular clearance of colloidal agents (2, 5). Since previous studies from our laboratory have suggested a glucoregulatory role for the RES in resistance to endotoxin shock (1, 5, 6, 7, 8, 9, 10), the present study evaluated the effect of lead-induced depression of the RES on glucose homeostasis and insulin dynamics.

MATERIALS AND METHODS

Male rats of the Holtzman strain were treated with either lead acetate (5 mg i. v.) or as a control - 0.9% saline or sodium acetate i. v. Crystalline insulin was supplied by the Eli Lilly Company (Indianapolis, Indiana). Using the methods described previously (5-10), the following measurements were obtained: sensitivity to insulin seizure deaths, glucose tolerance, *in vivo* and *in vitro* assessments of hepatic gluconeogenesis, *in vivo* and *in vitro* assessments of glucose oxidation and both basal and glycemic-stimulated serum immunoreactive insulin levels.

RESULTS

Effect of lead acetate on insulin lethality and glucose tolerance. The effects of lead acetate on lethality in convulsive seizures induced by insulin are presented in Table I. In contrast to low lethality to insulin at doses of 0.5, 0.75, 1.0 and 1.5 units per rat in control rats, lead treatment increased lethality in classic insulin convulsive seizures.

Lead treatment was also evaluated for effects on glucose tolerance (Table II). The marked decrease in the half-time for glucose disappearance, i. e., increased glucose tolerance, is suggestive of a functional hyperinsulinism.

Effects of lead acetate on gluconeogenesis and glucose oxidation in vivo and in vitro. As presented in Table III, lead acetate treatment depressed conversion of an alanine load to glucose. Furthermore, as presented in Table IV, hepatocytes

TABLE I

Insulin Seizure Lethality After Acute Lead Administration[a]

Group	Number of Rats	Insulin Dose (Units/Rat)	% Lethality
Control	20	0.50	0
	10	0.75	0
	20	1.00	5.0
	20	1.50	40.0
Lead Acetate	30	0.50	16.7
	10	0.75	30.0
	30	1.00	70.0[b]
	20	1.50	95.0[b]

[a]Overnight fasted rats received a 1 ml i. v. injection of either 5 mg/ml lead acetate or 0.9% saline (control) immediately followed by a 1 ml injection of insulin sc. Lethality was recorded at 24 hr

[b]$p < 0.001$ as compared to control groups using the X^2 test

TABLE II

Glucose Tolerance After Acute Lead Administration[a]

Group	Number of Rats	Basal Plasma Glucose[b] (mg/dl)	Half-Time of Glucose Disappearance (min)
Control	10	84 ± 3	49 ± 6
Lead Acetate	10	75 ± 4	24 ± 3
	p-value	N. S.	<0.001

[a]Overnight fasted rats received a 1 ml i. v. injection of either sodium acetate (control) or lead acetate (5 mg/ml) 4 hr before i. v. glucose tolerance testing
[b]Plasma glucose immediately before injection of 200 mg glucose i. v. at 0 min
N. S. = not statistically significant at $p < .05$ using Student's unpaired t test

isolated from lead-treated donor rats manifested depressed gluconeogenesis *in vitro* from the three major gluconeogenic precursors - lactate, pyruvate and alanine.

Thus, using both *in vivo* and *in vitro* assessments of hepatic gluconeogenesis, depression of the RES by lead salts produced decreases in the ability of the liver to transform precursors into glucose. Since the gluconeogenic process in fasted rats is especially sensitive to insulin depression, the data are consistent with a functional hyperinsulinism incident to RES depression.

Lead acetate was also evaluated for influences on glucose oxidation *in vivo* (Table V) and *in vitro* (Table VI). Glucose oxidation of rats treated with lead acetate was increased as reflected in the higher percentages of ^{14}C-glucose oxidized to $^{14}CO_2$. Similarly, epididymal fat pads from lead-treated donors showed increased glucose oxidation when incubated with ^{14}C-glucose *in vitro* (Table VI).

Thus, to summarize to this point, lead acetate depression of the RES was associated with sensitivity to exogenous insulin as well as with the conventional metabolic indices of a functional

TABLE III

Effect of Acute Lead Administration on Gluconeogenesis *In Vivo*[a]

Group	Number of Rats	Gluconeogenic Index[c] (% conversion of alanine to glucose)
Control	10	16.2 ± 1.4
Lead Acetate	10	9.2 ± 0.9[b]

[a]Overnight fasted rats (300 ± 10 gm) received 5 mg of lead acetate or sodium acetate i. v. 4 hr prior to 100 mg of alanine + 0.5 μCi of ^{14}C-alanine i. p. Thirty min later all rats were sacrificed and the conversion of ^{14}C-alanine to ^{14}C-glucose computed

[b]$p < .001$

[c]Gluconeogenic index calculated as:

$$\text{\% conversion to glucose} = \frac{\text{glucose space x glucose } ^{14}\text{C in blood}}{\text{injected dose of } ^{14}\text{C-alanine}} \times 100$$

hyperinsulinemic state, *viz*, increased glucose tolerance, depressed hepatic gluconeogenesis, and enhanced peripheral glucose utilization.

Effects of lead acetate on basal and glycemia-stimulated serum insulin levels. Table VII presents the effects of lead acetate on serum immunoreactive insulin levels. As indicated, basal serum insulin levels were increased 62% by lead treatment. Even more striking was the insulin response to a glucose challenge since lead treatment resulted in a 581% increase in insulin levels.

DISCUSSION

Endotoxin shock is characterized by a progressive, profound hypoglycemia due to a combination of depressed hepatic gluconeogenesis and enhanced peripheral glucose oxidation (1, 10). Our past studies have suggested that the glucoregulatory defect in endotoxicosis is due to hyperinsulinism (5, 6, 7, 8, 9, 10). The findings of the current study suggest that lead treatment shares the ability to induce a functional hyperinsulinism which is probably a reflection of a true hyperinsulinemia. Thus, lead salts sensitize to endotoxin due to their ability to undermine host glucoregulation in endotoxicosis. Since lead salts depress

TABLE IV

Effect of Lead Acetate on Gluconeogenesis in Isolated Hepatocytes[a]

Hepatocyte Donor Rats (N)	KRB	+	Glucose Production (µmoles of glucose/gm protein/120 min) 10mM Lactate	10mM Pyruvate	10mM Alanine
Control (8)	13 ± 1		159 ± 13	194 ± 32	132 ± 12
Lead Acetate (8)	18 ± 1		81 ± 12[b]	84 ± 14[b]	60 ± 5

[a]Overnight fasted rats (300 ± 10 gm) received either 5 mg of lead acetate or sodium acetate i. v. 5 hr prior to sacrifice for hepatocyte isolation and gluconeogenic evalution

[b]$p < .05$ as compared to control substrate group

TABLE V

Effect of Lead Depression of the RES on *In Vivo* Glucose Oxidation of Glucose to $^{14}CO_2$ (%)[a]

Group	Number of Rats	Glucose Oxidation to CO2 (Min) 30	60	90	120	180	240
Control	7	0.94 ±.05	4.41 ±.20	9.60 ±.34	15.24 ±.55	25.47 ±.83	33.23 ±.04
Lead Acetate	12	1.72[b] ±.17	7.81[b] ±.52	15.06[b] ±.90	22.05[b] ±1.15	33.38[b] ±1.23	41.38[b] ±1.14

[a]400 mg D-glucose + 20 µCi U-D-^{14}C-glucose i. p. at 4 hr after 5 mg lead or sodium acetate i. v. (controls). Data are expressed as percent of the injected glucose dose recovered as CO_2

[b]$p < .05$ as compared to respective control group

TABLE VI

Effect of Acute Lead Administration on Glucose Oxidation in Epididymal Fat Pads[a]

Donor Group	Number of Rats	Glucose Oxidation (DPM - $^{14}CO_2$/gram/hr)
Control	12	48,177 ± 3264
Lead Acetate	12	62,740 ± 4176[b]

[a]Overnight fasted rats (100 ± 10 gm) received 1.5 mg of lead acetate or sodium acetate i. v. 4 hr prior to sacrifice
[b]$p < .001$

TABLE VII

Effect of Lead Treatment on Basal and Glucose-Stimulated Insulin Levels[a]

Group	Number of Rats	Serum Glucose (mg/dl)	Serum Insulin (μU/ml)
Basal Insulin:			
Control	8	116 ± 2	9.4 ± 0.5
Lead Acetate	8	110 ± 3	15.2 ± 2.1
		N. S.[b]	0.018[b]
Glucose-Stimulated Insulin:			
Control	8	569 ± 9	34.6 ± 4.7
Lead Acetate	8	652 ± 27	235.5 ± 17.4
		0.011[b]	0.001[b]

[a]A 1 mo i. v. injection of 5 mg/ml lead acetate or sodium acetate was administered to fasted rats 4 hr before the time of blood sampling. For glucose-stimulated responses, blood samples were taken at 5 min after 400 mg glucose i. v.
[b]= p values

RES function (9), the findings are consistent with the theory that RES depression is a central event in the hyperinsulinemic state (5, 7, 8, 9).

Thus, it is suggested that a role of the RES in gluco-regulation is a key factor in host resistance to endotoxin shock and agents such as lead salts which interfere with RES function will sensitize to endotoxic deterioration of carbohydrate homeostasis and contribute to the pathogenesis of fatal endotoxin shock.

ACKNOWLEDGEMENTS

The collaboration of Bernard J. Buchanan, Robert P. Cornell and Angela M. Hadbavny in these investigations is gratefully recognized. This work was supported by USPHS Grant HL 08682.

REFERENCES

1. Buchanan, B. J. and Filkins, J. P. Circ. Shock 3 (1976) 267.
2. Cook, J. A., DiLuzio, N. R. and Hoffman, E. O. Crit. Rev. Toxicol. 3 (1975) 201.
3. Cornell, R. P. and Filkins, J. P. Proc. Soc. Exptl. Biol. Med. 145 (1974) 203.
4. Cornell, R. P. and Filkins, J. P. Proc. Soc. Exptl. Biol. Med. 147 (1974) 371.
5. Hadbavny, A. M., Buchanan, B. J. and Filkins, J. P. J. Reticuloendo. Soc. 24 (1978) 57.
6. Filkins, J. P. Proc. Soc. Exptl. Biol. Med. 142 (1973) 915.
7. Filkins, J. P. J. Reticuloendo. Soc. 20 (1977) 461.
8. Filkins, J. P. and Buchanan, B. J. J. Reticuloendo. Soc. 21 (1977) 389.
9. Filkins, J. P. and Buchanan, B. J. Proc. Soc. Exptl. Biol. Med. 142 (1973) 471.
10. Filkins, J. P. and Cornell, R. P. Am. J. Physiol. 227 (1974) 778.
11. Selye, H., Tuchweber, B. and Bertok, L. J. Bacteriol. 91 (1966) 884.

A METABOLIC COMPARISON BETWEEN HUMAN BLOOD MONOCYTES AND NEUTROPHILS

D. ROOS[1], M. REISS[1], A. J. M. BALM[1], A. M. PALACHE[1], P. H. CAMBIER[2] and J. S. VAN DER STIJL-NEIJENHUIS[1]

[1]Central Laboratory of the Netherlands Red Cross Blood Transfusion Service and Laboratory for Experimental and Clinical Immunology of the University of Amsterdam, P. O. Box 9190, Amsterdam (The Netherlands) and
[2]Laboratory for Electron Microscopy, University of Leiden, Leiden (The Netherlands)

The two most prominent types of phagocytic cells in the human circulation are the neutrophilic granulocytes and the monocytes. Both cell types are involved in host defense by their ability to move into the tissues to the site of an infection, to bind to foreign material, to ingest it, and to kill living microorganisms. The latter reaction is mediated to a large extent by the formation of toxic oxygen radicals.

Besides this apparent similarity between neutrophils and monocytes, there are also clear differences. Monocytes have a larger synthetic and digestive capacity than neutrophils do, and monocytes appear to be also involved in the lymphocytic reaction towards antigens. Neutrophils are short-living end-cells, monocytes develop into tissue macrophages with specialized functions. To characterize the circulating phagocytes, we have made a metabolic comparison between human blood neutrophils and monocytes.

First, we compared the capacity to generate microbicidal oxygen products during phagocytosis. Table I shows the reaction of the two cell types to serum-opsonized zymosan (5). Neutrophils not only generate more oxygen products than monocytes do, but also convert a larger part of the consumed oxygen into H_2O_2 (neutrophils: 89 ± 3% in the first 10 min, monocytes: 29 ± 5%).

This difference between H_2O_2 recovery of the two cell types might be due to a difference in the activity of H_2O_2-utilizing enzymes, such as catalase, myeloperoxidase, and glutathione peroxidase. Under our reaction conditions, however, azide (NaN_3) is present to inhibit catalase and myeloperoxidase. The activity of glutathione peroxidase was 6.2-13.6 (n=24) and 5.9-7.8 (n=10) in neutrophils and monocytes, respectively. Therefore, the low recovery in monocytes is probably not caused by a high utilization of H_2O_2 in these cells.

TABLE I

Oxygen Metabolism of Zymosan-Stimulated Cells

	Oxygen Consumption	Superoxide Generation	Hydrogen Peroxide[a] Production
Neutrophils[b]	3.8 ± 0.6	1.3 ± 0.2	4.5 ± 0.6
Monocytes[b]	1.4 ± 0.3	0.8 ± 0.1	0.7 ± 0.2
Ratio (%)	39 ± 6	62 ± 9	19 ± 5

[a]In the presence of 2 mM NaN_3.

[b]Maximal rates in nmoles/1 x 10^6 cells per min; mean ± S.E.M. of 8 paired experiments with neutrophils and monocytes from the same donor.

Another possible cause for the difference in H_2O_2 recovery might be that monocytes do not use all the consumed oxygen for the production of H_2O_2, as neutrophils do. Instead, monocytes might metabolize oxygen in other, non-H_2O_2-generating reactions, such as the oxidative phosphorylation, which takes place in the mitochondria and generates ATP. To check the possibility that monocytes display more mitochondrial activity than neutrophils, we have quantitated the number and the size of the mitochondria in the two cell types from electron microscopical photographs of cell sections. Table II shows that monocytes contain more and larger mitochondria than neutrophils do.

If monocytes do indeed increase the mitochondrial oxygen consumption during phagocytosis, this activity must be susceptible to inhibitors of the oxidative phosphorylation. Table III shows the effect of some of these agents on the stimulated oxygen consumption of the two cell types. NaN_3 and cyanide (KCN) increase the respiration of neutrophils. This effect is probably due to the inhibition of catalase, however, since this enzyme decomposes H_2O_2 to oxygen and water. Thus, inhibition of catalase increases

TABLE II

Mitochondria in Human Neutrophils and Monocytes

	Neutrophils (n=26)	Monocytes (n=26)
Number of mitochondria per cell section	8.2 ± 0.5	14.1 ± 1.0
Mitochondrial surface area (percentage of cell area)	0.61 ± 0.06	2.97 ± 0.20

the overall disappearance of oxygen from the medium, and seemingly stimulates the oxygen consumption.

$$O_2 \longrightarrow O_2^- \longrightarrow H_2O_2 \xrightarrow[\text{(catalase)}]{N_3^-,\ CN^-} H_2O_2 + \tfrac{1}{2}\,O_2$$

Therefore, any effect of N_aN_3 or KCN on the mitochondrial respiration will be masked by this effect on catalase. This probably explains the lack of a significant effect of these agents on the respiration of monocytes (Table III).

Antimycin A, which blocks electron transfer at the cytochrome b level, and Oligomycin, which inhibits the phosphorylation reaction, are more specific mitochondrial inhibitors. Table III shows that Antimycin A had no effect on neutrophil respiration but significantly inhibited this reaction in monocytes ($p<0.01$). The inhibiting effect of Antimycin A on the oxygen consumption of monocytes, contrary to the effect on neutrophils, is illustrated in Fig. 1. This Fig. also shows the effect of Antimycin A on the H_2O_2 generation by the two cell types. The inhibitor had no effect on the release of H_2O_2 by either cell type. It appears that the oxygen consumption of Antimycin A-treated monocytes is nearly equal to the H_2O_2 release by these cells. This indicates that the oxygen that is consumed in the Antimycin A-insensitive respiration is converted almost completely into H_2O_2, similar to the situation in neutrophils.

From the above-described results, we conclude that monocytes activate the oxidative phosphorylation reaction during phagocytosis. An obvious reason for the increase in the oxidative

TABLE III

Effect of Metabolic Inhibitors on the Oxygen Consumption of Zymosan-Stimulated Cells[a]

	NaN_3 (2 mM)	KCN (2 mM)	Antimycin (360 μM)	Oligomycin (15 μg/ml)
Neutrophils	110-146	115-130	106-112	n.t.
Monocytes	81-99	48-77	14-35	21-62

[a]Values in percentage of the oxygen consumption without inhibitors (range).

[b]n.t. = not tested.

phosphorylation activity by zymosan-stimulated monocytes is the generation of ATP needed for the process of particle ingestion. It must be realized, however, that small changes in the rate of the oxidative phosphorylation are not easily detected by oxygen determinations; yet, this may lead to large changes in the ATP formation, owing to the high efficiency of this process. Therefore, it cannot be concluded from the lack of effect of the inhibitors on the neutrophil respiration that these cells do not generate any ATP in the mitochondria.

We have tested, therefore, the effect of Antimycin A both on the uptake of the zymosan particles and on the ATP levels in the cells. Antimycin A caused a dose-dependent inhibition of zymosan uptake by monocytes, with total blocking at 360 μM (not shown). In contrast, this inhibitor had no effect on the uptake of zymosan particles by neutrophils at Antimycin A concentration below 150 μM. At higher concentrations clumping of the neutrophils occurred, thus preventing accurate measurements of the ingestion process. The phagocytosis by monocytes was inhibited for 40% at 150 μM. Antimycin A. These results indicate that monocytes depend more heavily on oxidative phosphorylation for particle uptake than neutrophils do.

It should also be noted that, although the ingestion of zymosan is totally inhibited by 360 μM Antimycin A, the generation of H_2O_2 is unaffected under these conditions. This means that phagocytosis of particles is not needed for the occurrence of the respiratory burst in monocytes. Apparently, attachment of the particles to the monocytes provides sufficient stimulus for the activation of the oxygen-reducing system in these cells. Similar observations have been made with neutrophils (1).

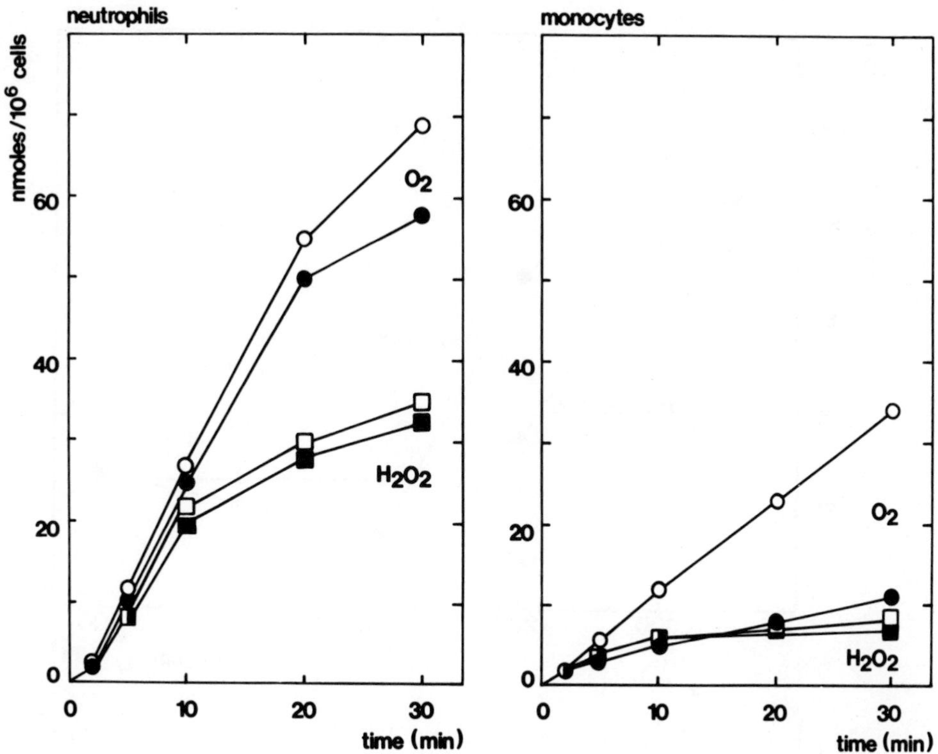

Fig. 1. Effect of Antimycin A on oxygen consumption and hydrogen peroxide release by zymosan-stimulated cells. O_2 consumption without (o——o) and with (●——●) 360 μM Antimycin A, and H_2O_2 generation without (□——□) and with (■——■) 360 μM Antimycin A, is given in nmoles per 10^6 cells.

The effect of Antimycin A on the level of ATP in the two cell types at rest is shown in Fig. 2. In both, neutrophils and monocytes, this inhibitor caused a dose-dependent decrease of the ATP level. Thus, also in neutrophils the ATP synthesis appears to be dependent on the process of oxidative phosphorylation in the mitochondria.

From the foregoing experiments, it appears that monocytes do increase the mitochondrial ATP synthesis during phagocytosis. Fig. 3 shows that, as a result, the ATP level in monocytes is hardly affected by the ingestion process. On the other hand, neutrophils do not, or to a minor extent, increase the mitochondrial synthesis

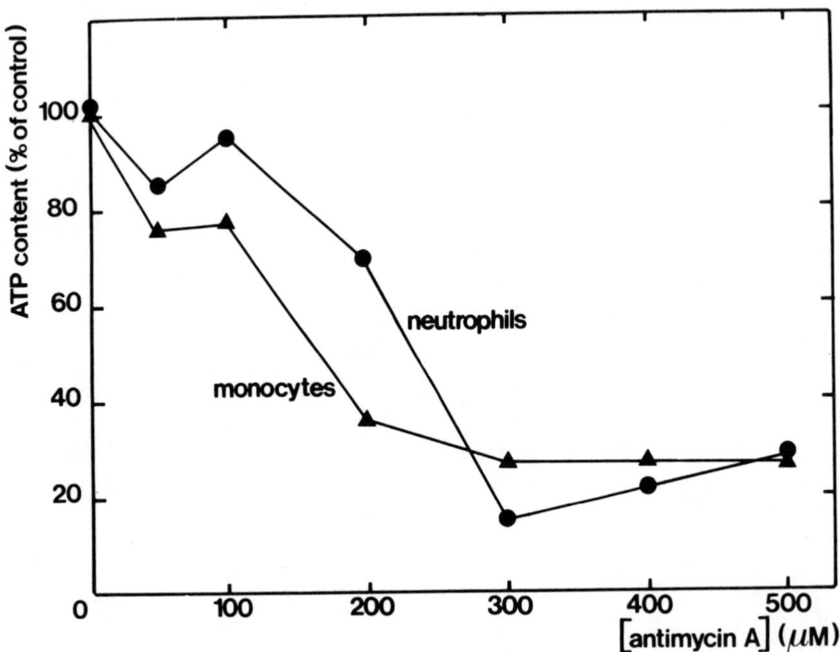

Fig. 2. Effect of Antimycin A on the ATP level in human neutrophils and monocytes.
Values in percentage of the ATP levels found without Antimycin A (in neutrophils, 100% = 1.1 ± 0.1 nmoles per 1 x 10^6 cells, n = 10; in monocytes, 100% = 1.4 ± 0.2 nmoles per 1 x 10^6 cells, n = 7).

during phagocytosis, although these cells depend on this process for most of their ATP synthesis at rest. Since phagocytosis is an energy-consuming process, it can be expected that the level of ATP in neutrophils will decrease during particle uptake. Some investigators, however, have reported an increased rate of anaerobic glycolysis in neutrophils during phagocytosis, especially during the first 15 min after particle addition (3,7). In principle, this may be of importance in maintaining ATP levels, although the anaerobic glycolysis is much less efficient in ATP generation than the oxidative phosphorylation is.

We have tested, therefore, the effect of zymosan phagocytosis on the ATP level in neutrophils. We also measured the lactate production by these cells at rest and during phagocytosis. Table IV

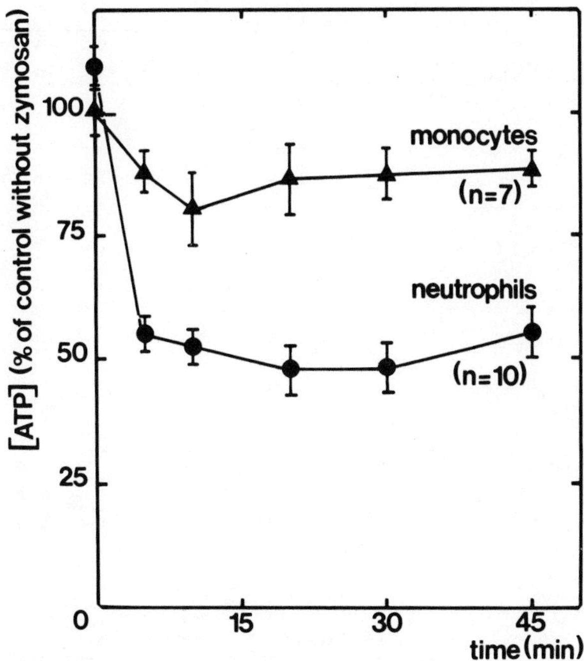

Fig. 3. Changes in the ATP level of human neutrophils and monocytes during zymosan ingestion.
Values in percentage of the ATP levels of resting cells (for 100% values, see legend to Fig. 2).

shows that neutrophils do not significantly enhance the lactate production during phagocytosis. This was found both for the first 15 min of phagocytosis and during longer periods. Thus, these cells do not enhance the ATP generation in either the aerobic or the anaerobic glycolysis. As a result, Fig. 3 shows that the level of ATP decreases in these cells during phagocytosis.

As Table IV shows, we did not find a significant difference in lactate production between resting and phagocytosing monocytes too. The higher rate of lactate production in monocytes as compared to neutrophils indicates that monocytes contain a carbodydrate metabolism which is in general more active than that of neutrophils.

Thus, we have found as others did (2,4,6,8), that human blood neutrophils and monocytes both generate microbicidal oxygen pro-

TABLE IV

Lactate Production by Human Neutrophils and Monocytes

	At Rest	During Zymosan Uptake
Neutrophils	70 ± 5 (n=10)	86 ± 7 (n=11)
Monocytes	164 ± 20 (n- 8)	192 ± 17 (n= 9)

Values in nmoles/1 x 10^6 cells per min (Mean ± S.E.M.).

ducts. Neutrophils are more active in this respect than monocytes are. We have also found that monocytes activate the mitochondrial ATP synthesis during phagocytosis, whereas neutrophils do not or to a much smaller extent. Since neutrophils do not activate the anaerobic glycolysis either, these cells seem to rely on presynthesized ATP for the ingestion process. As a consequence, the ATP levels in neutrophils decrease during phagocytosis in contrast to the situation in monocytes. It remains to be investigated whether these differences represent functional differences between the two cell types, such as the protein synthetic capacity, and/or this is only an indication of the pre-macrophage stage of the monocytes as opposed to the end-stage of the neutrophils. Perhaps, our results give an indication why monocytes show a much higher resistance towards external stress, such as during cell culturing or freeze-preservation.

REFERENCES

1. Goldstein, I. M., Roos, D., Kaplan, H. B. and Weissmann, G., J. Clin. Invest., 56 (1975) 1155.
2. Johnston, Jr., R. B., Lehneyer, J. E. and Guthrie, L. A., J. Exp. Med., 143 (1976) 1551.
3. Kakinuma, K., J. Biochem. (Tokyo), 68 (1970) 177.
4. Nelson, R. D., Mills, E. L., Simmons, R. L. and Quie, P. G., Infect. Immun., 14 (1976) 129.
5. Reiss, M. and Roos, D., J. Clin. Invest., 61 (1978) 480.
6. Sagone, Jr., A. L., King, G. W. and Metz, E. N., J. Clin. Invest., 57 (1976) 1352.
7. Sbarra, A. J. and Karnovsky, M. L., J. Biol. Chem., 234 (1959) 1355.
8. Weiss, S. J., King, G. W. and LoBuglio, A. F., J. Clin. Invest., 60 (1977) 370.

THE REGULATION OF MACROPHAGE ACTIVITIES: ROLE OF THE ENERGY-DEPENDENT INTRACELLULAR Ca^{2+} BUFFERING SYSTEMS

D. ROMEO, C. SCHNEIDER, R. GENNARO and C. MOTTOLA

Istituto di Chimica Biologica, Università di Trieste

Trieste (ITALY)

The central role played by phagocytic cells in immunological and inflammatory phenomena is related to their capacity of exhibiting a variety of physiological activities such as locomotion, endocytosis and secretion (8, 9, 18, 19, 22, 24, 28, 51, 53, 55). The mechanisms by which such diverse biological functions are regulated in these cells have only partially been clarified. Recent studies have suggested the possibility that changes in the fluxes of cations across the plasma membrane or other cell membranes, resulting in a variation in steady-state levels of these cations in the cytoplasm, may be involved in the initiation or control of the activity of the phagocytic cells. In particular, it has been demonstrated that an elevation of Ca^{2+} concentration in the cytoplasm of polymorphonuclear leukocytes and macrophages, catalyzed by the ionophore A23187 (35), promotes an increased directional motility, secretion of granule enzymes and O_2 reduction to bactericidal H_2O_2 (30, 35-39, 44, 46, 49, 50, 56, 58, 59). Furthermore, the exposure of polymorphonuclear leukocytes to the complement fragment C5a, to kallikrein or to formylmethionyl peptides, which are all able to stimulate chemotaxis, oxidative metabolism and secretion in these cells (3, 16, 17, 21, 23, 30, 45, 48, 49, 51), has been shown to cause a change in Ca^{2+} fluxes across the plasma membrane (4, 14, 29, 30).

These observations indicate that a study on the properties of the cell Ca^{2+} buffering systems might help elucidate the molecular mechanisms by which the great variety of Ca^{2+}-dependent activities of phagocytic cells are regulated.

While the concentration of Ca^{2+} in biological fluids is in the order of 10^{-3} M, the free Ca^{2+} concentration in the cytosol of

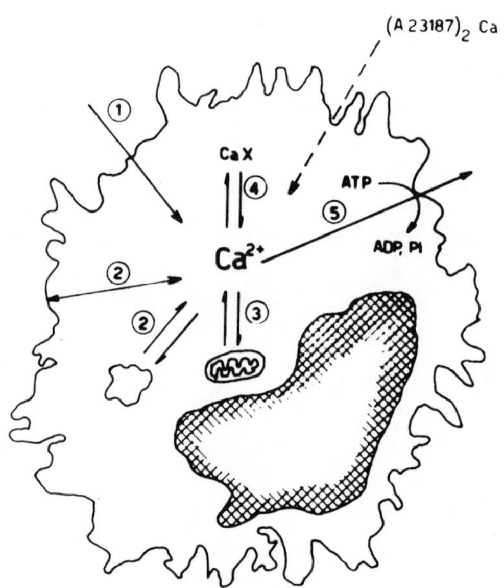

Fig. 1. Mechanisms involved in intracellular Ca^{2+} buffering.

cells at rest is in the order of 10^{-6} to 10^{-8} M (2, 5, 34). According to the current views various pathways and systems contribute to maintain this steady-state concentration (Fig. 1): 1) the non-specific Ca^{2+} leak through the plasma membrane downhill the ion concentration gradient; 2-3) the release of Ca^{2+} from, and uptake into, the plasma membrane and other organelles, particularly the mitochondria; 4) the dissociation of Ca^{2+} from, or association to, macromolecules and small molecules in the cytoplasm; 5) the cell extrusion of Ca^{2+} by an ATP-driven system localized at the cell boundary.

In view of its localization at the periphery of the cell, the latter system may be a suitable candidate for regulation of intracellular Ca^{2+} concentrations by cell surface-reactive compounds, thereby deserving a priority in any investigation dealing with these problems. The first part of this paper will indeed concern the description of a Ca^{2+}-dependent ATPase activity in the plasma membrane of alveolar macrophages, which might be a component of a Ca^{2+} transport system such as that discussed above.

<u>Ca^{2+}-dependent ATPase activity of alveolar macrophage plasma membrane</u>. We performed our studies on a plasma membrane fraction purified from lysates of BCG-induced rabbit alveolar macrophages by flotation through a discontinuous sucrose gradient (54). This fraction consists of vesicular structures of various sizes,

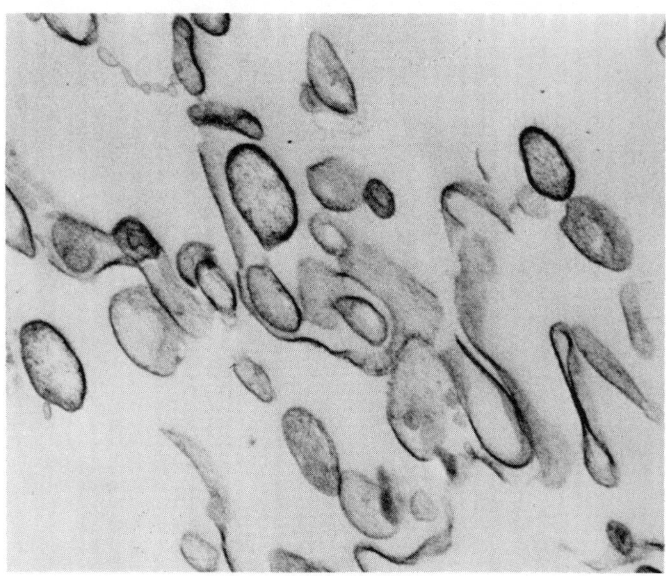

Fig. 2. Electron micrograph of the plasma membrane fraction isolated from BCG-induced rabbit alveolar macrophages (40,000 x).

characteristic of plasma membrane of other cells (Fig. 2). Although no specific experiment was carried out to control the efficiency of the resealing of the isolated membrane vesicles, it seems reasonable to assume that both inside and outside surfaces are available to the medium when the membrane is assayed for enzyme activities.

As shown in Table I, a consistent and large increase in the specific activity of the plasma membrane marker enzyme phosphodiesterase I is seen in the isolated vesicles over the cell lysate. In contrast, the specific activity of marker enzymes of mitochondria (succinate cyt. c reductase), lysosomes (β-glucuronidase) and endoplasmic reticulum (NADPH cyt. c reductase) significantly decreases in the plasma membrane fraction when compared to the original cell lysate. As indicated by the amount of phosphodiesterase I activity recovered in the plasma membrane fraction ($41.6 \pm 0.9\%$, mean of 7 individual preparations $\pm$ SEM), the yield of the membrane purification procedure is rather high.

Once verified the degree of purity of the plasma membrane fraction by morphological and biochemical criteria, we turned our attention to the analysis of the ATPase activity of the membrane. The activity of the ATP splitting enzyme(s) was assayed in the presence of the bivalent ion-chelator EGTA and the amounts of

TABLE I

Specific Activities of Marker Enzymes in Lysates and Plasma Membrane Fractions of Rabbit Alveolar Macrophages

	Lysates	Plasma Membrane Fractions
Alkaline Phosphodiesterase	65.6 ± 2.4	682.2 ± 20.9
Succinate Cytochrome c Reductase	40.8 ± 1.2	25.4 ± 2.0
NADPH Cytochrome c Reductase	10.7 ± 0.4	6.5 ± 0.3
β -Glucuronidase	146.6 ± 8.3	111.0 ± 7.7

The values represent the means of 7 individual preparations ± SEM. The activities of the enzymes, assayed at 37 C, are expressed as follows: alkaline phosphodiesterase I = nmoles p-nitropheno/mg protein/min; succinate cytochrome c reductase and NADPH cytochrome c reductase = nmoles cytochrome c reduced/mg protein/min; β - glucuronidase = nmoles 4-methyl umbelliferone/mg protein/15 min.

ionized calcium and magnesium present in the medium were calculated from the stability constants of the Ca^{2+}-EGTA or Mg^{2+}-EGTA complexes (33, 43).

As shown in Fig. 3, with Ca^{2+} in the medium at a concentration as little as 5 x 10^{-7} M there is already a 4-fold increase in the basal EGTA-ATPase activity (0.32 ± 0.03 µmoles Pi/mg protein/15 min). By gradually increasing the Ca^{2+} concentration, the enzyme activity rapidly rises and is about 10-fold higher than the basal value at 1.7 x 10^{-5} M Ca^{2+}. From this point up to 1 x 10^{-3} M Ca^{2+} the ATPase activity continues to increase, but the rate of increment is very much lower than that observed in the first part of the dose-activity curve.

The ATPase activity specifically stimulated by low concentrations of Ca^{2+}, with an apparent K_m (Ca^{2+}) of 1.1 x 10^{-6} M, will be referred to in this paper as Ca^{2+}-ATPase.

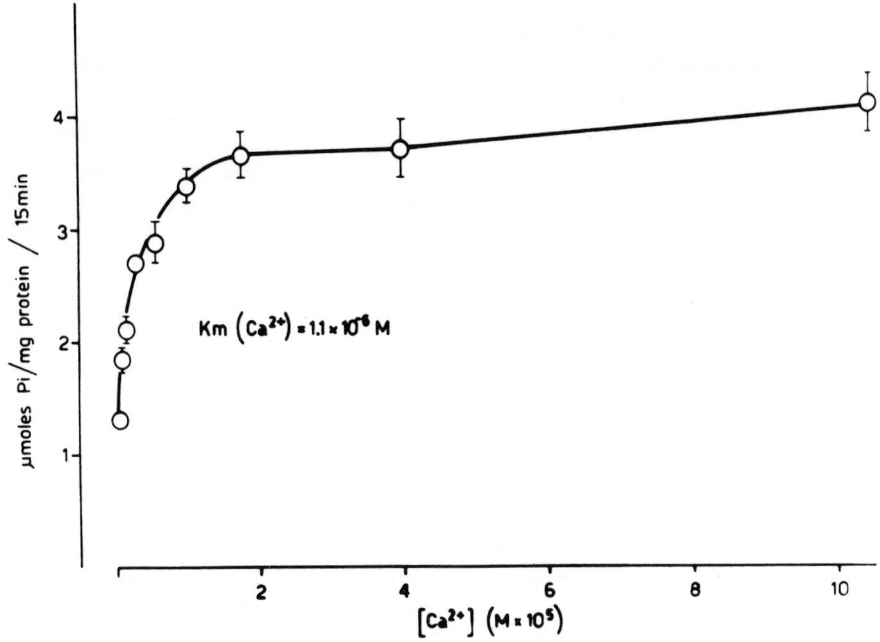

Fig. 3. Ca^{2+}-ATPase activity of alveolar macrophage plasma membrane as a function of free Ca^{2+} concentration.

That this enzyme is a component of the plasma membrane of macrophages is demonstrated by its relative purification in the isolated plasma membrane fraction (Table II). In fact, the specific activity of the Ca^{2+}-ATPase, assayed at pCa 5.5, is enriched about 8-fold in this fraction over the cell lysate. The specific activity of Mg^{2+}-ATPase and Na^+, K^+, Mg^{2+}-ATPase (27) also exhibits a several-fold enrichment. In contrast, the specific activity of K^+, EDTA-ATPase, associated to macrophage myosin (20), on the average increases only 1.3-fold.

The latter result, coupled to the observation that -SH group reagents, known inhibitors of myosin ATPase (1), have no influence on the Ca^{2+}-ATPase activity, strongly suggests that this enzyme is not bound to subplasmalemmal contractile structures but is a true component of the plasma membrane itself.

This conclusion is also supported by the observation that the exposure of the plasma membrane to detergents, such as Triton X-100 and deoxycholate, causes a decrease in the activity of the Ca^{2+}-ATPase, which is particularly evident with the non-ionic detergent (Fig. 4). The plasma membrane enzyme Mg^{2+}-ATPase is

TABLE II

Specific Activities of ATPase in Lysates and Plasma Membrane Fractions of Rabbit Alveolar Macrophages

	Lysates	Plasma Membrane Fractions
Ca^{2+}-ATPase	0.41 ± 0.02	3.10 ± 0.09
Mg^{2+}-AtPase	2.04 ± 0.04	12.60 ± 0.17
Na^+, K^+, Mg^{2+} ATPase	2.76 ± 0.11	17.32 ± 0.31
K^+, EDTA ATPase	0.017 ± 0.001	0.022 ± 0.002

The values represent the means of 5 individual experiments ± SEM. Activities are expressed as μmoles Pi/mg protein/15 min. The assay of K^+, EDTA-ATPase was carried out at 37 C in the medium described in reference 20. The basic medium for the assay of the other 3 ATPases contained 30 mM imidazole-HCl, pH 7.0, 0.2 M sucrose, 1 mM EGTA, 0.5 mM ATP and 3 to 20 μg or 1 to 8 μg of protein equivalent of cell lysate or plasma membrane fraction, respectively. In addition, the medium contained: Ca^{2+} at pCa 5.5 (Ca^{2+}-ATPase) or 1 mM Mg^{2+} (Mg^{2+}-ATPase) or 50 mM Na^+, 5 mM K^+ and 1 mM Mg^{2+} (Na^+, K^+, Mg^{2+} ATPase).

also inhibited by two surfactants, although in the case of deoxycholate the patterns of inhibition is different (Fig. 4).

A Ca^{2+}-dependent ATPase activity has been demonstrated to be present in the plasma membrane of other cells in addition to a Mg^{2+} dependent activity (10, 12, 15, 25, 31, 41-43, 47, 57), which has a pattern of Ca^{2+}-dependence similar to that reported here (43), most of the above enzymes are activated by Ca^{2+} at rather higher concentration. This sometimes does not permit establishment of whether the same enzyme is activated unspecifically by either Mg^{2+} or Ca^{2+}, although to a different degree, or 2 enzymes with different cation specifically exist in the membrane. A number of evidences suggest that the ATPase of macrophage plasma membrane, activated by Ca^{2+} at concentrations lower than about 1×10^{-5} M, is different from the Mg^{2+}-ATPase, with an apparent K_m (Mg^{2+}) of 0.5×10^{-3} M (Fig. 5). These evidences are the following: a) from 6×10^{-8} M to about 1×10^{-5} M Ca^{2+}, but not

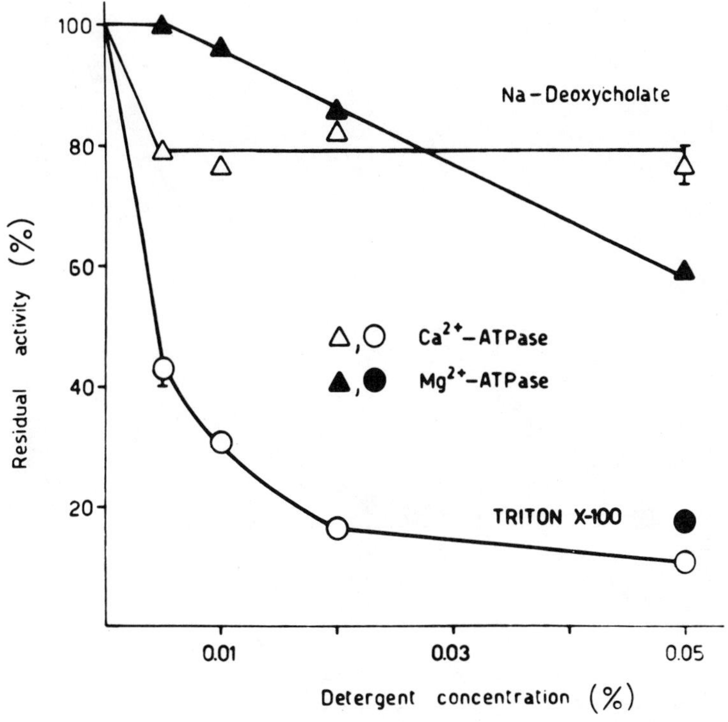

Fig. 4. Effect of detergents on the activity of macrophage plasma membrane Ca^{2+}-ATPase (pCa 5.5) and Mg^{2+}-ATPase.

Mg^{2+}, stimulates the enzymatic splitting of ATP (Fig. 5); b) the pattern of inhibition of the 2 enzymes of deoxycholate is different (Fig. 4); c) the Ca^{2+}-ATPase has a sharp pH optimum of 7, whereas the Mg^{2+} ATPase displays maximal activity around pH 7.8 (Fig. 6).

Another important parameter which permits distinguishing the Ca^{2+}-dependent from the Mg^{2+}-dependent ATPase activity is provided by the effect of Na^+ and K^+ on the 2 enzyme activities. In fact, while 50 mM Na^+ plus 5 mM K^+ enhance the Mg^{2+}-ATPase activity by about 40%, the same amounts of these ions causes an approximately 35% inhibition of Ca^{2+}-APTase activity. Parallel assays carried out with either alkali ion reveal that both ions inhibit the Ca^{2+}-ATPase, the inhibition of Na^+ being more marked than that of K^+. At 50 and 100 mM K^+, the Ca^{2+}-ATPase activity is decreased to 88 $\pm$ 5%, and 80 $\pm$ 6%, respectively; at 50 and 100 mM Na^+, the residual enzyme activity is 75 $\pm$ 5% and 63 $\pm$ 8%, respectively (means of 5 determinations $\pm$ SEM). The monovalent ion choline, at the same concentrations, has no effect on the Ca^{2+}-ATPase activity.

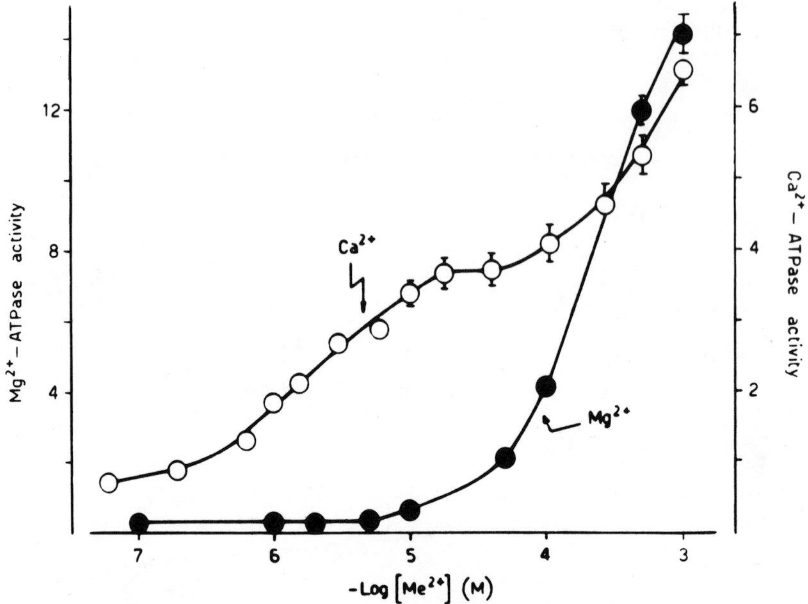

Fig. 5. Different stimulatory effects of Ca^{2+} and Mg^{2+} on the ATPase activity of macrophage plasma membrane (the activity is expressed as µmoles Pi/mg protein/15 min).

We have no direct evidence whether Ca^{2+}-ATPase identified in the plasma membrane fraction of the alveolar macrophages is a transport enzyme. The localization of the enzyme at the cell boundaries and its activation by free Ca^{2+} concentrations close to those presumably present in the cytosol of macrophages suggest, however, that the Ca^{2+}-ATPase may indeed by involved in active Ca^{2+} extrusion from the cell. In this assumption, the control of its activity would have a great relevance in the overall regulation of macrophage functions and may provide one of the mechanisms by which events such as locomotion, secretion, endocytosis and oxidative metabolism are activated.

Ca^{2+} uptake and Ca^{2+}-dependent secretion of granule enzymes by alveolar macrophages. Some evidence suggesting a role of the plasma membrane Ca^{2+} ATPase in the control of Ca^{2+} concentrations in macrophage cytosol is provided by experiments in which the Ca^{2+} uptake by alveolar macrophages was measured after their *in vitro* exposure to the antibiotic A23187 (46). This compound acts as an ionophore, equilibrating divalent cations across biological membranes (35). The treatment of the macrophages with the ionophore was carried out in the absence or in the presence of metabolic inhibitors, such as oligomycin, rotenone plus antimycin A or

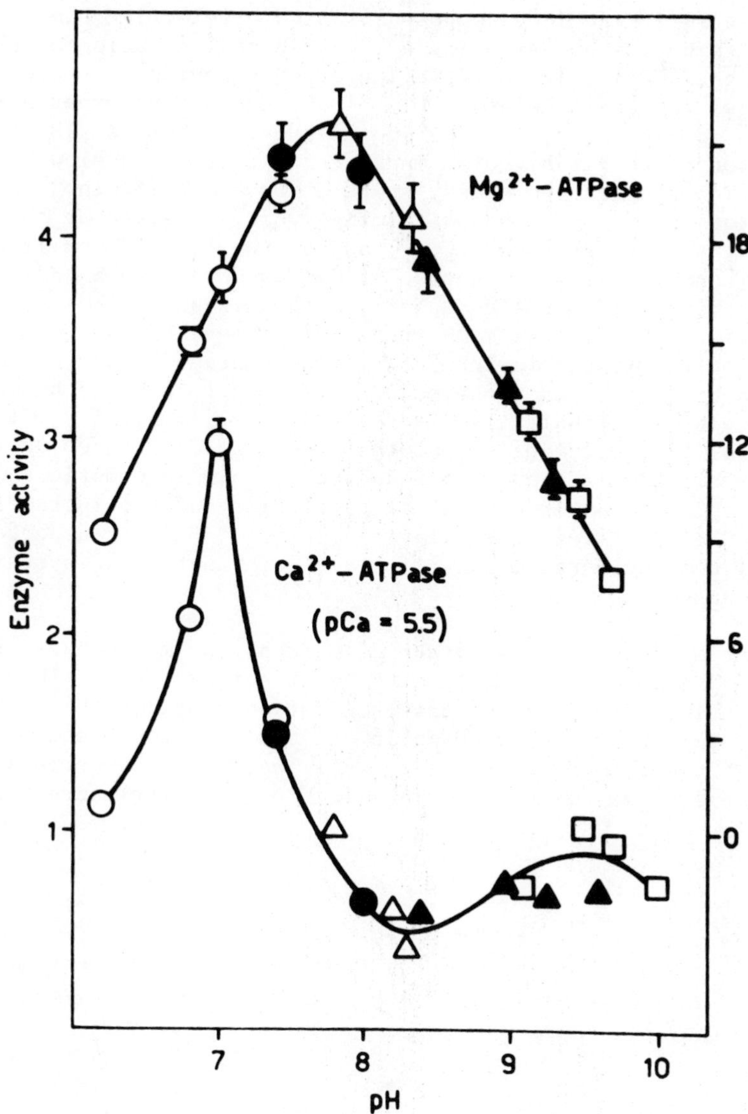

Fig. 6. Activities of macrophage plasma membrane ATPases as a function of pH (ordinates: μmoles Pi/mg protein/15 min; left: Ca^{2+}-ATPase; right: Mg^{2+}-ATPase).

cyanide, which prevent the mitochondrial energy utilization or completely block the electron transport chain (13, 26), thereby dramatically decreasing the ATP content of the cell.

The Ca^{2+} uptake by the alveolar macrophages was measured by a very sensitive device, composed of a Ca^{2+}-selective electrode and an amplifying system, allowing a 100-fold amplification of the electrode signal (46). The calibration of this device was made by additions of the Ca^{2+}-chelator EGTA at the end of the experiments. As shown in Fig. 7, after addition of the ionophore A23187 to a suspension of rabbit alveolar macrophages there is a slow uptake of Ca^{2+}, which reaches the steady-state after about 15 min. When the macrophages are first exposed to oligomycin, in spite of the marked drop in the cell ATP (see Fig. 9) and of the steep downhill gradient of Ca^{2+} concentration, no uptake of Ca^{2+} occurs. Upon addition of the ionophore to these ATP-depleted cells a rapid influx of Ca^{2+} is seen, which leads to the same steady-state levels observed in the absence of the metabolic inhibitor. The average amount of Ca^{2+} taken up by 1 x 10^6 macrophages is 12 nmoles. From the known value of cell water in rabbit alveolar macrophages, i. e., 1.67 µl/1 x 10^6 cells (52), it emerges that the amount of Ca^{2+} taken up is about 7-fold higher than that required for simple osmotic equilibration of the cation between the extracellular and the intracellular fluids. This implies that a large portion of Ca^{2+} transported into the cell becomes associated to intracellular buffering systems, as discussed above.

Concomitant with the uptake of Ca^{2+} by the macrophages there is an activation of secretion of granule enzymes (46). This is consistent with the notion that this cation provides the coupling between stimulus and exocytosis in various secretory cells (11, 30, 32, 37, 40, 49, 50, 58, 59). Fig. 8 illustrates the morphology of the process of exocytosis of granules from alveolar macrophages

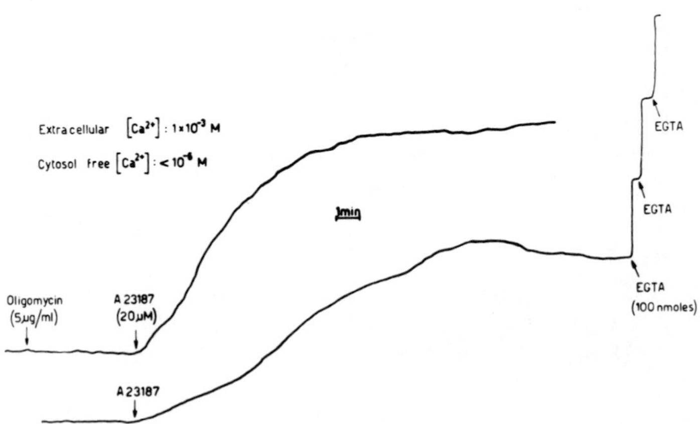

Fig. 7. Ca^{2+} uptake by rabbit alveolar macrophages exposed to the ionophore A23187 (medium: 123 mM NaCl, 5 mM KCl, 0.2 mM glucose, 1 mM $CaCl_2$ and 15 mM tris-HCl, pH 7.4; temperature: 37 C).

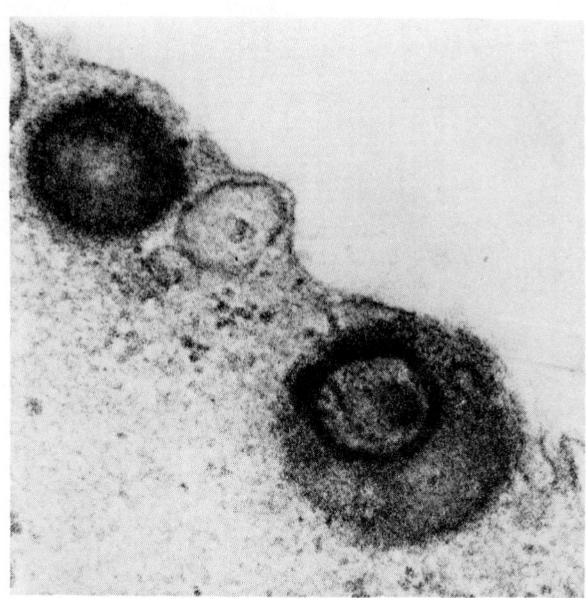

Fig. 8. Exocytosis of granules from rabbit alveolar macrophages induced by the ionophore A23187 in the presence of extracellular Ca^{2+} (120,000 x). The granule on the top left is approaching the plasma membrane, which is pushed out by the second granule and has already fused with the membrane of the third granule.

treated with the ionophore A23187 and Ca^{2+}, whereas Figs. 9 and 10 show the biochemical evaluation of the secretion.

When the macrophages are exposed to the ionophore and Ca^{2+}, some decrease in ATP occurs in the first 10-15 min of incubation (Fig. 9), very likely as a consequence of the uncoupling of mitochondrial oxidative phosphorylation (35). Under these conditions, some amount of the granule enzymes β -glucuronidase and lysozyme (7) is released from the macrophages. The appearance of the granule enzymes in the medium does not derive from disruption of the macrophages, since lactate dehydrogenase, a soluble cytoplasmic enzyme, remains confined to the cells. If in a parallel assay oligomycin is added at the tenth min, a rapid fall in ATP occurs with a simultaneous burst of exocytosis. As shown in Fig. 10, ATP depletion *per se* causes only a slight activation of exocytosis, which is several-fold amplified by the ionophore-induced Ca^{2+} influx from the extracellular space.

Some hypothetical considerations can be made by discussing these data in relation to the scheme of Fig. 1, illustrating the various systems that the macrophage very likely utilizes to

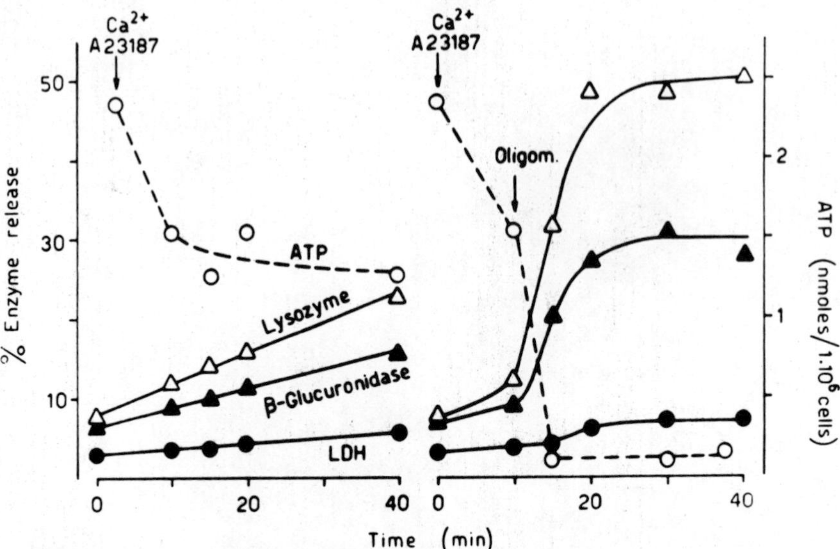

Fig. 9. Kinetics of enzyme release from rabbit alveolar macrophages exposed to the ionophore A23187 in the presence of extracellular Ca^{2+} (medium: as in Fig. 7; A23187: 20 μM; oligomycin: 5 μg/1 x 10^7 cells/ml; enzymes: % total cell activity appearing in the extracellular fluid; ATP: nucleotide concentrations in cells).

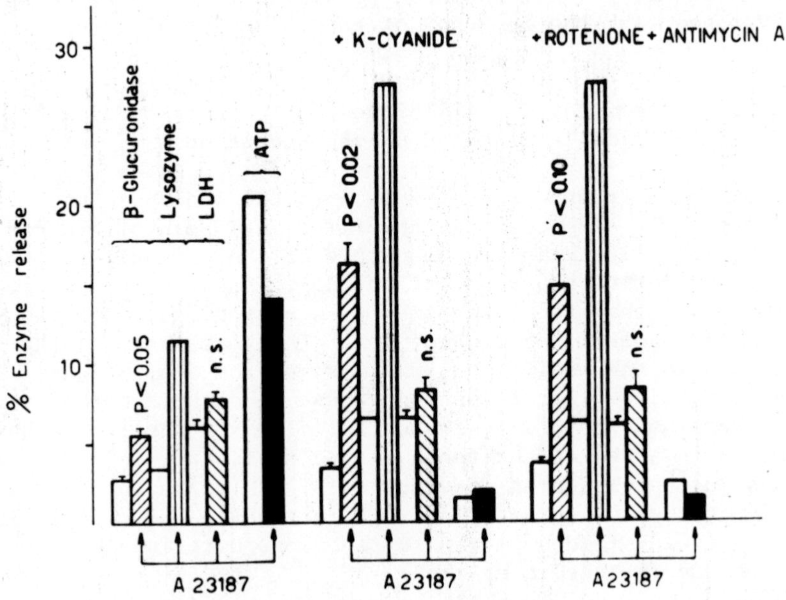

Fig. 10. Effect of metabolic inhibitors on the release of enzymes from alveolar macrophages in the presence of 1 mM extracellular Ca^{2+}, with and without the ionosphore A23187 (20 M). Incubation: 30 min at 37 C in the medium of Fig. 7.

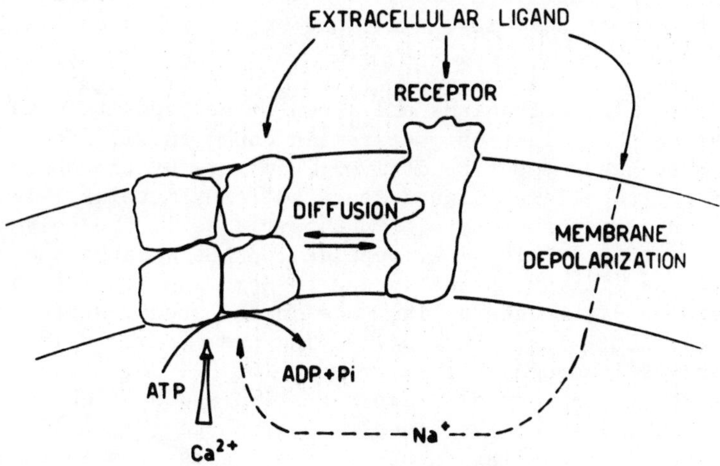

Fig. 11. Schematic illustration of possible mechanisms of control of the activity of the macrophage plasma membrane Ca^{2+}-ATPase.

maintain low concentrations of free Ca^{2+} in the cytosol and, therefore, to remain in a resting state. When the alveolar cells are treated with the Ca^{2+}ionophore the cation is transported into the cell but at the same time is also presumably extruded by the plasma membrane Ca^{2+}-ATPase. On account of the different nature and efficiency of the 2 transport systems, Ca^{2+} slowly accumulates in the cytosol and triggers some exocytosis of granules. When the macrophages are exposed to inhibitors of the mitochondrial activity, the buffering system provided by the mitochondria is inactivated (6), the functionality of the Ca^{2+}-ATPase at the plasma membrane is impaired, the Ca^{2+} concentration rises and secretion is slightly activated. If at the same time Ca^{2+} is transported intracellularly by the ionophore the exocytosis of granule enzymes is several-fold potentiated.

Although substances facilitating the downhill diffusion of extracellular Ca^{2+} into macrophages might exist _in vivo_, for example, at inflammatory sites, the experiments carried out with the Streptomyces ionophore A23187 should be regarded as _in vitro_ attempts aimed at emphasizing the role of Ca^{2+} and of the Ca^{2+} buffering systems in controlling the activity of the phagocytic cells. More physiological ways of elevating the concentrations of free Ca^{2+} in macrophages might be found in the mobilization of Ca^{2+} from the plasma membrane coupled to the inhibition of the Ca^{2+}-ATPase, ensuing from binding of extracellular ligands to the enzyme itself or to the adjacent receptors (Fig. 11). Further, since the plasma membrane Ca^{2+}-ATPase is particularly sensitive to Na^+, an increase in local Na^+ concentration caused by membrane depolarization might depress the enzyme activity, thus leading to Ca^{2+} accumulation in the cytosol.

Until similar mechanisms are shown to be present in macrophages, these possibilities must remain conjectural. Some support to these hypotheses might be derived, however, by the observed effects of extracellular ligands such as formylmethionyl-leucyl-phenylalanine on another type of phagocytic cell, the polymorphonuclear phagocyte. This small peptide induces a large and rapid increase in Na^+ influx, probably due to membrane depolarization, and simultaneously causes an increase in the steady-state level of intracellular Ca^{2+} (29), thus activating chemotaxis, oxidative metabolism and lysosomal enzyme release (3, 21, 30, 45, 48). Since formylmethionyl peptides also exert a stimulation of chemotaxis and oxidative metabolism of the alveolar macrophage (21, 45) it may be that they elicit a similar change of ion fluxes also in these cells utilizing the mechanisms postulated above.

ACKNOWLEDGEMENTS

This work was supported by grants from the National Research Council of Italy (No. 75.00607.04 and No. 76.01317.04) and from the University of Trieste. C. Mottola is grateful to the L. Stock Foundation for the support of her studies.

REFERENCES

1. Bailey, K. and Perry, S. V. Biochim. Biophys. Acta 1 (1947) 506.
2. Baker, P. F. Fed. Proc. 35 (1976) 2589.
3. Becker, E. L. Am. J. Pathol. 85 (1976) 385.
4. Boucek, M. M. and Snyderman, R. Science 193 (1976) 905.
5. Brinley, F. J. Fed. Proc. 32 (1973) 1735.
6. Carafoli, E. Malmström, K., Capano, M., Sigel, E. and Crompton, M. In: Calcium transport in contraction and secretion (Eds. E. Carafoli, F. Clementi, W. Drabikowski and A. Margreth) North-Holland, Amsterdam (1975) 53.
7. Cohn, Z. A. and Wiener, E. J. Exp. Med. 118 (1963) 991.
8. Dannenberg, A. M. Bacteriol. Rev. 32 (1968) 85.
9. Davies, P. and Allison, A. C. In: Lysosomes in biology and pathology (Eds. J. T. Dingle and R. T. Dean) Vol. 5, North-Holland, Amsterdam (1976) 61.
10. Dornand, J., Mani, J. C., Mousseron-Canet, M. and Pau, B. Biochimie 56 (1974) 1425.
11. Douglas, W. W. Brit. J. Pharm. 34 (1968) 451.
12. Dunham, E. T. and Glynn, I. M. J. Physiol. 156 (1961) 274.
13. Ernster, L., Dallner, G. and Azzone, G. F. J. Biol. Chem. 238 (1963) 1124.

14. Gallin, J. F. and Rosenthal, A. S. J. Cell Biol. 62 (1974) 594.
15. Garnett, H. M. and Kemp, R. B. Biochim. Biophys. Acta 382 (1975) 526.
16. Goetzl, E. J. and Austen, K. F. J. Clin. Invest. 53 (1974) 591.
17. Goldstein, I., Hoffstein, S., Gallin, J. and Weissman, G. Proc. Nat. Acad. Sci. USA 70 (1973) 2916.
18. Gordon, S. and Cohn, Z. A. Int. Rev. Cytol. 36 (1973) 171.
19. Green, G. M. Ann. Rev. Med. 19 (1968) 315.
20. Hartwig, J. H. and Stossel, T. P. J. Biol. Chem. 250 (1975) 5696.
21. Hatch, G. E., Gardner, D. E. and Menzel, D. B. J. Exp. Med. 147 (1978) 182.
22. Henseon, P. M. In: Lysosomes in biology and pathology (Eds. J. T. Dingle and R. T. Dean) Vol. 5, North-Holland, Amsterdam (1976) 99.
23. Kaplan, A. P., Kay, A. B. and Austen, K. F. J. Exp. Med. 135 (1972) 81.
24. Keller, H. U., Wissler, J., Hess, M. W. and Cottier, H. In: Movement, metabolism and bactericidal mechanisms of phagocytes (Eds. F. Rossi, P. Patriarca and D. Romeo) Piccin Medical Books, Padua (1977) 15.
25. Janis, R. A., Crankshaw, D. J. and Daniel, E. E. Am. J. Physiol. 232 (1977) C50.
26. Lardy, H. A., Johnson, D. and McMurray, W. C. Arch. Biochem. Biophys. 78 (1958) 587.
27. Mustafa, M. G., Cross, C. E. and Hardie, J. A. Life Sci. 9, part 1 (1970) 947.
28. Myrvik, Q. N. J. Reticuloendothel. Soc. 11 (1972) 459.
29. Naccache, P. H., Showell, H. J., Becker, E. L. and Sha'afi, R. I. J. Cell Biol. 73 (1977) 428.
30. Naccache, P. H., Showell, H. J., Becker, E. L. and Sha'afi, R. I. J. Cell Biol. 75 (1977) 635.
31. Parkinson, D. K. and Radde, I. C. Biochim. Biophys. Acta 242 (1971) 238.
32. Poisner, A. M. In: Biochemistry of simple neuronal models (Eds. E. Costa and E. Giacobini) Raven Press, New York (1970) 95.
33. Portzehl, H., Caldwell, P. C. and Rüegg, J. C. Biochim. Biophys. Acta 79 (1964) 581.
34. Rasmussen, H. Science 170 (1970) 404.
35. Reed, P. W. and Lardy, H. A. J. Biol. Chem. 247 (1972) 6970.
36. Romeo, D., Zabucchi, G., Miani, N. and Rossi, F. Nature 253 (1975) 542.
37. Romeo, D., Zabucchi, G. and Soranzo, M. R. In: Calcium transport in contraction and secretion (Eds. E. Carafoli, F. Clementi, W. Drabikowski and A. Margreth) North-Holland, Amsterdam (1975) 195.

38. Romeo, E., Zabucchi, G. and Rossi, F. In: Movement, metabolism and bactericidal mechanisms of phagocytes (Eds. F. Rossi, P. Patriarca and D. Romeo) Piccin Medical Books, Padua (1977) 153.
39. Root, R. K. and Metcalf, J. A. In: Movement, metabolism and bactericidal mechanisms of phagocytes (Ed. F. Rossi, P. Patriarca and D. Romeo) Piccin Medical Books, Padua (1977) 185.
40. Rubin, R. P. Pharm. Rev. 22 (1970) 389.
41. Sack, R. A. and Harris, C. M. Nature 265 (1977) 465.
42. Schatzmann, H. J. and Vincenzi, F. F. J. Phsyiol. 201 (1969) 369.
43. Schatzmann, H. J. and Rossi, G. L. Biochim. Biophys. Acta 241 (1971) 379.
44. Schell-Frederick, E. FEBS Letters 48 (1974) 37.
45. Schiffmann, E., Corcoran, B. A. and Wahl, S. M. Proc. Natl. Acad. Sci. USA 72 (1975) 1059.
46. Schneider, C., Gennaro, R., de Nicola, G. and Romeo, D. Exp. Cell Res. 112 (1978) 249.
47. Shami, Y. and Radde, I. C. Biochim. Biophys. Acta 249 (1971) 345.
48. Showell, H. J., Freer, R. J., Zigmond, S. H., Schiffmann, E., Aswanikumer, B., Corcoran, B. and Becker, E. L. J. Exp. Med. 143 (1976) 1154.
49. Showell, H. J., Naccache, P. H., Sha'afi, R. I. and Becker, E. L. J. Immunol. 119 (1977) 804.
50. Smith, R. J. and Ignarro, L. J. Proc. Nat. Acad. Sci. USA 72 (1975) 108.
51. Snyderman, R. and Mergenhagen, S. E. In: Immunobiology of the macrophage (Ed. D. S. Nelson) Academic Press, New York (1976) 323.
52. Tsan, M. F. and Berlin, R. D. Biochim. Biophys. Acta 241 (1971) 155.
53. Unanue, E. R. Adv. Immunol. 15 (1972) 95.
54. Wang, P., Shirley, P. S., DeChatelet, L. R., McCall, C. E. and Waite, B. M. J. Reticuloendothel. Soc. 19 (1976) 333.
55. Weissmann, G., Dukor, P. and Zurier, R. B. Nature New Biol. 231 (1971) 131.
56. Wilkinson, P. C. Exp. Cell Res. 93 (1975) 420.
57. Wins, P. and Shoffeniels, E. Biochim. Biophsy. Acta 120 (1966) 341.
58. Zabucchi, G., Soranzo, M. R., Rossi, F. and Romeo, D. FEBS Letters 54 (1975) 44.
59. Zabucchi, G. and Romeo, D. Biochem. J. 156 (1976) 209.

O_2^- AND H_2O_2 PRODUCTION DURING THE RESPIRATORY BURST IN ALVEOLAR MACROPHAGES

F. ROSSI, G. ZABUCCHI, P. DRI, P. BELLAVITE and G. BERTON

Istituto di Patologia Generale
Trieste (Italy)

It is known that the process of phagocytosis in polymorphonuclear leukocytes and in macrophages is associated with a dramatic change in oxidative metabolism. This change includes: an increase in oxygen consumption, in O_2^- and H_2O_2 generation and in glucose catabolism through the hexose monophosphate pathway (HMP) (3,7,9,10,13,20-23,29,31,44-46,49,56). These metabolic changes are referred to as the "respiratory burst" of phagocytic cells.

A similar stimulation of oxidative metabolism is induced also when phagocytic cells are exposed to membrane perturbing agents such as endotoxins (51), phospholipase C (30), phorbol myristate acetate (35), concanavalin A (40), antileukocyte antibodies (48), inophores (39,50), chemotactic fragments of complement (15,52), etc.

In general terms it appears that the stimulation of the oxidative metabolism has a variable intensity depending on cell type, on the sources of phagocytic cells, on the animal species, on the type of stimulant used, and, in macrophages (29), with the state of activation.

An analysis of the various events of the respiratory burst shows the following situation: 1) All the phagocytic cells so far investigated present an increase in the oxygen consumption and in HMP activity. As regards the oxygen consumption, by and large, it may be said that polymorphs and inflammatory peritoneal macrophages show the greatest stimulation, whereas the lung macrophages show a moderate extrarespiration. 2) The present status of our knowledge of the other aspects of the respiratory burst such as the mechanism and the amount of O_2^- and of H_2O_2 generation is not very clear. In general terms it may be said that the stimulation of the generation of these highly reactive compounds, and the amount that is measurable, presents a variability much greater than that of oxygen consumption and of HMP activity. The main reason of this variability is that O_2^- and H_2O_2 are intermediate products, which can be rapidly degraded by the cells.

Within this variability, two peculiar situations have been presented: the first one regards the polymorphs of chicken in which the phagocytic act would be accompanied by an increase in the respiration and in HMP activity but not in the production of O_2^- and of H_2O_2 (34).

The second situation is represented by alveolar macrophages of rabbit, rat and guinea pig where during the stimulation of the respiration no O_2^- and no, or only traces, of H_2O_2 would be produced (Table I).

In order to explain these results, the following hypotheses can be advanced: 1) The association between oxygen consumption and O_2^- and H_2O_2 production is not a general dogma of the metabolic burst of phagocytes. 2) In some type of cells only a very small part of oxygen consumed is reduced to H_2O_2. 3) In all the phagocytic cells the stimulation of oxygen consumption is associated with the general of O_2^- and H_2O_2 but in some cells these intermediates are degraded or utilized as fast as they are formed.

It is widely accepted that one of the purposes of the respiratory burst is to provide a battery of oxidizing agents that can be used in the phagocytic vacuole or in the extracellular environment for the killing and the destruction of microorganisms.

We have reinvestigated the respiratory burst of rabbit alveolar macrophages. In this paper, evidence will be provided that also in these cells the stimulation of O_2 consumption is associated with generation of O_2^- and H_2O_2.

MATERIALS AND METHODS

Preparation of the cells. Alveolar macrophages (AM) were obtained by tracheobronchial lavages from rabbits, 15 days after the intravenous injection of 10 mg of BCG (kindly supplied by Istituto Vaccinogeno Antitubercolare, Milano, Italy) suspended in 1 ml of physiological saline (37).

Polymorphonuclear leukocytes (PMNL) were obtained by injecting intraperitoneally 100 ml of 1% sterile sodium caseinate solution. The exudates were collected 14 hr later.

TABLE I

Reports of H_2O_2 and O_2^- Production by Alveolar Macrophages During the Respiratory Burst Induced by Phagocytosis

Authors	References	Species	O_2^-	H_2O_2
Paul *et al.*	(32)	rabbit	-	traces
Gee *et al.*	(13)	rabbit	-	traces
Klebanoff and Hamon	(24)	rabbit	-	traces
DeChatelet *et al.*	(9)	rabbit	no	-
		rabbit, BCG	no	-
Drath and Karnovsky	(10)	mouse	yes	-
		guinea pig	no	-
Gee and Khandwala	(12)	rabbit	no	-
Biggar *et al.*	(5)	rabbit	no	-
Bolen	(see ref. 29)	rabbit	-	traces
Tsan	(53)	rabbit	no	no
Biggar	(6)	rat	-	no
Lowrie	(25)	rabbit	yes	-

The cells were subjected to hypotonic treatment in order to lyse contaminating erythrocytes, and resuspended in Krebs Ringer phosphate buffer pH 7.4 (KRP) containing 5 mM glucose and 0.5 mM $CaCl_2$, and counted in an hemocytometric chamber.

Differential counts were carried out with May-Grunwald and Giemsa stained smears. On the average, alveolar lavages consisted of 87.6% macrophages, 8.5% lymphocytes and 3.9% polymorphs. The peritoneal exudates contained 93.5% polymorphs, 4.5% lymphocytes and 2.0% monocytes.

Metabolic assays. Oxygen consumption was measured polarographically with a Clark type oxygen electrode as previously described (38).

Superoxide anion was measured by the superoxide dismutase (SOD) inhibitable reduction of cytochrome c (2), on samples withdrawn from the electrode vessel, 4 min after the addition of the stimulatory agent. The experimental details have been described previously (11).

Hydrogen peroxide was measured flurimetrically by the homovanillic acid (HVA) method. This procedure is based on the conversion of the non-fluorescent compound homovanillic acid to the highly fluorescent 2, 2'dihydroxy3,3'dimethoxydiphenil5,5'diacetic acid, by horse radish peroxidase in the presence of H_2O_2 (17,18). In our hands, concentrations of H_2O_2 as low as 0.03 μM could be determined by this method. Three experimental procedures were employed: in the first one (method A) the H_2O_2 accumulated was measured on the supernatants of samples withdrawn from the electrode vessel, where oxygen consumption was being continuously recorded, 4 min after the addition of the stimulatory agent. Aliquots of such supernatants (10-100 μl) were added to a spectrofluorimetric cuvette containing in 2.5 ml of KRP, 0.02 mM HVA and 20 μg of HRP, and the increase of fluorescence was compared with appropriate standards of H_2O_2. The molecular extinction coefficient of H_2O_2 at 230 nm was determined on H_2O_2 solutions whose concentration was checked by titration with $KMnO_4$. The value obtained from four determinations was 0.0622 ± 0.00045 (SD) $cm^{-1}mM^{-1}$. In the second procedure (method B) HVA (0.8 mM) and HRP (20 μg/ml) were included in the incubation mixture, where oxygen consumption was being continuously recorded, and the fluorescence developed, indicating the H_2O_2 released and simultaneously trapped, was measured on the supernatants of samples withdrawn from the electrode vessel, 4 min after the addition of the stimulatory agent. In the third one, the kinetics of H_2O_2 release during the respiratory burst were carried out in a spectrophotofluirimetric cuvette, under continuous stirring, and the increase of fluorescence was followed with a CGA mod. DC3000 recording spectrophotofluorimeter.

Glucose oxidation: the rate of $^{14}CO_2$ production from 1-^{14}C-glucose was determined as described elsewhere (38).

Cell fractionation. The cells, sedimented and resuspended in 0.35 M sucrose (300-400x10^6/ml), were homogenized in a potter type glass homogenizer equipped with a teflon pestle, until more than 90% of the cells was broken as judged by light microscopic examination. The homogenate was then centrifuged at 100,000 g for 20 min and the pellet resuspended in 0.34 M sucrose to the original volume.

Enzyme assays. Superoxide dismutase activity was assayed according to the method of McCord and Fridovich (28), in the presence of 10 μM KCN in order to inhibit peroxidases and cytochrome c oxidase that would lead to an overstimulation of SOD activity (27).

Catalase activity was assayed by following the disappearance of H_2O_2 at 230 nm with an Hitachi-Perkin Elmer recording spectrophotometer was previously described (4).

Glutathione peroxidase and reductase activities were measured according to Gennaro *et al*. (14).

Peroxidase activity was assayed with the guaiacol test as described elsewhere (36).

RESULTS AND DISCUSSION

We began the investigation by comparing the various events of the respiratory burst of AM and PMNL.

The data of Table II show that the respiratory burst induced by phagocytosis in PMNL is associated with a substantial release of O_2^- and with a very small amount of H_2O_2 accumulated. On the contrary, the respiratory burst of AM is not accompanied by an accumulation of H_2O_2 while only traces of O_2^- are released. These results although in agreement with those reported by others (Table I) cannot be used as an evidence that AM do not produce H_2O_2. In fact in the experimental procedure employed, O_2^- was measured with cytochrome c present in the incubation medium, in such a way as the free radical is trapped as it is released from the cells. On the contrary, H_2O_2 was determined on samples withdrawn from the electrode vessel 4 min after the addition of bacteria. With this system only the aliquot of H_2O_2 that escaped the degradation was measured.

The reactions involved in oxygen consumption. Before describing the next data, in order to make clear the strategy of the experimental approaches and the results, it is worthy to indicate the reactions involved in O_2 consumption, in O_2^- and H_2O_2 formation and in H_2O_2 degradation (Fig. 1). Assuming that the reduction of O_2 essentially proceeds via a one electron pathway, in the first step (reactions 1, 1' of Fig. 1) O_2^- is formed. Evidences have been presented in our and in other laboratories that RH_2 is NADPH and that the reaction is catalyzed by an NADPH oxidase (20,1,8,19,33,47,55). O_2^- is a very reactive compound, that in the absence of oxidants, dismutates according to reaction 2. This reaction proceeds very fast either spontaneously with a rate constant of 1×10^5 M^{-1}, or catalyzed by SOD with a rate constant of 2×10^9 M^{-1} sec^{-1} (27). The H_2O_2 formed can be de-

TABLE II

O_2 Consumption, O_2^- Release and H_2O_2 Accumulation by Phagocytosing PMNL and AM from Rabbit

	PMNL (3)			AM (5)		
	Rest	Phag	Phag - Rest	Rest	Phag	Phag - Rest
O_2	31.5±5.4	166.7±17.8	135.2±13.8	116.0±13.3	194.9±14.3	78.9±7.6
O_2^-	9.2±8.1	124.6±33.4	115.4±39.6	0	4.5± 2.2	4.5±2.2
H_2O_2	0	10.1±3.0	10.1± 3.0	0	0	0

The values are expressed as nmoles/4 min/$1.5x10^7$ cells ± S.E.M.
Assay medium: $1-2x10^7$ PMNL or AM in 2 ml of KRP pH 7.4 containing 0.5 mM $CaCl_2$ and 5 mM glucose.
Opsonized B. mycoides were used as stimulatory agent (ratio cell/bacteria, 1/100).%= 37 C. O_2^- was measured by adding 400 μmoles of cytochrome c and, where required, 70 μg of SOD.
H_2O_2 was measured according to method A described in materials and methods.

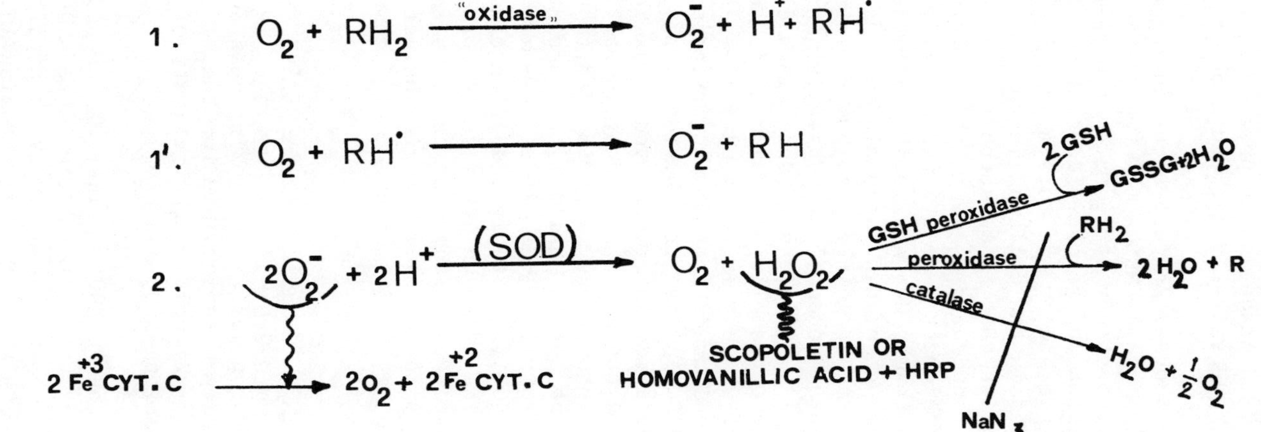

Fig. 1 - Scheme of the metabolic pathways involved in oxygen consumption, O_2^- and H_2O_2 production and degradation in phagocytes. The methods for O_2 and H_2O_2 measurement are also shown.

graded by different mechanism that is catalatic, where $\frac{1}{2}O_2$ is given back for each molecule of H_2O_2, or peroxidatic, where a reduced compound is oxidized and H_2O is formed. The main enzymatic reactions for H_2O_2 degradation in phagocytic cells are catalyzed by catalase, peroxidase and glutathione peroxidase.

Assuming that the above reactions occur during the activated metabolism of AM as well as in PMNL, it is worthy to stress the following points: 1) the steady state rate of oxygen consumption and O_2^- and H_2O_2 generation and recovery depends on the activity level of the O_2 reductase and on the rate at which O_2^- and H_2O_2 are released or utilized in the cell and in the surrounding medium. 2) The oxygen consumption that is measurable does not correspond to all oxygen that is reduced to O_2^- since this compound is not accumulated. The stoichiometric relationship between the actual oxygen consumed and O_2^- formed depends on the mechanism of H_2O_2 degradation and on the amount of H_2O_2 accumulated. 3) In many phagocytic cells, for example guinea pig, human, rabbit PMNL and in inflammatory peritoneal mononuclear phagocytes, part of O_2^- formed in reactions 1, 1', is released, and this aliquot undergoes dismutation in the extracellular medium or in the phagocytic vacuole. The amount of O_2^- that is released varies in different cell types. 4) In normal conditions of phagocytosis, that is when one allows that H_2O_2 follow its physiological fate, only a small aliquot of the peroxide is accumulated. 5) The amount of H_2O_2 that is accumulated can be increased by inhibiting the reations involved in its degradation. When impeded to be degraded H_2O_2 is released from the cells. 6) Only the amount of O_2^- and H_2O_2 that is released from the cells can be measured. For the first intermediate the SOD inhibitable reduction of cytochrome c or NBT can be used. The hydrogen peroxide is correctly measured by trapping as it is released or as it is formed by dismutation of O_2^-. This is achieved by using horseradish peroxidase (HRP) catalyzing the oxidation by H_2O_2 of compounds such as scopoletin or homovanillic acid.

Activities of the enzymes responsible for the formation and for the degradation of O_2^- and H_2O_2 in rabbit AM. In this group of experiments we try to answer the following questions: 1) is the NADPH oxidase the enzyme responsible for the reactions 1, 1' (Fig. 1) present in AM? 2) What is the activity of the enzymes involved in the degradation of O_2^- and H_2O_2?

Fig. 2 shows that the 20,000 g pellet of the postnuclear supernates of homogenates of resting AM, oxidize NADPH with formation of H_2O_2. This oxidizing activity is highly activated in the same fractions obtained from phagocytosing AM. This suggests that in these cells the enzymatic basis of the metabolic burst is similar to that described in PMNL (1,8,19,33,47,55). The

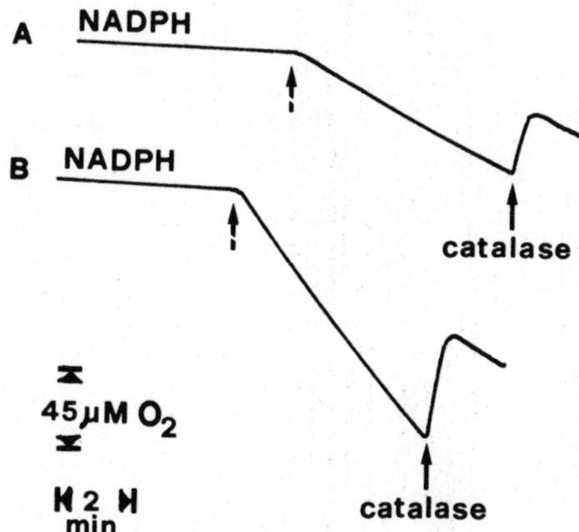

Fig. 2. Production of H_2O_2 during oxidation of NADPH by 20,000g sedimentable fractions isolated from resting (A) and phagocytosing (B) rabbit alveolar macrophages. Assay medium: 65mM Na, K-phosphate buffer pH 5.5, 125 mM sucrose, 0.5 mM $MnCl_2$, 1 mM NADPH. Final volume 2 ml T= 37 C. At the points indicated by broken arrows 80 µg of protein of 20,000g sedimentable fraction was added.

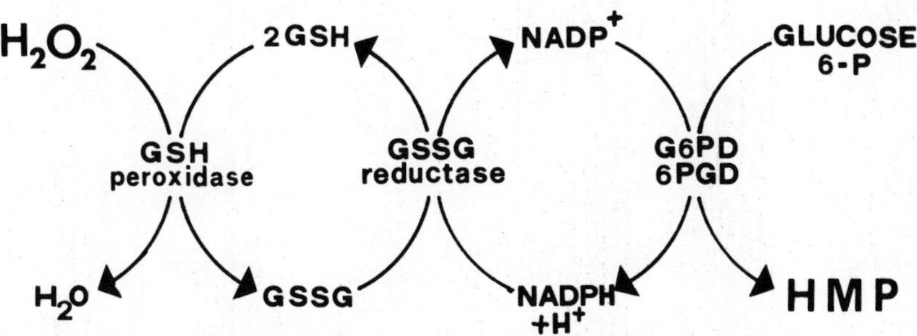

Fig. 3. Relationship between H_2O_2 degradation through the glutathione cycle and the hexose monophosphate pathway.

TABLE III

Enzyme Activities in Rabbit PMNL and AM

	PMNL (6)		AM (7)	
	*U/10^6 cells	specific activity	*U/10^6 cells	specific activity
GSH-PEROXIDASE[0]	0.62±0.19	36.5± 8.6	76.9±15.5	998.4±133.2
GSSG-REDUCTASE[0]	0.51±0.07	30.0± 7.2	4.5± 0.6	55.7± 6.6
CATALASE[0]	4.0 ±0.3	285.7±60.5	26.2± 3.1	340.3± 46.9
PEROXIDASE[□]	21.8 ±8.9	660.6±127.6	2.2± 0.4	21.5± 4.7
SOD[Δ]	0.13±0.03	2.6± 0.6	0.74± 0.12	4.31 0.5

The mean ± S.E.M. is reported. The number of experiments is given in parentheses.
* nmoles NADPH/min for GSH-peroxidase and GSSG-reductase, µmoles H_2O_2/min for catalase, nmoles tetraguaiacol/min for peroxidase. One unit of superoxide dismutase (SOD) is defined as the amount of enzyme that causes a decrease in the reduction of cytochrome c of 0.0125 OD/min.
[0]Measured on 1000,000g supernatant, [□]measured on 100,000g pellet, [Δ]measured on total homogenate.

results presented in Table III show that in AM, glutathione peroxidase, glutathione reductase, catalase and superoxide dismutase have activities much higher than those of PMNL. On the contrary, the peroxidase activity is higher in PMNL. From the pattern of the enzymatic activities, it appears that in comparison with PMNL, AM have very active mechanisms for H_2O_2 degradation. Since catalase has usually a low affinity for H_2O_2 and the activity of peroxidase is very low, it is likely that the main mechanism for H_2O_2 degradation in AM is linked to the activity of glutathione peroxidase coupled with that of glutathione reductase (glutathione cycle).

The utilization of H_2O_2 through the glutathione cycle is coupled with an increased activity of HMP, as shown in Fig. 3. On these basis the efficiency of the glutathione cycle can be investigated by measuring the effect of externally added H_2O_2 on $^{14}CO_2$ production from 1-^{14}C-glucose, that in these cells indicates the rate of glucose oxidation through the HMP.

The results reported in Fig. 4 show that the effect of exogenous H_2O_2 is much greater in AM than in PMNL. Furthermore, in AM the intensity of the stimulation of HMP activity by 0.05 mM H_2O_2 is very near to the maximal stimulation induced by phagocytosis.

This group of experiments indicate that in AM the respiratory burst is associated with H_2O_2 formation and that the peroxide is rapidly utilized as it is formed.

Attempts to increase the accumulation of H_2O_2. This was achieved by using two devices. The first one was that of inhibiting some of the reactions involved in H_2O_2 degradation, that is the heme enzymes catalase and peroxidase with NaN_3. The second way was that of trapping H_2O_2 as it is formed and released in NaN_3 treated alveolar macrophages, by adding HRP and homovanillic acid. The results presented in Table IV show that in the presence of NaN_3 (column II) the stimulation of O_2 consumption induced by phagocytosis in PMNL is associated with a marked accumulation of H_2O_2, while in AM, only traces of H_2O_2 are measurable. When the H_2O_2 trapping system is included in the incubation medium (column III) a definite amount of H_2O_2 becomes constantly measured during the respiratory burst of AM. By comparing the amounts of O_2 actually consumed and of H_2O_2 measured, it is evident that in AM the percentage of O_2 consumed, recovered as H_2O_2, is very low, while in PMNL is very high. These results clearly indicate that the main mechanism for H_2O_2 utilization involve reactions NaN_3-sensitive (catalase and myeloperoxidase) in PMNL, and reactions NaN_3-insensitive (glutathione peroxidase) in AM.

In subsequent experiments a continuous monitoring of H_2O_2

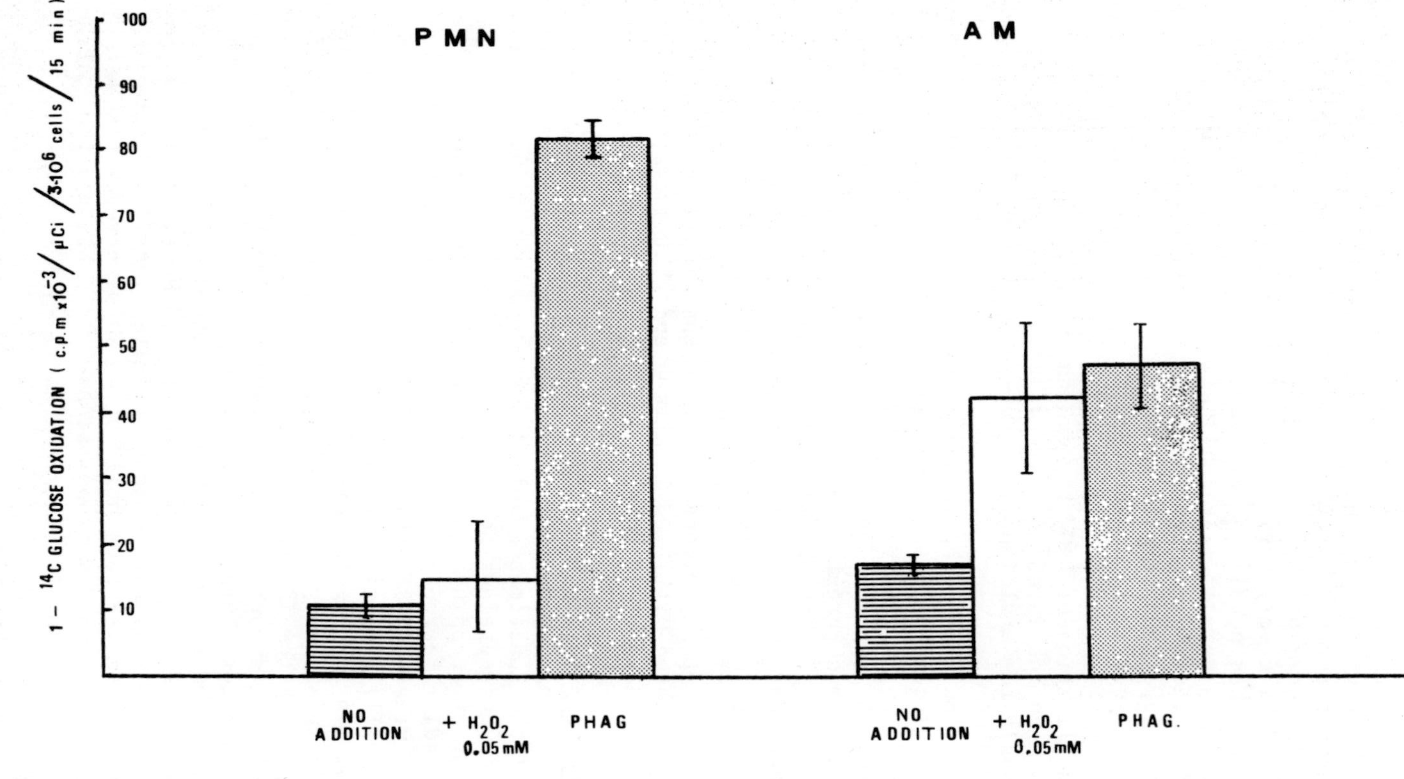

Fig. 4. Effect of bacteria and H_2O_2 addition on the activity of the hexose monophosphate pathway of rabbit PMNL and AM. Assay medium: $3x10^6$ cells in 1 ml of KRP pH 7.4 containing 0.5 mM $CaCl_2$, 0.2 mM glucose, 0.2 μCi of glucose-1-^{14}C. Opsonized <u>B. mycoides</u> was used as stimulatory agent (ratio cell/bacteria, 1/100). Vertical bars indicate S.E.M. T= 37 C.

TABLE IV

O_2 Consumption, O_2^- Release and H_2O_2 Accumulation by Phagocytosing PMNL and AM from Rabbit

	I		II + NaN_3		III + NaN_3 + HRP + HVA	
	PMNL (3)	AM (5)	PMNL (5)	AM (6)	PMNL (3)	AM (6)
O_2	135.2±13.8 (31.5± 5.4)	78.9± 7.6 (116.0±13.3)	195.9±12.9 (21.3± 5.6)	76.2±14.0 (111.7±18.5)	203.6±29.4 (18.8± 5.4)	71.3±12.8 (101.3±12.9)
O_2^-	115.4±39.5 (9.2± 8.1)	4.5± 2.2 (0)	105.9±20.7 (9.2±8.1)	6.0± 1.5 (0)	---	---
H_2O_2	10.1± 3.0 (0)	0	179.3±17.2 (6.2± 2.7)	0.2± 0.1 (0)	163.0±25.2 (7.8± 3.5)	7.1± 1.9 (0)
%O_2 recovered as H_2O_2	7.4	0	91.5	0.26	80.0	10.0

The differences between phagocytosing and resting cells are reported. The values are expressed as nmoles/4 min/1.5x10^7 cells ± S.E.M. Resting values are given in brackets.
Assay medium: 1-2x10^7 PMNL or AM in 2 ml of KRP pH 7.4 containing 0.5 mM $CaCl_2$ and 5 mM glucose. Opsonized B. mycoides were used as stimulatory agent (ratio cell/bacteria, 1/100). NaN_3, 2 mM. T= 37 C. O_2^- was measured as described in Table II. H_2O_2 was measured according to method A (columns I,II) and B (column III), described in materials and methods.

production during phagocytosis in NaN_3-treated AM and PMNL was employed. This was achieved by recording the change of fluorescence during the oxidation of homovanillic acid by HRP. A typical experiment is reported in Fig. 5. In the experiments performed with AM, only a small amount of H_2O_2 is detectable when the reactants for H_2O_2 measurement are added some min after addition of bacteria (trace B'). In contrast, when the reactants for trapping the peroxide are present at the beginning of the respiratory burst, H_2O_2 is detectable after a lag time of about 3-4 min. In the experiments performed by using PMNL a marked amount of H_2O_2 is measurable either when the reactants are present at the beginning of the metabolic burst or some min after addition of bacteria. These results are in agreement with those of Table IV and strengthen the conclusion that in AM, H_2O_2 is rapidly utilized even when catalase and peroxidase are inhibited.

This group of results permit the following conclusions: 1) By using appropriate devices it is possible to increase also in AM the amount of H_2O_2 that is measurable. 2) In any case the amount of H_2O_2 detectable represents a very low percentage of the O_2 actually consumed.

Effect of cytochalasin B on the production of O_2^- and H_2O_2 during phagocytosis. The results presented above introduce the problem of whether or not the small percentage of H_2O_2 accumulated represents the total amount that is formed or the aliquot that escaped the intracellular degradation. If the latter is the case it could be possible to increase this aliquot. This result was, at least partially, achieved by using cytochalasin B (CB), a drug that is known to increase the release of lysosomal enzymes and of O_2^- in phagocytic cells during the respiratory burst (16,42,43,57). Table V illustrates the effect of CB on oxygen consumption, O_2^- and H_2O_2 release during phagocytosis in NaN_3-treated AM and PMNL. The data show that: 1) CB induces a decrease of the intensity of the stimulation of oxygen consumption both in PMNL and AM. This effect is related to the inhibition of the rate of phagocytosis as shown in our and in other laboratories (26,41,43) and as it has been controlled in these experiments. 2) CB has also a great effect on the release of O_2^- both in PMNL and AM. In fact while CB induces a decrease of the total amount of oxygen univalently reduced, as it is shown by the decrease of measurable oxygen consumed, the aliquot of O_2^- released in comparison with the actual oxygen consumed is markedly increased either in PMNL and in AM. 3) CB increases the amount of the peroxide recovered in the extracellular medium of phagocytosing AM either as absolute value or as related to the extrarespiration. In fact, the percentage of oxygen actually consumed recovered as H_2O_2 rises from 10.0 to 25.0% in the presence of CB. In other words, by using CB we can see that a consistent aliquot of the oxygen consumed by AM during the respiratory burst is recovered as H_2O_2. This aliquot

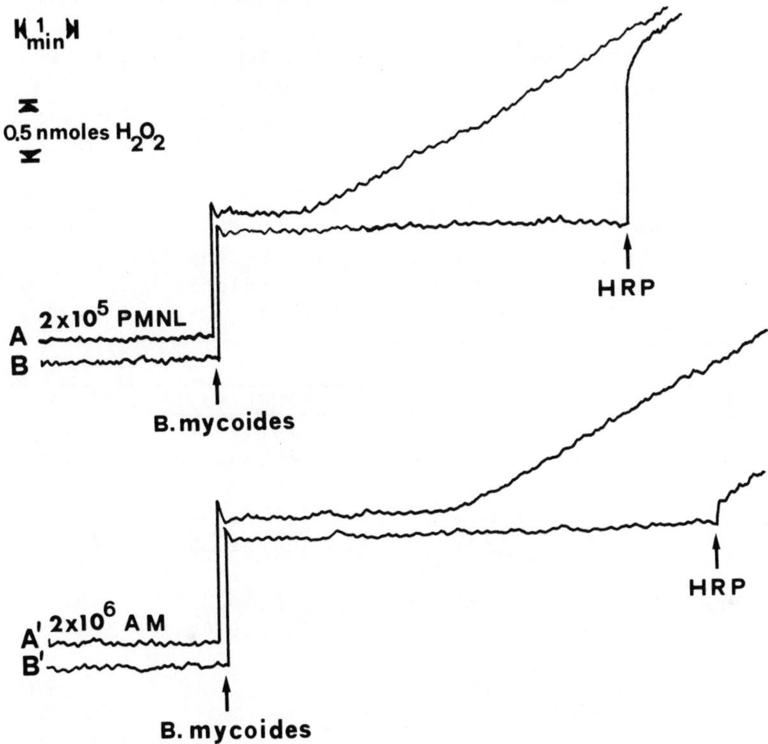

Fig. 5. Spectrophotofluorometric traces of H_2O_2 production by rabbit PMNL and AM during phagocytosis. Assay medium: 2.5 ml of KRP pH 7.4 containing 0.5 mM $CaCl_2$, 5 mM glucose, 2 mM NaN_3, 20 μM HVA and 20 μg HRP. A,A', complete system. B,B', HRP, omitted from the assay medium was added where indicated.

does not reach the values obtained in PMNL where 97.6% of oxygen consumed is recovered as H_2O_2 when CB is present.

Apart from the mechanisms by which CB causes these effects, that are in agreement with the results published by others (42, 43), the data presented in this group of experiments indicate that in AM the type of the metabolic burst is similar to that of granulocytes; that is, the univalent reduction of oxygen followed by formation of H_2O_2 is operative and substantial also in AM.

This conclusion has been further reinforced by the results obtained with another experimental approach.

TABLE V

O_2 Consumption, O_2^- and H_2O_2 Release by Phagocytosing PMNL and AM from Rabbit, in the Absence and in the Presence of Cytochalasin B

	-----		+ CB	
	PMNL (3)	AM (6)	PMNL (3)	AM (4)
O_2	203.6 ± 29.4 (18.8 ± 5.4)	71.3±12.8 (101.3±12.9)	79.3±8.7 (60.3±18.4)	38.1±5.7 (116.1±16.8)
O_2^-	105.9 ± 20.7 9.2 ± 8.1)	6.0±1.5 (0)	114.9±15.3 (24.7±0.4)	24.5±9.1 (6.2±3.1)
H_2O_2	163.0 ± 25.2 (7.8 ± 3.5)	7.1±1.9 (0)	77.4±28.8 (29.4± 4.5)	9.6±1.7 (3.6±2.6)
%O_2 recovered as H_2O_2	80.0	10.0	97.6	25.0

The differences between phagocytosing and resting cells are reported. The values are expressed as nmoles/4 min/1.5x10^7 cells ± S.E.M. Resting values are given in brackets.
Assay medium: 1-2x10^7 PMNL or AM in 2 ml of KRP pH 7.4 containing 0.5 mM $CaCl_2$ and 5 mM glucose. Opsonized B. mycoides were used as stimulatory agent (ratio cell/bacteria, 1/100). NaN_3, 2 mM. T= 37 C. CB, 10 μg in 2 μl DMSO. In control experiments, 2 μl DMSO were added.
O_2 was measured as described in Table II. H_2O_2 was measured according to method B described in materials and methods.

Effect of concanavalin A and CB. In an attempt to get an insight into the effect of CB and in order to avoid the effect of this drug on the respiratory increment due to inhibition of the phagocytic act, we employed as a stimulatory agent the Concanavalin A (ConA). First of all we have studied the metabolic burst induced by ConA, evaluated as H_2O_2 formation, in NaN_3-treated AM in the presence and in the absence of CB. The results presented in a typical experiment (Fig. 6) show that: 1) When ConA is added to CB-treated AM (trace B) a very rapid and marked increase of fluorescence takes place, indicating that in this condition a substantial amount of H_2O_2 is released from stimulated cells. A similar effect is obtainable when CB is added after ConA (trace C).

The amount of H_2O_2 measured in CB-treated AM was unexpectedly high in comparison to that detected in the experiments presented above. This fact prompted further experiments in order to investigate the effect of CB on all the events of the respiratory burst induced by ConA. The data on the contemporaneous measurements of oxygen consumption, of O_2^- and of H_2O_2 reported in Table VI show that: 1) ConA alone induces in PMNL an increase of oxygen consumption associated with O_2^- and H_2O_2 formation and release. In AM ConA alone induces an increase of oxygen consumption which is associated with a small production and release of O_2^- and H_2O_2. The relationship between these three events are similar to that observed when the stimulation is induced by phagocytosis (Table IV). 2) Both in PMNL and AM, CB markedly enhances the activation of the oxidative metabolism triggered by ConA measured as oxygen consumed and O_2^- and H_2O_2 formation and release. These results clearly suggest that the increased amount of O_2^- and H_2O_2 detected is due to a double effect of CB. The first one is a potentiation of the stimulatory activity of ConA with increased formation of O_2^- and H_2O_2. The mechanisms by which CB induces this stimulation is at present unknown. It is worthy to point out that CB does not modify the amount of ^{3}H-labeled lectin bound to the surface of the cell (results not presented here). The second effect consists in an increased availability in the extracellular medium of both the intermediate products of oxygen reduction. The mechanism of this increased availability might be related to an increased permeability of the cell membrane to O_2^- and H_2O_2 or to an inhibition of some of the mechanisms of their degradation. The latter possibility is unlikely since we have seen that CB does not modify in vitro the activities of SOD, catalase, peroxidase and glutathione peroxidase and reductase.

Although we need further investigations to clarify the mechanisms by which CB causes this double effect, the results obtained with this experimental model, that is ConA plus CB, show that also in AM it is possible to obtain a respiratory burst in which the values of the various parameters (oxygen consumed,

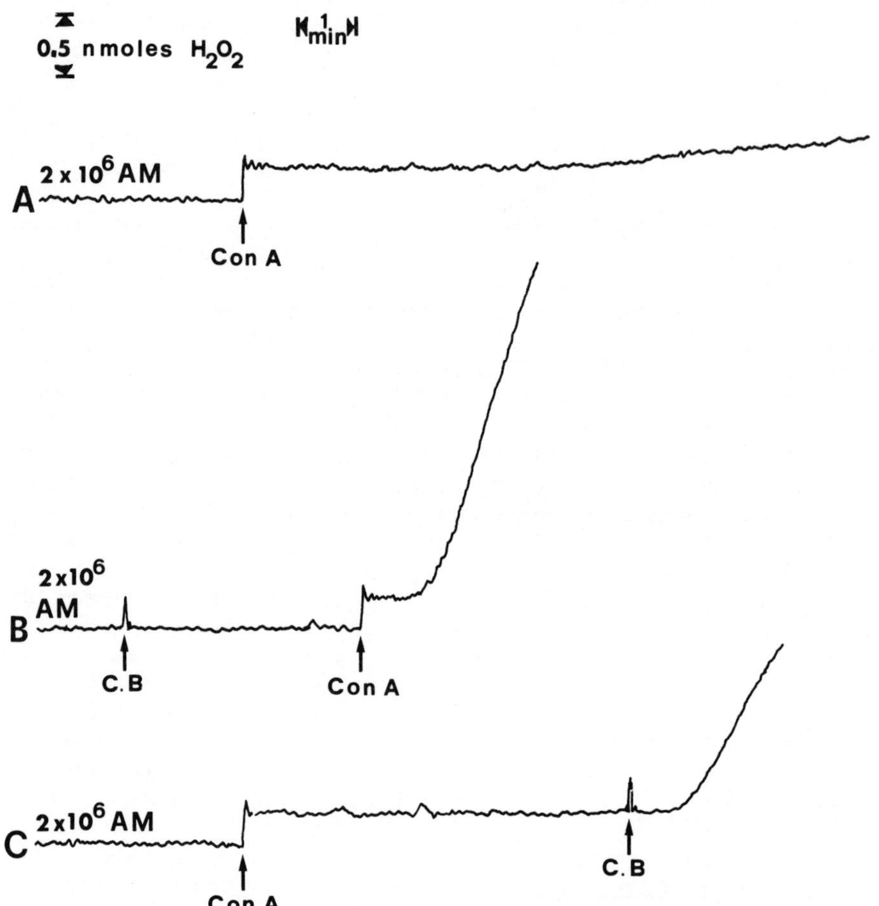

Fig. 6. Spectrophotofluorometric traces of H_2O_2 production by rabbit PMNL and AM stimulated by Con A, in the presence and in the absence of cytochalasin B. For experimental conditions see Fig. 5, Con A, 100 μg/ml. CB 12.5 μg in 2.5 μl DMSO. In A 2.5 μl DMSO were added.

O_2^- and H_2O_2 formed and released) and their quantitative relationship are in the range of the values obtained in the granulocytes of rabbit and of other mammalian species.

TABLE VI

O_2 Consumption, O_2^- and H_2O_2 Release by Rabbit PMNL and AM Stimulated by Concanavalin A in the Absence and in the Presence of Cytochalasin B

	Con A		Con A + CB	
	PMNL (3)	AM (4)	PMNL (3)	AM (4)
O_2	52.6±17.8 (18.8± 5.4)	24.3± 5.7 (101.3±12.9)	106.3±30.4 (60.3±18.4)	75.6± 6.9 (116.1±16.8
O_2^-	30.3±13.9 (9.2± 8.1)	3.7± 1.8 (0)	98.1±41.1 (24.7± 0.4)	48.4± 9.8 (6.2± 3.1)
H_2O_2	37.6±21.4 (7.8± 3.5)	2.1±1.5 (0)	93.4±42.7 (29.4± 4.5)	33.8± 2.2 3.6± 2.5)
%O_2 recovered as H_2O_2	71.5	8.6	87.8	44.7

The differences between phagocytosing and resting cells are reported. The values are expressed as nmoles/4 min/1.5x10^7 cells ± S.E.M. Resting values are given in brackets.
The experimental conditions are described in Table V. Concanavalin A (100 μg/ml) instead of bacteria was used as stimulatory agent.

CONCLUSIONS

The results presented in this paper can be summarized as follows: 1) In rabbit AM the respiratory burst is associated with the generation of O_2^- and H_2O_2. 2) These intermediate products of oxygen reduction are not accumulated in physiological conditions because these cells are equipped with very efficient systems for their transformation and degradation. 3) The main mechanism for the degradation of H_2O_2 in these cells is represented by the glutathione cycle in agreement with the results presented by others (54). By using appropriate experimental conditions, the intermediate products of oxygen reduction can be released at high rate and recovered in the extracellular medium.

In another paper elsewhere in this volume, experiments performed with chicken PMNL, will be presented. By following the same line of experimental approach, we obtained evidence that also in these phagocytic cells the respiratory burst is associated with the production of O_2^- and H_2O_2.

Thus we are provided with experimental evidence that allows the following conclusions: 1) Among phagocytic cells so far investigated, examples do not exist where the stimulation of oxidative metabolism is not accompanied by the formation of O_2^- and H_2O_2. 2) The possibility of detecting these compounds depends on the great differences found among the various types of phagocytic cells with respect to the efficiency of the mechanisms for their degradation and, also, on the experimental strategy employed. 3) These differences in the efficiency and in the type of the reactions for the degradation of intermediate products of respiration suggest that the phagocytic cells are heterogeneous, even as regards the defensive role played by the respiratory burst.

ACKNOWLEDGEMENTS

P. Bellavite is recipient of a fellowship from "Fondazione Anna Villa Rusconi", Varese, Italy. Supported by grant No 77.01481.04 from the National Council of Research (CNR) of Italy.

REFERENCES

1. Babior, B. M., Curnette, J. T. and Kipnes, R. S., J. Clin. Invest. 56 (1975) 1035.
2. Babior, B. M., Kipnes, R. S. and Curnutte, J. T., J. Clin. Invest. 52 (1973) 741.
3. Baehner, R. L., Gilman, N. and Karnovsky, M. L., J. Clin. Invest. 49 (1970) 692.
4. Bellavite, P., Dri, P., Bisiacchi, B. and Patriarca, P., FEBS Letters 81 (1977) 73.
5. Biggar, W. D., Buron, S. and Holmes, B., Infect. Immun. 14 (1976) 6.
6. Biggar, W. D. and Sturgess, J. M., Infect. Immun. 19 (1978) 621.
7. Curnutte, J. T. and Babior, B. M., J. Clin. Invest. 53 (1974) 1662.
8. DeChatelet, L. R., McPhail, L. C., Mullikin, D. and McCall, C. E., J. Clin. Invest. 55 (1975) 714.
9. DeChatelet, L. R., Mullikin, D. and McCall, C. E., J. Lab. Clin. Med. 85 (1975) 245.
10. Drath, D. B. and Karnovsky, M. L., J. Exp. Med. 141 (1975) 257.
11. Dri, P., Bellavite, P., Bergon, G. and Rossi, F., Molec.

Cell. Biochem. (1978) in press.

12. Gee, J. B. L. and Khandwala, A. S., J. Reticuloendothel. Soc. 19 (1976) 229.
13. Gee, J. B. L., Vassallo, C. L., Bell, P., Kaskin, J., Basford, R. E. and Field, J., J. Clin. Invest. 49 (1970) 1280.
14. Gennaro, R., Schneider, C., de Nicola, G., Cian, F. and Roemo, D., Proc. Soc. Exp. Biol. Med. 157 (1978) 342.
15. Goetzl, E. J. and Austen,K. F., J. Clin. Invest. 53 (1974) 591.
16. Goldstein, I. M., Roos, D., Kaplan, H. B. and Weismann, G., J. Clin. Invest. 56 (1975) 1155.
17. Guilbaut, G. G., Brignac, P., Jr. and Zimmer, M., Anal. Chem. 40 (1968) 190.
18. Guilbaut, G. G., Kramer, D. N. and Hackley, E., Anal. Biochem. 39 (1967) 271.
19. Hohn, D. C. and Lehrer, R. I., J. Clin. Invest. 55 (1975) 707.
20. Iyer, G. J. N., Islam, M. F. and Quastel, J. H., Nature (London) 192 (1961) 535.
21. Karnovsky, M. L., Physiol. Rev. 42 (1962) 143.
22. Karnovsky, M. L., Lazdins, J. and Simmons, S. R., In: Mononuclear Phagocytes (Ed. R. Van Furth) Blackwell Scientific Publications, Oxford, England (1975) 423.
23. Klebanoff, S. J. and Hamon, C. B., J. Reticuloendothel. Soc. 12 (1972) 170.
24. Klebanoff, S. J. and Hamon, C. B., In: Mononuclear Phagocytes (Ed. R. Van Furth) Blackwell Scientific Publications, Oxford, England (1975) 507.
25. Lowrie, D. B. and Aber, V. R., Life Sciences 21 (1977) 1575.
26. Malawista, S. E., Gee, B. J. and Bensch, K. G., Yale, J. Biol. Med. 44 (1971) 286.
27. McCord, J. M., Crapo, J. D. and Fridovich, I., In: Superoxide and Superoxide Dismutase (Ed. A. M. Michelson, J. M. McCord and I. Fridovich) Academic Press, London (1977) 11.
28. McCord, J. M. and Fridovich, I., J. Biol. Chem. 244 (1969) 6049.
29. Nathan, C. F. and Root, R. K., J. Exp. Med. 146 (1977) 1648.
30. Patriarca, P., Zatti, M., Cramer, R. and Rossi, F., Life Sciences 9 Part I (1970) 841.
31. Paul, B. B. and Sbarra, A. J., Biochim. Biophys. Acta 156 (1968) 168.
32. Paul, B. B., Strauss, R. R., Jacobs, A. A. and Sbarra, A. J., Infect. Immun. 1 (1970) 338.
33. Paul, B. B., Strauss, R. R., Jacobs, A. A. and Sbarra, A. J., Exp. Cell Res. 73 (1972) 456.
34. Pennial, R. and Spitznagel, J. K., Proc. Nat. Acad. Sci. USA 72 (1975) 5012.
35. Repine, J. E., White, J. G., Clanson, C. C. and Holmes, B. M. J. Lab. Clin. Med. 83 (1974) 911.

36. Romeo, D., Cramer, R., Marzi, T., Soranzo, M. R., Zabucchi, G. and Rossi, F., J. Reticuloendothel. Soc. 13 (1973) 399.
37. Romeo, D., Zabucchi, G., Jug, M. and Rossi, F., Cell. Immunol. 13 (1974) 313.
38. Romeo, D., Zabucchi, G., Marzi, T. and Rossi, F., Exp. Cell Res. 78 (1973) 423.
39. Romeo, D., Zabucchi, G., Miani, N. and Rossi, F., Nature 253 (1975) 542.
40. Romeo, D., Zabucchi, G. and Rossi, F., Nature New Biol. 243 (1973) 111.
41. Romeo, D., Zubacchi, G. and Rossi, F., In: Movement, Metabolism and Bactericidal Mechanisms of Phagocytes (Ed. F. Rossi, P. Patriarca and D. Romeo) Piccin Medical Books, Padova (1977) 154.
42. Roos, D., Homan-Miller, J. W. T. and Weening, R. S., Biochim. Biophys. Res. Commun. 68 (1976) 43.
43. Root, R. K. and Metcalf, J. A., In: Movement, Metabolism and Bactericidal Mechanisms of Phagocytes (Ed. F. Rossi, P. Patriarca and D. Romeo) Piccin Medical Books, Padova (1977) 185.
44. Root, R. K., Metcalf, J. A., Oshino, N. and Chance, B., J. Clin. Invest. 55 (1975) 945.
45. Rossi, F., Romeo, D. and Patriarca, P., J. Reticuloendothel. Soc. 12 (1972) 127.
46. Rossi, F., Zabucchi, G. and Romeo, D., In: Mononuclear Phagocytes (Ed. R. Van Furth) Blackwell Scientific Publications, Oxford, England (1975) 441.
47. Rossi, F. and Zatti, M., Brit. J. Exp. Pathol. 45 (1964) 548.
48. Rossi, F., Zatti, M., Patriarca, P. and Cramer, R., J. Reticuloendothel. Soc. 9 (1971) 67.
49. Sbarra, A. J. and Karnovsky, M. L., J. Biol. Chem. 234 (1959) 1355.
50. Schell-Frederick, E., FEBS Letters 48 (1974) 37.
51. Strauss, B. S. and Stetson, C. A., J. Exp. Med. 112 (1960) 653.
52. Tedesco, F., Trani, S., Soranzo, M. R. and Patriarca, P., FEBS Letters 51 (1975) 232.
53. Tsan, M. F., Blood 50 (1977) 935.
54. Vogt, M. T., Thomas, C., Vassallo, C. L., Basford, R. E. and Gee, J. B. L., J. Clin. Invest. 50 (1971) 401.
55. Zatti, M. and Rossi, F., Biochim. Biophys. Acta 99 (1965) 557.
56. Zatti, M., Rossi, F. and Patriarca, P., Experientia 24 (1968) 669.
57. Zurier, R. B., Hoffstein, S. and Weissmann, G., Proc. Nat. Acad. Sci. USA 70 (1973) 844.

BIOCHEMICAL AND BIOLOGICAL PROPERTIES OF LEUKOCYTE INTRACELLULAR INHIBITORS OF PROTEINASES

M. KOPITAR[1], T. GIRALDI[2], P. LOCNIKAR[1], and V. TURK[1]

[1]Department of Biochemistry, J. Stefan Institute
Ljubljana (Yugoslavia) and [2] Istituto di Farmacologia
Universita di Trieste (Italy)

Leukocyte proteinases are postulated to be involved in variety of physiological and pathological events (7,9). It has also been proposed that proteinases are involved in the process of malignant invasion and that they could be responsible for the altered growth control in tumor cells (14). In this context the so-called neutral proteinases - histonases are of interest. It has been suggested that the histone hydrolyzing proteinases remove histones, which are known to act as gene repressors by binding to the DNA double helix, and thus may cause the derepression which is followed by DNA synthesis and cell division (6). It has already been found that leukocyte, as well as spleen elastases and chymotrypsin-like neutral proteinases have the ability to catalyze the hydrolysis of histones (11). Relevant to this ability of neutral proteinases, proteinase inhibitors are of particular interest and many studies have appeared dealing with the effect of synthetic and protein inhibitors on neutral proteinases.

Recently, much attention has been paid to the intracellular inhibitors isolated from leukocytes (5,10,13). In the course of our continuing studies two types of specific inhibitors of neutral proteinases (I_1 and I_2) were isolated from leukocytes (11). These inhibitors differ in molecular weight (I_1 = 15,000, I_2 - 40,000), as well as in their inhibition ability against tested enzymes.

In the present study we investigated the inhibitory effect of I_1 and I_2 on the activity of elastase, chymotrypsin-like neutral proteinase, cathepsin B, papain and urokinase, as well as the inactivation of these inhibitors by cathepsin D.

MATERIAL AND METHODS

Leukocyte inhibitors were isolated from the soluble phase of disrupted pig peripheral leukocytes freed of nuclei and granules by differential centrifugation, named post-granular supernatant, as described previously (10,11). In the present work we used the inhibitor of molecular weight of about 15,000 designated as LNPI-1 (leukocyte neutral proteinase inhibitor) and the inhibitor of molecular weight 40,000 designated as LNPI-2 (11).

In the inhibition studies purified samples of elastase (E.C. 3.4.21.11), chymotrypsin-like neutral proteinase (E.C.3.4.21.-), cathepsin B (E.C.3.4.12.3) and cathepsin D (E.C.3.4.23.5), papain (E.C.3.4.22.2) and urokinase (E.C.3.4.99.26) were used.

The enzyme activity of elastase and chymotrypsin-like neutral proteinase was determined with haemoglobin and histones as substrates as reported earlier (11). Enzyme activity is expressed as the change in absorbance at 750 nm, after a period of incubation. The activity of cathepsin D was determined by the method of Anson (1). The activities of cathepsin B and papain were determined using N-benzoyl-DL-arginine-2-naphthylamide (BANA), according to Barrett's procedure (3). Urokinase activity was determined by Astrup's plate technique (2).

Protein was assayed by the method of Lowry (12). Polyacrylamide gel electrophoresis was performed at pH 8.5 in 8% gels (4).

RESULTS

Inhibitory characteristics of LNPI-1 and LNPI-2. In Fig. 1 are shown the gel electrophoregrams of LNPI-1 and LNPI-2, used throughout the experiments. Staining revealed one protein band for LNPI-2 and two protein bands for LNPI-1. In the first group of experiments the inhibition effect of LNPI-1 and LNPI-2 on proteinases was studied, in a system where the amount of enzyme was maintained at a constant level, in buffer solutions, with the addition of variable quantities of inhibitor.

Inhibition of elastase by increasing quantities of LNPI-1 and LNPI-2 is shown in Fig. 2. It is evident that LNPI-1 does not inhibit elastase even at the highest concentration, whereas LNPI-2 inhibits elastase completely (100%) at a volume ratio of 2(E): 1(L). The degree of elastase inhibition increases linearly with the concentration of inhibitor. Elastase consisted of 3 isoenzymes (3 protein bands), with no other impurities detectable by gel electrophoresis. For the purpose of calculation, however, this mixture of enzymes was assumed to be a single entity with a molecular weight of 27,000; whereas, the molecular weight of

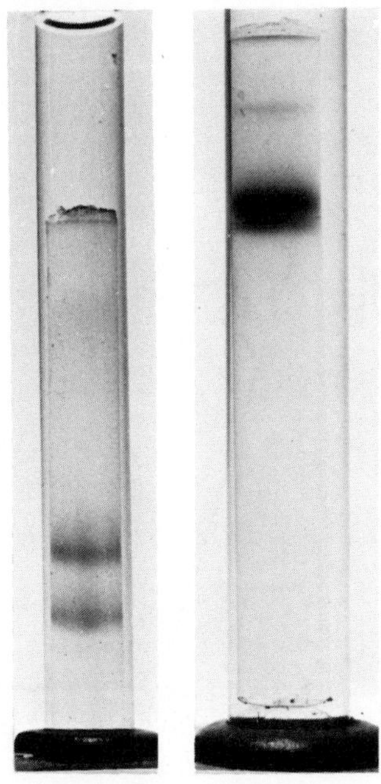

Fig. 1. Gel electrophoregrams of inhibitor sample (LNPI-1 and LNPI-2.

LNPI-2 was 40,000. Thus, the activity of elastase toward haemoglobin was completely inhibited by LNPI-2 in about 1:1 molar ratio.

Fig. 3 shows the inhibition of chymotrypsin-like neutral proteinase with increasing amount of LNPI-1 and LNPI-2, where histones were used as substrate. LNPI-1 shows higher inhibitory ability than LNPI-2. LNPI-2 at the highest concentration used of 210 μg (in 200 μl) inhibits chymotrypsin-like neutral proteinase 224 μg (in 200 μl) by only 70%, whereas LNPI-1 at the concentration of 230 μg (in 50 μl) already inhibits it by 95%.

We found that only LNPI-1 has inhibitory ability against cathepsin B. Fig. 4 shows the inhibition of cathepsin B (from spleen) by increasing quantities of LNPI-1. It is evident that the degree of inhibition increases linearly with concentration of the inhibitor to complete inhibition. At the volume ratio of 1(E): 1(1) (25 μl : 25 μl) inhibition was 80%. If the values

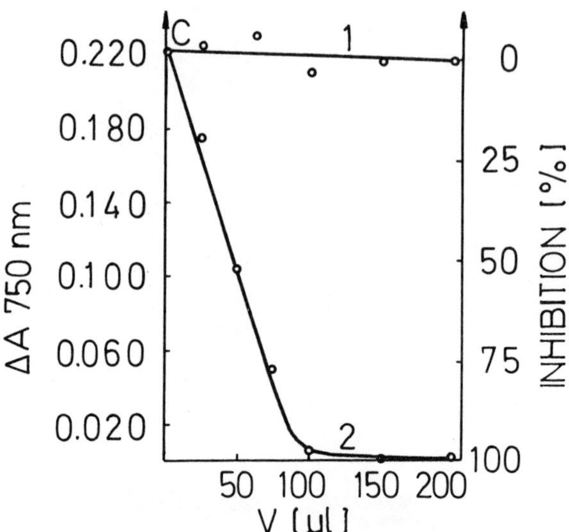

Fig. 2. Inhibition of elastase (200 μl) by addition of different quantities (25 - 200 μl) of LNPI-1 and LNPI-2. Preincubation time of the enzyme with the inhibitor was 10 min. Inhibition was measured after 2 hr digestion of hemoglobin; C - control LNPI-1 - 4.60 mg/ml; LNPI-2 - 1.05 mg/ml, elastase - 0.38 mg/ml.

are given in mcg then the corresponding quantities of cathepsin B and LNPI-1 are 3.2 μg : 19 μg. LNPI-1 also possesses the ability to inhibit papain, and in preliminary experiments we observed that LNPI-1 is also able to inhibit urokinase.

Another important characteristic of these inhibitors was observed, namely, the irreversibility of the enzyme inhibition by these inhibitors. The stability of the enzyme - inhibitor complex was not time dependent, and this was independent of the substrate used.

Interactions of LNPI-1 and LNPI-2 with cathepsin D. In our earlier studies we found that the inhibition ability of leukocyte post-granule supernatant was diminished to about 80% at acid pH from pH 3-5. From these results we concluded that post-granule supernatant inhibitors are unstable in this acid pH region. The results of the present work elucidate the mechanism of the acid

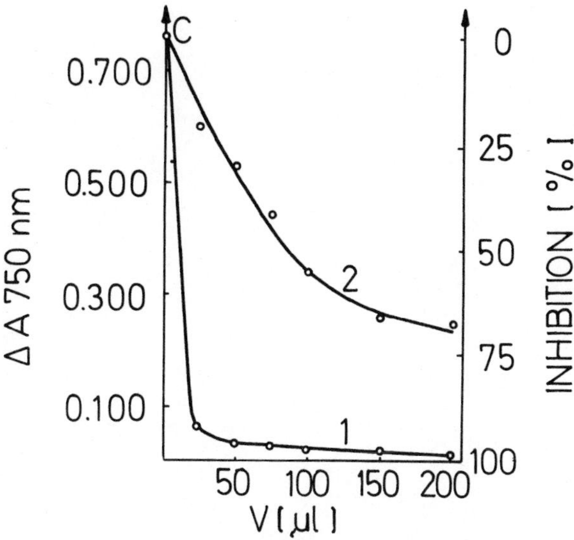

Fig. 3. Inhibition of chymotrypsin-like neutral proteinase (200 μl) by addition of different quantities (25-200 μl) of LNPI-1 and LNPI-2. Preincubation time of enzyme with inhibitor was 10 min. Inhibition was measured after 2 hr digestion of histone; c - control LNPI-1 - 4.60 mg/ml; LNPI-2 - 1.05 mg/ml, chymotrypsin-like neutral proteinase - 1.12 mg/ml.

inactivation of post-granule supernatant inhibition ability. Namely, when we determined the pH stability of highly purified LNPI-1 and LNPI-2 (as used in these experiments) we observed that the inhibitors are quite stable over the whole pH region from pH 3.5 to 7.0. These new data indicate that post granule supernatant inhibitory activity might be affected by an enzyme that is active in the acid pH region. The best known active enzyme at this acid pH is cathepsin D. Fig. 5 shows the effect of cathepsin D on the stability of LNPI-2, as a function of the preincubation time. A rapid decrease in the activity of the inhibitor, over 90%, was noted after only 5 min of preincubation with cathepsin (in molar ratio 1(D) : 20(1)). Complete loss of inhibitory activity was observed with a prolonged time of preincubation. On the other hand, cathepsin D has no ability for decreasing the activity of LNPI-2 when it is already complexed with elastase.

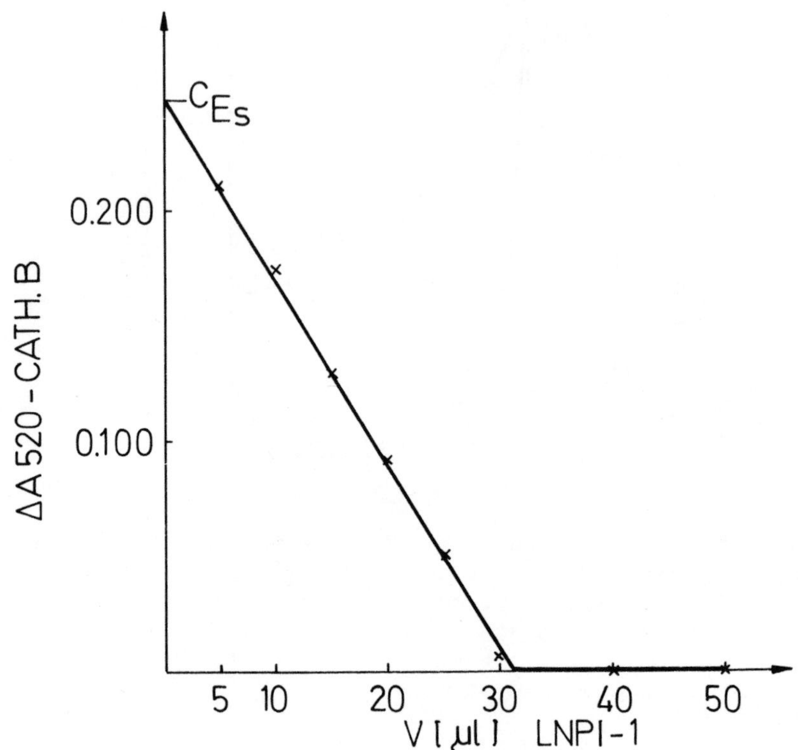

Fig. 4. Inhibition of cathepsin B from spleen (25 µl) by addition of different quantities of LNPI-1 (5-50 µ). Residual enzyme activity was assayed on BANA substrate. CE - enzyme control: 25 µl of cathepsin B + 475 µl of buffer of pH 6.0, were preincubated for 15 min at room temperature and then assayed on BANA substrate. LNPI-1 - 0.76 mg/ml; cathepsin B - 0.13 mg/ml.

We have already studied the effect of cathepsin D on LNPI-1. The reaction was completely different from the case of LNPI-2, as no change in activity of LNPI-1 was noted. However, the question of LNPI-1 stability in post granule supernatant at different pH values still remains unexplained. In this work we only determined that cathepsin D has no effect on the activity of LNPI-1.

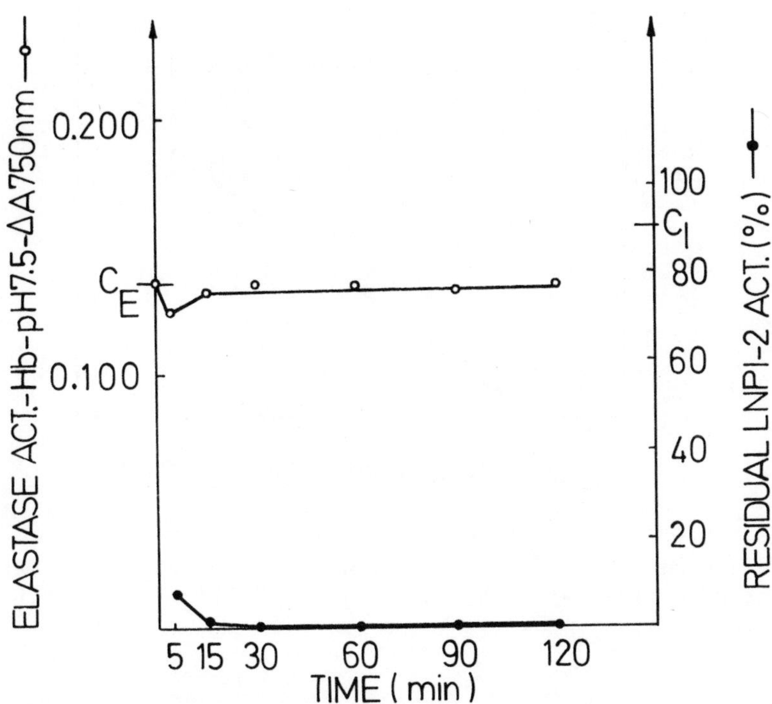

Fig. 5. Inactivation of LNPI-2 by cathepsin D. Samples (50 μl) of inhibitor (20 mol/mol cathepsin D) were incubated with cathepsin D in acetate buffer pH 3.5 (290 μl) at 38 C. At the time point indicated, to each tube elastase (50 μl) was added and samples were assayed for residual inhibitory activity toward elastase.
CE - enzyme control, CI - inhibitor control.

The regressive effect of leukocyte intracellular inhibitors on tumor growth and metastases formation has already been reported in a previous study (8). Fig. 6 shows the effect of leukocyte inhibitors on primary tumor growth. Leukocyte inhibitors significantly reduce the growth of the primary tumor in mice bearing Lewis lung carcinoma. The number of lung metastases found at sacrifice is also significantly reduced to about 64% with respect to the control, and their mass is significantly decreased.

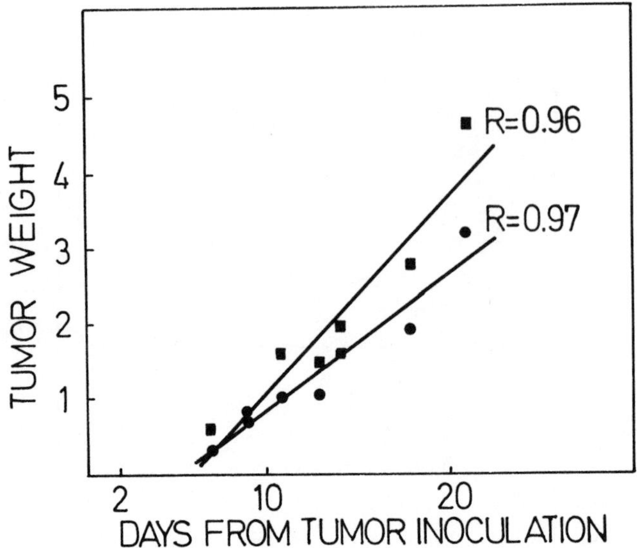

Fig. 6. Effects of LNPI on primary tumor growth. Linear-regression analysis of primary tumor growth in untreated (■) and LNPI-treated mice (●). The slope of the 2 lines is significantly different (t test, $p<0.01$).

CONCLUSION

From the results presented it is evident that LNPI-1 and LNPI-2, isolated from the cytoplasm of pig peripheral leukocytes, differ not only in their molecular weight and interactions with cathepsin D, but also in their ability to inhibit the tested enzymes. LNPI-1 inhibits chymotrypsin-like neutral proteinase, cathepsin B, papain and urokinase, whereas LNPI-2 inhibits only elastase and chymotrypsin-like neutral proteinase.

The biological significance of intracellular inhibitors is presently unknown. Janoff (9) has already proposed that a possible function of such agents might be preservation of nucleohistones from degradation by lysosomal proteases released during mitosis. Elastase and chymotrypsin-like neutral protease are enzymes with the ability to degrade histones.

From the present experiments, where we found that cathepsin D inactivates LNPI-2, it can be proposed that a temporary lowering of intracellular pH (during the process of phagocytosis) diminished the intracellular inhibitory ability (LNPI-2) and changed the intracellular equilibrium in favor of neutral proteinases. In this way, cathepsin D might be a potential regulator of intracellular proteinase activity.

ACKNOWLEDGEMENT

We thank Mgr. M. Stegnar from the Institute of Gerontology, Medical Faculty of Ljubljana, for the fibrinogen agar plate tests performed on urokinase. The excellent technical assistance of Mrs. M. Bozic and Mrs. J. Komar is gratefully acknowledged. Supported by the research grant from the Research Council of Slovenia and in part by NSF grant No. F7F030Y.

REFERENCES

1. Anson, M. L., J. Gen. Physiol, 22 (1939) 79.
2. Astrup, T., Sixtus, T., Med. Clin. North America, 56 (1972) 153.
3. Barrett, A. J., Analyt. Biochem., 47 (1972) 280.
4. Davies, B. J., Ann. N. Y. Acad. Sci., 121 (1964) 404.
5. Dubin, A., Europ. J. Biochem., 73 (1977) 429.
6. Fräki, J., Ruuskanen, O., Hopsu-Havu, V. K. and Kouvalainen, K., Hoppe Seylers Z. Physiol. Chem. 354 (1973) 933.
7. Fritz, H., Schiessler, A. and Geiger, R., Agents and Actions, 8 (1978) 57.
8. Giraldi, T., Kopitar, M. and Sava, G., Cancer Res., 37 (1977) 3834.
9. Janoff, A., Blondin, J., Sandhaus, R. A., Mosser, A. and Malemud, C. In: Proteases and Biological Control (Ed. E. Reich, D. B. Rifkin and E. Shaw), Cold Spring Harbor Laboratory, New York, (1975) 603.
10. Kopitar, M. and Lebez, D., Europ. J. Biochem., 56 (1975) 571.
11. Kopitar, M., Suhar, A., Giraldi, T. and Turk, V., Acta Biol. Med. German., 36 (1978) 1872.
12. Lowry, O. H., Rosenbrough, M. J., Farr, A. L. and Randal, R. J., J. Biol. Chem., 193 (1951) 265.
13. Steven, F. S., Milsom, D. W. and Hunter, J. A. A., Europ. J. Biochem., 67 (1976) 165.
14. Stubblefield, E. and Brown, R. L. In: 29th Annual Symposium of Fundamental Cancer Research, Growth Kinetics and Biochemical Regulation of Normal and Malignant Cells. M. D. Anderson Hospital, Houston, Texas (1976).

IMMUNOLOGICAL STUDIES OF INTRACELLULAR LEUKOCYTE PROTEINASE INHIBITOR BY GRANULAR EXTRACT AND CATHEPSIN D

J. BABNIK, M. KOPITAR and V. TURK

Department of Biochemistry
J. Stefan Institute
Ljubljana (Yugoslavia)

There are many reports in the literature (1) on the purification and properties of plasma proteinase inhibitors (i.e. alpha 1-antitrypsin, alpha 2-macroglobulin) and on attempts to make antisera, but so far there have been very few adequate reports on the isolation of intracellular leukocyte proteinase inhibitors and there have been no adequate reports on a specific anti-(LNPI) serum.

The inactivation effect of acid proteinases on extracellular inhibitors was recently reported by Sandhaus and Janoff (6) who showed that hepatocyte granule extract at acid pH produced degradation of alpha 1-antitrypsin within 1 hr, as monitored by immunoelectrophoretic analysis. Later Johnson and Travis (2) on the basis of biochemical analysis, confirmed that cathepsin B was the enzyme which inactivates alpha 1-antitrypsin by specific bond hydrolysis.

Kopitar and Lebez (4) described the purification and characterization of specific intracellular inhibitors of neutral proteinases. Two types of intracellular inhibitors of neutral proteinases were isolated, designated LNP-1 and LNPI-2 (5). These inhibitors differ not only in molecular weight but in inhibition ability against proteinases, and also in inactivation by cathepsin D. In studying the biochemical properties of these inhibitors we observed that cathepsin D inactivates LNPI-2 at acid pH. The inhibitor lost over 90% of its inhibition ability, after only 5 min of preincubation with cathepsin D (in molar ratio : 1(D) : 20(LNPI-2)). Complete loss of the inhibitor activity was observed with prolonged time of incubation. On the other hand, cathepsin D had no effect on LNPI-1, no inactivation being observed.

In the present paper we describe the preparation of specific antisera to leukocyte neutral proteinase inhibitors and detailed experiments on the immunological studies of inhibitor degradation by cathepsin D and leukocyte granular extract.

MATERIALS AND METHODS

Preparation of antiserum. The concentrated fraction of the electrophoretically pure intracellular inhibitors LNPI-1 and LNPI-2 isolated from pig leukocytes, with 3.5 mg of protein per ml, was used for immunological purposes. One ml of sample was divided into 4 portions and one portion was mixed with an equal volume of Freund's complete adjuvant and injected intramuscularly into the foot of a New Zealand rabbit. The procedure was repeated after 10, 20 and 30 days. Blood was taken 10 days after the final injection.

Immunoelectrophoretic (EP) analysis. Agar (Behringwerke A. G.) gels were prepared using 0.075 M Veronal buffer, ph 8.6. Gels were poured onto 2.5 x 7.5 cm glass slides. Two 5 µl wells and one 50 µl trough were cut, and 5 µl aliquots were placed in the wells for electrophoresis (7). Electrophoresis was carried out for 130 min in a water-cooled bath at a constant voltage of 8 V/cm (10 mA per gel). After electrophoresis, the troughs were filled with 50 µl of rabbit anti(LNPI) serum. After 48 hr in a refrigerator (T^{o} = 4 C) the IEP plates were extensively rinsed in 0.15 M NaCl and water, dried, stained with Coomassie blue and photographed.

RESULTS

IEP analysis of anti(LNPI) serum showed two precipitin lines against an antigen which contained a mixture of both inhibitors. In immunodiffusion plates (3) it was shown that whole pig serum and alpha 1-antitrypsin alone contain no crossreacting protein, which confirms that the two intracellular inhibitors used immunologically differ from serum inhibitors and that they belong to a specific type of proteinase intracellular inhibitor.

Anti(LNPI) serum gave a single precipitin line against pure LNPI-1 intracellular inhibitor with a lower molecular weight (Fig. 1) and a single precipitin line against pure LNPI-2 inhibitor with a molecular weight of 40,000 (Fig. 2). From these results it can be seen that these two inhibitors have different electrophoretic mobility on IEP plates, and that they do not differ only in biochemical but also in immunological properties, and that they are completely pure.

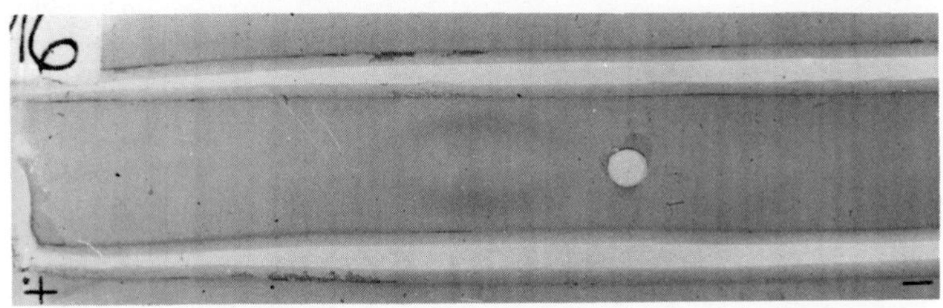

Fig. 1. Immunoelectrophoresis of anti(LNPI) serum against pure LNPI-1 inhibitor. The well contained 5 μg of inhibitor in 5 μl; the trough contained 50 μl antiserum.

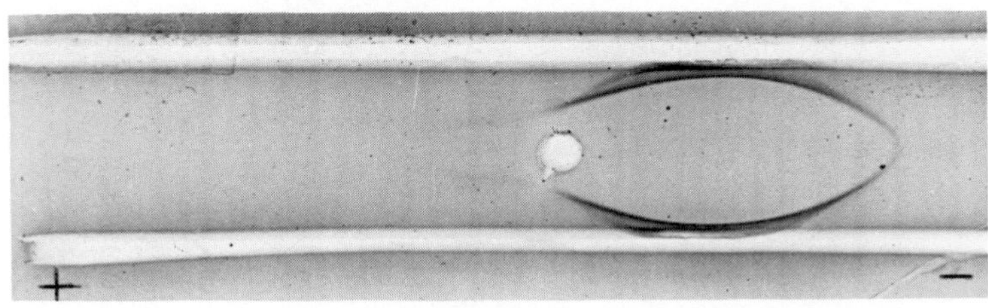

Fig. 2. Immunoelectrophoresis of anti(LNPI) serum against pure LNPI-2 inhibitor. The well contained 10.5 μg of inhibitor in 5 μl; the trough contained 50 μl of antiserum.

Degradation of pure LNPI-2 inhibitor by bovine cathepsin D. IEP plates were developed with rabbit anti(LNPI) serum and the inhibitor was degraded at pH 3.5 during incubation at 37 C with cathepsin D (8). The results obtained are shown in Fig. 3. It can be seen that the LNPI-2 present in the reaction mixture was degraded during incubation with cathepsin D. Small but visible degradation product was apparent within 30 min of incubation.

After these experiments, similar electropherograms were developed with a prolonged incubation time and with increased amounts of both reactants at pH 3.5. As can be seen from Fig. 4, a higher digestion occurred within 2 hr of incubation.

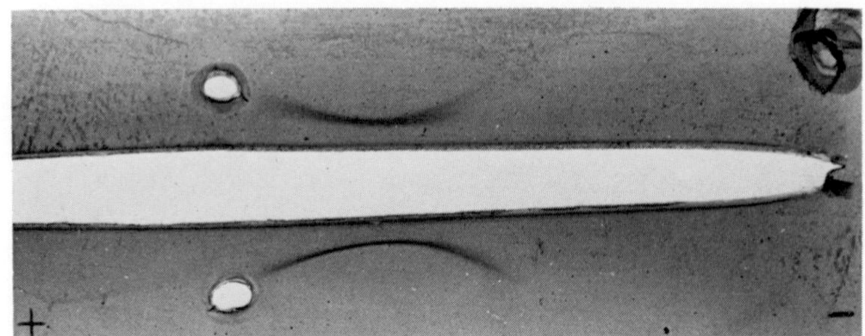

Fig. 3. Immunoelectrophoresis of anti(LNPI) serum against degradation products of inhibitor by cathepsin D. The reaction mixture (RM) was made up to a total volume of 37 µl and contained 5.1 µg of inhibitor, 1.2 µg of cathepsin D and buffer solution to give a final concentration of 0.1 N acetate buffer at pH 3.5; duration of incubation was 30 min at 37 C before IEP analysis. Control reaction mixture (C) containing inhibitor and buffer solution without cathepsin D was incubated at 37 C. 30 min. Top well (TW) = 5 µl of RM, bottom well (BW) = 5 µl of C.

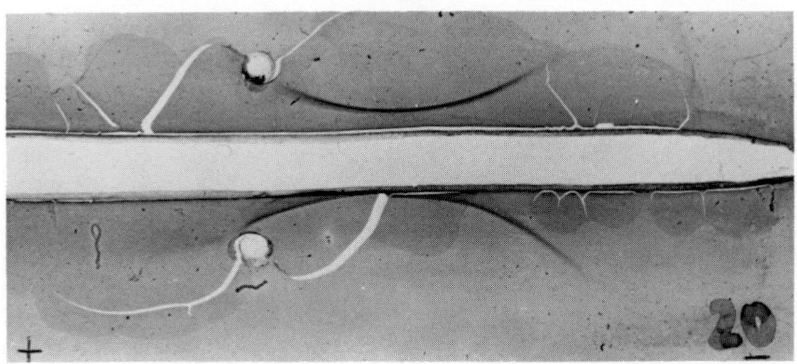

Fig. 4. IEP of anti(LNPI) serum against degradation products of inhibitor by higher concentration of cathepsin D at pH 3.5. Reaction mixture of 46 µl contained 10.2 µg of inhibitor, 4 µg of cathepsin D and buffer solution at pH 3.5. Incubation time was 2 hr at 37 C before analysis of IEP. CRM contained an identical amount of inhibitor and buffer but without cathepsin D, incubated at 37 C for 2 hr. TW = RM, BW = C.

Degradation of LNPI-2 inhibitor by granule extract from pig leukocytes. As can be seen from Fig. 5, the degradation of the inhibitor occurring in these experiments was much more pronounced; it is well known that granule extract contains, besides cathepsin D, also other proteinases and degradation can develop over a broader spectrum.

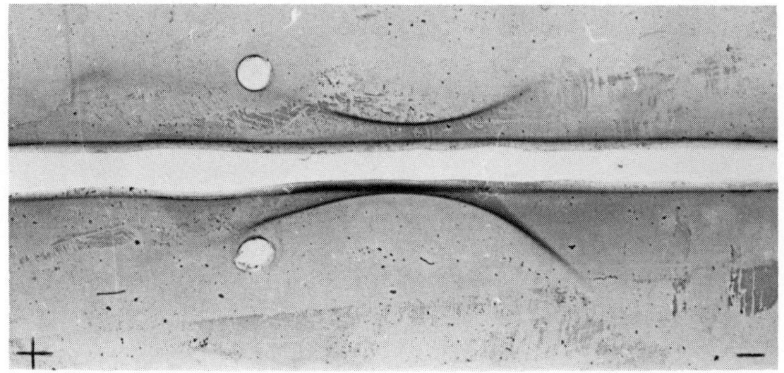

Fig. 5. IEP analysis of anti(LNPI) serum against degradation products of inhibition by granule extract. Reaction mixture was made to a total volume of 46 μl and contained 10.2 μg of inhibitor, 10 μg of granule extract protein and buffer solution to give a final concentration of 0.1 N acetate buffer at pH 3.5. These RM were incubated for 2 hr at 37 C before IEP analysis. Control reaction mixture containing inhibitor preparation without granule extract was incubated at 37 C 2 hr. TW = RM, BW = C.

DISCUSSION

On the basis of the experiments presented, it can be concluded that inhibitors designated LNPI-1 and LNPI-2 have different electrophoretic mobility on IEP plates, confirming that these two inhibitors are not only different in their biochemical, but also in their immunological properties. From the results shown (3), no cross reactivity with whole pig serum and with alpha 1-antitrypsin was observed. We confirm with these immunological studies that the two proteins belong to a specific type of intracellular proteinase inhibitor.

The foregoing *in vitro* studies showed that cathepsin D inactivates LNPI-2 at acid pH. Complete loss of the inhibitor activity was observed with prolonged time of incubation. On the contrary, cathepsin D has no ability for LNPI-2 when it is already complexed with the enzyme (Kopitar *et al.*, VIII International RES Congress, 1978). In the presented work we assumed that the inhibitor served as a substrate for the acid proteinase used. A different degree of inhibitor degradation occurred with the same amount of LNPI-2, as shown in Figs. 4 and 5, but with different enzyme samples. Pure cathepsin D caused a much lower degree of degradation in caomparison with granule extract. The higher effect of degradation of inhibitor by granule extract could be ascribed to the broader spectrum of proteolytic enzymes present in the extract. We believe that these immunological studies may help to elucidate the role of intracellular proteinases and their inhibitors in living systems.

ACKNOWLEDGEMENT

This research was supported by the Research Council of Slovenia (Yugoslovia) and in part by the NSF grant no. F7F030Y (USA).

REFERENCES

1. Fritz, H., Tschesche, H., Greene, L. J., and Truscheit, E., Proteinase Inhibitors. Proc. of the 2nd International Research Conference. Springer Verlag, Berlin-Heidelberg-New York (1974).
2. Johnson, D. and Travis, J., Biochem. J. 136 (1977) 639.
3. Kopitar, M., Babnik, J. Kregar, I. and Suhar, A., In: Movement, Metabolism and Bactericidal Mechanisms of Phagocytes (Eds. F. Rossi, P. Patriarca and D. Romeo), Piccin Medical Books, Padua (1977) 295.
4. Kopitar, M. and Lebez, D., Europ. J. Biochem. 56 (1975) 571.
5. Kopitar, M., Suhar, A., Giraldi, T. and Turk, V., Acta Biol. Med. Germ. 36 (1978) 1863.
6. Sandhaus, R. A., and Janoff, A., Am. Rev. Respir. Dis. 110 (1974) 263.
7. Scheidegger, J. J., Int. Arch. Allergy 7 (1955) 103.
8. Smith, R. and Turk, V., Europ. J. Biochem. 48 (1974) 245.

A COMPARATIVE STUDY OF THE BIOCHEMICAL PROPERTIES OF MYELOPEROXIDASE AND EOSINOPHIL PEROXIDASE

R. CRAMER, B. BISIACCHI, G. DE NICOLA and P. PATRIARCA

Istituto di Patologia Generale
Trieste (Italy)

Myeloperoxidase, the peroxidase of neutrophilic leukocytes, is genetically distinct from the eosinophil peroxidase as suggested by the absence of myeloperoxidase activity from neutrophils, but not eosinophils of subjects with inherited myeloperoxidase deficiency (6,8,13).

Several biochemical differences between the two peroxidases have been also reported (1,4,5,11). It has been estimated that the peroxidase activity of eosinophils is 4 to 10 times higher than that of neutrophils on a cell basis (5,10). This implies that the biochemical determinations of the myeloperoxidase of white blood cell preparations which contain even a small percentage of eosinophils may lead to significant overstimulation of this enzymatic activity. We found that this inconvenience is particularly serious when pedigree studies of families with genetic myeloperoxidase deficiency are carried out. In such instance in fact, the presence of the eosinophil peroxidase in the sample may obscure the occurrence of heterozygous subjects and may make totally deficient subjects to appear partially deficient. This led us to search for experimental conditions which would eliminate the interference of the eosinophil peroxidase. We therefore started a comparison of the biochemical properties of the two peroxidases and found that certain differences between the two enzymes might be exploited to minimize the interference of eosinophils with the assay of myeloperoxidase.

MATERIALS AND METHODS

Neutrophils. Human neutrophils were obtained from heparinized venous blood after dextran sedimentation of red cells. The blood was mixed with five volumes of 4.5 % (w/v) solution of dextran (Dextran type 200, Sigma, 240,000 m.w.). After gravity sedimentation of the erythrocytes for about 30 min at room temperature, the white blood cell rich plasma was centrifuged at 600 x g for 10 min. Leukocytes were found from contaminating erythrocytes by hypotonic lysis and were then resuspended in calcium-free Krebs-Ringer phosphate buffer, ph 7.4. The leukocyte preparations usually contained more than 85% polymorphs, as judged by differential counts on May-Grunwald Giemsa stained smears.

Eosinophils. These were obtained from a patient with eosinophilia of unknown origin (about 30% eosinophils in the blood). The heparinized venous blood was processed as described in the previous paragraph. The white cell rich plasma was then processed according to the method of Day (3) in order to separate the eosinophils from the other cell types. The plasma was then layered on top of sodium metrizoate (density 1.148) in 100 ml centrifuge tubes. The diameter of the tubes was 4 cm and the height of the metrizoate layer was 3 cm from the bottom of the tube. The tubes were then centrifuged at 400 x g for 40 min at room temperature in a swinging bucket rotor. The neutrophils banded at the metrizoate-plasma interface, whereas the eosinophils pelleted at the bottom of the tube. The cells were recovered and were exposed to a brief hypotonic treatment (30-60) sec) in order to lyse any erythrocytes. Finally, the cells were resuspended in Krebs-Ringer phosphate, pH 7.4.

Peroxidase assay. The kinetics of the peroxidation of guaiacol or o-dianisidine in the presence of H_2O_2 was recorded. The initial linear part of the trace recording was used for calculation. The optimal conditions for the measurement of the peroxidation of guaiacol have been established in a previous paper (12). They are as follows: 0.1 M phosphate buffer, pH 7.0, 13 mM guaiacol, 0.02% cetyltrimethylammonium bromide (CTAB) and about 2 x 10^4 cells (final volume's 3 ml). The reaction is started by adding 1 μmole of H_2O_2. The increase in optical density at 470 nm is recorded.

Preliminary experiments have shown that the optimal conditions to measure the peroxidation of o-dianisidine are as follows: 0.1 M citrate buffer, pH 5.5, 0.017% o-dianisidine, 0.02% CTAB and about 2 x 10^4 cells (final volume is 3 ml). The reaction is started by adding 0.24 μmoles of H_2O_2 and the increase in optical density at 450 nm is recorded.

Myeloperoxidase-deficient subjects. The homozygous subject

(F.M.) and the heterozygous subject (E.Z.) belong to two newly identified families with hereditary myeloperoxidase deficiency. These families will be described in more detail elsewhere. The neutrophils and the monocytes, but not the eosinophils, of F.M. were negative to histochemical staining for peroxidase, whereas all the three cell types of E.Z. reacted positively.

RESULTS

Table I shows the effect of increasing the percentage of eosinophils in the white cell preparation on the peroxidation of guaiacol and o-dianisidine, respectively. The peroxidation of both substrates increases with the increase of the number of eosinophils. The increase, however is much greater with guaiacol than with o-dianisidine, indicating that guaiacol is more sensitive than o-dianisidine to peroxidation by eosinophil peroxidase.

A practical consequence of this phenomenon is illustrated in Table II, which shows the results of the assay with the two methods of the residual peroxidase activity of white cell preparations from two subjects with different degrees of a genetically determined

TABLE I

Peroxidase Activity of White Blood Cell Samples Containing Varying Percentages of Eosinophils as Measured by the Peroxidation of Guaiacol and o-Dianisidine

Percent Eosinophils	Peroxidase Activity	
	Guaiacol[a]	O-Dianisidine[b]
<1	0.267	544
6	0.658	-
9	0.853	-
34	2.329	1,012
50	3.065	1,739
62	3.139	-
71	4.177	2,258

[a] µmoles tetraguaiacol/min/10^6 neutrophils + eosinophils

[b] o-dianisidine units/min/10^6 neutrophils + eosinophils. One o-dianisidine unit is defined as the amount of enzyme which causes an increase in optical density of 0.01/min.

TABLE II

Residual Myeloperoxidase Activity of the White Blood Cells of Homozygous (F.M.) and a Heterozygous Subject (E.Z.) for Myeloperoxidase Deficiency as Determined with Guaiacol or o-Dianisidine as Substrates[a]

Patient	No. of Eosinophils in the White Cell Preparation	Peroxidase Activity % of Normal Subjects	
	%	Guaiacol	o-Dianisidine
F.M.	4	50	1.6
E.Z.	4	98	50

[a]The average peroxidase activity of normal subjects was: 0.457 μmoles tetraguaiacol/min/10^6 cells±0.122 SD (9 subjects), and 5.222 o-dianisidine units/min/10^6 cells±0.735 SD (9 subjects).

myeloperoxidase deficiency. On the basis of the results of the guaiacol method the subject F.M. appears to have about 50% of the peroxidase activity of the control subjects, and therefore he should be classified as heterozygous. This result, however, does not fit with the finding that the neutrophils of this subject are completely unreactive to histochemical staining for myeloperoxidase. In fact, the neutrophils and monocytes of subjects with total hereditary myeloperoxidase deficiency do not stain for myeloperoxidase, whereas those of heterozygous subjects do (8). On the contrary, the results of the o-dianisidine assay indicate that this subject is homozygous for the defect in agreement with the unresponsiveness of his neutrophils to the histochemical reaction. Subject E.Z. would be considered normal with regard to myeloperoxidase activity on the basis of the guaiacol assay, whereas she appears to have about 50% of the myeloperoxidase activity of the control subjects on the basis of the o-dianisidine assay. Therefore, she should be designated as heterozygous.

Table III shows the effects of a cationic detergent, cetyltrimethylammonium bromide (CTAB), and a non-ionic detergent, Triton X-100, on the activity of myeloperoxidase and eosinophil peroxidase. In the presence of CTAB a higher activity (25-30%) than with Triton X-100 could be measured with both guaiacol and o-dianisidine as substrates in preparations containing less than 1% eosinophils. When the percentage of eosinophils is raised to 50 the activity in the presence of CTAB is about 2.7 times higher, with both guaiacol and o-dianisidine as substrates, than that measured with Triton X-100. This indicates that the eosinophil peroxidase has a stricter requirement for CTAB than myeloperoxidase in order for optimal activity to be displayed.

TABLE III

Effect of Cetyltrimethylammonium Bromide (CTAB) and Triton X-100 on the Peroxidase Activity of White Cell Samples with Different Percentages of Eosinophils

Percent Eosinophils	Peroxidase Activity			
	[a]Guaiacol		[b]o-Dianisidine	
	+CTAB	+TX-100	+CTAB	+TX-100
<1	0.267	0.206	544	430
50	3.065	1.134	1,739	644

[a]µmoles tetraguaiacol/min/10^6 neutrophils + eosinophils.
[b]o-dianisidine units/min/10^6 neutrophils + eosinophils. The o-dianisidine units are defined in the previous table.

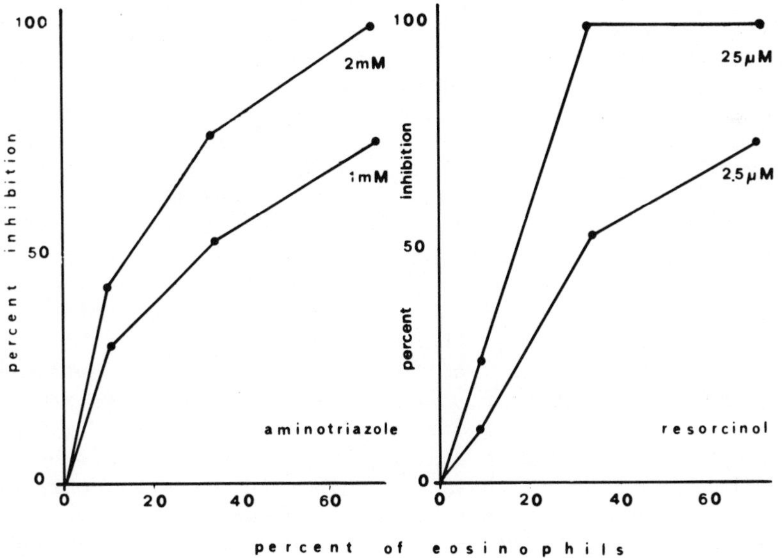

Fig. 1. Inhibition by resorcinol and 2,4-aminotriazole of the peroxidase activity of white blood cell samples as a function of the increasing percentage of eosinophils.

Fig. 1 shows the effect of 2,4-aminotriazole and resorcinol on the peroxidase activity of a mixture of neutrophils and eosinophils as a function of the increasing percentage of eosinophils. Both reagents inhibit the peroxidase activity, and this effect becomes more marked as the percentage of eosinophils in the sample increases, indicating that the eosinophil peroxidase is more sensitive to inhibition by 2,4-aminotriazole and resorcinol than myeloperoxidase.

Table IV shows the effect of aging on the peroxidase activity of white blood cell samples with different content of eosinophils. The peroxidase activity progresively decreases as the percentage of eosinophils increases during the first two days of storage in the cold room, whereas the activity of the sample without eosinophils is not affected by storage. After 4 days of storage the loss of peroxidase activity from the samples which contain eosinophils becomes more marked. At this time even the peroxidase activity of the sample without eosinophils begins to decline.

DISCUSSION

Myeloperoxidase is an essential component of the oxygen-dependent bactericidal system of polymorphonuclear leukocytes. A lack or a reduced level of this enzyme has been reported to occur at least in the following circumstances, a) hereditary myeloperoxidase deficiency (6,8,13), b) drug induced myeloperoxidase deficiency (7), c) acquired idiopathic refractory anemia (9), and d) myeloproliferative disorders such as chronic granulocytic leukemia (2). In these cases, therefore, a reduction in the bactericidal power of leukocytes is to be expected whose severity depends on the degree of the myeloperoxidase deficiency. In such circumstances, the identification of the molecular defect underlying the reduced bactericidal power requires the assay of myeloperoxidase activity. A quantitation of these enzymatic activity can be easily and quickly obtained by using biochemical assays which measure the peroxidation of a substrate in the presence of hydrogen peroxide. However, the presence of eosinophils in the white cell preparation may lead to significant overestimation of the myeloperoxidase activity, due to the high peroxidase activity of these cells. One could get rid of eosinophils by centrifuging the leukocyte preparation on a layer of metrizoate according to the method of Day (3), which allows to obtain virtually pure eosinophils at the bottom of the tube, whereas the neutrophils rest on top of the metrizoate layer. This procedure, however, is impractical for routine assay of several samples. The need therefore arises for a biochemical assay which allows at least to minimize the interference of eosinophil peroxidase with the assay of myeloperoxidase.

In this paper some biochemical differences have been shown to exist between myeloperoxidase and eosinophil peroxidase, which could be exploited to minimize the interference of eosinophil peroxidase with the estimation of myeloperoxidase. For example, a) aging of white cell preparations in the cold room for 48 hr leads to a major reduction of the eosinophil peroxidase activity, whereas the activity of myeloperoxidase is virtually unaffected; b) 2,4-aminotriazole and resorcinol are strong inhibitors of the eosinophil peroxidase, whereas they only partially affect the activity of myeloperoxidase; c) CTAB is required for optimal activity of the eosinophil peroxidase, whereas the activity of myeloperoxidase is not significantly different whether CTAB or Triton X-100 is used; d) the peroxidation of o-dianisidine seems to be less sensitive than the peroxidation of guaiacol to the eosinophil peroxidase. Particularly, the last difference offers a simple way of discriminating between the two peroxidase activities in mixed white blood cell populations. When the myeloperoxidase activity of pure neutrophils was measured with o-dianisidine and guaiacol as substrates, an average increase in optical density of 0.088 O.D. units/min and 0.065 O.D. units/min, respectively, was obtained using 2×10^4 cells in each assay. This indicates that the peroxidation of the two substrates has a comparable sensitivity to myeloperoxidase. By measuring the peroxidase activity of neutrophil preparations containing varying percentages of eosinophils it was found that the activity progressively increased over that of pure neutrophils by increasing the percentage of eosinophils with both methods. However, with the o-dianisidine assay, the increment was lower than that observed with the guaiacol assay. This indicates that the peroxidase activity of eosinophils is higher than that of neutrophils, and that the o-dianisidine assay is less sensitive than the guaiacol assay to the eosinophil peroxidase. On the basis of our data, we calculated that the peroxidase activity of eosinophils is 15 and 6 times higher than that of neutrophils when assayed with guaiacol or o-dianisidine as substrates, respectively. This implies that overestimation of the myeloperoxidase activity of neutrophil preparations containing even a small percentage of eosinophils would be much more marked when guaiacol is used as substrate instead of o-dianisidine. Specifically, we found substantially different results when the peroxidase activity of leukocyte preparations from subjects with hereditary myeloperoxidase deficiency was assayed using guaiacol or o-dianisidine. In this enzyme deficiency, myeloperoxidase is absent or reduced in neutrophils and monocytes but is normal in eosinophils. The guaiacol assay of the leukocyte preparation with 4% eosinophils from a subject whose neutrophils were unreactive to histochemical staining for peroxidase showed about 50% activity as compared to control subjects, which suggests that the subject was heterozygous for the defect. This conclusion, however, is in conflict with the histochemical data, since it is known that the neutrophils of heterozygous subjects react to histochemical staining for myeloperoxidase, whereas those of homozygous subjects do not. Furthermore, a heterozygous condition for this subject would not fit the pedigree of the family. The o-dianisidine assay showed that the myeloperoxidase activity of the leukocytes of this subject was 98.4% below the normal level. The residual myeloperoxidase activity may be safely attributed to contaminating eosinophils. Therefore, on the basis of the results of the assay with o-dianisidine, this subject is properly identified as homozygous for the deficiency of myeloperoxidase in accordance with the histochemical staining and the pedigree studies. We also found examples of subjects that should be classified as heterozygous on the basis on the o-dianisidine assay in agreement with the pedigree studies, but would appear to have a normal level of myeloperoxidase on the basis of the guaiacol assay.

We conclude that whenever the need arises of determining the activity of myeloperoxidase in leukocyte preparations containing even a small number of eosinophils the assay which employs the peroxidation of o-dianisidine is recommended in order to minimize the interference by the eosinophil peroxidase.

ACKNOWLEGEMENT

Supported by grant No 77.01481.04 from the National Council of Research (CNR) of Italy.

REFERENCES

1. Archer, G. T., Air, G., Jackas, M. and Morell, D. B., Biochim. Biophys. Acta, 99 (1965) 96.
2. Bainton, D. F., In: Unclassifiable Leukemias, (Ed. M. Bessis and G. Brecher), Springer, New York (1975).
3. Day, R. P., Immunology, 18 (1970) 955.
4. Desser, R. K., Himmeloch, S. R., Evans, W. H., Januska, M., Mage, M. G. and Shelton, E., Arch. Biochem. Biophys. 148 (1972) 452.
5. Fabian, I. and Aronson, M., J. Reticuloendothel. Soc. 17 (1975) 141.
6. Grignaschi, V. J., Sperperato, A. M., Etcheverry, A. J. and Macario, A. J. L., Rev. Asoc. Med. Arg., 77 (1963) 218.
7. Harkness, R. A. and Grant-Renz, M., In: Movement, Metabolism and Bactericidal Mechanisms of Phagocytes, (Ed. F. Rossi, P. Patriarca and D. Romeo), Piccin Medical Books, Padova, Italy (1977).
8. Lehrer, R. I. and Clinc, M. J., J. Clin. Invest., 48 (1969)

1478.
9. Lehrer, R. I., Goldberg, L. S., Apple, M. A. and Rosenthal, N. P., Ann. Int. Med., 76 (1972) 447.
10. Mage, M. G., Evans, W. H., Himmeloch, S. R. and McHugh, L., J. Reticuloendothel. Soc., 9 (1971) 201.
11. Migler, R., De Chatelet, L. R. and Bass, D. A., Blood, 51 (1978) 445.
12. Romeo, D., Cramer, R., Marzi, T., Soranzo, M. R., Zabucchi, G. and Rossi, F., J. Reticuloendothel. Soc. 13 (1973) 399.
13. Undritz, E., Blood, 14 (1966) 129.

GLUCOCORTICOID PROTECTION OF HEPATIC PHAGOCYTOSIS IN HYPOXIA

M. J. GALVIN and A. M. LEFER

Department of Physiology, Jefferson Medical College

Philadelphia, Pennsylvania (USA)

Although deterioration of the cardiovascular system has been the most obvious consequence of circulatory shock, the factors contributing to the circulatory collapse are complex (20). Recently, the liver has been recognized as a critical organ in the pathogenesis and metabolism, serving as a biological filter to the blood returning to the heart (23).

Furthermore, the reticuloendothelial system (RES), of which the liver comprises over 80%, has been reported to play a vital role in the responses to shock stimuli (7, 16, 17). In particular, alterations in the phagocytic activity of the RES have been reported following burn injury (18), whole body trauma (11, 19), hemorrhage (13, 14) and splanchnic artery occlusion (3). The depression of RES activity has been shown to parallel the accumulation of toxic products such as lysosomal enzymes (13) which have been implicated in the pathogenesis of shock (9, 10). In addition, inhibition of the RES has been demonstrated to increase the susceptibility of animals to various stressful stimuli (7, 17), whereas stimulation of the RES enhances resistance to shock (1, 14, 15).

Although a number of pharmacologic agents such as glucagon (12), beta adrenergic blockers (10), and glucocorticoids (10, 12) have been reported to be beneficial in animals experiencing circulatory shock, glucocorticoids have probably received the widest acceptance. In this regard, methylprednisolone (MP) has been reported to increase the resistance of animals to both hemorrhagic (10) and splanchnic artery occlusion (9) shock. The mechanisms proposed for the increase in resistance to shock afforded by glucocorticoids have included lysosomal stabilization, circulatory and metabolic effects and RES activation (12).

Because of the importance of impairment of hepatic function in the pathogenesis of circulatory shock, these experiments were designed to examine the effects of two shock-like stimuli, hypoxia and endotoxin in the presence and absence of steroids, on liver integrity *in vitro*. In particular, the changes in RES activity and lysosomal stability of liver cells were examined, uncomplicated by the presence of plasma factors or changes in pH, PO_2 or flow.

MATERIALS AND METHODS

Operative procedures. Cats of either sex weighing 2.5-3.5 kg which had been fed *ad libitum* were anesthetized intravenously with sodium pentobarbital (30 mg/kg). Heparin (Upjohn beef lung, 1000 units) was injected intravenously prior to laparotomy. The liver and its blood vessels were excised within 2-3 min after occlusion of the hepatic portal vein according to the technique of Carlson and Lefer (20). The liver was then placed in oxygenated Krebs-Henseleit solution and transferred to the perfusion apparatus.

Perfusion technique. Livers (60-100 gm) were placed in a jacketed lucite chamber. The portal vein cannula was connected to the inflow tubing and the inferior vena cava outflow catheter was connected to a reservoir-oxygenator containing 400 ml of perfusate. The osmolarity of the perfusate was 325 mOsm. The perfusate pH was maintained at 7.2-7.4 using 25 mM HEPES (2-N-hydroxyethylpiperazine-2-n'-ethanesulfonic acid). The ionic composition of the perfusate was the same as that used by Carlson and Lefer (20). Samples were collected from the outflow catheter at 0, 30, 60, 90, 120 and 150 min for determination of pH, and lactate dehydrogenase (LDH) and cathepsin D activities. Oxygen consumption was determined from PO_2 readings of samples taken at the inflow and outflow catheters at 0 and 150 min. A Haake constant-temperature circulator bath was used to maintain perfusate temperature at 37 $\pm$ 0.2 C at the inflow to the liver. Perfusate flow was adjusted to 1.4 ml/gm liver per min. Oxygenation of the system was maintained by a finely dispersed gas mixture of 95% O_2 + 5% CO_2 bubbled through the perfusate at a constant rate to achieve a PO_2 of 400 to 450 mm Hg. A 100-mesh nylon filter was placed in the circuit to remove particulate matter. To induce hypoxia, the gas mixture was replaced with a mixture of 95% N_2 + 5% CO_2. This resulted in a perfusate PO_2 of 25-35 mm Hg. *E. coli* endotoxin (Difco Laboratories, Detroit, Michigan, Np. 026:B6) was added to some perfusates at a concentration of 50-80 g/ml, which corresponds to a dose of 75 g/g liver just prior to the start of the experiment. In some experiments, either methylprednisolone (MP) or dexamethasone (Dex) was added to the perfusate 30 min prior to the induction of either hypoxia or endotoxemia.

Analytical procedures. An International Laboratories Model 313 blood gas analyzer was used to determine perfusate PO_2 in mm Hg. Samples were read immediately upon drawing. Oxygen consumption of the livers were calculated from the PO_2 between the portal vein and hepatic vein samples of the perfusate according to previously described methods (20).

LDH activity was determined in perfusate samples spectrophotometrically at 340 nm using pyruvate as substrate. Activities are expressed as change in absorbance units of NADH per min at 25 C (24). Samples of perfusate and liver were also assayed for cathepsin D activity according to the method of Anson (2) using bovine hemaglobin as substrate. Activities are expressed as milliequivalents of tyrosine x 10^{-4} produced per milliliter of perfusate per hr at 37 C. In addition, tissue samples were assayed for cathepsin D in the presence and absence of 0.1% Triton X-100.

Reticuloendothelial clearance techniques. Carbon particles (Gunther Wagner ink 11/1441A) were collected by centrifuging the ink preparation at 3,000 g for 15 min, which resulted in a homogenous supernatant containing carbon at 100 to 135 mg/ml. The suspension was stabilized by adding 1% gelatin at the time of the experiment, yielding a final carbon concentration of 50 mg/ml. Clearances were performed at 150 min by adding 1.2 mg of carbon/g tissue to a perfusate volume of 350 ml. Samples were taken at one min intervals and diluted 1:20 in 0.1% Na_2CO_3. Carbon concentrations were determined spectrophotometrically at 675 nm. The calculation of k (i.e., slope) of the disappearance curve of carbon was used as a measure of the rate of phagocytosis of the RES.

Statistical methods. Statistical comparisons were made using the Student's t test for unpaired data.

RESULTS

The perfusate lactic dehydrogenase activity following 150 min of perfusion for the 9 groups of livers are given in Table I. In the control groups, there was no difference in the perfusate LDH activity of the vehicle, MP or Dex treated livers. In both the hypoxia and endotoxin treated livers receiving vehicle there resulted in a significant increase in LDH activity of the vehicle treated liver increasing approximately 12- and 14-fold, respectively. In contrast, the addition of MP or Dex to the perfusate prior to hypoxia or endotoxin significantly retarded the accumulation of LDH activity in the perfusate, having perfusate levels at 150 min comparable to the control groups.

Table II lists the effects of glucocorticoids on the circulating cathepsin D activity following either hypoxia or administra-

TABLE I

Effect of Glucocorticoids on Perfusate Lactate Dehydrogenase Activity[a] Following 150 Min of Either Hypoxia or Endotoxin

Drug[b]	N	Treatment		
		Control	Hypoxia	Endotoxin
Vehicle	8	11 $\pm$ 32	120 $\pm$ 7.5[c]	43 $\pm$ 3.5[c]
Methylprednisolone	8	12 $\pm$ 4.1	23 $\pm$ 4.5	14 $\pm$ 3.2
Dexamethasone	8	11 $\pm$ 3.2	17 $\pm$ 3.5	10 $\pm$ 2.5

[a]Activities are expressed as changes in units of absorbance of NADH per min at 25 C X 10^2

[b]Methylprednisolone (10^{-3}M) or Dexamethasone (10^{-3}M) was added to the perfusate 30 min prior to either hypoxia or endotoxin (75 μg/g liver). N = number of observations in each treatment group

[c]$p < 0.01$ compared to control

tion of endotoxin. The three control groups had only modest perfusate cathepsin D levels following 150 min of perfusion and were not statistically different from each other. In contrast, both hypoxia and endotoxin resulted in significant increases in circulating cathepsin D activities exhibiting values approximately 4-fold that of the control vehicle-treated livers. Addition of MP or Dex to the perfusate blunted the appearance of cathepsin D in the perfusion medium with the final values for both the hypoxia and endotoxin treated steroid livers comparable to the control values.

The influence of glucocorticoids on the lysosomal integrity of control, hypoxia and endotoxin treated livers is shown in Table III. The three control groups exhibited free cathepsin D activities of 25-30% and were not significantly different from each other. However, in both the hypoxia and endotoxin treated livers, there was a significant increase in free cathepsin D activity to 60-65%. Similarly, these values were not significantly different from each other. In contrast, addition of Dex or MP to the perfusate resulted in significantly lower percent free cathepsin D values in both the hypoxia and endotoxin groups. Thus, both steroids significantly prevented the increase in lysosomal fragility usually induced by either hypoxia or endotoxin.

TABLE II

Effect of Glucocorticoids on Perfusate Cathepsin D Activity[a] Following 150 Min of Either Hypoxia or Endotoxin

Drug[b]	N	Treatment		
		Control	Hypoxia	Endotoxin
Vehicle	8	1.5 ± .35	6.5 ± .5[c]	6.1 ± .45[c]
Methylprednisolone	8	1.9 ± .25	2.2 ± .35	2.2 ± .35
Dexamethasone	8	1.8 ± .30	1.9 ± .31	2.1 ± .20

[a]Activities are expressed as milliequivalents of tyrosine x 10^{-4} produced per ml of perfusate per hr at 37 C. N = number of observations in each group
[b]Methylprednisolone (10^{-3}M) or Dexamethasone (10^{-3}M) was added to the perfusate 30 min prior to either hypoxia or endotoxin (75 µg/g liver)
[c]$p < 0.01$ compared to control

The changes in phagocytic function, a measure of RES function for the nine experimental groups, are listed in Table IV. In the control groups, the carbon clearances did not change significantly over the 2.5 hr perfusion period. In addition, neither glucocorticoid had a direct effect on the half time as there was no significant difference between the vehicle and steroid treated control groups. In the vehicle groups, both hypoxia and endotoxin treatments resulted in significant increases in half-time. Glucocorticoids prevented the hypoxia-induced RES depression, however, neither steroid had any influence on the endotoxin-induced impairment of RES clearance.

DISCUSSION

Glucocorticoids are useful agents for the treatment of a variety of types of circulatory shock (10, 11, 21). However, the mechanisms and sites of action of steroids have been difficult to establish because of the many complicating and interrelating factors of the circulatory shock state. Hepatic cellular integrity and RES phagocytic function are compromised in the perfused liver during hypoxia and endotoxin comparable to changes encountered in

TABLE III

Influence of Glucocorticoids on Percent Free Cathepsin D Activity Following 150 Min of Either Hypoxia or Endotoxin[a]

Drug	N	Treatment		
		Control	Hypoxia	Endotoxin
Vehicle	8	25 ± 4.2	60 ± 4.2[b]	65 ± 3.7[b]
Methylprednisolone	8	27 ± 3.1	33 ± 4.1	35 ± 3.2
Dexamethasone	8	29 ± 3.2	29 ± 2.1	34 ± 3.2

[a]Results are expressed as percent free cathepsin D activity of total cathepsin D activity. N = number of observations. Methylprednisolone (10^{-3}M) or Dexamethasone (10^{-3}M) was added to the perfusate 30 min prior to either hypoxia or endotoxin (75 µg/g liver)

[b]$p < 0.001$ compared to control

hemorrhagic, endotoxic, and other forms of shock (4, 13, 16). Our data indicate that the synthetic glucocorticoids, methylprednisolone and dexamethasone, in doses comparable to those employed in the treatment of myocardial ischemia and circulatory shock, can prevent much of the hepatic damage which occurs following either hypoxia or endotoxin administration. The preservation of hepatic cell integrity following hypoxia and endotoxin *in vitro* may represent an important pathway through which glucocorticoids exert beneficial actions in circulatory shock states.

A 10-fold increase in LDH activity over the appropriate control level was observed in the hypoxic and endotoxic treated vehicle livers. Similar increases in this cytoplasmic enzyme have been demonstrated during severe ischemia *in vivo* (6, 23) and following endotoxin administration (21, 22). The data suggest that both endotoxin and hypoxia adversely affect cell membrane integrity. Addition of either MP or Dex to the perfusion medium dramatically retarded the release of the cytoplasmic enzyme, LDH, induced by either endotoxin or hypoxia, suggesting a membrane stabilization by these steroids.

As an index of the increase in lysosomal fragility, perfusate and percent free cathepsin D activity were determined. Hypoxic

TABLE IV

Effect of Glucocorticoids on the Percent Change in Carbon Clearance[a] Following 150 Min of Either Hypoxia or Endotoxin

Drug[b]	N	Treatment		
		Control	Hypoxia	Endotoxin
Vehicle	8	5 ± 4	90 ± 10[c]	55 ± 4[c]
Methylprednisolone	8	8 ± 5	10 ± 7	65 ± 6
Dexamethasone	8	7 ± 4	12 ± 6	62 ± 5

[a]Values are the percent increase in half-time for the clearance of colloidal carbon from 0 to 150 min
[b]Methylprednisolone (10^{-3}M) was added to the perfusate 30 min prior to either hypoxia or endotoxin (75 μg/g liver). N = number of observations in each treatment group
[c]$p < 0.01$ compared to control

and endotoxin treated livers with only the steroid vehicle added to the perfusate, experienced a large increase in the circulating and percent free cathepsin D following 150 min of perfusion. Similar increases in lysosomal enzyme release have also been shown during experimentally induced ischemia (5). Addition of the glucocorticoids, MP or Dex, to the perfusate in the hypoxic or endotoxin treated livers prevented the increase in perfusate and in the percent free cathepsin D activity. These actions of the steroids are consistent with the hypothesis that glucocorticoids exert all or part of their therapeutic action via a lysosomal membrane stabilization (12, 13, 17).

The results on the clearance of colloidal carbon provide further insight into both the mechanism of RES depression induced by hypoxia and endotoxin and on the mechanism of glucocorticoid preservation of hepatic tissue. Both hypoxia and endotoxin caused a severe RE blockade in the liver with an approximate doubling of the carbon clearance half-times. However, addition of glucocorticoid reversed the RE blockade of the hypoxic groups but had no influence on the endotoxin induced impairment of phagocytosis. A similar preservation of RE function in hypoxia has been reported for methylprednisolone (5). These results suggest that the nature of the RE impairment in hypoxia and endotoxemia is due to differing mechanisms. In the hypoxic livers, the depression of RE function may be due to the disruption of cellular and lysosomal membranes induced by release of lysosomal hydrolases, leading to an impairment of cellular phagocytic capacity. In contrast, endotoxin may have both a direct cytotoxic action and perhaps after being phagocytized by RE cells, may produce additional impairment of phagocytosis. The steroids, though not influencing the RE clearance of endotoxin, which may induce the RE blockade, may prevent the lysosomal disruption following administration of endotoxin. The inhibition of phagocytosis by endotoxin in both vehicle and steroid treated livers suggests the possibility of this mechanism.

REFERENCES

1. Altura, B. M. and Hershey, S. C. In: Intermedes Proceedings: Combined injuries and shock (Eds. B. Schildt and L. Thoren) Forsvarets Forskingsanstalt, Stockholm (1965) 205.
2. Anson, M. L. J. Gen. Physiol. 20 (1936) 565.
3. Blattberg, B. and Levy, M. N. Amer. J. Physiol. 204 (1963) 899.
4. Carlson, R. P. and Lefer, A. M. Am. J. Physiol. 231 (1976) 1408.
5. Carlson, R. P. and Lefer, A. M. Inflammation 1 (1976) 347.
6. Farkouh, E. F., Daniel, A. M., Beaudoin, J. G. and MacLean, L. D. Surg. Gynecol. Obstet. 132 (1971) 832.
7. Gabrieli, E. R. In: Intermedes Proceedings: Combined injuries and shock. (Eds. B. Schildt and L. Thoren) Forsvarets Forskingsanstalt, Stockholm (1968) 165.
8. Galvin, M. J. and Lefer, A. M. Life Sci. 20 (1977) 1969.
9. Glenn, T. M. and Lefer, A. M. Circ. Res. 27 (1970) 783.
10. Glenn, T. M. and Lefer, A. M. Circ. Res. 29 (1971) 338.
11. Kaplan, J. E. and Saba, T. M. Am. J. Physiol. 230 (1976) 7.
12. Lefer, A. M. and Spath, J. A., Jr. Cardiovasc. Pharmacol. (Ed. M. Antonaccio) Raven Press, New York (1977) 377.
13. Loegering, D. J. Am. J. Physiol. 232 (1977) H283.
14. Pardy, B. J., Spencer, R. C. and Dudley, H. A. F. Surgery 81 (1977) 193.
15. Reichard, S. M. Radiology 89 (1967) 227.
16. Saba, T. M. Circ. Shock 2 (1975) 91.
17. Schildt, B. E. Ann. Chir. Gynecol. Fenn. 60 (1971) 165.
18. Schildt, B. E. and Bouveng, R. Life Sci. 10 (1971) 397.
19. Scovill, W. A., Saba, T. M., Kaplan, J. E., Bernard, H. and Powers, S. J. Trauma 16 (1976) 898.
20. Shanbour, L. L. In: Advances in experimental medicine and biology. (Eds. L. B. Hinshaw and D. G. Cox) Plenum Press, New York 23 (1972) 437.
21. Trejo, R. A., Crafton, C. G. and DiLuzio, N. R. J. Reticuloendo. Soc. 9 (1971) 299.

22. Vessel, E. S., Palmerio, C. F. P. and Frank, E. D. Proc. Soc. Exp. Biol. Med. 104 (1960) 403.
23. White, R. R., Mela, L., Bacalzo, L. V., Jr., Olofsson, K. and Miller, L. D. Surgery 73 (1973) 525.
24. Wroblewski, F. and LaDue, J. S. Proc. Soc. Exp. Biol. Med. 90 (1955) 210.

EVIDENCE THAT PHAGOCYTOSING CHICKEN POLYMORPHONUCLEAR LEUKOCYTES GENERATE HYDROGEN PEROXIDE AND SUPEROXIDE ANION

P. DRI, P. BELLAVITE, R. CRAMER, B. BISIACCHI, F. CIAN and P. PATRIARCA

Instituto di Patologia Generale
Trieste (Italy)

Polymorphonuclear leukocytes (PMN) are known to produce hydrogen peroxide during the respiratory stimulation associated with the ingestion of particles (9,10,19,24). The oxygen taken up by the cell is univalently reduced to superoxide anion (O_2^-) which, in turn, dismutates with formation of hydrogen peroxide. The fate of hydrogen peroxide in these cells is dual, a) it may be destroyed within the cell by enzymes such as myeloperoxidase, catalase or glutathione peroxidase, and/or b) it may leak out of the cell, the amount of peroxide released depending at least on the rate of formation and the efficiency of the intracellular H_2O_2 destroying systems.

It has been reported that production of H_2O_2 concomitant with the increment of respiration occurring during phagocytosis is not demonstrable in chicken PMN (16). On this basis it has been suggested that these cells also fail to produce or release O_2^- (16). This would set chicken PMN apart from all other types of phagocytes as far as the mechanism of metabolic activation during phagocytosis is concerned.

In the present paper the oxidative metabolism of chicken PMN leukocytes has been reinvestigated as compared to guinea pig PMN, thus representing a classical model for the study of the metabolic concomitants of phagocytosis. We conclude that the oxidative metabolism of PMN from both species is qualitatively similar including O_2^- and H_2O_2 generation.

MATERIALS AND METHODS

Cell preparation. Male adult chickens (Ubard strain) were injected intraperitoneally with 70 ml of 1% sterile sodium caseinate solution. The exudate was collected 5 hr later. The exudates contaminated with red cells were discarded. The cells were collected by centrifugation at 150 g for 7 min and were then resuspended in calcium-free Krebs-Ringer-Phosphate buffer (KRP) pH 7.4. The average differential count of the preparations used was: neutrophils 80-85%, mononuclear cells 11-20%, eosinophils 0-4%.

Guinea pig leukocytes were obtained as previously described (13).

Bacteria. *Bacillus mycoides* was used throughout the experiments. The bacteria were grown on nutrient agar, autoclaved and opsonized for 20 min at 37 C with fresh homologous serum.

Oxygen uptake. The rate of oxygen uptake by resting and phagocytosing leukocytes was measured at 37 C with a Clark oxygen electrode attached to a plastic chamber, as previously described (24).

Hydrogen peroxide production. The formation of H_2O_2 was assayed with three different methods, a) polarographic, b) colorimetric and c) fluorimetric.

In the polarographic assay (24) the oxygen consumption by phagocytosing cells was recorded for 3-4 min in the presence or absence of 1 mM cyanide. Excess catalase (from beef liver, Boehringer, Mannheim, GmbH, Germany) was then added into the electrode chamber, and a backward deflection of the recording trace was observed indicating that oxygen was released in the medium from H_2O_2.

The colorimetric method was that described by Thurman *et al.* (23). After recording the oxygen uptake of phagocytosing PMN leukocytes with a Clark oxygen electrode for various time intervals, 1 ml of the mixture was rapidly drawn from the electrode chamber and trichloroacetic acid was added to it at a final concentration of 10% (w/v). After centrifugation, the clear supernatant was used for assays.

Two different procedures were employed for the fluorimetric assay of H_2O_2. In one of these, the decay of scopoletin fluorescence following its oxidation by horseradish peroxidase in the presence of H_2O_2 was measured. The basic principle of this technique has been described by Root *et al.*(19). Briefly, while oxygen uptake by phagocytosing cells was being recorded with a Clark oxygen electrode, aliquots of the mixture were drawn at various time intervals from the electrode chamber and were immediately centrifuged in a 3,200 Eppendorf microcentrifuge. The clear supernatant was used for assays. The spectrophotofluorimeter cuvette contained 3 ml of KRP, 2.5 µM scopoletin (Sigma Chemical Co., St. Louis, Mo., USA) and 0.166 µM horseradish peroxidase (Sigma Chemical Co.). The volume of the samples that were added to the cuvette varied from 10 to 100 µl. The second procedure was based on the conversion of the nonfluorescent compound homovanillic acid to the highly fluorescent 2,2'-dihydroxy-3,3'-dimethoxybiphenyl-5,5'-diacetic acid by horseradish peroxidase in the presence of H_2O_2 (7,8). Concentrations of H_2O_2 as low as 0.03 µM could be determined by this method. This high sensitivity made it possible to perform kinetic measurements of H_2O_2 production by phagocytosing cells as follows. The spectrophotofluorimetric cuvette was filled with 2.5 ml of KRP containing 5 mM glucose, 0.5 mM $CaCl_2$, 20 µM homovanillic acid (Fluka AG, Buchs, Switzerland), 20 µg of horseradish peroxidase and 2 x 10^6 cells. The recorder was turned on. Usually resting cells did not cause any appreciable increase in fluorescence. After a baseline was established for resting cells, phagocytosis was started by adding 2.0 x 10^8 heat killed _B. mycoides_. The cuvette content was continuously stirred throughout the experiments.

Superoxide anion production. The assay was based on the superoxide dismutase inhibitable reduction of cytochrome c (1). The assay medium was the same as for oxygen uptake measurements plus 200 µM cytochrome c (from horse heart, grade VI, Sigma Chemical Co.) and, when required, 35 µg/ml of superoxide dismutase. The experimental details have been described elsewhere (6).

Cell homogenization and preparation of the granules. The leukocytes were incubated with or without bacteria in KRP containing 0.5 mM glucose for 5 min at 37 C. After dilution with ice-cold KRP, the leukocytes were sedimented at 150 g for 10 min so that most of the bacteria remained in the supernatant. The packed cells were suspended in ice-cold 0.34 M sucrose (buffered at pH 7.0 with Na-bicarbonate) to a concentration of 3-4 x 10^8 leukocytes/ml and homogenization was performed in a Potter type homogenizer equipped with a teflon pestle driven by a motor. The homogenization was stopped when 90% of the cells were broken as judged by light microscopy examination. Usually this process did not take more than 3-4 min. The homogenate was diluted with 0.34 M sucrose and centrifuged at 250 g for 7 min to remove nuclei, cell debris and unbroken cells. The supernatant fraction was centrifuged at 20,000 g for 20 min and sedimented granules were suspended in 0.34 M sucrose.

Determination of NADPH oxidase activity. The rate of NADPH oxidation was measured by determining the rate of O_2 consumption with a Clark type oxygen electrode as previously described (15,

13). Enzymatically reduced NADPH was purchased from Boehringer (Mannheim, GmbH, Germany).

RESULTS

Oxygen uptake, O_2^- and H_2O_2 Generation. The results of simultaneous determinations are shown in Table I. Chicken leukocytes respond to phagocytosis with an increased oxygen consumption as the PMN of all the other species so far tested do. The respiratory increment in chicken leukocytes was considerably lower than that observed in guinea pig cells. The oxygen uptake by phagocytosing chicken leukocytes was not significantly affected by azide, whereas guinea pig leukocytes showed a higher oxygen consumption in the presence of this inhibitor than in its absence.

Appreciable amounts of H_2O_2 could be measured in the incubation medium of phagocytosing chicken leukocytes, with or without azide, both by the scopoletin and thiocyanate method. The amount of H_2O_2 measured with phagocytosing chicken cells accounted for 37% of the oxygen consumed in the presence of azide. With phagocytosing guinea pig cells the amount of H_2O_2 that accumulated in the medium in the absence of azide was comparable to that observed with chicken cells under the same experimental conditions. However, if the guinea pig cells were let to phagocytose in the presence of azide the amount of H_2O_2 was several times higher than in absence of the medium of phagocytosing chicken leukocytes. The H_2O_2 measured with phagocytosing guinea pig cells accounted for about 99% of the oxygen taken up in the presence of azide.

A small but definite amount of superoxide anion was measured in the incubation medium of chicken phagocytosing leukocytes. The amount of superoxide anion released by phagocytosing chicken leukocytes was considerably lower than that released by phagocytosing guinea pig leukocytes.

Generation of hydrogen peroxide by phagocytosing chicken polymorphs could be detected also by polarographic techniques, as demonstrated by Fig. 1. This figure shows the recording traces of oxygen consumption by the cells and of oxygen liberation from H_2O_2 after addition of catalase. The backward deflection of the recording trace is therefore an index of H_2O_2 accumulation. Hydrogen peroxide could be detected in the medium of phagocytosing chicken leukocytes both in the presence and in the absence of cyanide, whereas no H_2O_2 was detectable with guinea pig cells in absence of the inhibitor.

Fig. 2 shows the generation of H_2O_2 by phagocytosing chicken PMN as determined by the homovanillic acid method. In this experiment the production of peroxide was followed kinetically

TABLE I

Oxygen Uptake and Generation of O_2^- and H_2O_2 by Chicken and Guinea Pig Polymorphonuclear Leukocytes During Phagocytosis[a]

	Chicken PMN		Guinea Pig PMN	
	---	+ NaN_3	---	+ NaN_3
O_2	19.8 ± 1.4(4)	14.3 ± 1.3(6)	73.2 ± 3.7(5)	103.3 ± 5.1(5)
O_2^-	9.0 ± 0.7(6)	not tested	71.7 ± 7.8(5)	not tested
H_2O_2	3.33 (2)[a] 3.12 (1)[b] 3.26± 0.2(3)[c]	5.03 ± 0.5(4)[a] 5.87 (2)[b] 5.31 ± 0.3(6)[c]	2.8 (2)	102.6 ± 2.3(5)

[a]The basic assay medium contained 2 ml KRP pH 7.4, 0.5 mM glucose and 0.5 mM $CaCl_2$. For O_2^- assay, 200 μM ferricytochrome c and, when required, 35 μg/ml of superoxide dismutase was added. Opsonized *B. mycoides* was the phagocytosable particle (ratio cell/bacteria, 1/100). Temperature 37 C NaN_3, 2 mM.

The results, given as differences between phagocytosing and resting cells, are expressed as nmoles/2min/2 x 10^7 cells ± S.E.M. Number of experiments in parentheses.

a, fluorimetric method. b, colorimetric method. c, mean of a and b.

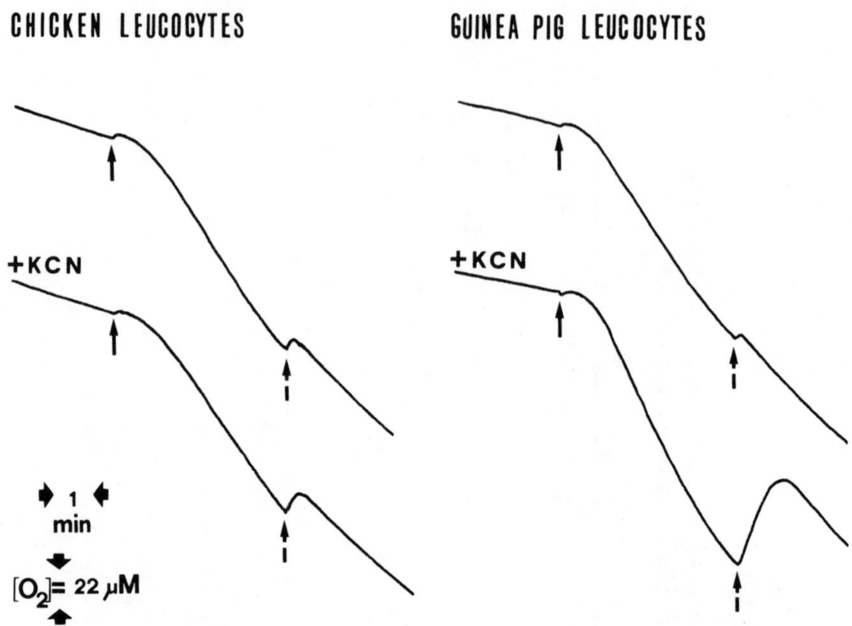

Fig. 1. Polarographic assay of oxygen uptake and H_2O_2 generation by chicken and guinea pig PMN. The basic assay medium was KRP pH 7.4 containing 0.5 mM glucose and 0.5 mM $CaCl_2$. Volume 2 ml. Temperature 37 C KCN, 1 mM. 9.5 x 10^7 chicken cells and 2.5 x 10^7 guinea pig cells were used in each assay. Opsonized _B. mycoides_ was added at the solid arrows (ratio cell/bacteria, 1/100). Excess catalase was added at the broken arrows.

during phagocytosis. The initial part of the recording traces is flat indicating that no appreciable amount of H_2O_2 was produced. This initial part of the recording trace was given by cells at rest. Phagocytosis was started by adding bacteria at the arrows. After a lag time of about 90 sec the recording traces begin to go upwards, in dictating that the non-fluorescent compound 2,2'-dihydroxy-3,3'-dimethoxybiphenyl-5,5'-diacetic acid. The appearance of fluorescence is specifically due to H_2O_2 as indicated by the addition of catalase which prevents further increase in fluorescence. Omission of either horseradish peroxidase or homovanillic acid prevented any appearance of fluorescence. The addition

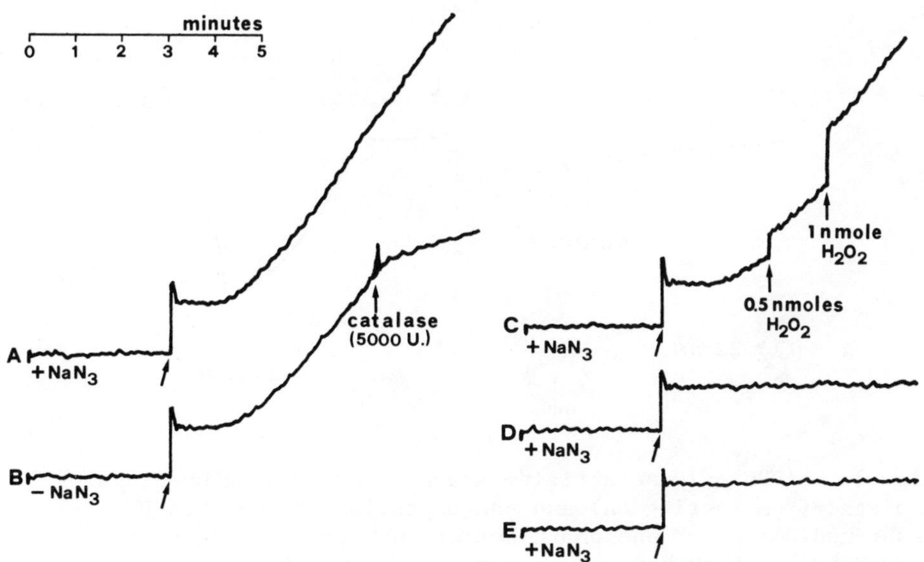

Fig. 2. Spectrophotofluorometric assay of H_2O_2 production by chicken PMN during phagocytosis. The basic assay medium was as follows: 2.5 ml KRP pH 7.4, 5 mM glucose, 0.5 mM $CaCl_2$, 20 μM homovanillic acid, 20 μg horseradish peroxidase, 2.0 x 10^6 cells and 2 mM NaN_3 where indicated. Opsonized B. mycoides was added at the arrows (ratio cell/bacteria, 1/100). In D and E homovanillic acid and horseradish peroxidase, respectively, were omitted from the assay medium.

of external standards of H_2O_2 during the recording of phagocytosis associated H_2O_2 production (curve C) shows that the fluorescence signal is a linear function of the amount of H_2O_2 added. Finally, it must be noted that the amount of H_2O_2 produced by phagocytosing chicken leukocytes is indentical in the presence and absence of sodium azide. In other animal species such as guinea pig, the amount of H_2O_2 measured in the presence of azide is much higher than in its absence. This difference is very likely due to the absence of the two H_2O_2-degrading enzymes catalase and myeloperoxidase from chicken polymorphs.

Oxidation of NADPH by chicken PMN granules. Fig. 3 shows that chicken leukocyte granules can oxidize NADPH and that this oxidation is higher in granules isolated from phagocytosing cells than from resting cells. The oxidation of NADPH was coupled with H_2O_2 production, the peroxide generated being stoichiometric to the oxygen consumed.

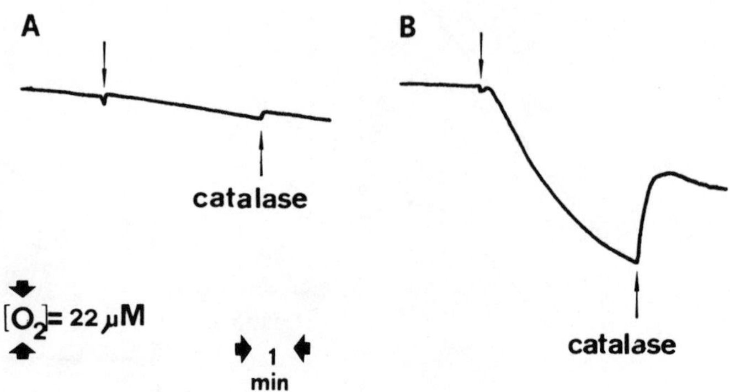

Fig. 3. NADPH oxidase activity and H_2O_2 production by granules isolated from resting (A) and phagocytosing (B) chicken PMN. Assay medium: 65 mM phosphate buffer, pH 5.5, 170 mM sucrose, 1 mM NADPH, 0.5 mM $MnCl_2$. Temperature 37 C. Granules isolated from 4 x 10^7 leukocytes were added at the arrows.

DISCUSSION

This paper shows that the metabolic burst of phagocytosing chicken leukocytes shares several features with that of phagocytosing guinea pig leukocytes. These include an increased oxygen consumption, an increased generation of superoxide anion and hydrogen peroxide and an activation of the NADPH oxidase of the granules which is coupled with an increased hydrogen peroxide production.

Some differences have been also observed between the two types of cell. A major one is that all the biochemical activities that have been recorded, are definitely lower in chicken cells than in guinea pig cells.

An increased respiration and hexose monophosphate shunt activity in phagocytosing chicken leukocytes has been already reported by Pennial and Spitznagel (16). These authors, however, failed to demonstrate generation of H_2O_2, and concluded that the inability of chicken leukocytes to produce H_2O_2 "sets these cells apart from the PMN of all other species". The original contribution of the present paper is that we were able to demonstrate generation and extracellular release of both superoxide anion and hydrogen peroxide in phagocytosing chicken leukocytes. Four different techniques were used to measure H_2O_2 production, including the sensitive scopoletin and homovanillic acid methods. The failure of Pennial and Spitznagel to demonstrate H_2O_2 using the technique of formate oxidation may be explained by the absence of catalase in chicken PMN (3,4). This technique, in fact, relies on the peroxidatic activity of catalase which converts formate into CO_2 concomitantly with the phagocytic production of H_2O_2 (2,10). Formate oxidation has been reported to be stimulated by addition of exogenous catalase at least in phagocytosing human leukocytes (11,12). Pennial and Spitznagel could not demonstrate formate oxidation by phagocytosing chicken leukocytes, even in the presence of exogenous catalase. This result cannot be obviously accounted for by catalase deficiency in chicken cells. Since the formate oxidation technique reveals only a small fraction of the peroxide produced (9,12), it might be that the failure of Pennial and Spitznagel to show formate oxidation by phagocytosing chicken leukocytes in the presence of exogenous catalase is attributable to the low sensitivity of the method employed. The authors failed to show H_2O_2 production even with the scopoletin method which, instead, we have employed with positive results. In our experiments a modification of the method as originally described by Root and Chance (19) has been used. In the original method the oxidation of scopoletin in the presence of horseradish peroxidase is measured concomitantly with phagocytosis. Operatively, the cuvette of the spectrophotofluorimeter is filled with both the reagents for the scopoletin reaction and leukocytes, and then the reaction is started by addition of the phagocytic particles. The rate of decay of scopoletin fluorescence is recorded and the linear part of the recording trace is used for calculation of the initial rate of H_2O_2 production. The number of human cells used for each assay in the method described by Root *et al.* (19) is 2.5×10^6/ml. In preliminary experiments we have shown that this cell concentration was too low for an evaluation of H_2O_2 produced by chicken leukocytes. On the basis of this fact a concentration of 5×10^7 leukocytes/ml was used and the cells were let to phagocytose for variable periods of time. The medium was then quickly separated from the cells and aliquots of variable size were used for the scopoletin assay of H_2O_2. This procedure offers two advantages, a) a large number of cells can be used, and b) the peroxide accumulated for the desired period of time can be measured. With this technique, accumulation of H_2O_2 in the medium of phagocytosing chicken leukocytes was detected both in the presence and in the absence of azide. With phagocytosing guinea pig leukocytes, only a small amount of H_2O_2 accumulated in the medium without the inhibitor, but it was about 40 times higher when the inhibitor was present. This difference might be explained by the presence in guinea pig leukocytes of two hydrogen peroxide destroying enzymes such as catalase and myeloperoxidase, which are both sensitive to azide, and by the lack of these enzymes from chicken leukocytes (3-5,17). In fact, we have recently shown that in phagocytosing guinea pig cells, about 90% of the H_2O_2 produced is degraded by catalase and myeloperoxidase (6).

A further demonstration that chicken leukocytes do produce hydrogen peroxide during phagocytosis was obtained by using the fluorimetric assay which employs homovanillic acid. With this technique the formation of a fluorescent compound is measured, at variance with the scopoletin method which measures the decrease of fluorescence. Furthermore, the fluorescent compound which is formed upon peroxidation of the homovanillic acid has a high fluorescence intensity which makes the method very sensitive. In fact, we could follow by this method the kinetics of H_2O_2 generation concomitant to phagocytosis with as low as 10^6 chicken cells/ml.

The enzymatic basis of the stimulated respiration in phagocytosing leukocytes, either polymorphs or macrophages, is still a debated issue (14,20,21). We have proposed in previous papers that the activation during phagocytosis of a NADPH oxidizing activity, which is bound to granules and is relatively insensitive to inhibition by cyanide, accounts for the increased respiration and H_2O_2 generation in either type of phagocyte (15,18,20-22). This paper shows that chicken leukocytes were able to oxidize NADPH. The 20,000 g fraction isolated from the homogenate of phagocytosing chicken cells had a higher NADPH oxidizing activity than the corresponding fraction isolated from resting cells. The final product of the granule catalized oxidation of NADPH was found to be hydrogen peroxide.

In conclusion, although the oxidative metabolism of chicken leukocytes is less active than that of guinea pig leukocytes, it seems to follow a pattern of oxidative response to phagocytosis similar to that of leukocytes from other species.

ACKNOWLEDGEMENTS

P. Bellavite is recipient of a fellowship from "Fondazione Anna Villa Rusconi", Varese, Italy. Supported by grant No. 77. 01481.04 from the National Council of Research (CNR) of Italy.

REFERENCES

1. Babior, B. M., Kipnes, R. S. and Curnutte, J. T., J. Clin. Invest. 52 (1973) 741.
2. Baehner, R. L., Gilman, N. and Karnovsky, M. L., J. Clin.

Invest. 49 (1970) 692.
3. Bellavite, P., Dri, P., Bisiacchi, B. and Patriarca, P., FEBS Letters 81 (1977) 73.
4. Breton-Gorius, J., Coquin, Y. and Guichard, J., Lab. Invest. 38 (1978) 21.
5. Brune, K. and Spitznagel, J. K., J. Infect. Dis. 127 (1973) 84.
6. Dri, P., Bellavite, P., Berton, G. and Rossi, F., Molec. and Cell. Biochem. (1978) in press.
7. Guilbaut, G. G., Brignac, P., Jr. and Zimmer, M., Anal. Chem. 40 (1968) 190.
8. Guilbaut, G. G., Kramer, D. N. and Hackley, E., Anal. Biochem. 39 (1967) 271.
9. Homan-Müller, J. W. T., Weening, R. S. and Roos, D., J. Lab. Clin. Med. 85 (1975) 198.
10. Iyer, G. Y. N., Islam, M. F. and Quastel, H. J., Nature (London) 192 (1961) 535.
11. Klebanoff, S. J. and Hamon, C. S., J. Reticuloendothel. Soc. 12 (1972) 170.
12. Klebanoff, S. J. and Pincus, S. H., J. Clin. Invest, 50 (1971) 2226.
13. Patriarca, P., Dri, P., Kakinuma, K. and Rossi, F., Molec. and Cell. Biochem., 12 (1976) 137.
14. Patriarca, P., Cramer, R. and Dri, P., In: Movement, Metabolism and Bactericidal Mechanisms of Phagocytes (Eds. F. Rossi, P. Patriarca and D. Romeo), Piccin Medical Books, Padova (1977) 167.
15. Patriarca, P., Cramer, R., Moncalvo, S., Rossi, F. and Romeo, D., Arch. Biochem. Biophys., 145 (1971) 255.
16. Pennial, R. and Spitznagel, J. K., Proc. Nat. Acad. Sci. USA, 72 (1975) 5012.
17. Rausch, P. G. and Moore, T. G., Blood 46 (1975) 913.
18. Romeo, D., Zabucchi, G., Soranzo, M. R. and Rossi, F., Biochem. Biophys. Res. Commun. 45 (1971) 1056.
19. Root, R. K., Metcalf, J., Oshino, N. and Chance, B., J. Clin Invest., 55 (1975) 945.
20. Rossi, F., Patriarca, P. and Romeo, D., In: The Reticuloendothelial System and Immune Phenomena (Ed. N. R. Di Luzio) Plenum Press, New York and London, (1971) 191.
21. Rossi, F., Romeo, D. and Patriarca, P., J. Reticuloendothel. Soc. 12 (1972) 127.
22. Rossi, F., Zatti, M. and Patriarca, P., Biochim. Biophys. Acta 184 (1969) 201.
23. Thurman, R. G., Ley, H. G. and Scholz, R., Eur. J. Biochem. 25 (1972) 420.
24. Zatti, M. and Rossi, F., Experientia 24 (1968) 669.

THE ROLE OF LEUKOCYTE EXTRACTS AND MYELOPEROXIDASE IN THE LYSIS OF STAPHYLOCOCCI AND THE INHIBITION OF BACTERIOLYSIS BY ANIONIC POLYELECTROLYTES AND BY INFLAMMATORY EXUDATES

I. GINSBURG, N. NEEMAN., M. LAHAV AND N. SELA

Department of Oral Biology, Hadassah School of Dental Medicine of Hebrew University (Founded by the Alpha Omega Fraternity) Jerusalem (Israel)

Although much is known today about the mechanisms by which leukocytes and their intracellular enzymes kill bacteria very little is known about the biochemical pathways of degradation of the ingested microbiota. It is accepted that soon after the uptake of bacteria by neutrophils (PMNs) and macrophages fusion of lysosomes with the phagosome occurs. This is followed by the intravacuolar discharge of lysosomal agents which lead to the killing and degradation of the intracellular bacteria (2).

Extensive studies in our laboratory have shown that extracts of human blood leukocytes, of purified PMNs and of macrophages contain factors which are capable of lysing *Staphylococcus aureus* and *Streptococcus faecalis* (4,5,7,8). Although the nature of these factors has not been fully defined they comprise a group of cationic substances which are capable of affecting the viability and integrity of the bacterial wall components leading to the rupture of the protoplast. It has also been shown that lysis of staphylococci by the leukocyte agents depends on the age of the culture (7). While young cells were lysed to a large extent older cells were highly resistant to degradation. These studies were also substantiated by in *in vivo* models where it was shown that while young staphylococci disappeared from the knee joints of rats at a fast rate, presumably due to bacteriolysis, older cells persisted for longer periods of time (5). More recent studies (7) have indicated that the leukocyte extracts cause lysis of the staphylococci indirectly by activating autolytic systems within the staphylococcal cells. This effect can also be obtained by a series of cationic proteins, by cationic antibiotics as well as by phospholipase A_2. Bacteriolysis is strongly inhibited by a variety of anionic polyelectrolytes, by certain dyes (trypan blue, congo red), by suramine, by phospholipids and by lipoteichoic acid (5,7). Studies from our laboratory have shown that staphylococci can be lysed by diluted serum and synovial fluid but are inhibited by concentrated serum or by Cohn's Fraction II (immunoglobulins). The serum lysis was not related to the complement system and was strongly inhibited by anionic polyelectrolytes.

The present communication shows that myeloperoxidase (MPO) of PMN's, which is a cationic protein, is highly lytic for S. aureus. This reaction takes place in the presence of KCN and NaN_3, which inhibit the MPO-halide-H_2O_2 bactericidal system of PMN's. It will also be shown that inflammatory exudates derived from pyogenic lesions strongly inhibit bacteriolysis induced by leukocyte extracts. The role played by inhibitory substances in the control of bacterial degradation in inflammatory sites will be discussed.

MATERIALS AND METHODS

A coagulase-positive strain of S.aureus was isolated from a pyogenic lesion of a patient. The bacteria were cultivated in brain heart infusion broth (Difco) which contained 0.1 μCi/ml of uniformly labeled ^{14}C-D-glucose specific activity 150-250 mCi/m mol (New England Nuclear, Boston, Mass, USA). The bacterial cells were harvested either from the logarithmic or stationary phases of growth and washed several times in saline. The bacterial cells were then resuspended in 0.1M acetate buffer pH 5.0 as described in detail elsewhere (7). Radiolabeled bacteria ($4x10^4$cpm/100 Klett Units/ml) were incubated for 12-18 hr at 37 C with: a) freeze and thaw extract of human blood leukocytes (7), b) a purified preparation of myeloperoxidase (MPO) kindly supplied by Dr. I. Olsson from the Department of Internal Medicine, University of Lund, Sweden, c) freeze and thaw extract derived from pyogenic exudates of patients with gingival granulomas and d) normal human serum. Following incubation, the tubes were centrifuged at 2000 g for 15 min and 50 μl aliquots of the supernatant fluids were assayed for soluble radioactivity as previously described (7). The results were expressed as percentage release of radioactivity from a standard bacterial suspension calculated after subtracting the radioactivity values released in buffer solutions alone.

RESULTS

Table I compares the lytic patterns of young and old staphylococci which had been subjected to leukocyte extracts and to MPO.

TABLE I

The Lysis of Young and Old Staphylococci by Leukocyte Extracts and by Myeloperoxidase

Test Preparation		% Release of Radioactivity from Staphylococci young	old
^{14}C-Staphylococci[a] +			
Acetate buffer		20	20
Leukocyte extract (ENZ)	10 μg	40	20
"	20 μg	75	30
"	50 μg	90	35
"	200 μg	95	45
"	200 μg + Heparine 100 μg	20	15
	" 100 μg	20	15
Myeolperoxidase	10 μg	27	20
	20 μg	50	30
	50 μg	60	30
	100 μg	70	35
	200 μg	86	40
	200 μg + Heparine 100 μg	20	20

[a] ^{14}C-labeled staphylococci were harvested either from the logarithmic or stationary phases of growth, were incubated for 15 hr at 37 C in 0.1M acetate buffer pH 5.0 with the various agents and the percentage of solubilization of radioactivity (measure of cell lysis) was determined on aliquots taken from the supernatant fluids.

TABLE II

The Lysis of Staphylococci by Leukocyte Extracts and by Purulent exudate

Test Preparation	Concentration mg protein/ml	Solubilization of radioactivity &	% Inhibitor
^{14}C-Staphylococci[a] +			
Acetate buffer		20	-
Leukocyte extract (ENZ)	0.02	75	-
"	0.1	90	-
"	0.5	95	0[b]
"	1.0	80	14
"	2.0	65	40
"	5.0	25	93
Purulent exudate (PUS)	0.05	60	-
"	0.1	80	0
"	0.5	76	7
	1.0	55	42
	2.0	38	70
	5.0	20	100
Leukocyte extracts	0.5 mg + Pus 2.0 mg	25	93
"	0.5 mg + Pus 5.0 mg	20	100
"	0.5 mg + DNA 1.0 mg	25	93
"	0.5 mg + Chondroitin sulfate 1.0 mg	30	87

[a]Radiolabeled staphylococci were incubated for 15 hr at 37 C with the various agents and the solubilized radioactivity was determined in the supernatant fluids.

[b]The percent inhibition of the solubilization of radioactivity was calculated on the basis of the maximal net release of radioactivity obtained by 0.5 mg of ENZ and 0.1 mg of pus following subtraction of the radioactivity values released by the buffer.

As shown, young cells were readily lysed by both agents and the specific activity of the leukocyte extracts was higher than that of MPO. It is also shown that old bacteria were extremely resistant to degradation by both agents. This Table also illustrates that heparin completely inhibited bacteriolysis. Since the lysis of staphylococci by both leukocyte extracts and by MPO was unaffected by KCN(10^{-2}M) or by NaN_3(5 x 10^{-2}M), known to interfere with the generation of H_2O_2 in the bactericidal system, it is suggested that MPO does not function as an enzyme but rather as a cationic protein. This assumption is further strengthened by previous findings that a series of cationic proteins and cationic antibiotics were equally effective in the activation of the autolytic systems in staphylococci which lead to the degradation of the bacterial cell wall components and to lysis. The finding that MPO is capable of doing so suggests that MPO may have an additional role in PMN's (7,8).

Since staphylococci induce purulent exudates rich in serum components and in degradation products of cells and tissues, it was of interest to test the effect of inflammatory exudates on the labeled staphylococci. Table II shows that the lysis of staphylococci by both leukocyte extracts and by purulent exudates assumes a bell-shaped curve. While small amounts of the agents are highly lytic, higher concentrations are practically non-lytic. It is also shown that purulent exudates strongly inhibit lysis of the bacteria by small amounts of leukocyte extracts. Both DNA and chondroitin sulfate strongly inhibit bacteriolysis induced by the leukocyte extracts. This effect, however, can be reversed to a large extent by the addition of cationic materials such as histone or protamine sulfate (not shown). When the bacteria were preincubated with large volumes of leukocyte extracts or with pus and then washed with buffer to remove excess unbound materials, the cells became completely resistant to lysis by small amounts of leukocyte extracts or by purulent exudates suggesting that a factor present in these fluids coated the bacterial cells and prevented the interaction of the bacterial surface with the lytic agents. Similar results were obtained with serum-coated bacteria (to be published). Other studies have shown that the globulin fraction of human serum contains a factor which is capable of coating staphylococci to render them resistant to degradation by leukocyte agents. This factor can be removed by adsorption with staphylococci but not with streptococci.

DISCUSSION

The data presented show that MPO isolated from PMN's can act as a bacteriolytic agent for staphylococci and that this agent may function not as an enzyme but as a cationic protein (see also

4,7,8). This may perhaps explain teleologically why PMN's synthesize so much of this cationic substance. Although the mechanism by which MPO brings about lysis of the staphylococci is not fully understood. It was postulated (7) that cationic substances may injure the cytoplasmic membrane which results in the activation of membrane-bound autolytic systems which lead to the degradation of the bacterial cell walls. Thus, activation of autolysins by leukocyte factors may constitute an indirect effect of leukocytes on bacteria. The bacteriolytic effect of MPO is strongly inhibited by heparin and by lipoteichoic acid derived both from staphylococci and streptococci (8) suggesting that a balance between anionic and cationic substances may determine the fate of bacteria in inflammatory sites. This assumption is further strengthened by the findings that both leukocyte extracts and purulent exudates, which can lyse bacteria, fail to do so in the presence of anionic polyelectrolytes. Furthermore, purulent exudates contain a factor which may interfere with the bacteriolytic effects of leukocyte extracts. It is thus postulated that bacteria suspended in inflammatory exudates may paradoxically be protected against bacteriolysis which may contribute to the survival of microbial constituents in tissues. This may lead to the development of chronic inflammatory reactions (5). Since macrophages are known to pinocytose anionic polyelectrolytes (2), and since several of the anionic polyelectrolytes have been shown to inhibit lysosomal enzymes, it is postulated that such macrophages when suspended in inflammatory exudates may lose their capacity to handle intracellular bacteria. This assumption is in accord with the findings of Hahn (3) who showed that macrophages which took up dextran sulfate were not capable of handling Listeria. Furthermore the uptake of bacteria which had been coated by immunoglobulins (1) have been shown to persist within leukocytes for prolonged periods suggesting that any substance which coats the bacterial surface (e.g. histone, leukocyte cationic proteins, antibodies, complement) may interfere with bacterial degradation (5). It is, therefore, suggested that studies on the interaction of leukocytes with bacteria be conducted not in a milieu which contains salt solutions and calf serum but in inflammatory exudates. These conditions may better mimic the natural events which take place within inflammatory sites (6).

ACKNOWLEDGEMENT

This study was supported in part by a research grant to the senior author by the Ministry of Health of the Government of Israel and by the Max Bogen Foundation (through the American Friends of the Hebrew University in the United States of America).

REFERENCES

1. Cohn, Z. A., J. Exp. Med. 117 (1963) 43.
2. Cohn, Z. A., Fed. Proceedings, 34 (1975) 1725.
3. Hahn, H., Infect. Immun., 10 (1974) 1110.
4. Ginsburg, I., Lahav, M., Neeman, N., Duchan, Z., Chanes, S. and Sela, M. N. Agents and Actions, 6 (1976) 292
5. Ginsburg, I. and Sela, M. N., Critical Reviews in Microbiology 4 (1976) 249.
6. Ginnsburg, I., Rheumatology and Rehabilitation 16 (1977) 161.
7. Lahav, M. and Ginsburg, I., Inflammation 2 (1977) 165.
8. Sela, M. N., Ofek, I., Lahav, M. and Ginsburg, I. Proc. Soc. Exp. Biol. Med. in press (1978)

BIOLOGICAL AND BIOCHEMICAL CHARACTERISTICS OF THE TETRAPEPTIDE TUFTSIN, THR-LYS-PRO-ARG

V. A. NAJJAR

Tufts University School of Medicine

Boston, Massachusetts (USA)

The naturally occurring tetrapeptide tuftsin (Thr-Lsy-Pro-Arg) was discovered on the basis of its ability to stimulate the phagocytic activity of the blood neutrophil (25, 32, 33). It is active only in the free tetrapeptide form. However, originally the molecule is covalently bonded to its parent carrier molecule leukokinin. The latter is a leukophilic γ-globulin that binds specifically to the blood neutrophil. In fact, under appropriate conditions, utilizing low ionic strength isotonic solutions, one can readily isolate blood granulocytes that possess a coat of γ-globulin all of which chromatographs in only 1 of the 4 peaks of serum γ-globulin, peak IV on phosphocellulose columns (9, 10, 49). Furthermore, even in the presence of normal physiological solutions such as Krebs-Ringer one can recover from purified neutrophils the leukokinin fraction which stimulates phagocytosis. This occurs after release of its tuftsin peptide by a specific enzyme on the outer surface of the membrane (26).

The presence of specific cytophilic bound γ-globulin is not unique to blood neutrophils. We were able to show earlier that circulating erythrocytes of man and dog are also coated with specific cytophilic γ-globulin (11, 12). More recently, it was shown by electron microscopy in Robinson's laboratory (40) that blood monocytes and lymphocytes also bind γ-globulin to the outer surface of their membranes.

THE ASSAY OF TUFTSIN

Several methods have been devised to assay tuftsin: (a) by its capacity to stimulate the engulfment of particles such as staphylococci or yeast cells (3, 14, 28), (b) through its ability to stimulate the reduction of nitroblue tetrazolium (44) - this latter is also secondary to the stimulation of phagocytosis of the dye that had been complexed with heparin or fibrin (42), (c) by a more quantitative radioimmunoassay method devised by Spirer et al. (45).

In all cases, the tetrapeptide must be set free from its carrier molecule by short treatment with trypsin or with the neutrophil membrane enzyme leukokininase, prior to assay by any of these methods (5, 26).

THE ENZYMES THAT RELEASE TUFTSIN FROM LEUKOKININ

Leukokininase. Our earlier studies indicated that upon binding of leukokinin to the outer membrane of the granulocyte, an enzyme leukokininase, present on the outer surface of the cell membrane, cleaves the tetrapeptide tuftsin at the amino end of the threonyl residue. The tetrapeptide is a part of the Fc fragment of the heavy chain (7). This single cleavage sets it free. This implied that tuftsin has a free arginine at its carboxy terminal. Indeed, if the whole leukokinin molecule is subjected to carboxypeptidase B action, the terminal residue arginine is released in quantities comparable to that of the tetrapeptide and the biological activity of leukokinin is destroyed (41). On the other hand, treatment with leucine aminopeptidase does not affect activity of leukokinin. This is clearly illustrated in Table I.

Tuftsin endocarboxypeptidase. Our earlier studies indicated that a few months after the removal of the spleen in dogs, tuftsin carrier leukokinin is still present and capable of specific binding to the blood neutrophil. However, it becomes inactive (29). Further studies on splenectomized humans confirmed the absence of any biological activity of isolated leukokinin. Nevertheless, chemical analysis of the leukokinin fraction indeed revealed the presence of the tetrapeptide (25). Unlike leukokinin from non-splenectomized human subjects, short trypsin treatment did not set free an active tetrapeptide (41). Clearly, the carboxyterminal arginine residue was still covalently linked to the next residue in the Fc portion of the heavy chain. Thus the presence of the spleen was necessary for cleavage at the arginyl residue. Consequently the splenic enzyme, tuftsin endocarboxypeptidase, would be required for such cleavage.

The neutrophil membrane enzyme leukokininase has been adequately studied and purified to a minor extent. It is highly active on its substrate leukokinin. It has a pH optimum of 6.8. The product tuftsin was identified by column chromatography and sequence analysis (32-34). The splenic enzyme is presently being studied.

TABLE I

Phagocytic Activity of Leukokinin (PC-IV) After Treatment with Carboxypeptidase-B(CP-B) or Leucine Aminopeptidase (LA-P) Phagocytosis Index[a]

Sample	CP Treated		LAP Treated	
	Cohn II	Fresh	Cohn II	Fresh
1	15	18	36	40
2	19	18	36	38
3	17	17	34	35
4	18	18	35	36
5	20	21	38	35
6	18	17	38	38
Reagent Control	18 ± 2	18 ± 2	18 ± 2	18 ± 2

[a]Six samples 1 mg each of phosphocellulose fraction IV (PC IV) containing leukokinin sufficient for maximal stimulation were prepared from fresh normal human γ-globulin (experiment I). Similarly, 6 samples were prepared from Cohn fraction II (experiment II). These were then treated with either leucine aminopeptidase in 0.05 M barbital buffer pH 8.5 containing 2.5 mM $MgCl_2$ or Carboxypeptidase B in 0.2 MN-ethylmorpholine acetate buffer pH 8.5 Each sample was then treated with leukokininase to free tuftsin at its amino terminal. The reaction mixture consisted of 4 μg of leukokininase, 1 mg of leukokinin (PC IV) in 0.25 ml of 0.1 M phosphate buffer at pH 6.8. After 30 min at 37 C, 1 ml of ethanol was added and centrifuged. The alcoholic supernatant was evaporated *in vacuo* and the residue dissolved in 0.25 ml of Krebs-Ringer medium. 50 μl was used for phagocytic assay.

THE BIOLOGICAL ACTIVITY OF TUFTSIN *IN VITRO*

The stimulation of the phagocytic activity of blood granulocytes by synthetic tuftsin has now been confirmed in several laboratories (8, 13, 16, 18, 23, 51, 52).

Granulocytes from various sources have been used successfully: human, dog, rabbit (3, 28, 32, 33), cow (8) and guinea pig (18). Equally sensitive to stimulation are macrophages from various sources such as mouse peritoneum, spleen and liver (23) and rabbit lung (3).

The sensitivity of both neutrophilic granulocytes and macro-

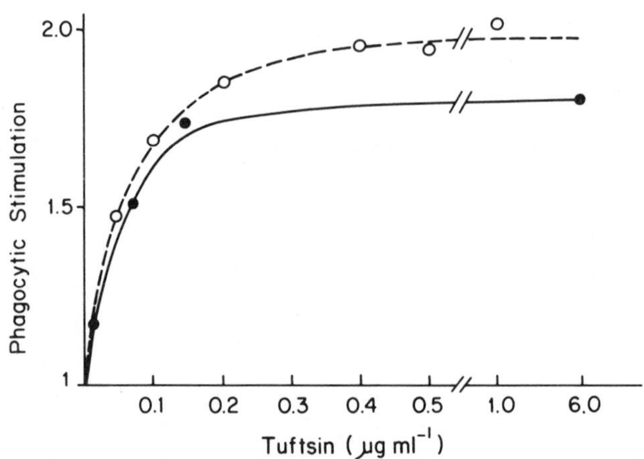

Fig. 1. This is a composite figure of phagocytosis assay using Staphylococcus aureus (3) and yeast cells (14). Both reactions involved blood polymorphonuclear leukocytes. Note the similarity of responses in both cases. For details refer to original articles.

phages is almost identical with a half maximal value of 50 ng ml^{-1}, i.e., 100 nM. In fact, definite stimulation was obtained with mouse peritoneal macrophages at 2.5, 5 and 10 ng ml^{-1} (23). This is well within the range of hormonal concentration. Fig. 1 shows 2 dose response curves representing phagocytic activity to various concentrations using Staphylococcus aureus (3) and yeast cells (14) as target particles.

Tuftsin stimulates pinocytosis by neutrophils most likely by the same mechanism as phagocytosis (3). Another biological effect of tuftsin is equally interesting. It exerts a definite chemotactic response (25, 33). Swarms of neutrophils migrate in a single band in glass capillary tubes towards tuftsin in the upper portion of vertically placed tubes (25, 33). This may be complicated by the stimulation of motility. However, no such chemotactic activity can be elicited in plastic chambers inasmuch as tuftsin prevents neutrophils from sticking to plastic surfaces. Utilizing Falcon dishes, we were able to show that a few nmol per ml cause a diminution of adherence of granulocytes to plastic surfaces. This is shown in Fig. 2. In fact, Goetzl has shown (25) that tuftsin is strongly inhibitory to chemotaxis presumably for the same reason. It is of special interest that tuftsin also exerts a strong chemotactic effect on Escherichia coli (52).

In the presence of tuftsin, the motility and survival time of neutrophils is considerably prolonged (25, 33). All the biological effects so far discussed are completely inhibited by a third of an equivalent of a pentapeptide analog of tuftsin possessing an additional proline residue, Thr-Lys-Pro-Pro-Arg.

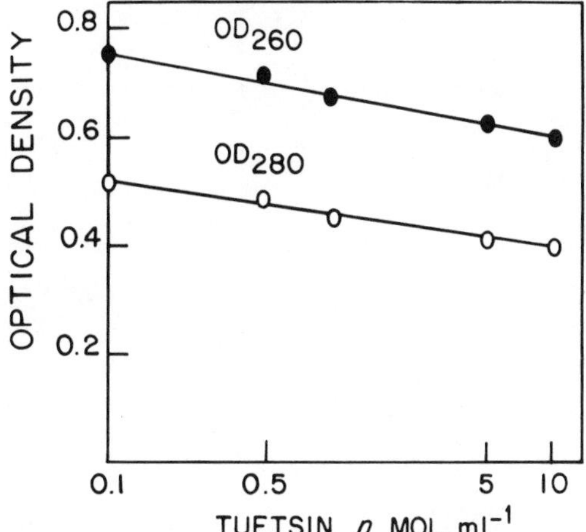

Fig. 2. Buffy coat was prepared from fresh dog blood as usual (5). 150 µl of this was mixed with 850 µl of Hank's medium and poured into a Falcon plastic tissue culture plate (35 mm x 10 mm). This was allowed to stand at 25 C for 30 min. The plate was then washed by dipping into 0.15 M NaCl 400 ml followed by 2 additional rinsings in 200 ml. The plate was inverted over tissue paper for complete drainage. One ml of 0.5 N NaOH was then added, mixed and allowed to stand for 20-30 min at 25 C. After centrifugation, the clear solution was then measured at 260 mµ and 280 mµ against 0.5 N NaOH.

Still another biological effect which has lately come to light and of singular interest is the ability of synthetic tuftsin to augment considerably the bactericidal activity of the macrophage. Martinez et al. (23) demonstrated that after prior exposure of peritoneal macrophages to tuftsin, up to 70% of ingested bacteria were killed after 15 min of incubation. By contrast, the control cells not exposed to tuftsin showed little or no killing of engulfed bacteria. Table II illustrates the bactericidal activity of the macrophage. This is particularly prominent during the first 15 min probably because the stimulatory effect of tuftsin does not last longer than that interval of time (3, 25, 32) because of its destruction by cell enzymes (38). A similar increase in the bactericidal activity was noted in spleen and liver macrophages of mice following an intravenous injection of bacteria (23).

A totally unexpected effect of tuftsin was shown recently by Luftig et al. (21). The addition of 1-100 nmol per ml of the tetrapeptide to cultured cells infected with Rauscher Murine leukemia virus, MuLV, resulted in a 3-fold increase in the release of MuLV as inferred by the 3-fold increase in the activity of the reverse transcriptase (21). Electron scanning micrographs of such cells shows a very marked increase in membrane budding presumably due to MuLV particles (20).

TABLE II

Bactericidal Activity of Tuftsin[a]

Listeria monocytogenes Killed, Percent of Count at Zero Time

Time of Incubation (min)	Control Mice		Tuftsin Injected Mice (i. p.) 10 mg/kg	20 mg/kg	
	I	II	II	I	II
15	0.0	5.2	49.8	57.3	68.6
30	30.5	20.0	63.0	55.8	71.8
60	46.9	29.6	63.8	75.4	72.2

[a]The effect of tuftsin on the intracellular bactericidal activity of mouse peritoneal macrophages against *Listeria monocytogenes* taken from Martinez et al (22, 23). Two experiments are shown. One ml of a suspension of *L. monocytogenes* 1-2 x 10^6 in gelatin Hank's medium with 10% fetal serum containing an amount of tuftsin corresponding to 0, 10 and 20 mg/kg of body weight was injected i. p. into mice. After 5 min the animal was sacrificed and 2 ml of saline solution was injected i. p. to harvest the macrophages. Cell suspensions were washed twice with cold gelatin Hank's solution and centrifuged at 100 g for 4 min. The number of macrophages was adjusted to 6-8 x 10^6 ml^{-1} of medium. One ml of each was incubated at 37 C. At intervals thereafter of 0, 15, 30 and 60 min, viable bacteria were determined. For this purpose, the cells were centrifuged 4 min at 100 g and 1 ml of distilled water was added to the sedimented cells containing cold bovine serum albumin. This was then frozen (-170 C) and thawed (37 C) 3 times and appropriate dilutions were then plated and viable bacteria scored. This table shows the percent of bacteria killed as a function of time, for control and for tuftsin at 10 mg and 20 mg/kg of body weight. In experiment I, tuftsin 20 mg/kg was injected 10 min before the injection of bacteria.

What led to the use of tuftsin in these experiments was the demonstration by Oroszlan *et al.* (36) that 1 of the components of the "gag" protein of MuLV, P12, has the tuftsin sequence Thr-Lys-Pro-Arg, 8 residues from the aminoterminal. The possibility that this might occur by chance is less than 1 in 600,000, i. e., 20^4. It is to be noted that Try-Lys-Pro, which would occur by chance in less than 1 in 8,000 does appear in 3 polypeptides: C-reactive protein (37), histone IV (35) and TSH-β (19).

Stimulation of motility of blood granulocytes was shown (32) in glass capillary tubes. More recently, stimulation of blood macrophages also in glass tubes has been shown by Nishioka (31) in a standard direct migration inhibition factor assay. Tuftsin also was shown to antagonize the migration inhibition effect of human malignant melanoma antigen (31).

THE BIOLOGICAL ACTIVITY OF TUFTSIN *IN VIVO*

The mechanism of action of tuftsin has not been explored. Suffice it to indicate at this time that it binds to the cell membrane very avidly at 4 C. At 37 C it is eventually taken into the cytoplasm of the cell and finally is fragmented into its constituent amino acids. Tuftsin degrading enzymes are present in the cytoplasm of the granulocyte but not in the membrane or granules (38). Degrading enzymes are also present in the soluble fraction of splenic extracts and in serum.

The rapid intravenous injection of up to 25 mg/kg body weight to rats does not reveal any systemic effects. Respiratory and cardiac rates remain at the preinjection level. Similarly, there is no change in animal's blood pressure and electrocardiograms (25).

Martinez and colleagues (22, 23) reported an increased rate o blood clearing of *E. coli*, *L. monocytogenes*, *S. aureus* and *Salmonella typhimurium*, following the intraperitoneal injection of tuftsin at a dose of 10 and 20 mg/kg body weight. This was the case both in normal and leukemic mice. Fig. 3 shows the rate of clearing of *E. coli* from normal mice with and without tuftsin. It was further shown (22) that after the injection of tustsin at 25 mg/kg body weight, mice survival following a near lethal injection of pneumococcus rose from 15% to 50%.

THE EFFECT OF TUFTSIN ON THE IMMUNOGENIC FUNCTION OF MACROPHAGES

In a recent study by Feldman, Fridkin, Spirer and their associates (50) it was reported that tuftsin augments considerably the antigen-specific macrophage dependent "education" of T lymphocytes.

Mouse peritoneal thioglycolate-induced macrophages were incubated with keyhole limpet hemocyanin (KLH) 50 μg per ml at 37 C with or without tuftsin at concentrations of 1-20 x 10^{-8}M. Excess antigen was then removed by thorough washing. Mouse spleen cells were then added to the antigen fed macrophage monolayers and incubated overnight. The nonadherent free cells were then exposed

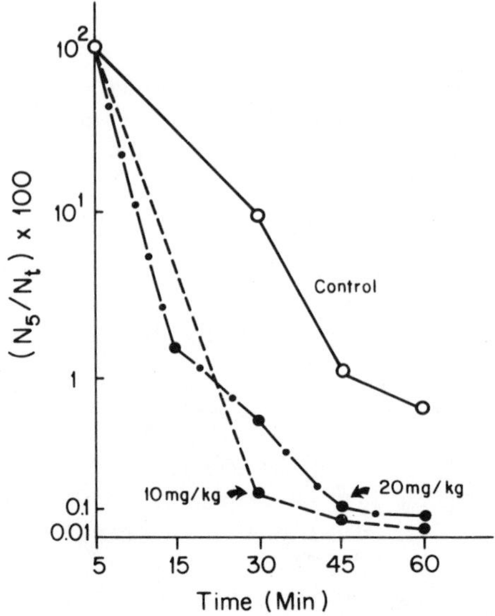

Fig. 3. The effect of tuftsin on bacterial clearing (23). Mice of CD-1 strain were injected intravenously (i. v.) with 0.25 ml of culture of E. coli. This was followed by an i. p. injection of tuftsin at 10 and 20 mg/kg body weight. At the indicated times, blood was obtained by cardiac puncture. The blood samples of the 3 animals were mixed, treated appropriately and inoculated on nutrient agar and counted. The number of bacteria was calculated on the basis of count ml^{-1} of blood. This type of experiment was repeated 3 times and apparently similar results were obtained under the same conditions. It was possible to assess the number of bacteria in the liver and spleen of these animals. In such cases, 4 animals were sacrificed by cervical dislocation after 5, 10 and 60 min. The organs were removed, homogenized in isotonic NaCl. The suspension was diluted and grown on nutrient agar and colonies counted (see text).

to X-ray, 1000 rads and injected into the foot pads of syngeneic mice. After 7 days a cell suspension was prepared from the popliteal lymph nodes and cultured in an appropriate medium with and without KLH antigen 0.05 and 0.5 μg. After 3 days of culture 2 μCi of tritiated thymidine were added. The incorporated radioactivity was measured in a scintillation counter after 4 hr of incubation.

Tufstin produced a significant concentration-dependent stimulation of the immunogenic function of macrophages with typical regulatory characteristics. Optimal stimulation of 700% of control was attained at $1.6 \times 10^{-8}M$ per 2×10^7 macrophages. On either side of the optimal concentration the effect was diminished. This activity could be obtained only when tuftsin is presented at the same time of antigen processing. The high stimulatory potency of tuftsin is specific and depended on the integrity of the amino acid sequence. Modification of either terminals leads to reduction loss or inhibition of macrophage activation. Replacement of threonine by serine or its deletion resulted in an inhibitory activity. Substitution of the guanido function of the arginine residue with methyl or a nitro group or its replacement by lysine resulted in an inactive or inhibitory analog. Amidation of arginine or its replacement by D-arginine however did not affect activity. Augmentation of activity was obtained if glycine was added to the terminal or if alanine replaces threonine at the aminoterminal. Furthermore, Thr-Lys-Pro, Thr-Lys-Arg and Thr-Lys-Leu-Arg showed greatly reduced or no activity.

TUFTSIN RECEPTOR SITES

Fridkin, Spirer and their colleagues (50) prepared radioactive tuftsin through the incorporation of tritium labeled arginine. This was done by coupling N-hydroxysuccinimide ester of the protected tripeptide Thr-Lys-Pro (47) to radioactive arginine. Stabinsky *et al.* (48) showed that binding to polymorphonuclear leukocytes (PMN) and monocytes was specific, rapid saturable and reversible. Dissociation constants (K_d) for these phagocytes were 130 and 125 nM, respectively , binding sites per cell approximately 50,000 and 100,000, respectively. The K_d values are remarkably close to the K_m observed for phagocytosis (5, 14) (see Fig. 1). Lymphocytes showed only threshold binding and no binding could be detected to erythrocytes.

Fudenberg's groups (24) also studied binding of labeled tuftsin with ^{14}C or ^{125}I by appropriate addition of labeled residues at either C- or N-terminals. Neutrophils bound 72 $\pm$ 10% of labeled tuftsin in the incubation medium. This binding was specific as well as that obtained for monocytes and lymphocytes although the extent of binding was lower than that obtained for PMN cells.

Horsmanheimo *et al.* (15) studied the effect of tuftsin on leukocyte migration. They showed with the agarose migration test that monocyte migration was significantly enhanced. No effect on PMN migration was observed. However, Nishioka (30) observed a definite stimulation using Boyden chamber. This contrasts with the large stimulation of PMN migration in glass tubes so readily demonstrable (33). It is quite possible that small impurities in the tuftsin samples used might account for the differences observed by the 2 laboratories (see below).

THE AUGMENTATION BY TUFTSIN OF THE ABILITY OF THE MACROPHAGES TO DESTROY CANCER CELLS

The killing effect of nonspecifically activated macrophages on tumor cells is well known. I have documented the activating effect of tuftsin on macrophages at hormonal concentrations. Our laboratory is currently engaged in studying the effect of tuftsin on the ability of macrophages to destroy cancer cells. My former student and colleague (30) already has preliminary evidence for a definite effect on cancer cells.

L1210 mouse leukemia cells, DBA mice. Ten control mice received 1 x 10^5 leukemia cells by i. p. injection. The experimental group (10 mice) were injected with the same number followed by 0. 2 μg of tuftsin. While all mice which received tumor cells alone died in 11 days (mean survival 9.2 days), those that received leukemia cells plus tuftsin showed 50% survival for over 30 days. This experiment has since been repeated twice with similar statistically significant differences in survival curves between the control and tuftsin injected groups.

Cloudman S-91 melanoma cells DBA mice. A control group of 4 mice received 2.5 x 10^5 melanoma cells subcutaneously in each hind leg. The experimental group, also 4 mice, was in addition injected with 10 μg of tuftsin together with the cells. These 2 groups were compared for tumor growth by measuring the size of the melanoma. Again a statistically significant slower growth was observed in the tuftsin injected group.

In vitro cytotoxicity enhancement by tuftsin was also examined. This was performed by following (^{3}H)-proline release assay (39). L1210 leukemia cells and peritoneal exudate cells of DBA mice were incubated at a ratio of 1:50, respectively. Tuftsin (10 μg/ml) activated macrophages showed statistically significant enhanced cytotoxicity (32%) as compared to control. This experiment was repeated 3 times. Statistically significant cytotoxicity enhancements were obtained in all experiments.

Cytotoxicity enhancement of human neutrophils by tuftsin was also examined using an established human melanoma cell line, 26-5, with peripheral granulocytes purified by Ficoll-Hypaque gradient and lysis of erythrocytes with NH_4Cl. With the same (^{3}H)-proline labeled L1210 cells, in the range of tuftsin concentration of 2-20 g, 13-23% of cytotoxicity enhancement by tuftsin has been obtained (statistically significant in repeated experiments). During this study release of chemiluminescence from neutrophils upon incubation with tuftsin with particle-free filtered isotonic buffer was observed (30).

TABLE III

The Biological Activity of Tuftsin Analogs

Tuftsin Analogs	Relative Activity[a]	Inhibitory[b]	Reference
Thr-Lys-Pro-Arg	1.0		3,8,16,17,25,44,51
Thr-Lys-Pro-Lys	0.3-0.5	0	18,38
Lys-Pro-Arg	0.0	+	14, 32 - 34)
Thr-Lys-Pro	0.0	0	32 - 34
Lys-Pro-Pro-Arg	0.0	+	17, 26
Thr-Lys-Pro-Pro-Arg	0.0	+	32 - 34
Lys-Lys-Pro-Arg	0.0-0.3	0	13, 14
Ser-Lys-Pro-Arg	0.0-0.2	+	13, 14
Tyr-Lys-Pro-Arg	0.0	0	13, 14
Val-Lys-Pro-Arg	0.0-0.5	+	13, 14, 18
Ala-Lys-Pro-Arg	0.0	+	13, 14
Thr-Lys-Pro-Ala	0.7	nd	17, 18
Thr-Lys-Pro-Arg-NO_2	0.0	0	13, 14
Thr-LysOAla-Arg	0.5	nd	17, 18
Thr-Orn-Pro-Arg	0.5	nd	17, 18
Thr-Orn-Pro-Ala	0.4	nd	17, 18
Thr-Ala-Val-Arg	0.7	nd	17, 18
Thr-Ala-Arg-Lys	0.6	nd	17, 18
Thr-Gly-Gly-Lys	0.1	nd	17, 18
Thr-Lys-Lys-Ala	0.7	nd	17, 18
Thr-Lys-Ala-Ala	0.1	nd	17, 18
Acetyl-Thr-Lys-Pro-Arg	0.0	+	13, 14
ρ-aminopenylacetyl tuftsin	0.0	+	13, 14
$(Lys)_{3,4,6,20}$	0.0	0	13, 14

[a]Relative activity of 1.0 is taken as the activity in the particular laboratory for the tretrapeptide tuftsin. That obtained by the analog is the fraction obtained relative to tuftsin in the same laboratory.

[b]0 = no inhibition; + = inhibition; nd = not done

ANALOGS OF TUFTSIN

Numerous analogs of tuftsin have been prepared in several laboratories. A study of the biological activity of these analogs revealed that the structure of tuftsin is unique. Any alteration however small results in reduced activity or confers on the polypeptide a definite inhibitory effect on the phagocytic stimulating action of tuftsin.

Table III shows the structure of the polypeptides and their relative effects, along with appropriate reference to the authors.

The analog Thr-Lys-Pro-Pro-Arg exerts a strong inhibitory effect on phagocytic stimulation and inhibits the chemotactic migration of blood granulocytes. Eight nmol/ml completely obliterated the stimulation of chemotactic migration by 25 nmol/ml of tuftsin (33).

CONGENITAL TUFTSIN DEFICIENCY

We have studied a total of 6 families, 4 of which have been reported (4, 5, 27). These were secured over a 2 yr period with little effort. This is intended to convey the feeling that this deficiency is not uncommon. In all families studied it was found that 1 of the parents, father or mother, was affected. In all cases studied thus far, the affected individual yielded peptide extracts that were not only inactive but also inhibitory to the stimulatory effect of tuftsin.

An additional family with tuftsin deficiency has since been reported in Japan (16). The clinical manifestations of repeated severe infections of the respiratory tract, skin and lymph nodes paralled in severity the symptoms and signs shown in our most severe case (27). Again, the peptide extracted from the γ-globulin of the patient and his father were inactive and strongly inhibitory to tuftsin activity.

ACQUIRED TUFTSIN DEFICIENCY

The first demonstration of an acquired deficiency in tuftsin activity was shown in splenectomized dogs (29). Further studies on human subjects that had undergone elective splenectomy for various reasons showed an almost complete loss of tuftsin activity (6, 28). Peptide extracts from their γ-globulin, in contrast to those obtained from cases with the congenital syndrome, showed no inhibition of synthetic tuftsin activity. It is noteworthy that subjects that had been splenectomized following accidental rupture of the spleen showed near normal values (6, 28).

Spirer and his colleagues (45, 46) using a radioimmunoassay for tuftsin showed that normal subjects yielded values of 256 $\pm$ 10 ng ml^{-1}. This compares with near normal values in splenectomized subject following accidental rupture of the spleen of 234 $\pm$ 10 ng ml^{-1}. While patients with elective splenectomy showed much lower values than either, 118 $\pm$ 8 ng ml^{-1}.

DISCUSSION

The results obtained in several laboratories indicate that each residue in the structure of tuftsin, L-threonyl-L-lysyl-L-prolyl-L-arginine, is strictly and uniquely necessary for activity. Any alteration however minor such as the substitution of serine for threonine greatly diminishes the biological activity. Other substitutions also diminish this activity more or less depending on the substituent residue. As can be seen in Table III, the majority of tuftsin analogs that had been tested are indeed tuftsin inhibitors as well.

The results obtained with nuclear magnetic resonance (2) indicate that both tuftsin and the pentapeptide inhibitor analog in aqueous solution do not possess a rigid structure. This is comforting in that both can adjust to the binding site to cause stimulation or inhibition. Had tuftsin been in a rigid 1-4 β turn as postulated by Konopinska _et al._ (17) it would be difficult to rationalize the strong inhibitory effect of the pentapeptide.

Tuftsin is active only in the free tetrapeptide state. In order to be released from the carrier parent molecule, it undergoes 2 enzymatic cleavage steps, 1 at the carboxyterminal arginine. This occurs in the spleen. The second cleavage step occurs at the target cell, the phagocyte. Here a membrane enzyme cleaves the tetrapeptide at the amino side of threonine. The tetrapeptide is therefore liberated in the intimate vicinity of the phagocyte membrane and consequently at an effective high concentration where it exerts its biological effect. One cannot wish for a better arrangement for this system, inasmuch as the tetrapeptide is not very stable in the blood due to the presence of leucine aminopeptidase and carboxypeptidase B. Either of these activities results in an inactive tripeptide (28, 32, 33).

In all these characteristics the tuftsin system is remarkably similar to that of the angiotensin II system. Here, the carrier molecule is also a plasma globulin. Similarly, 2 enzymatic steps are required to release angiotensin II. The first is a cleavage at the carboxyterminal leucine of the decapeptide angiotensin I. This occurs in the kidney through renin action. A second enzyme releases the terminal dipeptide histidyl-leucine to yield active angiotensin II. This occurs primarily in the lung (43).

The main biological effects of tuftsin, the stimulation of phagocytosis, is exerted equally well on the granulocyte as on the macrophage. Blood clearing of bacteria is stimulated by tuftsin. This is a natural consequence of increased rate of phagocytosis by both granulocytes and macrophages. However, there is an additional effect, namely the stimulation of the bactericidal activity of the macrophage. This is a most interesting phenomenon that deserves in-depth study. It is possible that the stimulation of the shunt, as deduced from increased reduction of nitroblue tetrazolium, increases the killing effect on the bacteria be it from increased halogenation, increased peroxide formation, OH radical or superoxide O_2^-, remains to be seen. All these may be directly involved in bacterial killing (1).

The additional ability of tuftsin at a 16 nM optimal concentration to augment the antigen-specific macrophage dependent programming or "education" of T lymphocytes (50) places it in a special category. It appears to exert effects which are uniquely oriented towards defensive mechanisms of the body. This defensive posture may well include more effective immune surveillance against tumorigenic body cells.

The presence of tuftsin, 8 residues from the amino terminal of P12 of MuLV, is of singular interest. In particular, the addition of tuftsin to the carrier cells of this virus increases the budding and release of the virus (20). This effect along with the other membrane effects of tuftsin on pinocytosis, phagocytosis, chemotaxis and motility strongly suggest that tuftsin may exert its primary effect first on the membrane. Other activities then follow. Consequently, tuftsin might be primarily a membrane active peptide that augments whatever function can be generated normally through membrane activity of the phagocyte.

It appears certain that phagocytes in general and macrophages in particular are capable of influencing the immune response. Upon activation, macrophages seem to augment the immune response to a considerable degree. This has been shown after activation with several bacteria or bacterial products and other nonphysiological compounds. This is the principle behind the adjuvant effect. We have seen how tuftsin can activate the macrophage of varied species of animals whatever the compartment source. This activation is expressed in increased phagocytosis of target particles, increased immunogenic activity of the macrophage with presumably an augmentation of antibody production.

The macrophage has also been implicated in a seek and destroy mission against errant cells such as cancer cells. It is no wonder then that the activation of the macrophage can prevent the implantation and growth of leukemic or cancer cells. Our current efforts and those of others are directed along those lines. It appears that tuftsin might wield a double-edged sword. On one hand, it increases the immunogenic response and on the other it activates the macrophage to render it more destructive of tumor cells (30).

In a recurrent state of bacterial infection it is probably that there is a consequent activation of host macrophages. Besides combating the particular infection, this would also upgrade their mission against mutant cells that probably arise continuously. Bacterial invasion of the host must then be looked upon as a blessing in disguise; the more frequent the infection the more susceptible is the budding cancer cell to the killing effect of the activated macrophages.

WARNING

It is noteworthy that most published work on tuftsin has emanated from laboratories where it was synthesized and purified. It has come to our attention lately that purchased tuftsin was not as active as it should be. Consequently, we and others (30) found that most, if not all, available tuftsin from biochemical suppliers is notoriously impure as analyzed by TLC, phenol:water 3:1 (32). As we and others have found (see Table III), most substitution of tuftsin is either inactive or inhibitory to tuftsin activity. It is strongly urged that future users of purchased material should test its purity and if necessary purify it (32, 33).

ACKNOWLEDGEMENTS

This work was supported by Public Health Service Grant 5R01 AI 096116, National Science Foundation Grant PCM76-23008, and the National Foundation March of Dimes 1-556.

REFERENCES

1. Babior, B. M. New Engl. J. Med. 298 (1978) 659.
2. Bluminstein, M. and Najjar, V. A. Unpublished observations.
3. Constantopoulos, A. and Najjar, V. A. Cytobios 6 (1972) 97.
4. Constantopoulos, A. and Najjar, V. A. Acta Paediat. Scand. 62 (1973) 645.
5. Constantopoulos, A., Najjar, V. A. and Smith, J. J. J. Pediat. 80 (1972) 564.
6. Constantopoulos, A., Najjar, V. A., Wish, J. B., Necheles, T. H. and Stolbach, L. L. Am. J. Dis. Children 125 (1973) 663.
7. Edelman, G. M., Cunningham, B. A., Gall, W. E., Gottlieb, P. D., Rutishauser, U. and Waxdal, M. J. Proc. Natl. Acad. Sci. US 63 (1969) 78.
8. Erp, E. E. and Fahrney, D. Arch. Biochem. Biophys. 168 (1975) 1.

9. Fidalgo, B. V. and Najjar, V. A. Biochemistry 6 (1967) 3386.
10. Fidalgo, B. V. and Najjar, V. A. Proc. Natl. Acad. Sci. US 57 (1967) 957.
11. Fidalgo, B. V., Katayama, Y. and Najjar, V. A. Biochemistry 6 (1967) 3378.
12. Fidalgo, B. V., Najjar, V. A., Zukoski, C. F. and Katayama, Y. Proc. Natl. Acad. Sci. US 57 (1967) 665.
13. Fridkin, M., Stabinsky, Y., Zakuth, V. and Spirer, Z. In: Peptides. (Ed. A. Loffet) Editions de l'Universite de Bruxelle, Belgique (1976) 541.
14. Fridkin, M., Stabinsky, Y., Zakuth, V. and Spirer, Z. Biochim. Biophys. Acta 496 (1977)203.
15. Horsmanheimo, M., Horsmanheimo, A. and Fudenberg, H. H. Clin. Immunol. Immunopathol. (1978) In press.
16. Inada, K., Nemoto, N., Nishijima, A., Wada, S., Hirata, M. and Yoshida, M. In: Proceedings of the international symposium on phagocytosis. Tokyo, Japan (1977).
17. Konopinska, D., Nawrocka, E., Siemion, I. Z., Szymaniec, St. and Slopek, S. In: Peptides (Ed. A. Loffet) Editions de l' Universite de Bruxelle, Belgique (1976) 535.
18. Konopinska, D., Nawrocka, E. Siemion, I. Z., Slopek, S., Szymaniec, St. and Klonowska, E. Int. J. Peptide Protein Res. 9 (1977) 71.
19. Li, C. H. Perspect. Biol. Med. 21 (1978) 447.
20. Luftig, R. B. Personal communication.
21. Luftig, R. B., Yoshinaka, Y. and Oroszlan, S. J. Cell Biol. 25 (1977) 397a.
22. Martinez, J. In: These docteur de science physiques, academie de Montpellier, Universite des Sciences Techniques de Langeudoc (1976) 1.
23. Martinez, J., Winternitz, F. and Vindel, J. Eur. J. Med. Chem. Chimica Therapeutica 12 (1977) 511.
24. Nair, R. M. G., Ponce, B. and Fudenberg, H. H. Immunochemistry. (1978) In press.
25. Najjar, V. A. Adv. Enzymol. 41 (1974) 129.
26. Najjar, V. A. In: Biological membrane (Ed. D. Chapmen, D. F. Wallach) Academic Press, New York 3 (1976) 191.
27. Najjar, V. A. Exp. Cell Biol. 46 (1977) 114.
28. Najjar, V. A. and Constantopoulos, A. J. Reticuloenthel. Soc. 12 (1972) 197.
29. Najjar, V. A., Fidalgo, B. V. and Stitt, E. Biochemistry 7 (1968) 2376.
30. Nishioka, K. Personal communication.
31. Nishioka, K. Gann 69 (1978) In press.
32. Niskioka, K., Constantopoulos, A., Staoh, P. S., Mitchell, W. M. and Najjar, V. A. Biochim. Biophys. Acta 310 (1973) 217.
33. Nishioka, K., Satoh, P. S., Constantopoulos, A. and Najjar, V. A. Biochim. Biophys. Acta 310 (1973) 230.
34. Nishioka, K., Constantopoulos, A., Staoh, P. and Najjar, V. A. Biochem. Biophys. Res. Commun. 47 (1972) 172.

35. Ogawa, Y., Quagliarotti, G., Jordan, J., Taylor, C. W., Starbuck, W. C. and Busch, H. J. Biol. Chem. 244 (1969) 4387.
36. Oroszlan, S., Henderson, L. E., Stephenson, J. R., Copeland, T. D., Long, C. W., Ihle, J. N. and Gilden, R. V. Proc. Natl. Acad. Sci. US 75 (1977) 1404.
37. Osmand, P., Gewurz, H. and Friedenson, B. Proc. Natl. Acad. Sci. US 74 (1977) 1214.
38. Rauner, R. A., Schmidt, J. J. and Najjar, V. A. Mol. Cell. Biochem. 10 (1976) 77.
39. Saal, J. G., Rieber, E. P., Riethmuller, G. Scand. J. Immunol. 5 (1976) 455.
40. Saravia, N. G., Derrebery, S. and Robinson, G. Mol. Cell. Biochem. (1978) In press.
41. Satoh, P. S., Constantopoulos, A., Nishioka, K. and Najjar, V. A. In: Chemistry and biology of peptides (Ed. J. Meinhoffer) Ann Arbor Science Publisher, Michigan (1972) 403.
42. Segal, A. W. and Levy, A. J. Clin. Sci. Mol. Med. 45 (1973) 817.
43. Skeggs, L. T., Jr., Dorer, E. F., Kahn, J. R., Lentz, K. E. and Levine, M. Am. J. Med. 60 (1976) 737.
44. Spirer, Z., Zakuth, V., Bogair, N. and Fridkin , M. Eur. J. Immunol. 7 (1977) 69.
45. Spirer, Z., Zakuth, V., Gllander, A., Bogair, N. and Fridkin, M. J. Clin. Invest. 55 (1976) 198.
46. Spirer, Z., Zakuth, V., Diamant, S., Mondorf, W., Stefanescu, T. Stabinsky, Y. and Fridkin, M. Brit. Med. J. 2 (1977) 1574.
47. Stabinsky, Y., Fridkin, M., Zakuth, V. and Spirer, Z. Int. J. Peptide Protein Res (1978) In press.
48. Stabinsky, Y., Gottlieb, P., Zakuth, V., Spirer, Z. and Fridkin, M. Biochem. Biophys, Res. Commun (1978) In press.
49. Thomaidis, T. S., Fidalgo, B. V., Harshman, S. and Najjar, V. A. Biochemistry 6 (1967) 3369.
50. Tzehoval, E., Segal, S., Stabinsky, Y., Fridkin, M., Spirer, Z. and Feldman, M. Proc. Natl. Acad. Sci. US (1978) In press.
51. Vicar, J., Gut, V., Fric, K. and Blaha, K. Collection Czechoslav. Chem. Commun. 41 (1976) 3467.
52. Yajima, H., Ogawa, H., Watanabe, H., Fujii, N., Kurobe, M. and Miyamoto, S. Chem. Pharm. Bull. 23 (1975) 371.

ANGIOTENSIN CONVERTING ENZYME: INDUCTION IN RABBIT ALVEOLAR MACROPHAGES AND HUMAN MONOCYTES IN CULTURE

E. SILVERSTEIN, J. FRIEDLAND and C. SETTON

Laboratory of Molecular Biology, Departments of Medicine and Biochemistry, State University of New York, Downstate Medical Center, Brooklyn, New York (USA)

The biochemical complexity of mononuclear phagocytes and its regulation by various chemical signals, as well as the rich molecular regulatory interchange among these and other cell types, has become increasingly recognized in recent years (20). Angiotensin converting enzyme (ACE) (E.C. 3.4.15.1, peptidyl dipeptidase) is a glycoprotein of about 150,000 daltons which catalyzes the cleavage of the carboxy-terminal dipeptide of the decapeptide angiotensin I to form the biological potent pressor octapeptide, angiotensin-II, as well as a similar cleavage which inactivates bradykinin (19). ACE has been shown in the rabbit to be localized predominantly at the lumenal surface of endothelial cells (10), and is strkingly increased in the pathological tissues and sera of patients with sarcoidosis (8,14-16) and Gaucher's disease (9,12,18), which are associated with proliferation of mononuclear phagocytes. This observation suggested that ACE may be abundant in sarcoidosis epithelioid cells and Gaucher cells as the cause of the ACE elevation in these conditions. This hypothesis (11, 16) has been born out by our recent localization by immunofluorescence of abundant ACE in these cells but not in other granulomatous controls using an anti-human lung ACE antibody prepared in rabbits with the aid of purified human lung ACE (2,13).

ACE was assayed with the substrate hippuryl-L-histidyl-L-leucine fluorimetrically (5) except for tissue homogenates which were assayed spectrophotometrically (1). ACE abundance in sarcoidosis epithelioid cells and Gaucher cells is not a manifestation of a general abundance of ACE in mononuclear phagocytes since mouse, rat and rabbit peritoneal and alveolar macrophages contained only minute quantities of ACE in comparison with lung (Table I). Furthermore, elevated ACE content does not appear to be due simply to macrophage activation since mouse thioglycollate stimulated peritoneal macrophages contained scant ACE on isolation and in culture (Tables I and II). Exposure of rabbit alveolar macrophages in culture to endotoxin stimulation similarly failed to result in the appearance of abundant ACE in these cells (Table III). Freund's adjuvant granulomas in rats were not enriched for ACE compared to control tissues, indicating that elevated ACE is not a function of granulomas generally (17).

TABLE I

Angiotensin-Converting Enzyme in Macrophages and Lungs of Mice, Rats and Rabbits[b]

	Macrophages				
	Peritoneal			Alveolar[a]	Lung
	Nonactivated		Thioglycollate-Activated		
Mouse	0.150	(4)	0.130 (7)	---	245
	0.220	(2)			
Rat	0.173±0.047[a]	(3)		0.058±0.024 (4)	166
Rabbit	----			0.314±0.085 (9)	216

[a]Values are means±standard error of the mean.

[b]See Silverstein, et al. (17) for experimental details (By permission of Israel Journal of Medical Sciences). Values in the Table are mean activities of angiotensin converting enzyme in $nmol \cdot min^{-1} \cdot mg\ protein^{-1}$. The numbers of animals from which the macrophages were pooled are shown in parentheses.

We therefore looked for specific control mechanisms for ACE synthesis in mononuclear phagocytes. Glucocorticosteroids caused a striking induction of ACE in rabbit alveolar macrophages in culture (Fig. 1). ACE was increased up to 16-fold in comparison with control values in 3 days at maximal stimulation. Rabbit alveolar macrophages were exquisitely sensitive to the glucocorticosteroid stimulation of ACE synthesis since maximum, half-maximum and modest stimulation was obtained at 4 nM, 0.6 nM and 0.003 nM (Fig. 2). The dependence of the increase in ACE activity on RNA synthesis-dependent new enzyme synthesis was indicated by significant inhibition of ACE induction by actinomycin D (0.1 μg/ml) and cycloheximide (1 μM). Colchicine had no significant effect on ACE (3) although it stimulates the secretion of several neutral proteinases (7).

TABLE II

Angiotensin Converting Enzyme in Mouse Peritoneal Macrophages in Culture[a]

Hours in Culture	Cells (nMol min^{-1} mg $Protein^{-1}$) Unactivated	Cells (nMol min^{-1} mg $Protein^{-1}$) Activated[b]	Medium (nMol min^{-1} ml^{-1}) from: Unactivated Cells	Medium (nMol min^{-1} ml^{-1}) from: Activated[b] Cells
Dulbecco's Medium (5% fetal calf serum)				
0	-	0.360	-	0.720
48	-	0	-	0.586
71	0.120	0.170	0.561	0.494
95	-	0.017	-	0.463
RPMI 1640 medium (10% fetal calf serum)[c]				
0	0.150	0.130	0.874	1.08
48	-	0	-	1.28
72	0	0.025	1.15	1.34
94		0	-	0.98

[a]See Silvertstein, et al. (17) for experimental details (By permission of Israel Journal of Medical Sciences).

[b]Cells were activated by thioglycollate.

[c]The higher angiotensin converting enzyme activity in RPMI 1640 medium can be explained by the doubled fetal calf serum concentration.

ACE inducer activity was limited to compounds possessing glucocorticosteroid activity, suggesting that very specific binding to a receptor is involved in the induction. The steroids aldosterone, β-estradiol, progesterone, and testosterone were not inducers, in contrast to the glucocorticosteroid dexamethasone (all concentrations were 0.45 μM except for progesterone which was up to 10 μM). Steroids with glucocorticoid activity, such as cortisone, dexamethasone, hydrocortisone, corticosterone, 11-β-

TABLE III

Angiotensin Converting Enzyme Activity of Rabbit Alveolar Marophages in Culture: Effect of Macrophage Activation by *Salmonella typhosa* Endotoxin[a]

Hours in Culture	Control	Endotoxin (100 μg/ml)	Control	Endotoxin (1 μg/ml)	Endotoxin (0.1 μg/ml)
Angiotensin converting enzyme in cells (nMol min^{-1} mg $protein^{-1}$)					
0	0.151	0.151	0.055	0.055	0.055
22	0.140	0.196			
47			0.207	0.196	0.176
70	0.890	0.187	0.241	0.233	
94	1.56	0.240	0.380	0.159	0.299
Angiotensin converting enzyme in culture medium (nMol min^{-1} ml^{-1})					
0	0.610	0.610	0.097	0.097	0.097
22	0.680	0.643			
47			0.236	0.168	0.183
70	1.24	0.820	0.402	0.188	0.273
94	2.25	0.910	0.497	0.478	0.526

[a]See Silverstein, *et al*. (17) for experimental details (By permission of Israel Journal of Medical Sciences).

hydroxyprogesterone and prednisone were inducers at 0.45 μM. Glucocorticosteroid activity appeared to be correlated with ACE inducer activity. Thus, 11-hydroxyprogesterone which has weak glucocorticosteroid activity had relatively weak inducer activity. 11-ketoprogesterone, 11-deoxycorticosterone and 17-α-hydroxyprogesterone (all at 0.45 μM) were inactive. Progesterone at a concentration more than 100-fold higher than dexamethasone failed to affect the induction of ACE significantly. Steroids without glucocorticosteroid activity tended to depress cellular concentrations of ACE below control levels when used in the absence of a glucocorticosteroid inducer. Cyclic 3'5' AMP (0.1 mM) and cyclic 3'5' GMP (0.1 mM), indomethacin (2.4 μM) and vitamin D3 (5 μM) were inactive as inducers. Prostaglandin E2 (13 μM), and F2α (6 μM), angiotensin I (3 μM) and bradykinin (1.5 μM) were inactive. Prostaglandin E2 and F2α at concentrations 13-fold higher than dexamethasone failed to inhibit ACE induction by dexamethasone (0.45 μM).

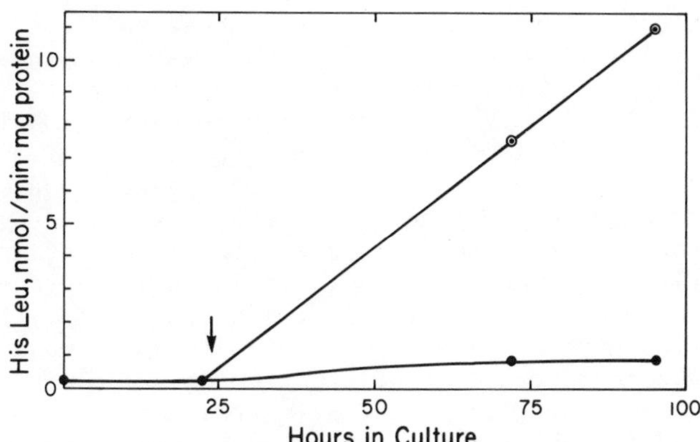

Fig. 1. Induction of angiotensin converting enzyme in rabbit alveolar macrophages by dexamethasone. All cultures contained 0.043% ethanol after 24 hr of incubation (arrow), at which time dexamethasone was added. (o) 0.45 μM dexamethasone; (•) control. (Reproduced from Friedland *et al.* (3).

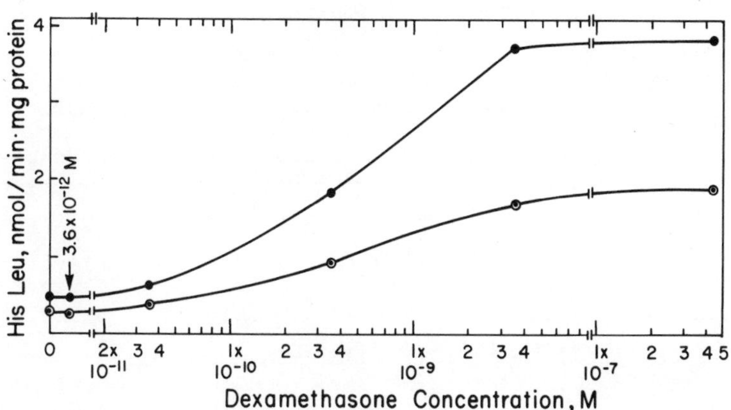

Fig. 2. Effect of dexamethasone concentration on the induction of angiotensin converting enzyme in rabbit alveolar macrophages. Dexamethasone was added after 22 hr of cell culture along with ethanol at a final concentration of 0.043%. (o) At 46 hr of cell culture; (•) at 70 hr of cell culture. (Reproduced from Friedland *et al.* (3).

The human monocyte normally contains only barely perceptible levels of ACE (Table IV). After 6 days in culture, however, a marked induction was evident. Glucocorticosteroid and autologous serum potentiated the induction, which was as high as at least 700-fold. Human lymphocytes did not appear to be induced for ACE (Table V) but were required for substantial ACE induction in monocytes. The level of ACE achieved in the cultured monocytes varied directly with the number of lymphocytes cultured with them. In preliminary experiments a soluble factor elaborated by cultured lymphocytes could substitute for lymphocytes in promoting ACE induction in cultured human monocytes. The catalytic properties of monocyte ACE were as expected for lung ACE (Table VI). The molecular properties of human serum, monocyte, lung and monocyte culture medium ACE as revealed by polyacrylamide gel electrophoresis, sepharose 6B gel filtration and trypsin treatment were similar to those described for the rabbit system, suggesting that the enzyme exists in a larger cellular particulate form which is susceptible to protease cleavage to a smaller soluble form similar to that present in serum, monocyte culture medium and cell cytosol (minor form).

TABLE IV

Angiotensin Converting Enzyme Activity in Monocytes in Cultures[a]

	No serum		20% Serum	
	Control	Dexamethasone	Control	Dexamethasone
	Cells, nMols min^{-1} mg $protein^{-1}$			
Initial	0.12	0.12	0.12	0.12
6 days attached	7.25	17.6±0.1[b]	8.3±1.0	24.3±6.2
6 days unattached	0.03	6.4±2.4	0.76±0.31	3.9±0.5
	Total (cells + medium), nMol min^{-1} $culture^{-1}$			
Initial	0.02	0.02	0.02	0.02
6 days	0.70	1.61±0.10	3.24±0.37	5.08±0.86

[a] 1×10^7 cells/plate. See Friedland, *et al.* (20) for experimental details. (By permission of Biochemical and Biophysical Research Communications.)

[b] Standard error of the mean.

TABLE V

Angiotensin Converting Enzyme Activity in Lymphocytes in Culture[a]

Treatment	Time in Culture (hr)	Enzyme Activity nMol min^{-1} mg $protein^{-1}$ ±SEM
None	0	0
None	89.5	0.50±0.09, n=3
0.45 μM dexamethasone	89.5	0.38±0.12, n=3

[a] 4×10^6 non-adherent lymphocytes were cultured in test tubes in 2 ml of RPMI 1640 containing 15% autologous serum at 37 C in 5% CO_2. Dexamethasone or ethanol vehicle alone were added for the last 66.5 hr of culture. See Friedland *et al*. (4) for experimental details (By permission of Biochemical and Biophysical Research Communications).

Our investigations have indicated that mononuclear phagocytes are under exquisite control for ACE synthesis. They normally contain only minute levels, but are capable of a vastly increased synthesis in response to appropriate signals *in vitro* and pathologically *in vivo* in such conditions as sarcoidosis and Gaucher's disease. Lymphocytes and their secretory products, glucocorticosteroids, and possibly other serum factors appear to exert significant control over ACE synthesis in mononuclear phagocytes.

ACE appears to have an important function in the conversion of the biologically inactive peptide angiotensin I to the biologically potent octapeptide angiotensin II, and in inactivating the vasodepressor peptide bradykinin (2). It has been assumed that these molecular transformations take place predominantly at endothelial cell surfaces where the enzyme has been ultrastructurally localized in the rabbit (10). ACE has now been shown to be an inducible enzyme in the mononuclear phagocytic system which pervades the entire organism. The marked nature of the induction and its exquisite control suggests a physiological function which remains to be elucidated. Perhaps ACE in this system may have a role in cellular defense, inflammation and tissue catabolism and in specific transformations of biologically active peptides which are known as well as those yet to be discovered.

ACKNOWLEDGEMENTS

This work was supported in part by grants from the National Institutes of Health, United States Public Health Service.

REFERENCES

1. Cushman, D. W. and Cheung, H. S., Biochem. Pharmacol., 20 (1971) 1637.
2. Friedland, J., Drooker, M., Setton, C. and Silverstein, E., Clinical Research,26 (1978) 634A.
3. Friedland, J., Setton, C. and Silverstein, E., Science, 197 (1977) 64.
4. Friedland, J., Setton, C. and Silverstein, E., Biochem. Biophys. Res. Commun.,83 (1978) 843.
5. Friedland, J. and Silverstein, E., Am. J. Clin. Path., 66 (1976) 416.
6. Friedland, J. and Silverstein, E., Fed. Proc. 37 (1978) 1332.
7. Gordon, S. and Werb, Z., Proc. Natl. Acad. Sci. USA, 73 (1976) 872.
8. Lieberman, J., Am. J. Med. 59 (1975) 365.
9. Lieberman, J. and Beutler, E., N. Engl. J. Med., 294 (1976) 1442.
10. Ryan, U. S., Ryan, J. W., Whitaker, C. and Chiu, A., Tissue and Cell 8 (1976) 125.
11. Silverstein, E., Med. Hypoth. 2 (1976) 75.
12. Silverstein, E. and Friedland, J., Clin. Chim. Acta 74 (1977) 21.
13. Silverstein, E., Friedland, J., Kim, D. S. and Pertshuk, L. P., Sarcoidosis pathogenesis. Mechanism of angiotensin converting enzyme elevation: epithelioid cell localization and induction in macrophages and monocytes in culture, In: Eithth International Conference on Sarcoidosis and Other Granulomatous Disorders, Cardiff, abstract, Proceedings (1978) 25 in press.
14. Silverstein, E., Friedland, J., Kitt, M. and Lyons, H. A., Isr. J. Med. Sci., 13 (1977) 995.
15. Silverstein, E., Friedland, J. and Lyons, H. A., Isr. J. Med. Sci. 13 (1977) 1001.
16. Silverstein, E., Friedland, J., Lyons, H. A. and Gourin, A., Proc. Natl. Acad. Sci. USA 73 (1976) 2137.
17. Silverstein, E., Friedland, J. and Setton, C., Isr. J. Med. Sci. 14 (1978) 314.
18. Silverstein, E., Friedland, J. and Vuletin, J. C., Am. J. Clin. Path. 69 (1978) 467.
19. Soffer, R. L., Annu. Rev. Biochem. 45 (1976) 73.
20. Unanue, E. R., Am. J. Path. 83 (1976) 396.

EFFECT OF PROTEINASES ON EA (IgG)-BINDING RECEPTORS OF RAT MACROPHAGES

G. BOLTZ-NITULESCU and O. FÖRSTER

Institute of General and Experimental Pathology
University of Vienna
Vienna (AUSTRIA)

Reports about the proteinase sensitivity of macrophage receptors for IgG (Fc-receptor) are equivocal. Sorkin (10) studying binding of cytophilic antibody to rabbit splenic macrophages found the binding diminished after treatment with proteolytic enzymes. Other authors, however, found an enhanced (1, 2) or unchanged (4, 7, 9) Fc-receptor activity after proteinase treatment of macrophages from various species. On mouse macrophages 2 different Fc-receptors for rabbit IgG were reported, 1 for aggregated IgG being trypsin resistant, another for monomeric mouse IgG_{2a} being sensitive to digestion by trypsin (3, 11).

In most of these studies the conditions were restricted to a single concentration of enzyme and 1 time of incubation. These conditions, however, varied from author to author. Therefore, the results obtained by different investigators are not really comparable. The aim of our study was to clarify whether variations in the conditions of incubation of macrophages with proteolytic enzymes could account for differences in their effect on Fc-receptors.

MATERIALS AND METHODS

Macrophages. Alveolar (AM) and peritoneal (PM) macrophages were obtained from male rats of a Sprague-Dawley deprived strain (Him:OFA(SPF)) 4 days after intraperitoneal injection of 10 ml 10% proteose-peptone by bronchial or peritoneal lavage with Hanks-BBS containing 0.25% Na_2-EDTA and 5% FCS. After incubation of the cells (1×10^6/ml) in Hepes buffered RPMI 1640 medium (Flow Laboratories) + 10% FCS in plastic Petri dishes (Nunclon, A/S Nunc, Roskilde, Denmark) for 1 hr at 37 C in 95% air + 5% CO_2 non-adherent cells were removed and adherent cells collected with a rubber policeman, washed 3 times in RPMI 1640 and suspended to 2 x 10^6 cells/ml. The cells consisted of more than 98% macrophages as tested by morphology and nonspecific esterase staining. The viability of AM was always higher than 80%, of PM 50-80%.

Enzymes and inhibitors. The following preparations were used: bovine pancreatic trypsin, TPCK treated, lyophilized, 2.0 U/mg or 3.5 U/mg (Merck); bovine pancreatic δ-chymotrypsin, TLCK treated, lyophilized, 45 U/mg (Merck), pronase E, lyophilized, 70000 PUK/g (Merck); trypsin inhibitor from soy bean (SBI) (Merck); cycloheximide (Sigma).

Enzyme treatment of macrophages. AM and PM were used in a final solution of 2 x 10^6 cells/ml in hepes-buffered RPMI 1640 without FCS. Enzymes were dissolved in the same medium and added to the cell suspension at the desired concentration, followed by incubation at 37 C. At the end of the incubation period the enzyme activity was stopped by addition of 15-20 volumes of cold (4 C) RPMI 1640 medium. When trypsin or chymotrypsin was used for digestion SBI in a concentration equivalent to the amount of enzyme was incorporated in the medium. The cells were then washed 3 times in cold medium, suspended to 2 x 10^6 cells/ml in RPMI 1640 + 10% FCS and used for the rosetting reaction. To inhibit resynthesis of receptor protein cycloheximide was added to a final concentration of 100 µg/ml in some of the experiments.

Anti-SRBC-IgG. A pooled rabbit antiserum against boiled sheep erythrocyte (SRBC) stromata (Anti-Forssman-serum), dialyzed against 50 mM ethylenediamineacetate buffer, pH 7.2, was chromatographed on a QAE-Sephadex column (Pharmacia, Uppsala, Sweden) equilibrated with the same buffer. The protein containing fractions eluted with starting buffer were pooled, concentrated and dialysed against phosphate buffered saline, pH 7.2 (PBS). This preparation contained pure IgG as tested by immunoelectrophoresis and antiglobulin reaction. The final preparation had a hemagglutinating titer of 1:200 against a 2% SRBC-suspension.

EA-rosetting reaction of macrophages. Equal volumes of a 2% suspension of washed SRBC in PBS and subagglutinating dilutions of anti SRBC-IgG were mixed and left at room temperature for 30 min. Two different concentrations of antibody, 1:400 and 1:3200, were used, yielding highly sensitized (HS) and lowly sensitized (LS) SRBC. Sensitized SRBC (EA) were washed 3 times in RPMI 1640 medium + 10% FCS and finally suspended in this medium to a concentration of 1% 0.2 ml macrophage suspension (2 x 10^6/ml) was mixed with 0.2 ml 1% EA in Kahn tubes, centrifuged at 150xg for 2-3 min, and kept on ice overnight. Immediately after removal from the ice bath the tubes were rotated at 22 rpm for 1 min, 1 drop of cell suspension was stained with toluidine blue and

TABLE I

Effect of Trypsin Treatment on EA (IgG)-Binding of Rat Macrophages (% RFC)

Source of Macrophage	Sensitivity of SRBC	Incubation Time (min)	Trypsin Concentration (mg/ml)				
			-	0.1	1.0	2.5	5.0
AM	HS	0	80	0	0	0	0
		5-15[a]	-	98	98	97	97
		30	82	98	97	86	80
		300	79	84	75	49	37
AM	LS	0	60	-	-	-	-
		5-15	-	95	93	90	84
		30	61	93	78	65	49
		300	59	82	65	46	32
PM	HS	0	79	-	-	-	-
		5-15	-	90	92	87	86
		30	81	84	81	76	72
		300	79	69	54	36	22
PM	LS	0	9	-	-	-	-
		5-15	-	38	41	40	35
		30	9	35	28	27	21
		300	7	29	21	19	15

[a]Highest percentage of RFC observed at 5, 10 or 15 min of incubation

mounted on siliconized glass slides with cover slips sealed with paraffin wax. The slides were kept on ice until counting the rosettes under the microscope. All macrophages binding 3 or more SRBC were counted as rosette forming cells (RFC).

RESULTS

Before incubation with proteolytic enzymes AM bound 70-90% of HS-SRBC, but only 60-80% of LS-SRBC, PM bound 60-80% of HS-SRBC, but only 8-20% of LS-SRBC.

Trypsin treatment. Incubation of both AM and PM with high doses of trypsin over a period of 5 hr showed a biphasic response (Table I). An early enhancement was followed by loss of Fc-receptor activity. This loss was most evident when the untreated macrophage population contained a high percentage of RFC (AM rosetting with HS- and LS-SRBC, PM with HS-SRBC). When the initial number of RFC was low, as was the case with PM-rosetting with LS-SRBC, an enhancement could be observed at all doses of trypsin even after 5 hr treatment. The same was true when AM were treated with a low dose of trypsin (0.1 mg/ml). Even in these instances, however, some decrease of Fc-receptor activity was observed as compared to the peak of RFC in the early phase of enzyme-treatment. While the degree of enhancement was approximately the same with all doses of trypsin, a dose-dependency could be observed in the second phase leading to decrease of receptor activity.

δ-chymotrypsin-treatment. Similarly to trypsin, treatment of rat macrophages with δ-chymotrypsin leads to an early enhancement of Fc-receptor activity, which is similar in extent at all doses studied (Table II). The subsequent decrease in number of RFC, however, is slower than with trypsin mainly when the effect of high doses of the enzymes are compared. Therefore, the dose dependency of the loss of receptor activity is less pronounced than with trypsin and only in some instances the percentage of RFC is significantly below the control level after 5 hr incubation (e. g., AM and LS-SRBC at 2.5 and 5.0 mg/ml chymotrypsin, PM and HS-SRBC at all doses).

Effect of cycloheximide on the degradation of Fc-receptor activity by trypsin and chymotrypsin. To prevent possible resynthesis of a protein essential for Fc-receptor activity during digestion with proteolytic enzymes, cycloheximide (100 μg/ml) was added (Table III). The reduction of RFC by both trypsin and chymotrypsin was much faster when cycloheximide was present. With both enzymes the number of RFC was below 10% in all experiments after 4 hr incubation.

Pronase-treatment. In these experiments only binding of HS-SRBC was studied. When AM or PM were incubated with pronase, a dose dependent loss of EA-binding activity was observed. This loss was much faster than that seen with trypsin or chymotrypsin in the later phases of incubation, even when cycloheximide was added to those enzymes. The initial rate of receptor disappearance was higher for AM than for PM in most experiments. After 2 hr the percentage of RFC was reduced to less than 10% with both AM and PM incubated with 1.4 mg/ml pronase (Table IV). An early phase of enhancement of Fc-receptor activity could rarely be observed with pronase digestion.

When macrophages after depletion of Fc-receptors by 90 min

TABLE II

Effect of δ-Chymotrypsin Treatment on EA (IgG)-Binding of Rat Macrophages (% RFC)

Source of Macrophage	Sensitivity of SRBC	Incubation Time (Min)	δ-Chymotrypsin Concentration (mg/ml)				
			-	0.1	1.0	2.5	5.0
AM	HS	0	85	-	-	-	-
		5-120[a]	-	96	98	100	99
		180	87	95	92	90	89
		300	81	82	81	79	78
AM	LS	0	68	-	-	-	-
		5-120	-	90	96	95	90
		180	71	82	79	77	72
		300	70	71	67	65	62
PM	HS	0	79	-	-	-	-
		5-120	-	91	92	88	86
		180	79	84	79	77	75
		300	76	69	63	61	55
	LS	0	19	-	-	-	-
		5-120	-	67	76	75	69
		180	18	58	46	39	37
		300	16	47	36	28	18

[a]Highest percentage of RFC observed at 5, 10, 15, 30, 60 or 120 min of incubation

incubation with pronase (1.5 mg/ml) were washed and incubated in fresh medium RPMI 1640 containing 10% FCS, they rapidly regained receptor activity at 37 C, more slowly at 25 C. The rate of reappearance of Fc-receptor was higher with AM than with PM at both temperatures. AM attained the original level of activity at 2 hr, PM at 4 hr incubation at 37 C. No receptor activity reappeared at 15 C (Table V). Cycloheximide (100 μg/ml), when added to the incubation medium together with pronase, enhanced the rate of disappearance of Fc-receptor only slightly. The reappearance of receptor activity after depletion by pronase digestion (1.5 mg/ml, 90 min), subsequent washing and incubation in fresh RPMI 1640 medium + 10% FCS was effectively inhibited only when cycloheximide was present both during digestion and regeneration, not if added after digestion (Table IV).

TABLE III

Effect of Cycloheximide on Modulation of Fc-Receptors on Rat Macrophages by Proteolytic Enzymes (2.5 mg/ml) (% RFC)

Source of Macrophage	Sensitivity of SRBC	Incubation Time (Min)	Trypsin		δ-Chymotrypsin	
			-C[a]	+C[b]	-C	+C
AM	HS	0	88	88	82	82
		5-15[c]	97	94	96	95
		30	93	75	95	93
		120	69	25	87	75
		240	62	5	79	6
	LS	0	73	73	71	71
		5-15	90	88	88	87
		30	77	45	86	85
		120	61	18	77	57
		240	53	3	67	1
PM	HS	0	81	81	79	79
		5-15	88	87	93	89
		30	79	68	92	89
		120	67	29	78	48
		240	59	6	69	8
	LS	0	8	8	11	11
		5-15	44	42	43	41
		30	44	38	41	39
		120	36	16	33	11
		240	21	3	21	1

[a]No cycloheximide
[b]With cycloheximide (100 μg/ml)
[c]Highest percentage of RFC observed at 5, 10, or 15 min of incubation

DISCUSSION

While the sensitivity of the receptor of mouse macrophages for mouse IgG_{2a} has been clearly established (3, 11), Fc-receptors for other types of IgG and of macrophages from other species have generally been thought to be resistant to proteolytic enzymes

TABLE IV

Effect of Pronase Treatment on EA (IgG)-Binding Activity of Rat Macrophages (% RFC with HS-SRBC)

Pronase Concen-tration mg/ml	Source of Macro-phage	Incubation Time (Min) 0	15	30	60	120
0,125	AM	88	85	81	71	42
	PM	79	79	71	58	35
0,50	AM	88	81	70	62	13
	PM	79	65	57	53	12
1,5	AM	88	73	55	42	5
	PM	79	62	37	29	4
3,0	AM	88	48	29	15	3
	PM	79	53	22	12	2
None	AM	88	89	90	89	88
	PM	79	81	82	81	80

TABLE V

Reappearance of Fc-Receptor Activity (% RFC) After Depletion by Pronase (1.5 mg/ml, 90 min)

Source of Macrophage	Depletion Before	After	Incubation Tempera-ture (C)	Incubation Time (Min) 30	60	120	240
AM	75	8	37	34	46	72	n.d.
			25	20	30	38	58
			15	9	11	12	11
PM	61	3	37	8	28	41	58
			25	6	10	24	42
			15	3	5	5	5

TABLE VI

Effect of Cycloheximide (100 μg/ml) Added at Different Times on Recovery of Fc-Receptor Activity of Rat Macrophages (% RFC)

Source of macro-phage	Cycloheximide Present During		Digestion		Incubation Time (Min) Recovery Phase			
	Digestion	Recovery	Before	After	30	60	120	240
AM	-	-	81	6	43	57	64	76
	-	+	81	6	37	51	55	63
	+	+	81	2	10	9	7	6
PM	-	-	62	2	17	28	41	58
	-	+	62	2	16	27	38	45

(1-5, 7, 8, 9, 11). Only few authors reported about loss of receptor activity after proteinase treatment (6, 10). In some cases an enhancement of IgG-binding was observed (1, 2).

Our results show clearly that Fc-receptors for rabbit IgG are removed from rat macrophages by treatment with various proteinases. Pronase was the most active enzyme in this respect, trypsin and δ-chymotrypsin showed lower activity. These 2 enzymes regularly produce an increase of the number of rosette forming cells in an early phase of the incubation. When low enzyme concentrations were employed or when macrophages with low initial rosetting capacity (like PM with LS-SRBC) were used, this enhancement lasted during the entire period of incubation (5 hr).

The apparently lower activity of chymotrypsin compared to trypsin in reducing Fc-receptor activity seemed to be due to higher stimulation of receptor-resynthesis by this enzyme. When protein biosynthesis was blocked by addition of cycloheximide during the digestion, the number of RFC approached zero after 4 hr incubation with each of both enzymes.

Also, pronase digestion provided a strong stimulus for resynthesis of Fc-receptor. When receptor activity was almost completely removed by 90 min incubation of macrophages with pronase, and cycloheximide added after the enzyme had been removed, EA-binding activity reappeared at almost the same rate as when these depleted cells were incubated in medium without inhibitor. When cycloheximide, however, was present also during the digestion period, no receptor reappeared on the cell surface. This shows that sufficient receptor protein was synthesized during the digestion phase to almost completely replace the digested receptor. Incubation of macrophages with cycloheximide and without pronase up to 8 hr did not significantly alter receptor activity (data not shown). This suggests that turnover of Fc-receptors is low without addition of proteolytic enzymes.

When pronase was used to deplete Fc-receptor activity, the initial rate of depletion was lower for PM than for AM in most experiments. There seemed to be a lag phase before digestion of receptors on PM went into full speed. This suggests a difference between Fc-receptors on AM and PM, either structural (2 different receptors) or in the position of the receptor within the plasma membrane. In addition, the rate of resynthesis of Fc-receptor was slower on PM than on AM. These observations present additional features of receptor heterogeneity on different types of macrophages.

SUMMARY

Pronase, trypsin and δ-chymotrypsin deplete rat alveolar peritoneal macrophages of EA (IgG)-binding activity. Trypsin and δ-chymotrypsin show an initially - under certain conditions long lasting - enhancement of receptor activity. Cycloheximide, an inhibitor of protein biosynthesis, accelerated the loss of Fc-receptors and inhibited their reappearance. There are differences between alveolar and peritoneal macrophages in the rate of loss as well as of regeneration of Fc-receptors.

ACKNOWLEDGEMENTS

We wish to thank Miss Irene Kothbauer for technical assistance and Drs. Deitrich Kraft, Otto Scheiner and Helmut Rumpold for helpful discussions. This study was supported by Grant No. 3026 of the Austrian Research Council and by Grant No. 1170 of the "Jubiläumsfonds der Österreichischen Nationalbank."

REFERENCES

1. Arend, W. P. and Mannik, M. J. Exp. Med. 136 (1972) 514.
2. Davey, M. J. and Asherson, G. L. Immunology 12 (1967) 13.
3. Heusser, C. H., Anderson, C. L. and Grey, H. M. J. Exp. Med. 145 (1977) 1316.
4. Howard, J. G. and Benacerraff, B. Brit. J. Exp. Pathol. 47

(1966) 193.
5. Huber, H., Polley, M. J., Linscott, W. D., Fudenberg, H. H. and Müller-Eberhard, H. J. Science 162 (1968) 1281.
6. Knutson, D. W., Kijlstra, A. and van Es, L. J. Exp. Med. 145 (1977) 1368.
7. Lay, W. H. and Nussenzweig, V. J. Exp. Med. 128 (1968) 991.
8. LoBuglio, A. F., Cotran, R. S. and Jandl, J. H. Science 158 (1967) 1582.
9. Steinman, R. M. and Cohn, Z. A. J. Cell Biol. 55 (1972) 616.
10. Sorkin, E. Int. Arch. Allergy 25 (1964) 125.
11. Unkeless, J. C. J. Exp. Med. 145 (1977) 931.

ENDOTOXIN-INDUCED SAA ELEVATION IN THE MOUSE - LACK OF A ROLE FOR COMPLEMENT OR ACID PROTEASES

Y. LEVO[1], P. D. GOREVIC[2], P. CHATPAR[2], E. C. FRANKLIN[2] and B. FRANGIONE[2]
Department Medicine A, Hadassah University Hospital[1] Jerusalem (Israel)
New-York University Medical Center[2], New-York, New York (USA)

Amyloidosis is a disease characterized by widespread tissue deposition of abnormal proteins grouped under the name amyloid. The protein which characterizes primary amyloidosis is the AL protein which is the degradation product of immunoglobulin light chains; whereas, the one which characterizes secondary or experimental amyloidosis is the A protein which seems to be the degradation product of the recently defined serum protein SAA (16,17).

Many investigators have suggested, mainly, on the basis of histological and ultrastructural studies, that the reticuloendothelial system (RES) may play a major role in the pathogenesis of amyloidosis (8,19). These suggestions have been recently substantiated by the *in vitro* study of Lavie, Zucker-Franklin and Franklin (10). They observed that monocytes in culture degrade SAA by a two-step DFP-inhibitable mechanism in which AA is being produced as an intermediate.

Endotoxin is one of the most potent agents for the induction of murine amyloidosis (1), and its administration generates a greater than 100-fold increase in serum SAA within the 24 hr period following injection (11). Endotoxins are known to activate a variety of mediation systems such as the classical and alternative pathways of complement, coagulation and fibrinolysis and to induce the release of effector substances including proteolytic enzymes from platelets, neutrophils and the cellular elements of the RES (6,7,12). The amyloidogenic properties of endotoxin might be attributed to release and or modulation of proteolytic activities of the RES.

In this report, the effects of endotoxin on the generation

of SAA and acid proteolytic activity in the sera of injected mice will be presented.

RESULTS AND DISCUSSION

First, we studied the SAA generating effect of endotoxin in comparison with other amyloidogenic and nonamyloidogenic proteins in various strains of mice by a specific radioimmunoassay (15) (Table I). Regardless of strain or inducing agent, SAA level peaks at 18-22 hr and returns to baseline (<50 μg/ml) by 48 hr. Peak levels of SAA following subcutaneous injection of 300 μg Escherichia Coli endotoxin (lipopolysaccharide-LPS) were 615 μg/ml compared to those resulting from 25 mg casein - 292 μg/ml, bovine serum albumin (BSA) - 240 μg/ml, or ovalbumin 75 μg/ml. The generation of SAA by casein, BSA and ovalbumin might have been the result of endotoxin-like contaminants (3). Indeed, the pyrogen-free human serum albumin (HSA/USP) failed to raise SAA levels. It is not yet known whether the effect of endotoxin on SAA level reflects the release of a preformed precursor with rapid serum turnover or de-novo synthesis. It is of interest that endotoxin (LPS) fails to raise SAA levels in C3H/HeJ mice (7). These mice are resistant to the effects of LPS in vivo, and their macrophages as well as their B lymphocytes are unresponsive to its effects in vitro (18,20).

Next, we tried to purify SAA from endotoxemic sera. Mice were exsanguinated 18-24 hr following the injection of endotoxin, the sera were pooled, dialyzed against water, brought to a concentration of 10% formic acid and applied to a Sephadex G-100 column (9,17).

As seen in Fig. 1, the elution pattern of these sera differed from that of control, uninjected, mice by the appearance of two retarded peaks (A & B). These peaks were further purified on Sephadex G-75 and were found to have a molecular weight of 12,000 and 3,000 dalton determined by SDS polyacrylamide gel electrophoresis. Peak A, with an approximate yield of 1 mg/ml serum, was identified by N-terminal amino acid sequencing as SAA (9), whereas, peak B consisted of the 24-amino terminal residues of mouse serum albumin (Fig. 2). Albumin isolated from acidified endotoxemic sera (the product of peaks 1 & 2 of G-100 column, Fig. 1, purified by zone electrophoresis in starch medium) yielded a major sequence beginning with isoleucine which is homologous to the sequence of human and bovine albumin starting at position 25 (Fig. 2) (2,4). No sequence corresponding to that of intact albumin up to residue 25 was detected; hence, all albumin in acidified endotoxemic serum was cleaved at leucine-isoleucine to release the 24-residue fragment. This fragment corresponds to the "asp" fragment of albumin produced by pepsin digestion at pH 3.0 (13,14), thus, suggesting the generation of serum acid protease activity following

TABLE I

SAA Generation[a] by Amyloidogenic and Nonamyloidogenic Substances

Inducer	LPS	Casein	BSA	Ovalbumin	HSA	Saline
Amount injected	300 μg	25 mg	25 mg	25 mg	25 mg	0.5 ml
SAA level (μg/ml)	615	292	240	75	50	<50

[a]All substances were injected subcutaneously 18-24 hr prior to determination of serum SAA level by RIA.

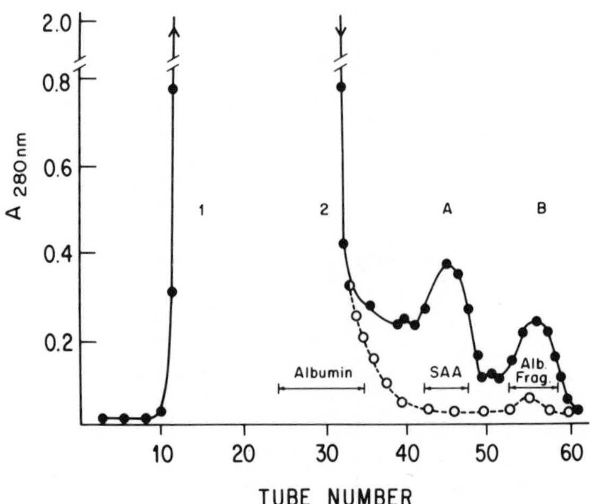

Fig. 1. Gel filtration on Sephadex G-100 of 7 ml serum dialyzed overnight against distilled water and diluted to a concentration of 10% formic acid just prior to application. Solid line (●——●) indicates the elution pattern of serum from groups of mice injected SC with 300 μg LPS and exsanguinated 18-20 hr later. Broken line (o- - -o) shows the elution pattern of equal amount of serum from control uninjected mice. Peaks 1 & 2 are composed mainly of IgG and Albumin; SAA elutes as peak A and the albumin fragment as peak B.

										10										20
HUMAN	Asp-	Ala-	His-	Lys-	Ser-	Glu-	Val-	Ala-	His-	Arg-	Phe-	Lys-	Asp-	Leu-	Gly-	Glu-	Glu-	Asn-	Phe-	Lys
BOVINE	—	Thr	—	—	—	—	Ile	—	—	—	—	—	—	—	—	—	—	His	—	—
MOUSE	Glu	—	—	—	—	—	Ile	—	—	( )	Asp-	( )	—	—	—	—	( )	His	( )	( )
FRAGMENT	Glu	—	—	—	—	—	Ile	—	—	—	Asp-	( )	—	—	—	—	—	His	—	—

				↓						30										40			
HUMAN	Ala-	Leu-	Val-	Leu-	Ile-	Ala-	Phe-	Ala-	Gln-	Tyr-	Leu-	Gln-	Glu-	Cys-	Pro-	Phe-	Asp-	Glu-	His-	Val-	Lys-	Leu-	Val
BOVINE	Gly	—	—	—	—	—	—	Ser	—	—	—	—	Gln	—	—	—	—	—	—	—	—	—	—
MOUSE	—	—	—	—	( )	—	( )																
FRAGMENT	Gly	—	—	—																			
ALBUMIN (-)					25 —	—	—	Ser	—	—	—	—	Lys	—	( )	( )	—	—	—	( )	—	—	—

Fig. 2. Amino terminal sequences of human, bovine and C57 BL/6 mouse albumins. These are compared to the amino terminal sequence of albumin isolated from acidified endotoxemic mouse serum by starch zone electrophoresis (Albumin-) and Peak A (Albumin Fragment). ↓ denotes the presumed point of cleavage by acid protease generated during endotoxemia.

TABLE II

The Effect of Enzyme Inhibitors and Decomplementation on Endotoxin-Induced SAA and Albumin Cleavage

	Saline	LPS	C5-Deficient Mice	CVF	Pepstatin		Leupeptin-Antipain	
					In Vivo	In Vitro	In Vivo	In Vitro
SAA								
RIA[a]	<50	615	600	1002	660	660	660	660
G-100[b]	-	+	+	+	+	+	+	+
Albumin fragment								
G-100[b]	±	+	+	+	-	-	+	+

[a]SAA levels (μg/ml) determined by RIA

[b]The presence (+) or absence (-) of SAA (Peak A) or albumin fragment (Peak B) assessed by chromatography on sephadex G-100 column.

the administration of endotoxin. The requirement of acid pH for the generation of SAA and the albumin fragment was established by the absence of peaks A and B when endotoxemic serum was chromatographed on G-100 under neutral conditions.

The acid proteolytic activity was further studied by various enzyme inhibitors. In vivo, pretreatment with pepstatin, a specific acid protease inhibitor, suppressed the appearance of the albumin fragment but had no effect on the generation of SAA. Albumin cleavage was also inhibited in vitro, by preincubation of endotoxemic serum with pepstatin. No inhibition was obtained with inhibitors of neutral proteases, i. e. antipain and leupeptin (Table II).

Since many of the biological effects of endotoxin are mediated via the activation of complement (6), we wanted to examine whether the endotoxin induced generation of SAA and acid proteolytic activity was complement dependent. Therefore, these effects were studied in a) congenital C5-deficient mice (CF1) and b) mice rendered C3-deficient by serial injections of Cobra Venon Factor (5). It was found that hypocomplementemic mice did not differ from normocomplementemic controls (Table II).

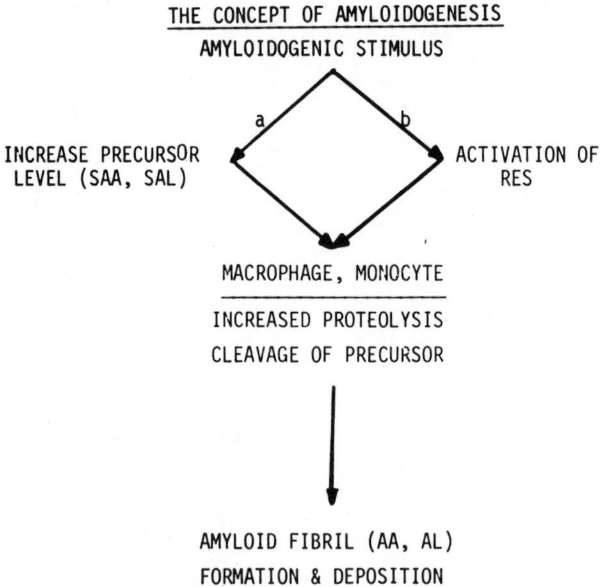

Fig. 3. Schematic representation of the suggested concept of amyloidogenesis (see text).

The present results show that administration of endotoxin, a most potent amyloidogenic substance, is associated both with a great increase in serum SAA level and with generation of serum acid proteolytic activity evidenced by albumin cleavage. These effects are unrelated to each other and are complement independent.

The dual effect of endotoxin, observed in the present study, might not only explain its amyloidogenic properties but also supports current concepts of amyloidogenesis in general.

According to this concept (Fig. 3) any amyloidogenic stimulus should have a dual effect, namely, a) it should increase amyloid precursor level (SAA, immunoglobulin light chain, or any other suitable protein) and b) it should enhance the degradative conversion of this precursor to the amyloid protein (AA, AL, etc.) presumably via direct activation of the RES. The amyloid protein, being produced in excess is then converted into fibrils which get deposited in the affected tissues and organs.

ACKNOWLEDGEMENT

This study was supported in part by USPHS Research Grants Nos. AM 01431, AM 02594 and AG 00458, The Irvington House Institute, The Michael and Helen Schaffer Fund and the Arthritis Foundation.

REFERENCES

1. Barth, W. F., Willerson, J. T., Asofsky, R., Sheagren, J. N. and Wolff, S. M., Arth. Rheum., 12 (1969) 615.
2. Behrens, P. Q., Spiekerman, A. M. and Brown, J. R., Fed. Proc., 34 (1975) 591.
3. Bito, L. Z., Science 196 (1977) 83.
4. Brown, J. R., Fed. Proc. 35 (1976) 2141.
5. Cochrane, C. G., Muller-Eberhard, H. J. and Aiken, B. J., J. Immunol. 105 (1970) 55.
6. Elin, R. J. and Wolff, S. M., Ann. Rev. Med., 27 (1976) 127.
7. Frank, M. M., May, J. E. and Kane, M. E., J. Infect. Dis., 128 (1973) S176.
8. Franklin, E. C. and Zucker-Franklin, D., Adv. Immunol. 15 (1972) 249.
9. Gorevic, P. D., Levo, Y., Frangione, B. and Franklin, E. C., J. Immunol. (1978) in press.
10. Lavie, G., Zucker-Franklin, D. and Franklin, E. C., Clin Res., 26 (1978) 517A.
11. McAdam, K. P. W. J. and Sipe, J. D., J. Exp. Med., 144 (1976) 1121.

12. McGevney, A. and Bradley, S. G., Fed. Proc., 36 (1977) 1052.
13. Peters, J., Jr., and Blumenstock, F. A., J. Biol. Chem., 242 (1967) 1574.
14. Peters, T. and Hawn, C., J. Biol. Chem 242 (1967) 1966.
15. Rosenthal, C. J., and Franklin, E. C., J. Clin. Invest., 55 (1975) 746.
16. Rosenthal, C. J. and Franklin, E. C., Recent advances in Clinical Immunology (Ed. R. A. Thompson) Churchill-Livingstone (1977).
17. Rosenthal, C. J., Franklin, E. C. Frangione, B. and Greenspan, J., J. Immunol. 116 (1976) 1415.
18. Ryan, J. L., Glode, L. M. and Nathan, C. F., Fed. Proc. 36 (1977) 1263.
19. Shirahama, T. and Cohen, A. S., Am. J. Pathol. 81 (1975) 101.
20. Sultzer, B. M. Infect. Immun. 5 (1972) 107.

DIFFERENTIAL EFFECT OF POLYCATIONS ON UPTAKE AND DESULPHATION OF HEPARIN

I. FABIAN, I. BLEIBERG and M. ARONSON

Department of Histology and Cell Biology, Sackler School of Medicine, Tel-Aviv University
Ramat Aviv, ISRAEL

Due to its potent anticoagulant effect, heparin is widely used both in the prevention and treatment of thrombosis (6). Since heparin is rapidly removed from the blood, continuous intravenous infusion of this material is required to maintain therapeutic blood levels.

Very little is known about the metabolic fate of heparin in the various body tissues. The uptake and desulphation of heparin by macrophages have been investigated recently in our laboratory (5). We have shown that heparin associated with histones, poly-amino-acids, protamine and eosinophilic basic protein is eliminated from the maintenance medium by mouse macrophages much more rapidly than is free heparin. The polyamino-acid-associated heparin was the most effectively eliminated. As is known, basic polyamino-acids are considered highly potent membrane agents which increase phagocytosis in leukocytes (2) and stimulate albumin uptake by tumor cells in culture (10). Their mode of action, however, is not clear although considerable importance is attributed to the electric surface charge in endocytosis (8). The possibility of membrane activation *per se* was also advanced. It was therefore deemed of interest to ascertain whether the increased heparin uptake by macrophages in the presence of polyamino-acids is due to the neutralization of the negative charge of the heparin molecule or, rather, to potentiation of the macrophage membrane.

In addition, the effect of various concentrations of serum on heparin uptake was investigated because it is known that heparin binds to various blood constitutents and that serum (in contrast to plasma) decreases the anticoagulatory activity of heparin (7). It has also been shown that serum albumin reduces latex uptake by polymorphonuclear leukocytes (PMN). Polystyrene latex spherules possess surface charges owing to sulphate groups originating from the method of preparation (1). The present communication deals essentially with the effect of polycations and serum on the uptake and desulphation of heparin by macrophages.

MATERIALS AND METHODS

N-sulphonate-^{35}S heparin (specific activity of 43.8 mCi/g) was purchased from Radiochemical Centre (Amersham, England). Before use the heparin was diluted with saline to 10 μCi/ml-1μCi/ml. Poly-DL-lysine HBr (mol. wt. 32,300) and poly-L-ornithine HBr (mol. wt. 20,400) were purchased from "Miles-Yeda", Israel. L-lysine monohydrochloride was purchased from Sigma Chemical Company (USA) and DL-ornithine monohydrochloride was purchased from Fluka A. G. (Switzerland).

Macrophage preparations from mice. Enriched macrophage suspensions were obtained by harvesting the peritoneal exudate of mice previously injected with 1 ml of 2.5% thioglycollate (Difco, USA). The collected cells (1.6 x 10^7 cells/mouse) were maintained in 10 cm Petri dishes in Medium 199 containing 15% calf serum and 2.5 x 10^7 cells were cultured in 10 ml of medium for 72 hr in a 5% CO_2 incubator before starting the experiments. The medium was replaced 24 hr after seeding. In the experiments designed to test the effect of serum on heparin uptake, the cells, following an initial 3 day incubation, were washed with Medium 199 and placed in maintenance medium containing 1/6M Na-lactate and M 199 (5:1) v/v or in M 199 + 15% or 30% calf serum. The cells were then incubated for 60 min at 37 C, following which heparin was added. Determination of heparin uptake and desulphation by cultured macrophages was carried out by a method previously described (5).

Preparation of cell extracts and enzyme assays. Cell extracts were obtained by a method previously described (4). Enzyme assay: the supernatant (1 ml comprising 3.2 x 10^7 cells) was used in the desulphation experiments together with 8.1 ml of 0.03 M sodium acetate buffer at pH 5.0 and 0.9 ml of a mixture of (^{35}S) heparin (1.2 x 10^6 cpm - 1.2 x 10^5 cpm) and 3 μg - 30 μg of poly-ornithine. After 24 hr of incubation at 37 C the amount of $^{35}SO_4$ was determined.

RESULTS

Uptake of heparin by cultured macrophages in the presence of polycations. Poly-DL-lysine and poly-L-ornithine and also monomers of the 2 were tested for their effect on the heparin uptake (during 24 hr) by macrophages. While there was but slight increase of

TABLE I

Uptake of Heparin in the Presence of Mono- and Poly-Amino Acids[a]

Amino-Acid Added	cpm
Heparin only	7,000 ± 250
L-lysine	11,000 ± 750
poly-DL-lysine	480,000 ± 27,000
DL-ornithine	10,800 ± 650
poly-L-ornithine	520,000 ± 40,000

[a]The reaction mixture contained ^{35}S heparin (1.2×10^6 cpm) and 30 μg of the various amino-acids. Incubation time: 24 hr.

heparin uptake in the presence of mono-amino acids, the polycations, in marked contrast, increased the heparin uptake by at least 30-fold and in some experiments by as much as 70-fold. A typical experiment run in triplicate is given in Table I.

The effect of reciprocal concentrations of heparin and poly-ornithine on heparin uptake. Uptake of increased amounts of heparin was tested in the presence of varying quantities of poly-ornithine. A typical table is given in Table II. Since the absolute values varied from one experiment to other, the results were not pooled. Each experiment served as its own control. Increasing the amount of heparin by 10-fold resulted in only slight (2-fold) increase of heparin uptake so long as the amount of poly-ornithine remained unchanged. If, however, both heparin and poly-ornithine were increased 10-fold, a corresponding 9-fold increase of heparin uptake by the cells was recorded. The highest uptake occurred when a constant ratio between heparin and poly-ornithine was maintained.

Effect of serum on heparin uptake by macrophages. Uptake of heparin was determined in the presence of various serum concentrations. It can be seen from Table III that serum has an adverse effect on heparin uptake, because in the absence of serum the amount of heparin taken up by the cells was about 10-fold that in the presence of 15% or 30% serum.

TABLE II

Uptake of Heparin in the Presence of Reciprocal Concentrations of Heparin and Poly-Ornithine[a]

Amount of Heparin (cpm)	Amount of Poly-Ornithine (μg)	cpm
1.2×10^6	30	80,800 ± 7,000
12×10^6	30	164,000 ± 25,000
12×10^6	300	700,000 ± 35,000
1.2×10^6	300	116,000 ± 9,500

[a]Results of 1 experiment done in triplicate. Incubation time: 2 hr.

TABLE III

Uptake of Heparin in the Presence of Various Concentrations of Serum[a]

Maintenance Medium	cpm
199 M + lactate	3100 ± 100
199 M + 15% calf serum	350 ± 50
199 M + 30% calf serum	300 ± 30

[a]Average of 2 different experiments done in triplicate. Incubation time: 60 min.

Desulphation of heparin by cultured macrophages and by macrophage extract. Previous results had shown that although the poly-amino-acids, histones and other polycations stimulated both heparin uptake and desulphation, the 2 processes were not related. In the presence of poly-ornithine there was marked increase in heparin uptake but a low rate of desulphation as compared to those in the presence of histone, which suggested the possibility that poly-ornithine inhibits heparin desulphation (5). Hence, it was deemed interesting to investigate the extent of inhibition of heparin desulphation in the presence of increasing amount of poly-ornithine. No corresponding increase in the release of ($^{35}SO_4^{=}$) occurred at 10-fold increased heparin concentrations (in the presence of a constant poly-ornithine concentration). Nor did increased inhibition of heparin desulphation occur upon 10-fold increase of the poly-ornithine concentration. Additionally, the process of heparin desulphation by macrophage extracts was also investigated. As shown in Fig. 1, poly-ornithine inhibited the release of ($^{35}SO_4^{=}$) from heparin and this inhibition occurred through the range of heparin-polycation concentrations studied.

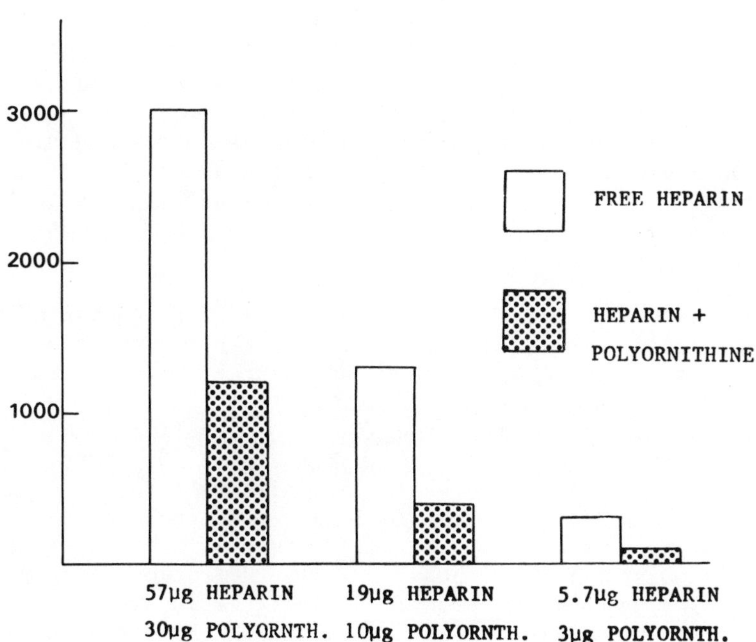

Fig. 1. Effect of poly-ornithine on desulphation by macrophage extracts. Results of 2 different experiments done in duplicate. Incubation time: 24 hr; uptake of (^{35}S) heparin (cpm).

DISCUSSION

The present study investigated the mechanism whereby poly-amino acids activate heparin uptake by macrophages. Poly-DL-lysine and poly-L-ornithine were found to accelerate heparin uptake to a much greater extent than the corresponding monomeric amino-acids. Our results are in agreement with those of Ryser and Hancock (10) and Deierkauf et al. (1), who found that poly-amino acids increase the uptake of negatively-charged molecules like albumin or latex particles by tumor cells and rabbit PMN, respectively.

Our experiments show that in order to obtain high heparin uptake, it is important to maintain a constant ratio between the heparin and poly-ornithine concentration. This finding suggests that at least where poly-ornithine is involved partial or complete neutralization of the negative charge of the heparin molecule rather than membrane stimulation is responsible for the uptake. Whether this is true also in the case of other polycations is now being investigated.

The decrease in heparin uptake in the presence of increasing serum concentrations indicate that the uptake is strongly influenced by 1 or more components of the maintenance medium, and that possibly heparin binds to some serum factors and thus becomes less available to the macrophages. Previous results have shown that poly-ornithine inhibits heparin desulphation by cultured macrophages. In the present study, increasing the amount of poly-ornithine did not result in additional inhibition of heparin desulphation. Presumably poly-ornithine being a charged molecule must become neutralized in order to be accessible to the cell in a manner similar to heparin. Hence, excess of the polycation was ineffective.

The discrepancy between the high uptake of the heparin-poly-ornithine complex and the low level of heparin desulphation merits some comments.

Our results suggest that the studied polycations inhibit the desulphation reaction, presumably by blocking $SO_4^{=}$ groups. This suggestion is supported also by the experiments with cell-free homogenates in which free heparin desulphated much faster than did the ornithine-complexed heparin. This result was obtained with different concentrations of heparin while the ratio of heparin to poly-ornithine was kept constant. Similar results were obtained in other experiments (unpublished data) in which increasing amounts of poly-ornithine were added to a constant amount of heparin. In these experiments the extent of inhibition was invariably proportional to the quantity of the polycation.

The metabolic fate of heparin in the body also deserves comment. It is now generally accepted that heparin functions as an anticoagulant by directly enhancing the inhibitory reaction which takes place between antithrombin III and the thrombin or factor Xa (7). There is also evidence that heparin binds to lysyl residues on the inhibitor (9). Such binding of heparin to lysyl residues is of considerable interest in that we have found poly-DL-lysine and poly-L-ornithine to accelerate mouse macrophage uptake of heparin from the incubation medium. The relatively brief sojourn of heparin in the blood has caused various investigators to speculate that heparin might be transferred to some extravascular compartment like the reticuloendothelial system (3) rather than be degraded enzymatically or eliminated via tubular secretion. Our findings lead us to suggest that in the vascular system heparin binds to cationic macromolecules and is subsequently removed by an active mechanism and, at least partly, by the cells of the macrophage system. The influence of antithrombin and other blood components on heparin uptake from the maintenance medium by cultured macrophages is now being investigated.

SUMMARY

Previous work has established that macrophages in culture release sulphate from heparin. We now report that increased uptake and desulphation of heparin occurred in the presence of polycations (poly-L-ornithine and poly-DL-lysine) and that the increase in heparin uptake was by about 30-fold. The desulphation was less related to uptake than to the nature of the bound polycation. Serum was found to have an inhibitory effect on heparin uptake while polycations inhibited heparin desulphation by macrophage extracts.

ACKNOWLEDGEMENT

This research was supported by the Chief Scientist Office, Ministry of Health, Israel.

REFERENCES

1. Deierkauf, F. A., Beukers, H., Deierkauf, M. and Riemersma, J. C. J. Cell Physiol. 92 (1977) 169.
2. DeVries, A., Salgo, Y., Matoth, A., Nevo, A. and Katchalski, E. Arch. Int. Pharmacodyn. 104 (1955) 1.
3. Estes, J. W. Curr. Therapeu. Res. 18 (1975) 45.
4. Fabian, I., Bleiberg, I. and Aronson, M. Biochim. Biophys. Acta 437 (1976) 122.
5. Fabian, I., Bleiberg, I. and Aronson, M. Biochim. Biophys.

(1978) In press.
6. Kakkar, V. V., Field, E. S., Nicolaides, A. N. and Flute, P. T. Lancet II (1971) 669.
7. Marciniak, E. J. Lab. Clin. Med. 84 (1974) 344.
8. Nagura, H., Asai, J., Katsumata, Y., Kojima, K. Acta Path. Jap. 23 (1973) 279.
9. Rosenberg, R. D. and Damus, P. S. J. Biol. Chem. 248 (1973) 6490.
10. Ryser, H. J. P. and Hancock, R. Science 150 (1965) 501.

THE PURIFICATION OF PLASMA MEMBRANES FROM GUINEA PIG PERITONEAL MACROPHAGES

G. CHAUVET, A. ANTEUNIS and R. ROBINEAUX

Centre de Physiologie et d'Immunologie Cellulaires,
INSERM U.104, CNRS and Ass.Cl.Bernard, Hôp. St-Antoine
Paris (France)

The plasma membrane undoubtedly plays an important role at the intracellular level as well as in the relationship of the cell with the surrounding environment. Therefore, it is of considerable interest to separate this membrane from other subcellular organelles before studying its specific function. The majority of mammalian cell membrane preparations described in the literature are generally obtained from organs, particularly the liver. Several authors have employed homogeneous cell suspensions (6). Nachman *et al*. (11) described a method for isolating plasma membranes from rabbit alveolar macrophages. It is known that macrophages participate in the defense of the organism, e.g. in inflammatory processes and in immune responses. The participation of the cell membrane in these biological phenomena is often recognized but ill-defined. Since we are interested in macrophage surface receptors, it is of great importance to work with purified membrane preparations. So we decided to initially develop a technique for the fractionation of guinea pig peritoneal macrophages, modifying the experimental procedure of Nachman *et al*. (11).

MATERIALS AND METHODS

Cell fractionation. Ten female "Hartley" guinea pigs weighing between 300 and 400g were intraperitoneally injected with mineral oil (15 ml/animal) three days prior to sacrifice. This was done in order to obtain an increased number of macrophages. Mineral oil was chosen after an ultrastructural study of macrophages performed in our laboratory (12). Animals were sacrificed by decapitation in the absence of anesthesia. Cells in the peritoneal cavity were recovered as described by Anteunis et al. (1) and were cultured in Roux bottles containing Earle-based Medium 199 (Institut Pasteur, Paris) supplemented with 5% newborn calf serum in an atmosphere of 5% CO_2 (about 10^6 cells/ml). After a 2 hr incubation at 37 C, the adherent cells were harvested and washed with phosphate-buffered saline. Light microscopy demonstrated that the vast majority of these cells was indeed macrophages. The yield was about 1 x 10^8 macrophages per guinea pig.

The following manipulations (Fig. 1) were all performed at 4 C. The cell pellet was homogenized in 26 ml of distilled water with three back-and-forth strokes in a Dounce homogenizer fitted with a tight pestle. An equal volume of 60% (w/v) sucrose was then added and 45 ml of this homogenate were gently layered on 36 ml of 45% (w/v) sucrose. After 40 min centrifugation at 200 g, the upper layer and a portion of the boundary were decanted and again layered on 36 ml of 45% sucrose. Centrifugation was performed as above. The two lower layers were successively harvested and combined to form fraction I. The upper layer was again decanted and diluted with distilled water to obtain a final sucrose concentration of 20% (w/v). In some experiments, 2 mg of digitonin was then added per 1 x 10^9 homogenized macrophages, i.e. per approximately 100 mg of protein, and was left in contact with the cell fraction for 15 min. An amount of digitonin stoichiometrically equivalent to cholesterol content increases the equilibrium density of plasma membranes in a sucrose gradient, as described for rat liver by Thinès, et al. (13). The cell fraction, whether or not treated with digitonin, was then immediately centrifuged at 20,200 g for 1 hr. The supernatant was recovered and named fraction II. The pellet was resuspended in 10% (w/v) sucrose in a Dounce homogenizer with a loose-fitting pestle and was called fraction III. Carefully, 4.8 ml of fraction III were layered on a linear 20 to 75% (w/v) sucrose gradient (1.6 ml of fraction per tube of Beckman SW 25.1 rotor), and centrifuged at 25,000 rpm for 4 hr. From each tube 18 equal volume fractions were then recovered by injecting a dense fluorinert solution in the bottom of the tube. A saccharimeter was used to measure the density of each fraction.

Biochemical analysis. The composition of fractions I, II and III as well as those of the linear gradient was defined with chemical and enzymatic determinations. The crude homogenate was also assayed in order to verify the recovery in each of the fractions analyzed. Inosine diphosphatase was measured according to Ernster et al. (8) and 5'-nucleotidase as described by Emmelot et al. (7). The technique of Beaufay et al. (3) was used to assay acid phosphatase. Succinic dehydrogenase determinations were performed according to Green et al. (9), with cytochrome C as electron acceptor. DNA was determined by means of the Burton method (4) and protein content as described by Lowry et al. (10)

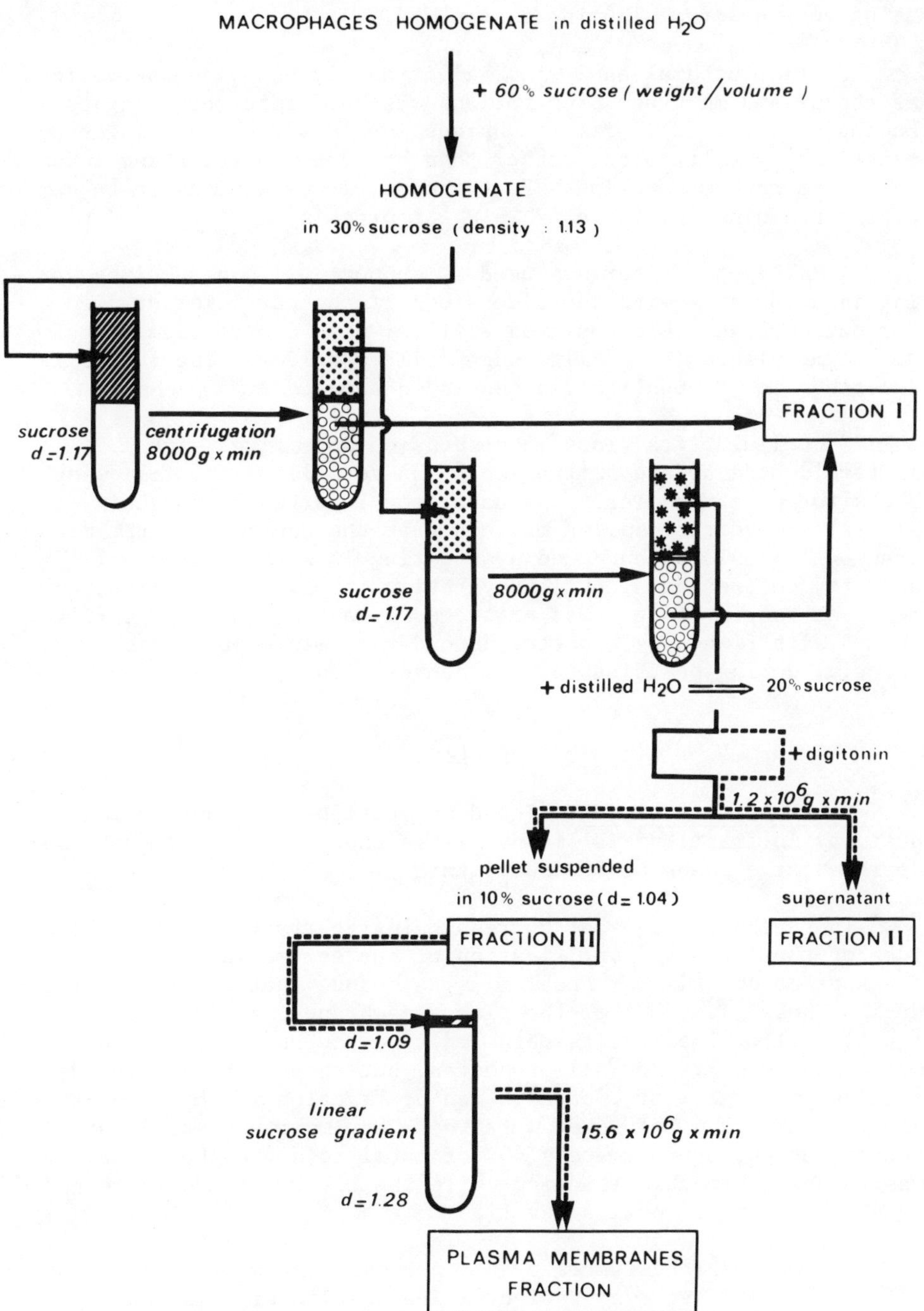

Fig. 1. Cell fractionation procedure.

using bovine serum albumin as standard.

Ultrastructural analysis. Electron microscopic observation of the plasma membrane preparations was performed according to Baudhuin *et al.* (2). This technique involves concentrating the fractions by filtration, rather than by centrifugation and leads to a true random sampling. Furthermore, it is applicable to samples containing as little as 25 μg of protein.

A Millipore filter was used as support, with pore sizes varying in accordance with the dimensions of the particles studied. For our membranes, we employed a filter with a pore diameter of 0.025 μm, placed in a "Filterfuge" filter holder. The latter is described in the publication mentioned above.

Subcellular fractions in suspension were fixed with 1.5% glutaraldehyde before filtration. The details of the following steps for electron microscopy have been reported by Baudhuin *et al.* (2). Nevertheless, we may add that the contrast of the membrane film could be enhanced by treating it with 0.5% uranyl acetate, before the alcohol dehydration steps. In addition, the membrane-bearing filter was protected by another Millipore filter coated with fixed erythrocytes in order to minimize losses of material during postfixation and dehydration.

RESULTS

Biochemical analyses. The distribution of 5'-nucleotidase activity in fractions I, II and III is shown in Fig. 2; the results represent the means of 12 experiments.

The height of the bar corresponding to fraction III gives an idea of the degree of purification of the enzyme in this fraction. The surface of this bar enables us to deduce that about 60% of 5'-nucleotidase, i.e. 60% of the plasma membranes, is located in fraction III. The results obtained from the assays of the other marker enzymes are not all presented, but they enabled us to determine the degree of contamination of fraction III by other cellular components. Lysosomes were the most important source of contamination, approximately 40% of total acid phosphatase activity was recovered in this fraction while the other enzymes represented only 20% of their total activities.

Plasma membranes were further purified by layering fraction III on a linear sucrose gradient. The results of this density equilibration experiment are shown in Fig. 3, where the ordinate represents the ratio of enzyme concentration to its initial concentration; the latter is calculated by dividing the total enzyme

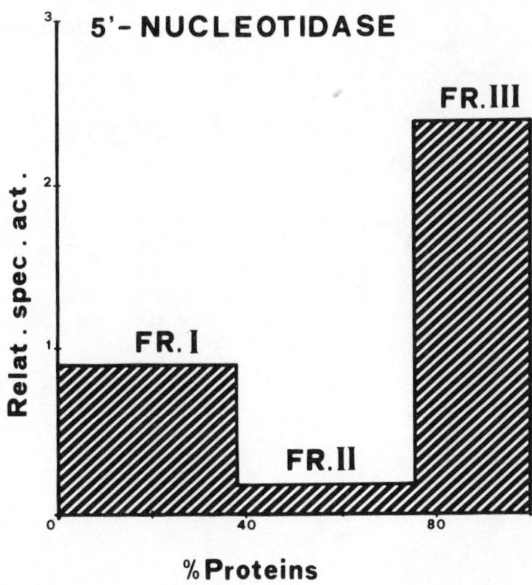

Fig. 2. Homogenate fractionation. With respect to the initial homogenate, the sum of 5'-nucleotidase activities recovered in the three fractions was 91%.

activity in the gradient by gradient volume. The abscissa represents the fractions in the order in which they have been recovered from lightest to heaviest.

The 5'-nucleotidase distribution resembles that of acid phosphatase, both enzymes equilibrate at median density of 1.14 g/cm^3. The low quantities of DNA, succinic dehydrogenase and inosine diphosphatase found in fraction III have different distributions in the gradient, with mean equilibrium densities greater than 1.14 g/cm^3. Lysosomes thus remain the major contaminant of our plasma membrane preparations.

Fig. 4 shows the distributions of 5'-nucleotidase and acid phosphatase activities in a linear sucrose gradient after a prior exposure of plasma membranes to a low concentration of digitonin as mentioned above. It can be seen that acid phosphatase again equilibrates at a median density of 1.14 g/cm^3, as in the experiments without digitonin, but that the 5'-nucleotidase peak is displaced towards higher densities: mean equilibrium density is now 1.16 g/cm^3. The distribution profiles of the other marker enzymes remain unchanged.

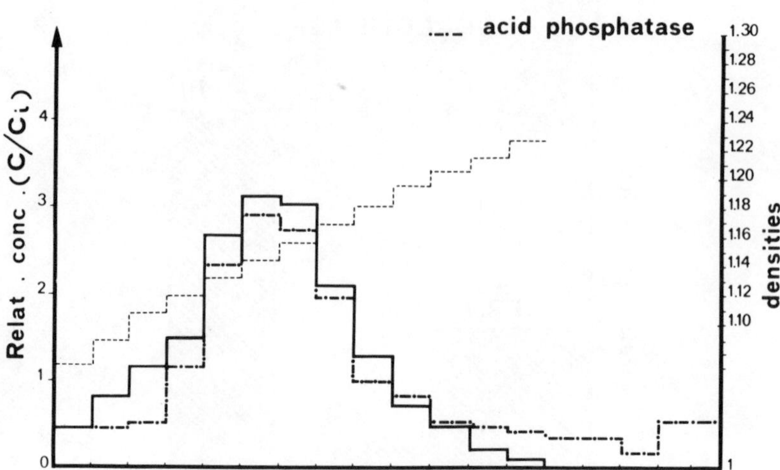

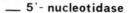

Fig. 3. Density equilibration of fraction III in a continuous sucrose gradient. The dotted line gives the shape of final density gradient after centrifugation 4 hr in SW 25.1 rotor. With respect to fraction III, the sum of activities recovered in the 18 fractions was respectively 86% for 5'-nucleotidase and 85% for acid phosphatase.

A more satisfactory purification of plasma membranes can thus be obtained by contact with an amount of digitonin stoichiometrically equivalent to that of cholesterol present in the cells.

Ultrastructural observations. A photomicrograph of the plasma membranes recovered in fraction III, without digitonin treatment, is shown in Fig. 5. It can be seen that they are contaminated, particularly by lysosomes. The membranes are predominantly in the form of large vesicles and the trilaminate aspect can be noted in several places. We can also observe cytoplasm adhering to these membranes.

Purified plasma membranes which have been exposed to digitonin (2 mg digitonin/10^9 macrophages) are shown in Fig. 6. No contaminating material could be detected after observing the entire surface and thickness of the membrane film (Fig. 6a). In comparison with the untreated membranes, those treated with digitonin exhibit structural changes: the membranes appear more rigid and

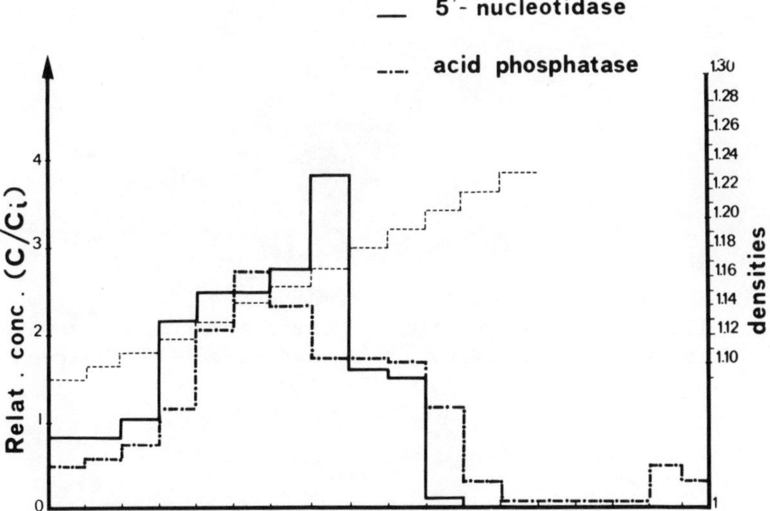

Fig. 4. Density equilibration of fraction III in a continuous sucrose gradient after digitonin treatment. With respect to fraction III, the sum of activities recovered in the 18 fractions was respectively 80% for 5'-nucleotidase and 90% for acid phosphatase.

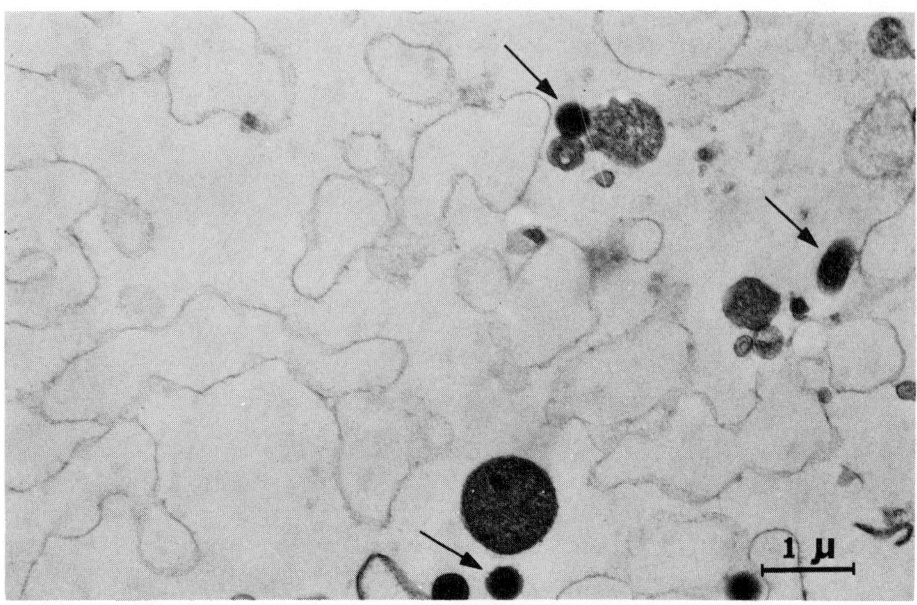

Fig. 5. Appearance of the plasma membranes collected from fraction III, without digitonin. These membranes are seen as large vesicles. Contamination by lysosomes can be observed (arrows).

take on an elongated shape. The trilaminate aspect is still visible, but the leaflets are dissociated and the membranes are often seen in the form of simple leaflets (Fig. 6b).

CONCLUSIONS

According to available data in the literature, alveolar macrophages are quite different from the peritoneal ones. In addition, Nachman et al.(11) worked with rabbits and not guinea pigs, and their animals were previously injected with BCG. We were thus led to modify their technique and the results obtained have been slightly different.

Thus, Nachman et al. (11) fixed their cells with glutaraldehyde before homogenization. According to these authors, 50 to 80% of the marker enzymes were destroyed by this treatment. They

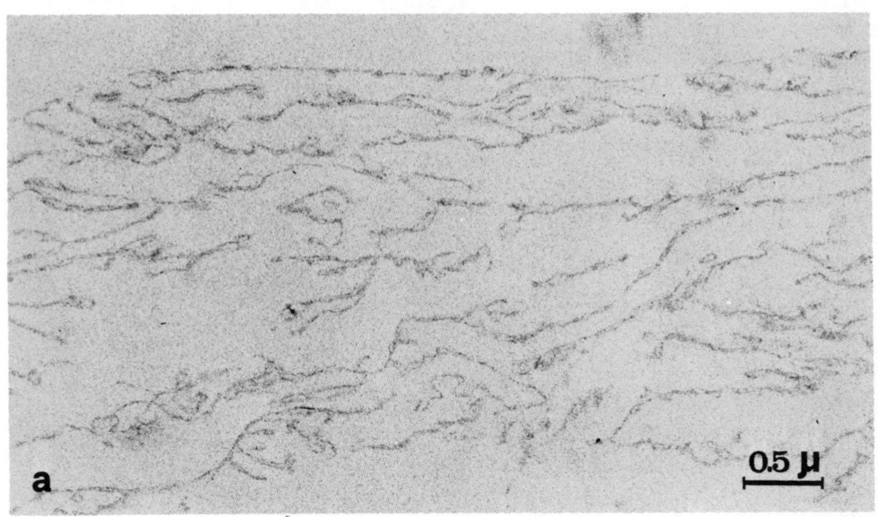

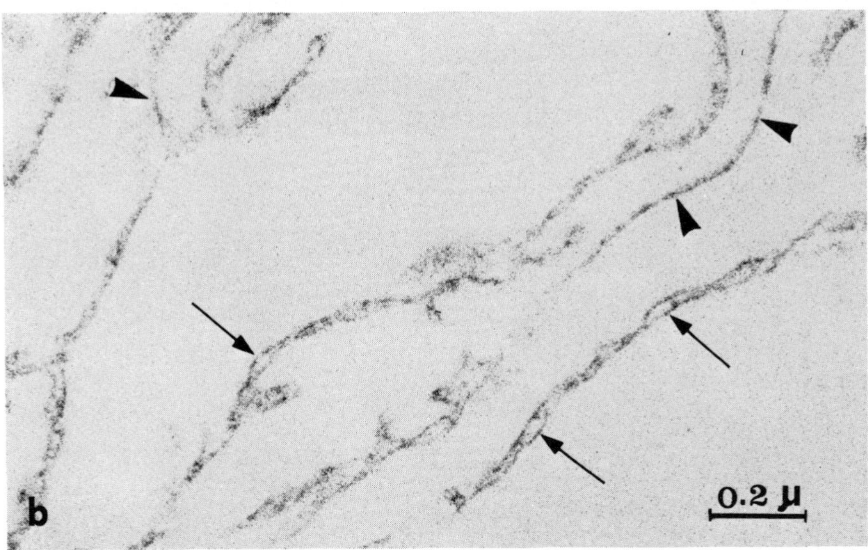

Fig. 6. Influence of digitonin treatment on the morphology of the plasma membranes fraction. a) in ultrathin section the membranes seem to be broken, presenting a rather rigid appearance. No contamination is observed over the entire thickness of the membrane film. b) detail of (a) showing spacing between the two leaflets of the plasma membranes (arrows); they are often seen as simple leaflets (pointers).

were forced to use glutaraldehyde, however, since rabbit alveolar macrophages require rather harsh conditions of homogenization. We also observed this deleterious effect of glutaraldehyde, especially on mitochondrial enzymes. Since guinea pig peritoneal macrophages are broken more easily, they were homogenized without prior fixation in order to retain intact the marker enzyme activities used to judge the purity of the various fractions.

Concerning the results obtained, whereas plasma membranes of rabbit alveolar macrophages equilibrate at a density of 1.20 g/cm^3 the membranes from guinea pig peritoneal macrophages were found at 1.14 g/cm^3. Since lysosomes also equilibrate at this density, we have exposed plasma membranes to a low concentration of digitonin in order to shift them towards a region of higher density. The amount of digitonin was determined after assaying the cholesterol content of our macrophages. We could thus eliminate a large proportion of contaminating lysosomes from our plasma membranes fraction.

Moreover, the representative nature of the ultrastructural technique used, enabled us to confirm the purity of the plasma membranes isolated.

Finally, we may note that our biochemical results are not reported as specific activities, but as histograms which is a more complete and faithful representation (5).

ACKNOWLEDGEMENTS

We wish to thank M. Auclair and M. Vial for their technical assistance, G. Develay for the accurate preparation of the micrographs and J. Dornic for the preparation of this manuscript.

REFERENCES

1. Anteunis, A., Robineaux, R., Bona, C. and Bernier, A., Ann. Inst. Pasteur 123 (1972) 69.
2. Baudhuin, P., Evrard, Ph. and Berthet, J., J. Cell Biol. 32 (1967) 181.
3. Beaufay, H., Bendall, D. S., Baudhuin, P., Wattiaux, R. and de Duve, C., J. Biochem. 73 (1959) 628.
4. Burton, K., J. Biochem. 62 (1956) 315.
5. de Duve, C., J. Cell Biol. 50 (1971) 20D.
6. De Pierre, J. W., and Karnovsky, m. L., J. Cell Biol. 56 (1973) 275.
7. Emmelot, P., Bos, C. J., Bennedetti, E. L. and Rümke, Ph., Biochim. Biophys. Acta 90 (1964) 126.
8. Ernster, L. and Jones, L. C., J. Cell Biol. 15 (1962) 563.

9. Green, D. E., Mii, S. and Kohout, P. M., J. Biol. Chem. 217 (1955) 55.
10. Lowry, O. H., Rosebrough, N. J., Farr, A. L. and Randall, R. J., J. Biol. Chem. 193 (1951) 265.
11. Nachman, R. L., Ferris, B. and Hirsch, J. G., J. Exp. Med. 133 (1971) 785.
12. Robineaux, R., Anteunis, A. and Bona, C., Ann. Inst. Pasteur 120 (1971) 329.
13. Thinès-Sempoux, D., Wibo, M. and Amar-Costesec, A., Arch. Int. Physiol. Biochim, 78 (1970) 1012.

CYTOLOGICAL CHARACTERISTICS OF BONE MARROW RETICULAR CELLS, TISSUE MACROPHAGES AND MONOCYTIC CELL LINE

M. KOJIMA and T. SATO

Department of Pathology
Fukushima Medical College
Fukushima (Japan)

The bone marrow consists of a loose stroma made up of a wide meshwork of reticular cells which are a supporting element closely related to bone marrow hematopoiesis, while fixed tissue macrophages also stretch their long cytoplasmic processes, participate in formation of the reticular mesh and show avid phagocytosis (3, 7).Together with the sinus endothelia these kinds of cells constitute the reticuloendothelial system of the bone marrow. In the reticular meshworks, there exist hematopoietic cells, including monocytic cells which also have phagocytic capacity (3). However, there is little or no precise knowledge regarding the relationship of these stromal cells and phagocytic cells.

This investigation was designed to make clear cytological characteristics of the reticular cells, tissue macrophages and monocytic cells, the nature and origin of the bone marrow phagocytic cells and relationship of the stromal cells to fat cells or fibroblasts.

MATERIALS AND METHODS

The materials used for the experiments were comprised of femur marrows taken from Wistar rats weighing 150 - 200 g and of bone marrows of rat fetus.

As for the perfusion fixation of rat bone marrows, the animals were injected into the abdominal aorta for 15 min with 1.5% glutaraldehyde in 0.067 M cacodylate buffer pH 7.4 containing 1% sucrose. The bone marrows harvested from the animals were cut into small pieces, fixed 2 hr in 1% OsO_4 in cacodylate buffer adjusted at pH 7.4, dehydrated in a graded series of ethanol and embedded in Epon 812.

As for the phagocytosis experiments, animals were injected with carbon (Günter-Wagner Co.), 16 mg/100 g body weight, into their tail vein and 30 min after the injection, bone marrows of these animals were fixed by the perfusion technique. In a group of animals administered with a large dose of carbon, similar injections were repeated 3 times at one day interval. Rats were injected in the tail vein with 0.1 ml/100 g or 0.35 ml/100 g of latex (0.81 μ) and were sacrificed 30 min and 24 hr after the injection for examination of their bone marrow.

Whole body irradiation with 1000 rad of Co^{60} was made on rats who had been injected with carbon through their tail vein and these animals were sacrificed 3 and 5 days after the irradiation.

For cytochemical demonstration of endogenous peroxidase activity, the bone marrows fixed by the perfusion technique were reacted for 60 min at room temperature in a medium with 0.1% DAB, 0.01 - 0.02% H_2O_2 and 0.05 M Tris-HCl buffer pH 7.6 containing 6% sucrose, according to the method of Daems _et al_. (2).

For tissue culture, femur or tibia marrows and peritoneal cells taken from Wistar rats, 150 - 200 g body weight, were used. Floating bone marrow cells (1×10^7/ml) were cultured for 2 hr in Leighton tubes and attached to the plastic cover slip according to the method of van Furth _et al_. (5). A part of the bone marrows examined was treated by 0.1% collagenase (Sigma Chemical Co. Type I 130 units/ml) for 30 min at 37 C. Cultivation of cells adhering to the cover slip contained by one month. For a comparison, peritoneal cells, 2×10^6/ml, were cultured in the same procedures.

For light microscopy, the materials were dried in air and stained with May-Giemsa staining. Enzyme cytochemically, acid phosphatase and naphthol AS-D chloroacetate esterase stains were employed. As for the detection of membrane receptors, IgGEA, IgMEAC and E rosette formation tests were done. In the phagocytosis experiments, carbon (0.1 mg/ml) or latex particles (more than 20/cell) were incubated 1 hr at 37 C in the culture medium with or without addition of serum. Up-take of ^{3}H-thymidine was tested according to the method of van Furth _et al_. (6); methyl ^{3}H-thymidine (specific activity 6.7 Ci/mmol NEN) 0.1 μCi/ml was added to the culture medium and incubated 2 hr. Radioautography was done on adhesive cells cultured for variable periods, after air drying and methanol fixation. Emulsion used was Sakura NR-M_2 and exposure time was 3 weeks.

For ultrastructural demonstration of endogenous peroxidase activity in cultured cells, bone marrow cells ($2 - 4 \times 10^7$/ml) were cultured in the plastic culture dish and attached to the dish wall, and the peroxidase activity was detected at 2, 6, 24 and 48 hr of cultivation according to the method of Bodel *et al.* (1) and Deames *et al.* (2).

RESULTS

Ultrastructural cell morphology. Reticular cells: This kind of cell distributed throughout the intersinus spaces of bone marrow, particularly around the venous sinuses and extended long slender, partly broad cytoplasmic processes in every direction among blood cells to connect with each other to form reticular meshworks. The reticular cells had a spindle, polygonal or ovid nucleus in their scant cytoplasm. Fine structurally, these cells somewhat resembled fibroblasts. On occasions, hairy projections were present in the cytoplasmic processes. Between the adjacent cytoplasmic processes, minor junctional apparatus was infrequently seen. In the cytoplasmic process or cytoplasm, a small number of bundles of fibrils were found and appeared in places to be collected densely just like minor dense patches. Similar bundles of fibrils were also found extracellularly, often attaching to the cell cytoplasm, but the bone marrow reticular cells never attached to or embraced any thick bundles of collagen fibers in their cytoplasm as seen in the reticulum cells of lymph nodes (3). In the fetal stage, similar reticular cells already developed forming loose reticular meshworks in the bone marrow anlage before the initiation of medullary hematopoiesis. Such fetal reticular cells contained abundant glycogen particles in their cytoplasm and possessed minor junctional apparatus between the cytoplasmic processes.

Tissue macrophages: These cells were also distributed throughout the bone marrow parenchyma and participated in formation of the reticular meshes in cooperation with the reticular cells by extending their cytoplasmic processes among blood cells to connect with the cytoplasmic processes of the reticular cells or tissue macrophages. Occasionally, the tissue macrophages were situated in the center of clusters of erythroblasts, a finding which has been named erythroblastic islands. The macrophages usually had a round nucleus in the copious cytoplasm which contained well-developed. Golgi complexes, rough endoplasmic reticulum, pinocytic vesicles. Variable sized phagosomes and phagocytic granules were found prominently. Between the neighboring cytoplasmic processes, minute junctional apparatus was also seen seldomly.

Monocytes: Monocytes existed within the reticular meshes formed by the above mentioned reticular cells and tissue macrophages and were freely round with a horseshoe-shaped and indented nucleus. The cell cytoplasm was relatively copious and contained well-developed Golgi complexes on the concave side of the indented nucleus. A number of round, oval or rod-shaped, electron-dense granules were dispersed in the cytoplasm which seemed to correspond to Azur granules. Numerous short cytoplasmic processes were projected from the cell surface.

Phagocytosis. The reticular cells, especially those situated near the venous sinuses, took up carbon particles as early as 30 min after intravenous (i.v.) injection of carbon, 16 mg/100 g body weight, to rats, but the degree of phagocytosis was very slight in these cells when compared with the phagocytic activity of sinus endothelial cells. Following repeated i.v. injection of carbon, the phagocytic capacity was not so increased in most of the reticular cells but reticular cells without ingested carbon particles were also found.

Shortly after a single i.v. injection of carbon, tissue macrophages showed slight phagocytosis of carbon particles which did not exceed the degree of phagocytosis of the sinus endothelial cells. After repeated i.v. injection of carbon, however, most of the tissue macrophages were stuffed with carbon particles and swollen by taking actively up the injected carbon and occasional swollen macrophages became freely rounded. On the other hand, monocytes ingesting carbon particles were scattered in and around the venous sinuses, some of which were seen passing through the gaps of sinus endothelial cells and entering in the sinusal lumen. However, there were no ultrastructural transitions between monocytes and tissue macrophages.

No latex phagocytosis of these above-mentioned cells existing in the intersinus spaces was observed, because latex particles, 0.81 μ in diameter, are too large to pass through the sinus wall to enter the intersinus spaces of bone marrow.

Endogenous peroxidase activity. In the tissue macrophages, endogenous peroxidase activity was demonstrated in the perinuclear cistern and rough endoplasmic reticulum, but the reticular cells showed no localization of endogenous peroxidase activity in these organelles. In monocytes, localization of endogenous peroxidase activity was confined to intracytoplasmic granules but it is not proved in the perinuclear cistern and rough endoplasmic reticulum. Similar localization pattern of this enzyme activity was also confined in immature monocytes in mitosis.

Co^{60} irradiation. After whole body irradiation of rats with 1000 rad of Co^{60}, rat cells appeared rapidly in the bone marrow of the irradiated animals. Rats which had already been injected i.v. with carbon prior to the irradiation were sacrificed 3 and 5 days after the irradiation, and the bone marrow from them was examined. As the results, many small fat droplets appeared in the cytoplasm of the reticular cells with a small amount of ingested

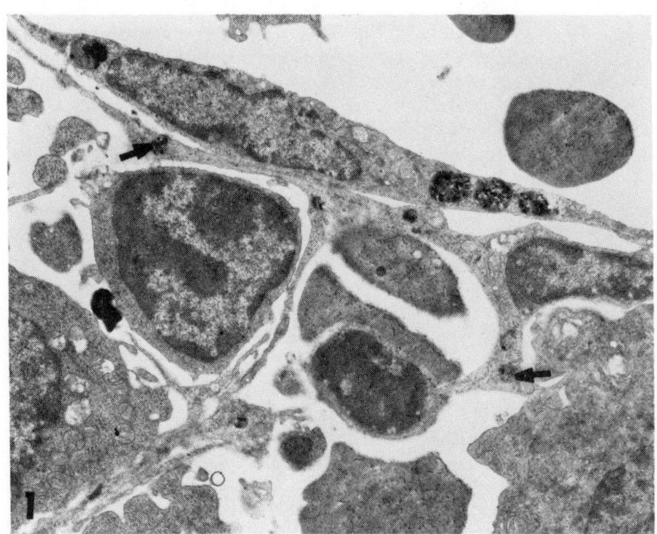

Fig. 1. Reticular cell situated beneath the venous sinus. In the long cytoplasmic processes, a small amount of carbon (two arrows) is ingested, 30 min after carbon injection (X 3,000).

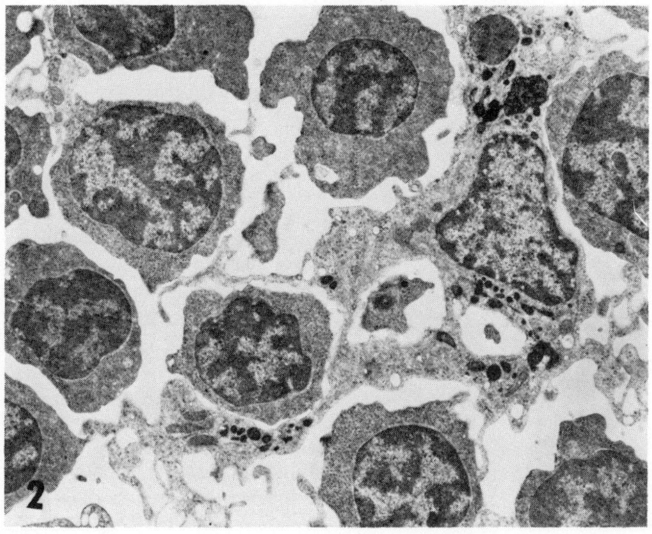

Fig. 2. Tissue macrophages exhibiting avid phagocytosis are surrounded by erythroblasts (X 2,500).

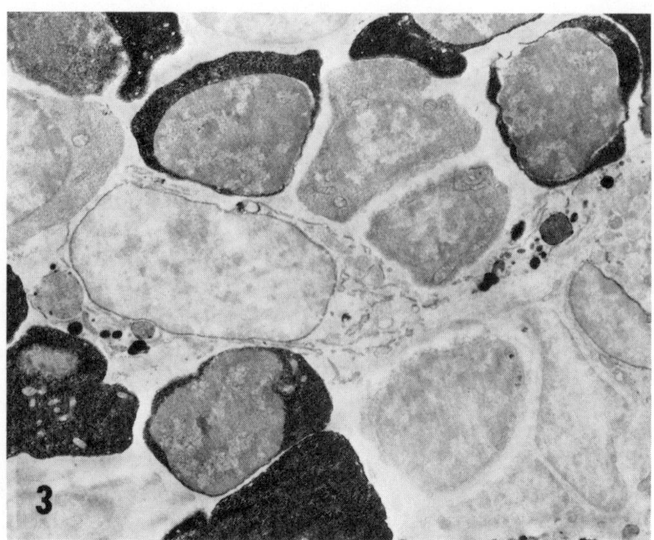

Fig. 3. Tissue macrophages. Endogenous peroxidase activity is found in the perinuclear cistern and rough endoplasmic reticulum. (Unstained X 2,500).

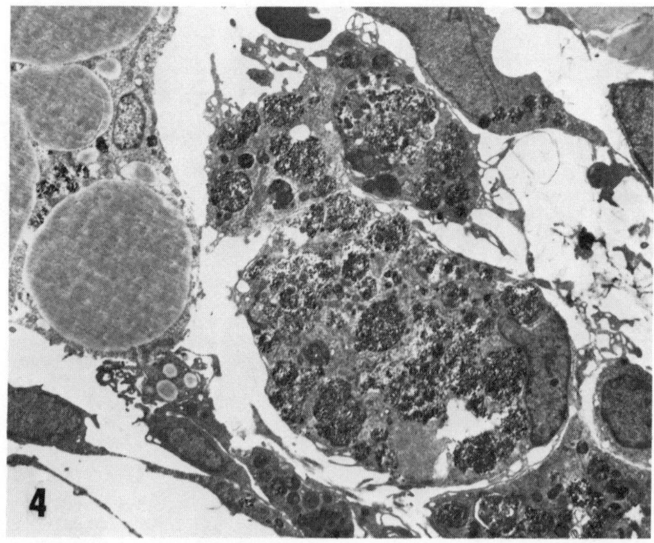

Fig. 4. 5 days after the Co^{60} irradiation, small amount of carbon is ingested in the fat cells and tissue macrophages become freely rounded, vigorously ingesting carbon particles (X 1,300).

carbon particles and simultaneously the rough endoplasmic reticulum became well developed. Many of these cells were rapidly transformed into mature fat cells. In such reticular cells and mature fat cells, endogenous peroxidase activity was observed in the perinuclear cistern and rough endoplasmic reticulum, as well as around the fat droplets. On the other hand, tissue macrophages became freely rounded and displayed vigorous phagocytosis of carbon particles. A small number of fat droplets also appeared in the cytoplasm of the macrophages but these cells did not transform into fat cells. Bone marrow monocytes were highly radiosensitive and were rapidly reduced in number and disappeared after the irradiation.

Tissue culture. At 2 hr of cultivation, monocytic cells were counted 50 - 70% of total bone marrow cells which adhered to the plastic cover slip. In the remaining 30 - 50% of the cultured adhesive cells, granulocytic cells, erythroblast, lymphocytes and megakaryocytes were included, all of which gradually disappeared with the time when the culture experiments continued further. Besides these various cells, a small number of tissue macrophages and reticular cells were observed.

Reticular cells: Adhering to the plastic cover slip, a small number of cells with a scant cytoplasm and long slender, dendritic cytoplasmic processes were found, some of which stretched their processes among blood cells when situated in blood cell clusters. These cells were about 8 - 10 μ in transverse axis with a round or ovoid nucleus. The extended cytoplasmic processes measured approximately 34 - 86 μ in length. In the culture experiment of bone marrows taken from the animals previously injected i.v. with carbon, it was shown that phagocytosis of carbon particles was weaker in this kind of cells than the tissue macrophages or monocytes. Based on the cell morphology and phagocytic activity, these cells seemed to be correspond to the reticular cells of bone marrow described in the preceeding section of cell morphology. Such reticular cells were less than 0.1% of the total adhesive cells in the early stage of cultivation and were slightly increased in number after the treatment with collagenase. With the lapse of cultivation time, the cytoplasm of these cells gradually appeared more abundantly, their nucleus became more rounded with appearance of one to a few nucleoli and with increasing basophilia of the cytoplasm, and mitosis was also often found in them. By the first week, these appeared small clusters of spindle cells transformed from the reticular cells. One month later, spindle cells predominated except certain numbers of remaining macrophages. From the second week, varying numbers of fat droplets began to be developed in the cytoplasm of reticular cells and transformation of these cells into fat cells was confirmed.

As for the membrane characters, it was shown that the reticular cells lacked Fc and C_3 receptors and did not form E rosette on the cell surfaces. These cells could not take up any latex particles but showed a slight carbon phagocytosis. Acid phosphatase was weakly positive and naphthol AS-D chloroacetate was esterase negative.

Tissue macrophages: The macrophages adherent to the cover slip were large and mostly round and measured 21 - 65 μ in diameter. They contained mostly a round nucleus in the copious cytoplasm which stained pale or was finely vacuolated in May-Giemsa staining. Occasional macrophages were found to ingest blood cells in their cytoplasm. Some of tissue macrophages were found in clusters of erythroblasts and were often seen phagocytizing erythroblasts, a finding which closely resembles the picture of erythroblastic islands usually seen in the bone marrow. Adherence rate of tissue macrophages on the cover slip was less than 1% of total adhesive cells and most of the adherent tissue macrophages became degenerated and disappeared by 2 days of incubation.

Endogenous peroxidase activity in the cultured tissue macrophages was unstable similar to the tissue macrophages in the bone marrow but it was enzyme ultracytochemically demonstrated in the perinuclear cistern and rough endoplasmic reticulum. As to the membrane characters, the cultured macrophages showed a high rate of IgGEA and IgMEAC rosette formation as compared to cultured bone marrow monocytes in the early stage of incubation. Almost all the tissue macrophages were positive for these rosette forming tests and vigorously ingested sheep red cells in the tests. However, E rosette formation was negative. Carbon or latex phagocytosis was also observed remarkably in these macrophages. Acid phosphatase activity was prominent but naphthol AS-D chloroacetate was negative.

Monocytic cells: Adherence rate of cultured monocytic cells reached approximately 100% in 48 hr-old culture, along with elimination of poorly adherent cells. Among the monocytic cells adhering to the cover slip, large immature monocytes were seen occasionally intermixed.

Immature monocytes measured about 15 - 20 μ in diameter and were generally larger than mature monocytes. These large immature cells had a large, round, ovoid or horseshoe-shaped nucleus with marked indentations and their cytoplasm stained more basophilic with May-Giemsa stain. When ^{3}H-thymidine was added to the culture medium before 2 hr, thymidine grains were demonstrated within the nucleus of these large immature monocytes. From these findings, the large immature cells are regarded as promonocytes. In the promonocytes, there were a small number of fine intracytoplasmic granules which are considered to be Azur granules. The majority

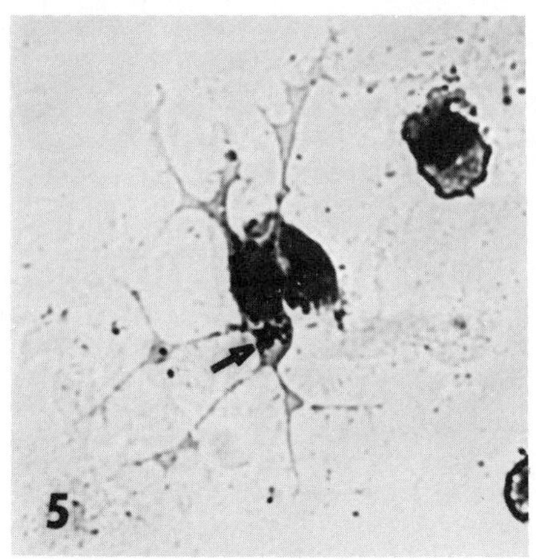

Fig. 5. A small amount of carbon (arrow) is ingested in the adhesive reticular cell of 6 hr cultivation (X 400).

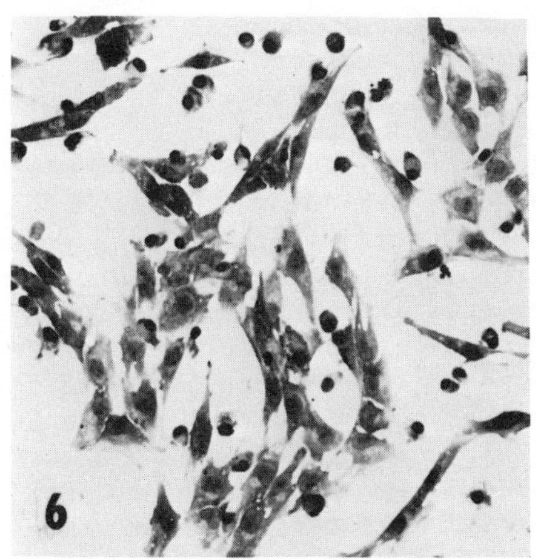

Fig. 6. In 7 day-old culture, there are small clusters of proliferating reticular cells (X 200).

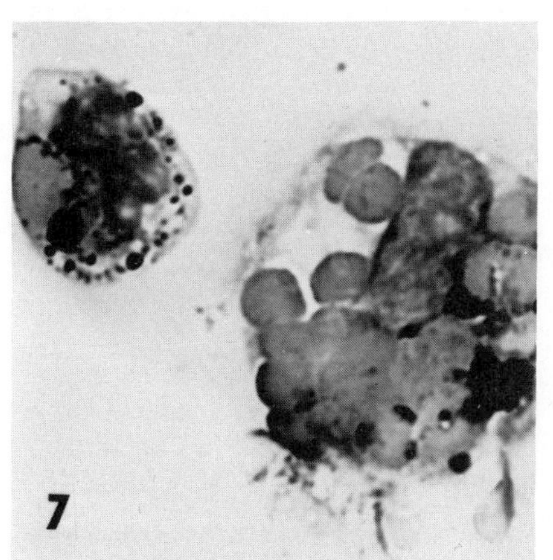

Fig. 7. Carbon phagocytosis and IgGEA rosette formation of tissue macrophage (right) and monocyte (left) in 6 hr-old culture. The tissue macrophage shows prominent phagocytosis of carbon particles and erythrocytes (X 1,000).

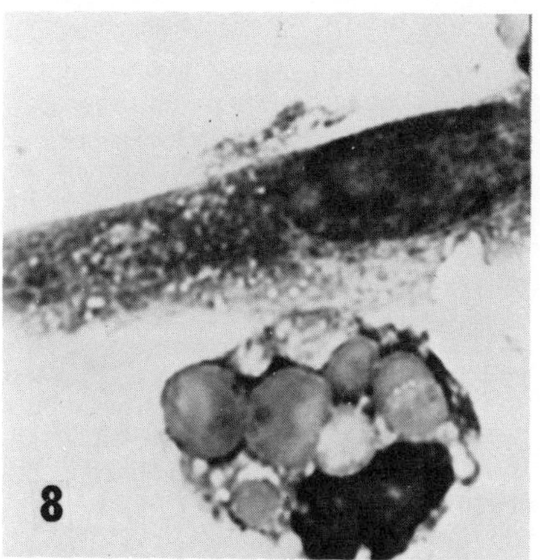

Fig. 8. Reticular cell (upper) and monocyte (lower) in 3 day-old culture. IgGEA rosette-forming test. Reticular cell lacks Fc receptor (X 1,000).

of promonocytes lacked Fc and C_3 receptors and showed a slight latex or carbon phagocytosis. Acid phosphatase was moderately positive and naphthol AS-D chloroacetate esterase was negative or faintly positive. Endogenous peroxidase activity was consistently substantiated to be localized only in a small number of Azur granules but not in the perinuclear cistern and rough endoplasmic reticulum, although this enzyme activity was found in the perinuclear cistern, rough endoplasmic reticulum and specific granules of cultured immature granulocytes. Such promonocytes were counted 10 - 12% of the total adhesive monocytic cells in 2 hr-old culture but they were gradually reduced in number with the lapse of incubation time and disappeared until 48 hr. On the contrary, mature monocytes were 80 - 90% of the total adhesive monocytic cells in 2 hr-old culture and reached approximately 100% at 48 hr. In 2 or 6 hr-old culture, none of the mature monocytes were labelled with ^{3}H-thymidine added to the culture medium. At 24 hr of incubation, however, a small number of labelled mature monocytes were observed. These data suggest that maturation process of promonocytes into mature monocytes exists in the bone marrow.

Mature monocytes measured 11 - 15 μ in diameter and contained a markedly indented nucleus in a pale blue cytoplasm with irregularly uneven or undulated cell margins. With incubation time, monocytes were activated and became gradually enlarged by increasing volume of their cytoplasm and their nucleus became round or ovoid. During the cultivation, these cells showed increasing rate of IgGEA and IgMEAC rosette formation, enhanced immunophagocytosis and carbon or latex phagocytosis, as well as increasing activity of acid phosphatase, so that within 2 or 3 days of cultivation, mature monocytes turned to cells of which cell morphology and functions are almost compatible to those of peritoneal macrophages. Such monocyte-derived macrophages were maintained until one month-old culture.

Interesting enough, in 6 hr-old culture, localization of endogenous peroxidase activity in not only Azur granules but also the perinuclear cistern and rough endoplasmic reticulum was demonstrated in about 10% of adhesive monocytes. Appearance rate of such a peroxidase localization pattern was increased to 20 - 30% of the monocytes in the IgGEA rosette-forming test. In 24 hr-old culture, endogenous peroxidase activity disappeared in the perinuclear cistern and rough endoplasmic reticulum but preserved only in Azur granules of these monocytes. From this, the above mentioned peculiar localization pattern of the peroxidase activity in monocytes is a transient phenomenon. Unlike the monocytes, localization of the enzyme activity in promonocytes cultured for 6 hr was confirmed to be confined only to Azur granules.

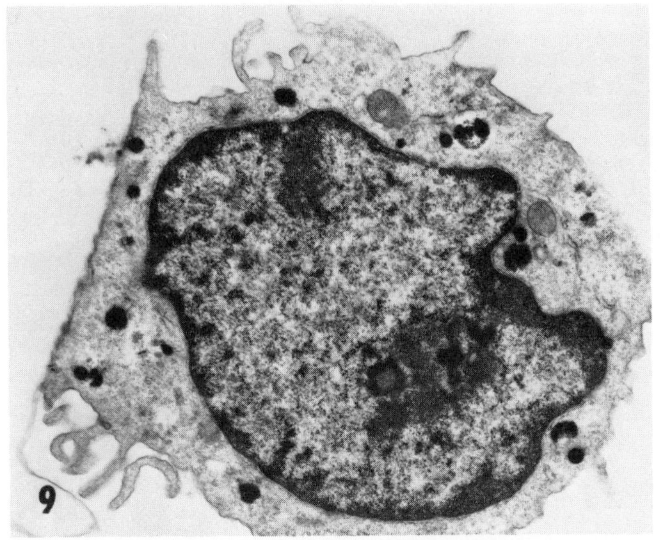

Fig. 9. Plastic-adhering promonocyte in 6 hr-old culture. Endogenous peroxidase is confined to Azur granules (X 6,500).

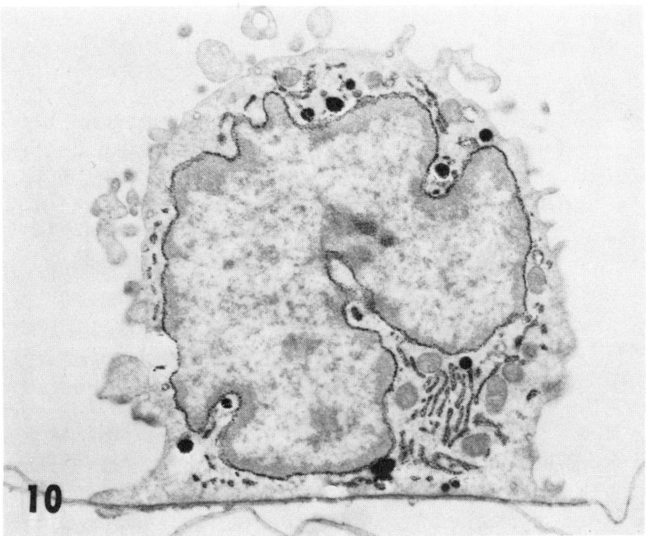

Fig. 10. In 6 hr-old culture, monocyte adhering to the plastic shows endogenous peroxidase activity in the perinuclear cistern, rough endoplasmic reticulum and Azur granules (Unstained. X 6,500).

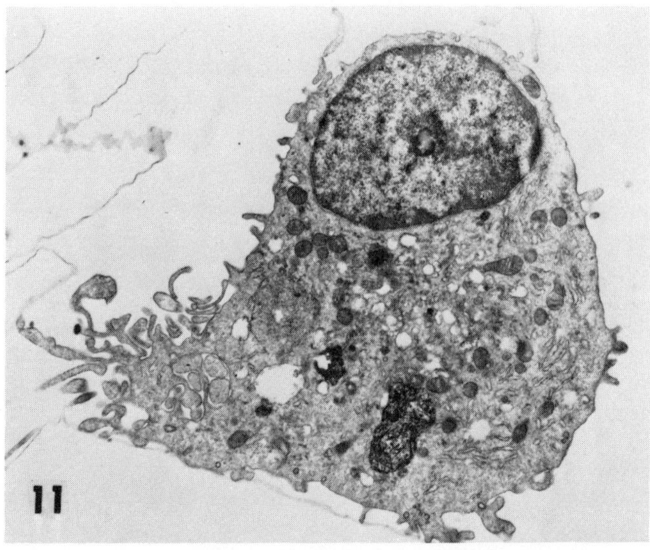

Fig. 11. In 48 hr-old culture, monocyte-derived macrophage shows no endogenous peroxidase activity in the perinuclear cistern and rough endoplasmic reticulum (X 4,200).

DISCUSSION

The present *in vivo* and *in vitro* observations have revealed cytological and enzyme cytochemical characteristics, membrane characters and phagocytic function of the reticular cells, tissue macrophages and monocytes existing in the bone marrow, as well as transformation or maturation processes of these cells under certain experimental conditions.

Among various kinds of bone marrow cells, the reticular cells are the major cell constituent forming reticular meshworks of the bone marrow and are poorly phagocytic fixed cells distributing throughout the intersinus marrow spaces, particularly around the venous sinuses. The reticular cells have a scant cytoplasm and somewhat resemble fibroblasts. However, they have long slender cytoplasmic processes extended in every direction among blood cells to form reticular meshes and are characterized by bundles of intracytoplasmic fibrils often with minor dense patches, hairy projections from the cytoplasmic processes, small junctional apparatus between the adjacent cytoplasmic processes and by occasional and partial attachment of a small amount of extracellular fibrils to the cell surfaces. In these cells, no localization of endogenous peroxidase activity was observed. In the process of transformation of the reticular cells to fat cells following Co^{60} irradiation, however, localization of this enzyme activity was proved in the perinuclear cistern and rough endoplasmic reticulum, as well as around fat droplets. In the fetal stage, similar reticular cells exist forming reticular meshes in the bone marrow anlage prior to the development of hematopoietic foci, and contain abuneant glycogen in their cytoplasm. In the experiment in vitro, the cultured reticular cells adhering to the plastic cover slip lacked Fc and C_3 receptors and showed no prominent phagocytosis. Acid phosphatase activity is weakly positive.

In the irradiation experiment, the reticular cells are rapidly transformed into fat cells. In tissue culture, the cultured reticular cells are gradually transformed into fibroblast-like cells which further divide and grow with the lapse of incubation time. During the cultivation, fat droplets appear in the cultured cells which are transformed into fat cells. In this way, the cytological, enzyme cytochemical and phagocytic functions of the reticular cells obviously differ from those of the bone marrow tissue macrophages or monocytes, and the reticular cells are considered to be interstitial cells constituting the supporting tissue of bone marrow and to be capable of transforming into fat cells or fibroblasts-like cells in the bone marrow according to certain alterations of its intramedullary circumstances.

Tissue macrophages, otherwise called "histiocytes" (3,4), are highly phagocytic fixed mononuclear cells which distribute in the intersinus marrow spaces, particularly being numerous in the areas distant from the venous sinuses and which stretch many cytoplasmic processes among blood cells to form reticular meshworks together with the reticular cells. Minor junctional apparatus is infrequently present between the cytoplasmic processes of such macrophages. In contrast to the monocytes, the tissue macrophages show localization of endogenous peroxidase activity in the perinuclear cistern and rough endoplasmic reticulum, and low radiosensitivity. Occasional macrophages in vivo are surrounded by many erythroblasts, forming erythroblastic islands. In the culture experiments, erythroblasts and erythrocytes surround cultured tissue macrophages and attached to their cell surfaces closely resembling the picture of erythroblastic islands in the bone marrow. Such a phenomenon may be characteristic of the tissue macrophages along with their prominent adhesiveness.

Under various experimental conditions, such as phagocytosis, irradiation or tissue culture, tissue macrophages become easily rounded and free and show avid phagocytosis. However, the present observation in various experiments has provided no evidence to support transition of the tissue macrophages into fibroblasts or fat cells. Although the macrophages possess Fc and complement receptors, show adhesiveness to the plastic cover slip and are intensely positive for acid phosphatase, identity between the tissue macrophages and monocytes is hardly recognized on the basis of the above-mentioned findings of the macrophages.

In the monocytes, ultracytochemical localization of endogenous peroxidase activity is usually demonstrated only in Azur granules, a finding which obviously differs from that of the tissue macrophages. In distinction to the tissue macrophages, the bone marrow monocytes are highly radiosensitive and rapidly disappear in a short period after the irradiation. In the present culture experiment, it was confirmed that immature monocytes or promonocytes matured into mature monocytes which were further transformed into macrophages several days later. In such promonocytes, Fc and C_3 receptors are mostly absent and phagocytosis of carbon or latex particles is slight. However, endogenous peroxidase activity is confined to Azur granules in the promonocytes, like mature monocytes. The cultured mature monocytes have Fc and C_3 receptors on their cell membrane and are gradually transformed into macrophages with prominent immunophagocytosis, latex or carbon phagocytosis and intense acid phosphatase activity. In such monocyte-derived macrophages, however, endogenous peroxidase activity is negative in the perinuclear cistern and rough endoplasmic reticulum.

In agreement with the results of their culture studies by Bodel and associates (1), we reconfirmed that about 10% of monocytes adhering to the plastic surface in 6 hr-old culture showed localization of endogenous peroxidase activity not only in Azur granules but also in the perinuclear cistern and rough endoplasmic reticulum. However, such a localization pattern of this endogenous peroxidase in monocytes seems to be a transient phenomenon and actually it was not observed in 24 hr-old culture. In this way, it may be obvious that the persistent localization of endogenous peroxidase activity is different between the monocyte-derived macrophages and tissue macrophages or histiocytes.

As discussed above, it is a fact that there are some noteworthy differences in cytology, enzyme cytochemistry and functions among the reticular cells, tissue macrophages and monocytes. However, for elucidation of the mutual relationship of these three kinds of cells, particularly of the nature and origin of tissue macrophages and monocytes, there remain further problems to be solved, on which subsequent studies will be required from various aspects.

REFERENCES

1. Bodel, P. T., Nichols, B. A. and Bainton, D. F., J. Exp. Med., 145 (1977) 264.
2. Daems, W. Th. and Brederoo, P., Z. Zellforsch., 144 (1973) 247.
3. Kojima, M., Recent Advances in RES Research, 16 (1976) 1.
4. Kojima, M., Acta Path. Jap., 26 (1976) 273.
5. van Furth, R. and Cohn, Z. A., J. Exp. Med., 128 (1968) 415.
6. van Furth, R. and Diesselhoff-den Dulk, M. M. C., J. Exp. Med., 132 (1970) 813.
7. Weiss, L., Anat. Rec., 186 (1976) 161.

LEUKOCYTE ENZYME ASSAYS BY FLOW CYTOPHOTOMETRY

L. S. KAPLOW

Laboratory Service Veterans Administration Hospital, West Haven, Ct. and Departments of Pathology and Laboratory Medicine, Yale University School of Medicine, New Haven, Connecticut (USA)

Flow-cytophotometers are optical electronic devices which measure a variety of physical characteristics of individual cells in suspension as they flow, one at a time, past a laser beam of a particular wavelength. Some instruments measure fluorescent emission at different wavelengths and light scattered from each cell detected at a narrow angle. Other instruments measure both narrow angle light scatter and axial light-loss (extinction) due to impingement of the cell on the light path as it traverses the laser beam. The studies to be described will refer only to instruments of the latter type.

By means of photodiode sensors, light scatter and transmission intensities are converted to voltages which are displayed as a scattergram on an oscilloscope screen (Fig. 1a). Each dot on the screen represents the coordinates of the scatter and extinction signals for a single cell. In addition, with most instruments, one can obtain pulse-height distribution curves based on signals from any one of the sensors for the population of cells under study (Fig. 1b). With more sophisticated equipment, it is possible to obtain a three-dimensional, two parameter contour histogram, in which, for example, extinction signals are plotted on the x-axis, scatter signals on the y-axis, and number of cells on the z or height axis. With such a system, sub-populations of cells with similar characteristics tend to form mounds or peaks.

Some instruments have the added capability of physically sorting sub-populations of cells, permitting positive identification of oscilloscope clusters and allowing for further biochemical, biophysical and immunologic studies on specific cell types.

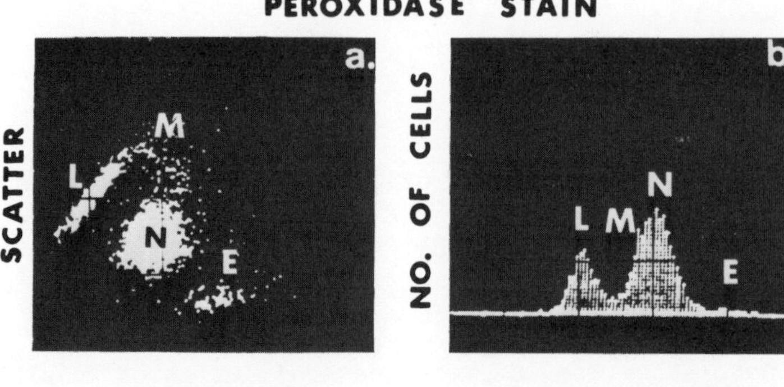

Fig. 1 (1a). Scattergram of human blood stained for peroxidase activity. Clusters are identified as lymphocytes (L), monocytes (M), neutrophils (N) and eosinophils (E). (1b) Histogram of same sample for light-loss signals.

Scatter signals from unstained cells are primarily dependent upon cell size and to a lesser extent on internal structure. As would be expected, stained cells transmit less light than unstained cells and hence exhibit greater axial light-loss signals. Stained cells also scatter less light than unstained cells. Axial light-loss signals are conventionally plotted on the x-axis and scatter signals on the y-axis. As a consequence of the effect of size and staining on scatter and axial light-loss, small unstained cells tend to locate on the oscilloscope screen as a cluster close to the origin, whereas large unstained cells cluster high on the y-axis and only slightly to the right on the x-axis. Stained cells tend to be located further away from the origin on the x-axis but closer to the origin on the y-axis than unstained cells.

These observations led to the development of a strategy for quantitating enzyme activity in various intact peripheral blood leukocytes which did not require physically separating differing cell types from one another or from plasma and obviated the need for performing classical biochemical assay procedures.

Empirical studies have demonstrated that cell populations which exhibit an all or none staining reaction appear as isolated clusters on the oscilloscope screen. Unstained leukocytes group as an inclined linear population of cells with relatively low axial light-loss signals. This is well demonstrated by the appearance of lymphocytes (L) after exposure to the peroxidase stain, as shown on Fig. 1. Since all neutrophils (N) normally stain fairly uniformly for peroxidase, they appear as a separate round cluster. Eosinophils (E) stain most intensely and also appear as an isolated cluster.

The results are quite different with bloods stained for neutrophil alkaline phosphatase (NAP) activity. Since neutrophils are the only leukocytes which stain for this enzyme and usually vary considerably in activity, they do not appear as a discrete cluster but rather as an extension from the unstained cell population. Examples of flow-cytophotometric oscilloscope displays of six stained human blood samples with varying NAP activity are illustrated in Fig. 2. Note the progressive increase in light-loss signals and decrease in scatter signals for cells of increasing staining activity. Blood sample #6, from a patient with bacterial pneumonitis, demonstrated unusually high activity and, since all neutrophils stained, the cluster appeared arc-shaped with almost complete separation from unstained cells (Fig. 2).

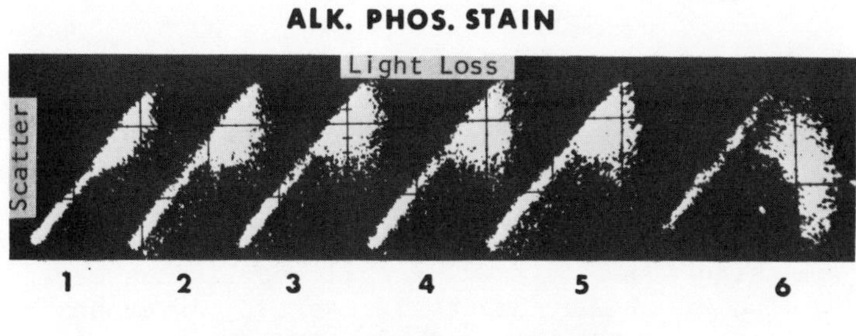

Fig. 2. Examples of Cytograf scattergrams of six random blood samples from hospitalized patients, stained in suspension for leukocyte alkaline phosphatase activity arranged in order of increasing enzyme activity from left to right.

MATERIALS AND METHODS

Technics were developed for staining peripheral blood leukocytes in suspension for myeloperoxidase (5), nonspecific esterase (6,8), alkaline phosphatase (7) and more recently for naphthol AS-D chloroacetate esterase activity. Peroxidase was originally demonstrated using benzidine dihydrochloride and more recently with 4-chloro-1-naphthol as the hydrogen donor. Hydrolytic enzymes were stained by modifying traditional azo dye technics as usually applied to tissue sections or blood smears. In all cases, cells were unfixed prior to staining and only 0.1 ml of blood was required for analysis. Incubation times varied from a low of 45 sec for peroxidase (4-chloro-1-naphthol) to 20 min for alkaline phosphatase. The reactions were stopped by addition of reagents which simultaneously lysed erythrocytes, inhibited further enzyme activity and partially or completely fixed the stained suspended intact leukocytes. Hydroxylamine hydrochloride-cetyltrimethyl ammonium bromide solution or acetic acid were used as the lysing-fixative agents for peroxidase and esterase stains. The high pH of the alkaline phosphatase incubation mixture caused lysis of all red cells without destroying the white cells. Stained cell suspensions were introduced into a Model 6300 Cytograf flow-cytophotometer (Ortho Diagnostics, 410 University Avenue (Westwood, MA). Flow rates were set at 0.4 ml per min resulting in measuring rates of approximately 300 cells per second. Thus, it was possible to analyze 18,000 leukocytes in less than one min. The unit was adjusted for maximum sensitivity (highest internal gain setting) and patterns of at least 10,000 cells were visualized on a storage oscilloscope. Platelets remained intact but because of their small size could be eliminated from the display along with residual red cell membranes by adjustment of an electronic lower threshold control.

The axial light-loss signals for all cells were stored in a Model 2100 Distribution Analyzer (Ortho Diagnostics, Raritan, N. J.) with single parameter histogram capability. Unfortunately, single parameter histograms are often difficult or impossible to accurately interpret if all or portions of two or more cell populations are so aligned as to fall within similar histogram channels. In such situations, differing cell populations may be difficult to resolve or may be completely masked. An economical, hard-wired, electronic device was fabricated which permitted 360 degree rotation of the entire scatterplot allowing selection of a rotational position which would yield optimum cluster separation as shown in Fig. 3 (9). The appearance of a scattergram and histogram of a peroxidase stained blood sample after rotation for maximum cluster separation is illustrated by Fig. 4. Note the improved resolution as compared to the same specimen unrotated as shown in Fig. 1.

The pulse-height distribution analyzer was interfaced to a Wang model 2200 microprocessor for storage and data manipulation. Utilizing a custom designed software computer program, arbitrary values were assigned to stained cells dependent upon the magnitude of their rotated axial light-loss signals. Cells were given progressively higher rating values dependent upon their histogram channel number (that is, distance from origin). The sum of the

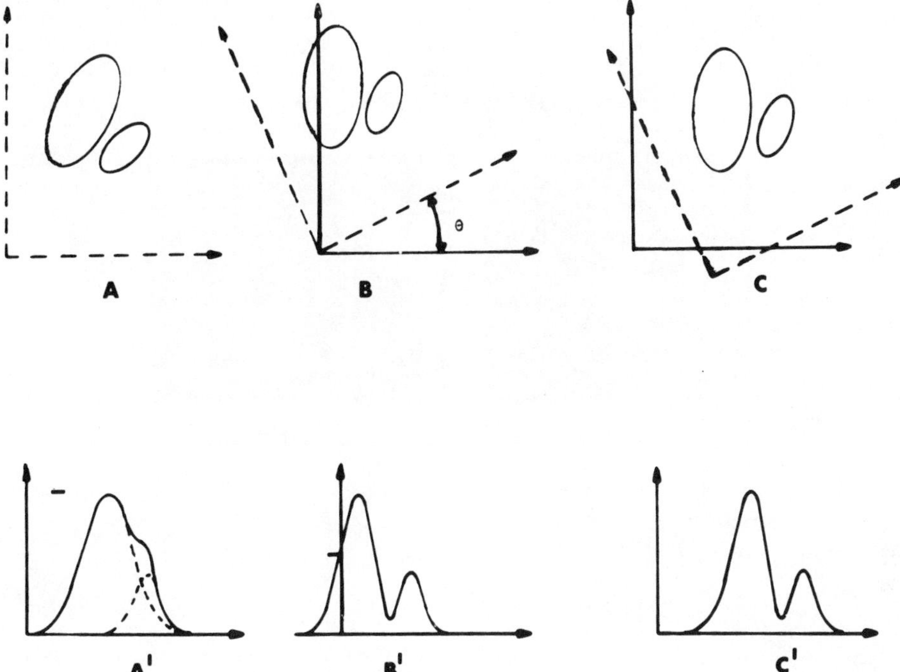

Fig. 3. Diagrammatic scattergrams and corresponding histograms of blood sample stained for non-specific esterase activity showing appearance before rotation (A,A'), after being rotated by angle θ (B,B') and final appearance (CC') after repositioning so that all data are relocated to original sector.

ratings was multiplied by a constant to yield a "score" representing average enzyme activity for the specified cell population in a particular blood sample. Similar studies were carried out on Ficoll-Hypaque mononuclear leukocyte preparations.

The reproducibility and accuracy of the instrument in discriminating and counting specific cell populations was assessed by comparing the results of duplicate or replicate analyses of the same blood sample and by comparing machine data with counts derived from manual differential white cell counts. Similarly, the reliability of assaying nonspecific esterase enzyme activity was determined by comparing instrument results with a manual scoring method (4). Flow-cytophotometric interpretations of neutrophil alkaline phosphatase activity were also compared to a manual scoring technique (3) and in addition to biochemical assays on concentrated leukocytes (10).

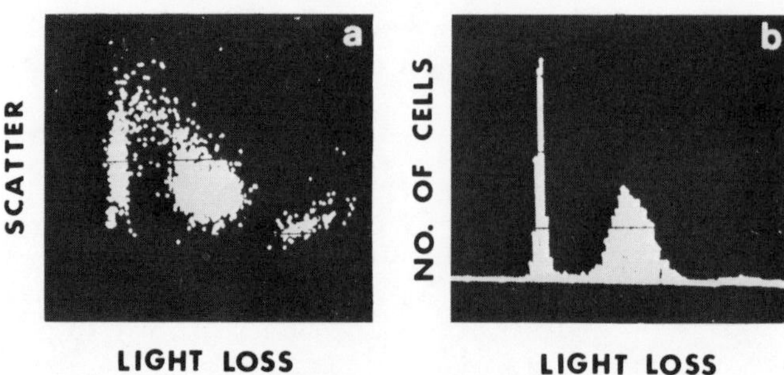

Fig. 4. Scattergram and histogram of peroxidase stained leukocytes after rotation for maximum cluster separation. Compare with appearance before rotation as shown in Fig. 1.

RESULTS

The methods proved to be highly reproducible. Comparisons of scores derived from replicate staining mixtures indicated coefficients of variation of less than 5% and the stained cell suspensions were stable for as long as 2½ hr after addition of the lysing-fixative reagents.

A summary of the reliability in discriminating and counting various cell types and in assessing average enzyme activity in specific sub-populations of leukocytes is given in Table I.

The precision and accuracy in counting sub-populations of leukocytes or in assessing enzyme activity was dependent upon a number of variables. Studies on the influence of the anticoagulant used indicated that ethylenediaminetetracetate (EDTA) was the preferred agent. However, the use of heparinized blood resulted in higher scores for alkaline phosphatase activity than did the use of samples collected with EDTA. Neutrophil alkaline phosphatase is considered to be a zinc dependent enzyme and the reduced activity associated with EDTA blood has been attributed to removal of zinc by chelation with EDTA (12). Studies indicated that this decrease in activity could not be reversed by adding zinc ions to the incubation mixture (7). The interval between blood collection and analysis did not significantly alter the results, provided the samples were analyzed within 5 hr.

TABLE I

Accuracy Studies: Coefficients of Correlation (r)

Assay	Enzyme Stain	Reference Method	(r)
% Neutrophils	Peroxidase	Manual 500 cell differential	0.93
% Lymphocytes	Peroxidase	Manual 500 cell differential	0.94
% Eosinophils	Peroxidase	Manual 500 cell differential	0.96
% Monocytes	Peroxidase	Manual 500 cell differential	0.40
% Monocytes	α-naphthyl acetate	Manual 300 cell differential	0.95
Esterase Activity	α-naphthyl acetate	Manual scoring	0.86
Phosphatase Activity	α-naphtyl phosphate	Manual scoring	0.83
Phosphatase Activity	α-naphthyl phosphate	Biochemical assay	0.89

The use of different lots of substrates or diazonium salts had only minimal effects on quantitation of enzyme activity by this technique. The Cytograf itself was found to be quite stable. It was possible to run the instrument continuously for at least as long as 6 hr with no appreciable adverse effects.

Preliminary efforts to devise a method for cytochemically demonstrating naphthol AS-D chloroacetate esterase in cells in suspension were encouraging. Under appropriate staining conditions, this enzyme localizes almost exclusively within the cytoplasm of neutrophils and mast cells. Scattergrams of such stained preparations differ from scattergrams of peroxidase stained blood cells by absence of an eosinophil cluster and by a sparse cluster in the region associated with monocytes. However, cells forming this latter cluster have not yet been identified with confidence.

The appearance of such scattergrams is illustrated in Fig. 5.

In addition to studies on whole human blood, preliminary studies were performed on guinea pig blood and on mononuclear cell concentrates prepared by Ficoll-Hypaque density gradient techniques. When appropriately diluted, such material was found to be as satisfactory as whole human blood. Examples of scattergrams of concentrated human mononuclear cells stained for non-specific esterase are shown in Fig. 6.

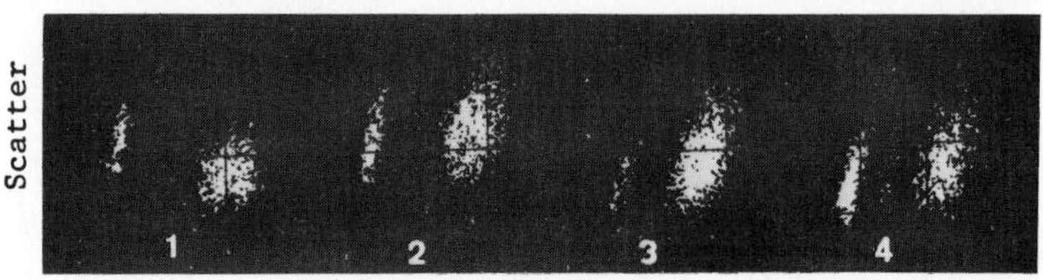

Fig. 5. Examples of Cytograf oscilloscope displays of four different bloods stained for naphthol AS-D chloroacetate esterase activity.

DISCUSSION

Interest in flow-systems for studying intact suspended cells has centered primarily on flow-cytophofluorophotometers. These instruments measure light scatter and, with appropriately stained material, also derive data concerning nuclear and/or cytoplasmic fluorescence. Such applications have been especially fruitful in cell cycle analysis studies and in investigating the effects of drugs on various stages of the cycle (2).

Non-fluorescence detecting flow-systems have received considerably less attention. Pioneer work in this area was done by a group of investigators associated with the Technicon Corp. (1, 11) in developing an automated differential white cell counter (Hemalog D^R). Some of the staining methods described in this study are modifications of techniques developed for the Hemalog D but considerably altered to suit the requirements of the Cytograf. The Hemalog D is an inflexible instrument, limited to

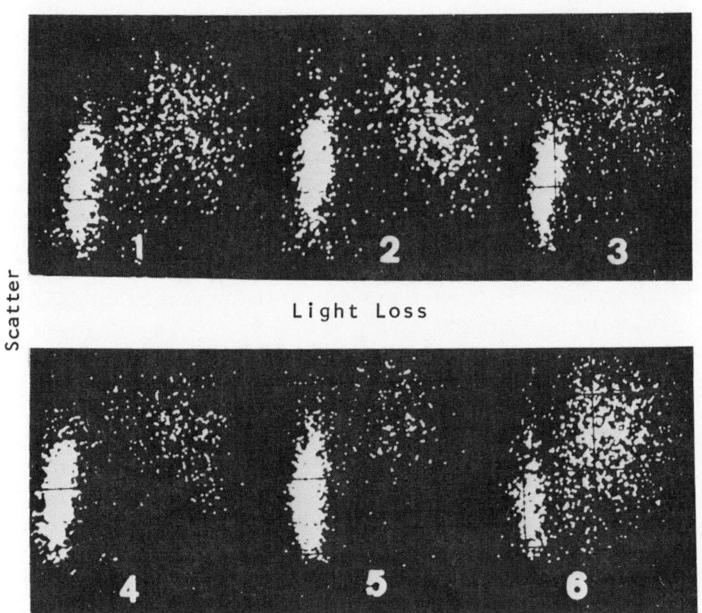

Fig. 6. Rotated Cytograf oscilloscope patterns of six different Ficoll-Hypaque mononuclear cell concentrates stained for non-specific (α-naphthyl acetate) esterase. The dense vertical clusters represent lymphocytes and the less dense irregular clusters represent monocytes.

specific stains and especially designed to discriminate and enumerate the major leukocyte groups. It cannot be easily adapted for enzyme assay studies.

Flow-systems examine cells one by one at remarkably high flow rates. Cell populations can be individually studied, even when present in a mixed cell population, without resorting to separatory techniques. Furthermore, cells may be examined intact and under suitable conditions may even be viable. Harsh disruptive techniques are not required. These attributes make flow-systems particularly attractive devices for studying minority cell populations in a heterogenous cellular "gemisch". The studies described here on blood monocytes, would be extremely difficult and time consuming to perform by other methods. Studies on basophils and eosinophils would be even more difficult to carry out.

In staining human blood cells for peroxidase, we have noted varying shapes for the eosinophil cluster. This could be due to variations in cell volume or in granule content. It could also represent variability in average granule peroxidase activity. The significance of such variability is not known. But the answers to such questions could not even have been approached prior to the availability of these instruments. Similarly, the significance of differences in monocyte nonspecific esterase activity is also uncertain and we are currently studying this problem. Our original approach involved the microscopic examination of 50 or 100 esterase-stained monocytes on a slide and subjective assessment of staining intensity. Aside from the subjectivity involved, the problem of simply locating 100 monocytes would tax most of us. By means of flow-cytophotometry, we were able to obtain objective data on 10,000 esterase stained monocytes from one patient in less than 5 min.

Our preliminary studies on granulocyte naphthol AS-D chloroacetate activity indicate variations in this enzyme system from patient to patient. This can be inferred from Fig. 5 which demonstrates a greater distance from the center of the lymphocyte cluster to the center of the neutrophil cluster for patients 1 and 2 as compared to patients 3 and 4.

The applications noted above are not limited to whole blood nor to blood cells. The esterase technique was applied to Ficoll-Hypaque lymphocyte preparations and served as a simple means of determining contamination by monocytes. Such contamination may be considerably greater than one might conclude from examining Wright's stained preparations (13). Similarly, lymphocyte preparations stained for peroxidase could quickly and accurately indicate the extent of contamination by granulocytes.

It should be emphasized that these approaches to the study of blood cells are adaptable to suspended tissue culture material or to disaggregated solid tissues. Isolated intact nuclei can be similarly studied. However, such applications present additional problems, relating to preservation of cell integrity and avoidance of debris.

Cells of the reticuloendothelial (RE) system are particularly suited for analysis by flow-cytophotometers. Blood and lymph require no preliminary preparative steps other than dilution. Solid tissues of the RE system can be more readily disaggregated into cell suspensions than most other parenchymal tissues. The heterogeneity of RE cells, their primary role in immune functions and the intracellular alterations which they undergo in many disease processes make them especially attractive candidates for investigation by flow-cytophotometry. The information to be derived from such studies will depend, to a great extent, upon the availability of new staining methods and on our ingenuity in their application.

ACKNOWLEDGEMENT

Supported by the Medical Research Service of the Veterans Administration.

REFERENCES

1. Ansley, H. and Ornstein, L., Adv. Automated Anal. 1 (1971) 437.
2. Horan, P. K. and Wheeless, L. L., Jr., Sci. 198 (1977) 149.
3. Kaplow, L. S., Am. J. Clin. Path. 39 (1963) 439.
4. Kaplow, L. S., Acta Cytol. 19 (1975) 358.
5. Kaplow, L. S. and Eisenberg, M., Leukocyte differentiation and enumeration by cytochemical-cytographic analysis, In: First International Symposium on Pulse-Cytophotometry, (Eds. C. A. M. Haanen, H. F. P. Hillen and J. M. C. Wessels), European Press Medikon, 262 (1975).
6. Kaplow, L. S. and Lerner, E., J. Histochem. Cytochem. 25 (1977) 590.
7. Kaplow, L. S. and Soman, S., Fed. Proc. 37:1234 (1978) 444.
8. Kaplow, L. S., Dauber, H. and Lerner, E., J. Histochem. Cytochem. 24 (1976) 363.
9. Kaplow, L. S., Gershman, R., Weiner, I. and Soman, S., J. Histochem. Cytochem. 26 (1978) 214.
10. Peacock, A. C., Brecher, G. and Highsmith, E. M., Am. J. Clin. Path. 29 (1958) 80.
11. Saunders, A. M., Clin. Chem. 18 (1972) 783.
12. Trubowitz, S., Feldman, D., Benate, C. and Kirman, D., Proc. Soc. Exp. Biol. Med. 95 (1957) 35.
13. Zucker-Franklin, D., Arch. Intern. Med. 135 (1975) 55.

Part II
Immunopharmacology of the Reticuloendothelial System

One of the most recent areas in the biomedical sciences to occupy the center of interest is that dealing with Immunopharmacology. Classical pharmacology has now been combined with many areas of immunology to generate exciting new information and concepts. Many of the "factors" involved in immune reactivity can certainly be considered as pharmacologically active substances. In addition, those agents which affect a known pharmacological activity of the living organism are now known to obviously have effects on RE cell systems. In this section a wide variety of agents and treatments which can influence metabolic and functional activities of macrophages are described and discussed. In particular, the effects of natural substances including bacterial extracts and polysaccharides (e.g., glucan) on macrophage activity and anti-infectious or anti-tumor immunity are described. Recently, it has been shown by a number of investigators, including those from more classic areas of immunology, that substances derived from microorganisms can markedly influence lymphoid cell responsiveness. The "natural" adjuvant within BCG, for example, appears to be a muramyl dipeptide, which can be synthesized *in vitro*. Thus, data demonstrating that components of mycobacteria, corynebacteria, and the gram-negative rods can influence antibody formation and cellular immunity, have been related to specific immunopharmacologically active moieties derived from these organisms or from analogues of natural substances. It is obvious that this field of investigation will also expand very rapidly over the next few years.

ALTERATIONS OF RAT LIVER LYSOSOMES AFTER TREATMENT WITH PARTICULATE β 1-3 GLUCAN FROM *SACCHAROMYCES CEREVISIAE*

P. J. JACQUES and F. LAMBERT

Laboratory of Cytological Biochemistry
Université de Louvain (Belgium)

The possible interactions between lysosomes and the activin-immunoamplifier glucan from yeast are numerous: a) glucan treatment might influence some properties of the lysosomes present in a given organ (e.g., the liver), either through alteration of preexisting lysosomes, through changing the cellular composition of the organ provided that the lysosomes be different in the various cell populations at stake, or by a combination of these two phenomena; b) if glucan particles reach the lysosomes proper and if their slow *in vivo* degradation (7) occurs there, lysosomal effectors would alter glucan molecules; this probable phenomenon is of such great importance that a hypothesis considering glucan as a rather inert drug-precursor requiring chemical activation within lysosomes has already been formulated on the basis of some indirect experimental evidence (7); c) oxidative enzymes associated with lysosomes or related structures (e.g., the plasma membrane) of all cell types (e.g., mono- or "poly"-nucleated phagocytes, lymphocytes) involved in the cellular part of both nonspecific and specific immunity are thought to play a determinant role in the major and ultimate host-defense act, which is the killing of intracellular (infectious) or extracellular (tumor cells, parasitic worms...) parasites (Fig. 1). In addition, hydrolytic enzymes in lysosomes would intervene in a latter stage, in the biodegradation of the intravacuolar bodies (and antigens) of killed parasites. Thus, lysosomes of white inflammatory cells appear as the major executive agents operating at the last step of the chain of events accelerated by glucan and other immunoadjuvants, e.g., killing of parasites and disposal of their remnants.

This study deals with the effect of glucan treatment on

lysosomes. Rat liver was chosen in this biochemical study, because its lysosomes are by far the best known as regard enzymatic equipment and biophysical versus morphological properties; also, because the liver is one of the major targets for glucan action, even in normal rodents (1,11) and the place of residence for some parasites, e.g., the exoerythrocytic forms of plasmodia causing malaria (10), which are susceptible to benefit from glucan administration.

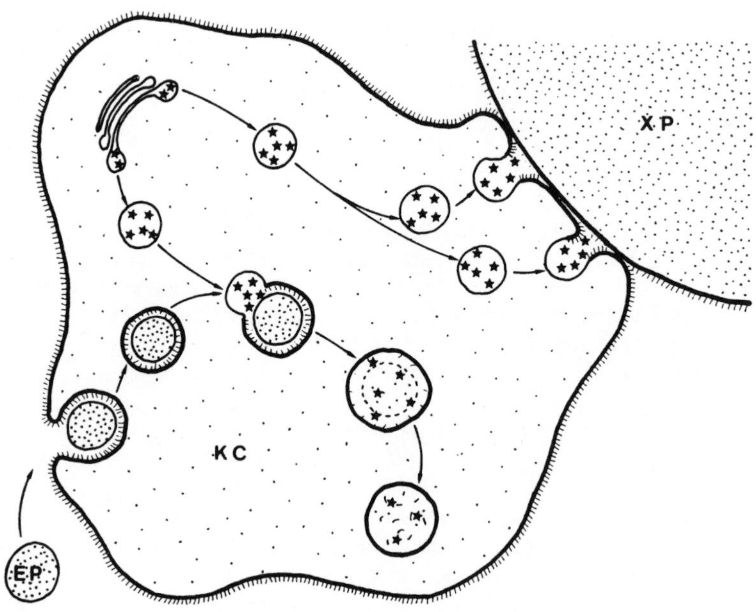

Fig. 1. Lysosomes and immunological killing.
Intravacuolar killing of endocytozable parasite (EP) and contact killing of extracellular parasite (XP) by lysosomal effectors (★) of inflammatory killer cell (KC).

Two lysosomal marker enzymes were used throughout the present study, e.g. acid µ-glycerophosphatase and acid deoxyribonuclease, which are more concentrated in hepatocytes and in Kuppfer cells (14), respectively. Their levels were compared in liver homogenates from control and glucan-treated rats, as well as the degree of distribution of their respective container-vacuoles. Their distribution was also followed after fractionation of the whole homogenate by differential pelleting in 0.25 M sucrose, and subfractionation of the thus obtained fraction gathering the larger cytoplasmic organelles, by isodensity equilibration in discontinuous gradients of hypertonic sucrose.

MATERIALS AND METHODS

Particulate β 1-3 glucan (batch DL-102777) from *Saccharomyces cerevisiae* was obtained as suspensions in saline, from Dr. N. R. Di Luzio (Tulane University, New Orleans). It was administered intravenously to normal adult male Wistar rats, usually at a single dose ranging from 1 to 40 mg/kg. Control animals received the same amount of saline. One to 20 day(s) later, the animals were fasted overnight and bled by careful section of the neck vessels, under light ether anesthesia. The liver, spleen, lungs and kidneys were dissected out and weighed.

Liver homogenates were prepared in 0.25 M sucrose, using a manually operated a 11-glass Dounce homogenizer. Fractionation of the whole homogenate by differential pelleting in 0.25 M sucrose was previously described (5), except that the two fractions (M and L) gathering most of the large cytoplasmic organelles remained combined. That combined (M + L) fraction was then subfractionated by isodensity equilibration in discontinuous gradients of hypertonic sucrose in H_2O and D_2O (13,15), with extreme densities 1.15 and 1.38.

Total proteins, acid β-glycerophosphatase and acid deoxyribonuclease were measured in the homogenates, their fractions and subfractions. In addition, the ratio of free to total activity of both lysosomal enzymes was measured in the homogenates, as an index for integrity of the corresponding lysosome subpopulations.

RESULTS

In a first experimental series (Fig. 2), the animals were sacrificed on day 7 after single injection of glucan. Drug dosage was varied between 1 mg/kg and the highest value (40 mg/kg), which was tolerated with this specific batch of glucan (DL-102777). The concentration of the nuclease (Fig. 2a) was appreciably increased by treatment, whereas those of the phosphatase (Fig. 2a) and of total proteins (Fig. 2c) were slightly decreased. Glucan treatment also increased the ratio of free to total activity of the two lysosomal enzymes (Fig. 2b) and liver wet weight (Fig. 2c). If the effect on concentration of the two enzymes was qualitively different (Fig. 2a), that on the degree of disruption of their carrier-organelle in the homogenate differed only from the quantitative viewpoint (Fig. 2b). All these effects increased with dosage.

For that reason, the maximal dosage of 40 mg/kg was selected for the second experimental series, which aimed at observing the influence of time after injection on the same biological parameters. Grossly speaking, the effects of glucan administration reported for day 7 (Fig. 2) could be observed during all the experimental period, e.g. from day 1 to 50 (Fig. 3). However, treatment effect on phosphatase concentration (Fig. 3a) and degree of disruption of its carrier-lysosomes in tissue homogenate (Fig. 3b) showed a tendency to reverse at a larger stage, when compared to controls. Qualitative and/or quantitative differences in response to treatment could also be observed for tissue concentration of nuclease and phosphatase (Fig. 3a), and for the level of disruption of their respective subpopulations of container-lysosomes (Fig. 3b). In addition, treatment effect on the ratio of free to total acid deoxyribonuclease (Fig. 3b) and on liver weight (Fig. 3c) peaked on day 7 after glucan injection.

Above results reveal an influence of glucan treatment on the concentration of two lysosomal hydrolases in the liver, and on the ratio of their free to particle-bound activity in the homogenate. The question then arises as to whether the residual intact lysosomes recovered in the homogenate were normal or not. The problem was approached through prospecting the possible influence of treatment on the distribution of the two acid hydrolases, considered as markers for lysosomes, in two centrifugal systems of biochemical cytology : differential pelleting and isodensity equilibration. The former approach is sensitive to changes in size of the sedimenting particle and, to a lesser extent, to its density in the fractionation medium (e.g. isotonic sucrose), whereas the latter would evidence changes in the matrix density of the organelles, since the fractionation was performed in hypertonic gradients.

Fig. 4 depicts the distribution of the two lysosomal markers in 6 experiments of differential pelleting. Distribution patterns obtained after fractionation of liver homogenates from untreated animals (thin linings) fully agree with those previously obtained (5) for the two marker enzymes; namely, nuclease was more concentrated than phosphatase in heavier fractions.

Administration of glucan (40 mg/kg) one day prior to the experiment (Fig. 4, left part) had no discernible effect on distribution of phosphatase but led to shifting of an appreciable amount of nuclease from the ML to the microsomal (P) fraction. When that ML fraction was subfractionated on discontinous gradients of sucrose, no difference could be observed in the distri-

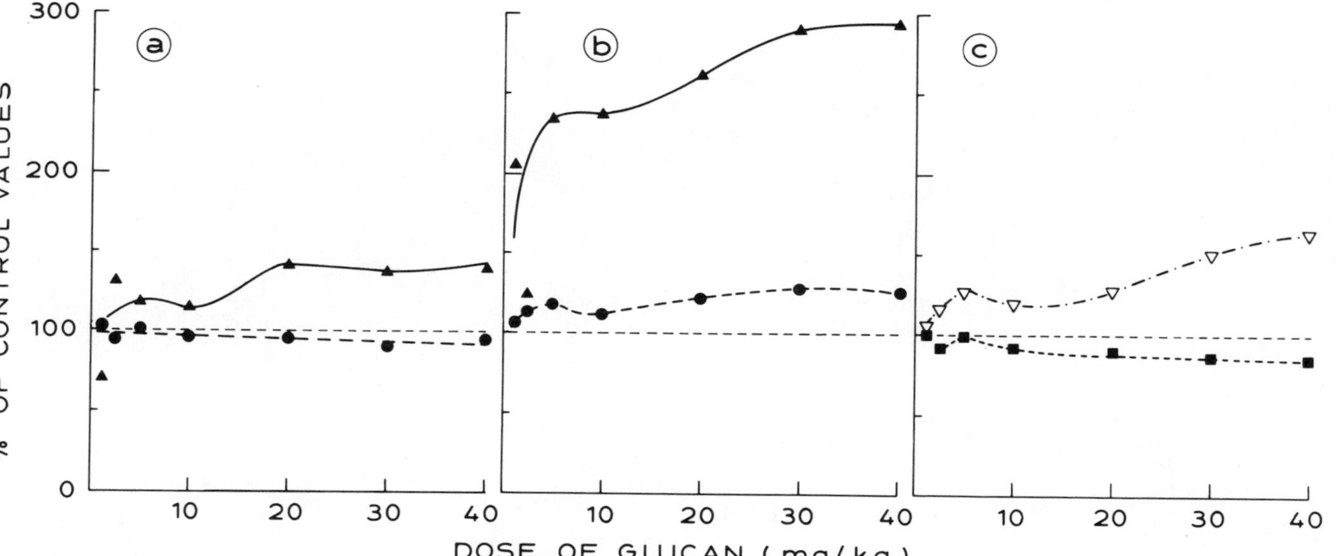

Fig. 2. Various biological parameters on day 7 after single intravenous administration of glucan as functions of dosage (1 to 40 mg/kg).
2a : Concentration of lysosomal deoxyribonuclease (▲) and β-glycerophosphatase (•) in liver homogenate. 2b : Ratio of free to total activity of the nuclease (▲) and the phosphatase (•) in the homogenate. 2c : Concentration of total proteins (■) in the homogenate, and liver wet weight (▽). Each value averages 3 observations, and is expressed as percentage of average from 3 corresponding controls.

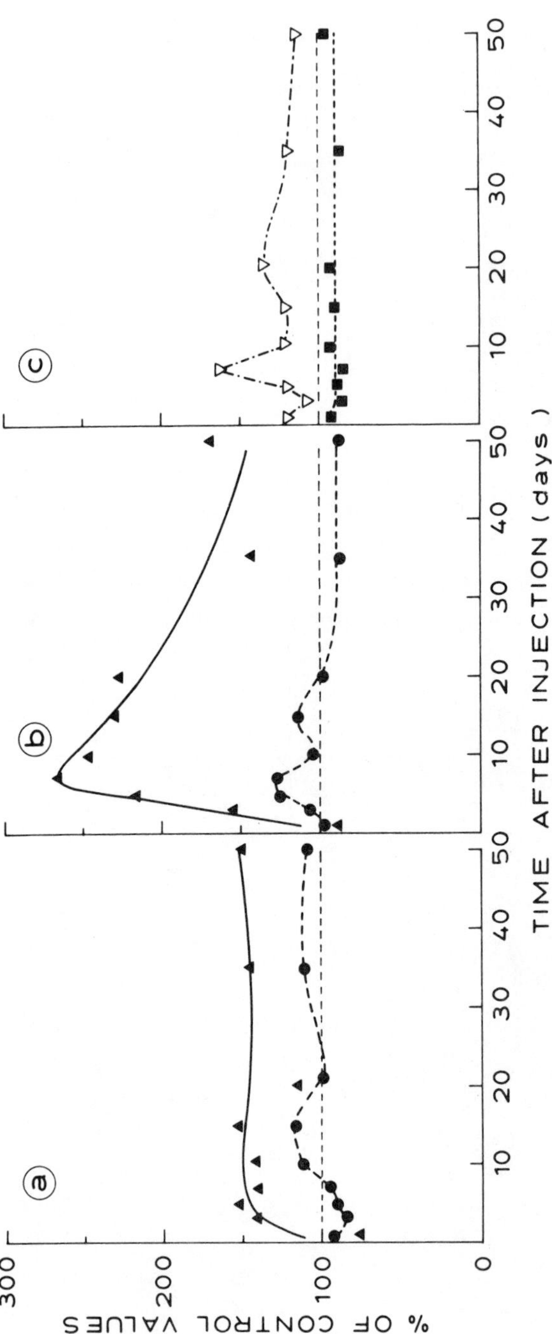

Fig. 3. Various biological parameters as functions of time (1 to 50 days) after single intravenous administration of glucan (40 mg/kg).
3a : Concentration of lysosomal deoxyribonuclease (▲) and β-glycerophosphatase (●) in liver homogenate. 3b : Ratio of free to total activity of the nuclease (▲) and the phosphatase (●) in the homogenate. 3c : Concentration of total proteins (■) in the homogenate, and liver wet weight (∇). Each value averages 3 observations, and is expressed as percentage of average from 3 corresponding controls.

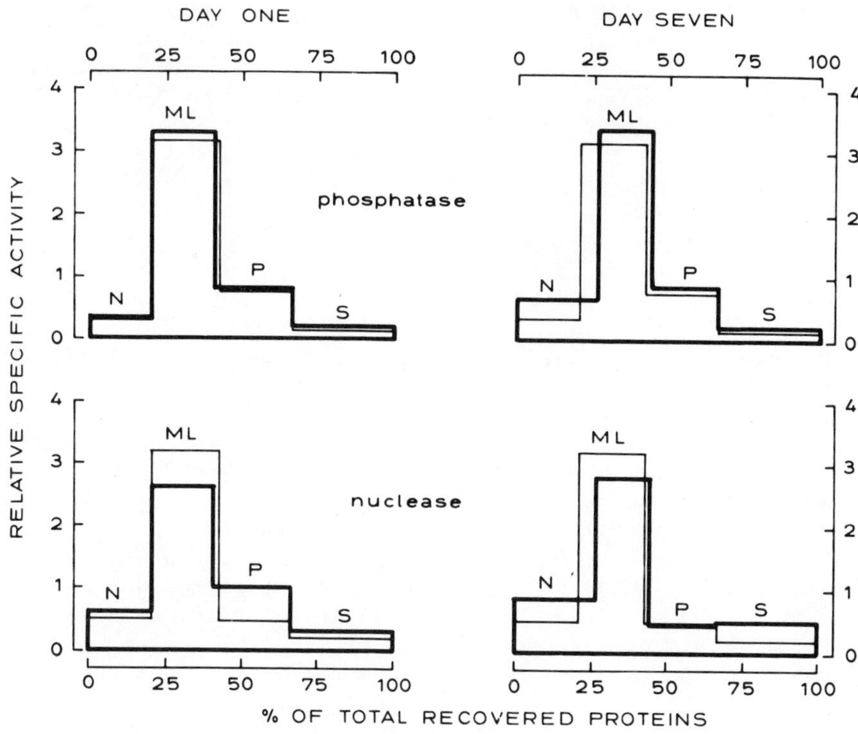

Fig. 4. Distribution of lysosomal acid deoxyribonuclease and acid β-glycerophosphatase, after differential pelleting of liver homogenates.
Thin lines : average of 2 control livers ; thick lines : average of 2 livers from glucan treated rats. Exp. on day 1 : 40 mg/kg on day 0 ; exp. on day 7 : 40 mg/kg on day 0, followed by 20 mg/kg on day 3 and 5.

bution of the marker enzymes obtained from treated or from control animals.

Confronted with the almost complete lack of treatment effect on the behavior of the residual lysosomes after single administration of the maximal intravenous dose of that glucan, we decided, in view of a similar experiment to be performed on day 7, to increase glucan dosage through administering 40 mg/kg on day 0 as usual, and then 20 mg/kg on days 3 and 5. In this case (Fig. 4, right part), the distribution pattern of the enzymes was strikingly altered, especially that of the nuclease. In both instances, a considerable fraction of carrier-organelles which was present in the ML fraction of the controls, sedimented with the nuclei after glucan treatment. In addition, the percentage of soluble nuclease was approximately doubled, whereas that of the phosphatase was not significantly increased. However, subfractionation of the ML fraction in density gradients did not evidence influence of treatment on matrix density of the lysosomes.

DISCUSSION

Present results clearly establish that there is an important influence of glucan treatment, on the liver lysosomes of normal (e.g. non-infected, non-tumor-bearing) rats. Indeed, total activity of both acid deoxyribonuclease and β-glycerophosphatase per liver were considerably increased (Figs. 2a and 3a), so was the amount of extracorpuscular nuclease, as measured by its ratio of free to total activity (Figs. 2b and 3b) and of its non-sedimentable to total (Fig. 4, right part), in the homogenate; in the same experiments, only the dose-response curve of the phosphatase (Fig. 2b) showed a similar but very slight tendency. Finally, the average sedimentation coefficient of the lysosomes in isotonic sucrose was considerably increased (Fig. 4, right part).

One is tempted to establish a causal relationship between the increased hydrolytic capacity of the liver, and its apparently increased ability to control parasitic diseases like cancer metastases (8,9) and malaria (10); parallel changes for other lysosomal enzymes like lysozyme and especially myeloperoxidase would however be necessary to establish that relationship on a firmer basis. As to the mechanism of that increased hydrolytic activity, several hypotheses can be put forward, which histology of the liver should help ascertain. It must first be pointed out that even transient specific multiplication of the Kuppfer cells, as observed in mouse liver soon after yeast glucan administration (1,6), might explain (or at least contribute to) the earlier and more important increase of nuclease concentration compared to that of phosphatase (Figs. 2a and 3a), and perhaps also the initial decrease of average sedimentation coefficient of the nuclease-rich lysosomes, one day after glucan administration (Fig. 4, left part). However, it should be kept in mind that liver weight rapidly increased as a result of treatment (Fig. 3c) and that a large part of that response is probably explained by infiltration of the organ by inflammatory cells. In this respect, our results indicate that changes in cellular composition of the liver do not affect the concentration of phosphatase, and in contrast, parallel that of nuclease; in other words, the relative concentration of phosphatase and nuclease in liver-invading cells must be closer to that of Kuppfer cells rather than to that of hepatocytes.

Various phenomena might cause increased levels of free lysosomal enzymes in the liver homogenate (Figs. 2b and 3b), as well as higher concentrations of soluble nuclease (Fig. 4, right part). All depends on whether this effect related to a lysosomal disruption prevailing _in vivo_, or it took place during homogenization and/or subsequent _in vitro_ manipulations. The first situation would be encountered if extensive damage should be caused to liver cells by glucan treatment, or would result from death of a large population of short-lived lysosome-rich invader-cells (e.g. polymorphs); but histology of rodent liver after glucan treatment did not evidence such phenomena with sufficient intensity. More likely is the second situation, that would involve mechanical disruption of the lysosomes during homogenization and/or decreased stability in the isotonic sucrose solutions utilized for measurement of free activity, and as medium for fractionation by differential pelleting. Increased size of the lysosomes present in the liver after glucan treatment would indeed lead to such artifacts. Besides, it would inevitably take place, should glucan particles reach the lysosomes after phagocytosis and especially be slowly degraded therein. Indeed, cytoplasmic vacuoles containing glucan particles are larger than usual in rodent liver (1), and intravacuolar water-soluble polysaccharides produced from the particles should, at a later stage, cause osmotic swelling of their container-vacuoles, much in the same way as treatment by sucrose (4, 12,16) and other concentrated solutes (2,3) does in liver cells. In addition, that still hypothetical swelling of the lysosomes, which is now being searched by means of photon-and electron-microscopy, would explain the increase of sedimentation coefficient of the lysosomes in isotonic sucrose (Fig. 4, right part); indeed, size is the major parameter of sedimenting particles which increases their sedimentation rate in a given medium.

At first sight, the high density of glucan particles and water-soluble polysaccharides in general ($\rho \simeq 1.6$) renders very surprising the lack of detectable increase of lysosomes density in gradients of hypertonic sucrose. However several factors might explain that negative observation. Firstly, the gradient which was used was discontinuous and thus lacked most of the fair sensitivity of continuous gradients towards slight changes in the density of equilibrating particles. Secondly, the subfractionation involved the ML fraction, from which the lysosomes that had been mostly modified by glucan treatment and had nevertheless resisted the critical step of homogenization, were discarded and rejoined the heavier N fraction, during the step of differential pelleting necessary to isolate the ML fraction. Finally, it may be that glucan dosage was insufficient or administered according to a non-optimal time-sheet.

ACKNOWLEDGEMENTS

The authors are greatly indebted to Mrs. M. Guiot and Mr. E. Dermience for precious and skillful assistance, and to Belgian Fonds de la Recherche Fondamentale Collective (contract n° 2.4542. 76-F) for financial and moral support. One of us (P. J. Jacques) holds tenure at Maître de Recherche from the Belgian Fonds National de la Recherche Scientifique.

REFERENCES

1. Ashworth, C. T., Di Luzio, N. R. and Riggi, S. J., Exp. Molec. Pathol., Supp. I, (1963) 83.
2. Aterman, K., Lab. Invest., 7 (1958) 577.
3. Aterman, K., Liver Function (Ed. R. W. Brauer), Amer. Inst. Biol. Sci., Washington, 4 (1958) 153.
4. Brewer, D. B. and Health, D., J. Pathol. Bacteriol., 87 (1964) 105.
5. de Duve, C., Pressman, B. C., Gianetto, R., Wattiaux, R. and Appelmans, F., Biochem. J., 60 (1955) 604.
6. Diller, I. C. and Mankowski, Z. T., Acta Unio Intern. Contra Cancrum, 16 (1960) 584.
7. Di Luzio, N. R. and Riggi, S. J., J. Reticuloendothelial Soc., 8 (1970) 465.
8. Di Luzio, N. R., Kuppfer Cells and Other Liver Sinusoidal Cells (Eds. E. Wisse and D. L. Knook), Elsevier/North-Holland, Amsterdam (1977) 397.
9. Di Luzio, N. R., Cook, J. A., Cohen, C., Rodrigue, J. and Jones, E., The Macrophage and Cancer (Eds. K. James, B. McBride and A. Stuart), Econoprint, Edinburgh (1977) 188.
10. Gillet, J., Jacques, P. J. and Herman, H., (1978) in press.
11. Hennekinne, M. F., Song, M. and Jacques, P. J., Arch. Intern. Physiol. Biochim., 85 (1977) 983.
12. Jacques, P. J., Epuration Plasmatique de Protéines Etrangéres, leur Capture et leur Destinée dans l'Appareil Vacuolaire du Foie, Librairie Universitaire, Leuven (1968).
13. Jacques, P. J., Huybrechts-Godin, G. and Smeesters, C., Biochem. Soc. Trans., 3 (1975) 155.
14. Munthe-Kaas, A. C., Berg, T. and Seljelid, R., Exp. Cell Research, 99 (1976) 146.
15. Thinès-Sempoux, D., Lysosomes in Biology and Pathology (Ed. J. T. Dingle), North-Holland, Amsterdam, 3 (1973) 278.
16. Wattiaux, R., Etude Expérimentale de la Surcharge des Lysosomes, Duculot, Gembloux (1966).

SUPPRESSOR CELL INDUCTION AND RETICULOENDOTHELIAL CELL ACTIVATION PRODUCED IN THE MOUSE BY β 1-3 GLUCAN

F. J. LEJEUNE, A. VERCAMMEN-GRANDJEAN,
P. MENDES da COSTA, D. BRON and V. DEFLEUR

Laboratory of Oncology and Experimental Surgery
Department of Surgery, Institut Jules Bordet
Centre des Tumeurs de l'Université Libre de
Bruxelles, Bruxelles (Belgium)

The insoluble polysaccharide β 1-3 glucan was shown to be the active component of zymosan for producing hyperplasia and hyperfunction of the reticuloendothelial (RE) system (9). Moreover, it was found to increase the protection against tumor grafts, bacterial and parasitic infections (2,3,7). Most of previous studies on the mechanisms whereby glucan seems to be an immunostimulant were performed after two or several injections of glucan (1,2,3). In order to evaluate the sequence of qualitative changes in RE system, and their reversibility, we used a single injection of glucan. The intravenous (i.v.) and intraperitoneal (i.p.) routes were compared in the study of functional changes of T and B lymphocytes and of mononuclear phagocytes.

MATERIAL AND METHODS

Glucan. β 1-3 glucan 35 mg/ml batch n°9/29/76 (donated by N. R. Di Luzio, Tulane University, New Orleans) was diluted appropriately with saline. The usual dosage was 50 mg/kg i.v. or 1 mg/mouse and 15 mg or 50 mg/kg, 300 μg or 1 mg/mouse i.p.

Mice. Three month-old C57BL and BDF_1 mice of both sexes were obtained from Charles River Inc. (USA) via the NCI Liaison Office of the Institut Jules Bordet (Brussels).

Spleen cells. Mechanical suspensions of spleen cells were centrifuged onto LYMPHOPREP (Nyegaard, Oslo) cushion for removing erythrocytes and polymorphs. They were seeded at a concentration of 2×10^6 cells/ml into Nunc microwells, in RPMI

1640 medium + 15% heat inactivated FBS (Gibco, Grand Island, N. Y.).

Response to mitogens in vitro. PHA (Wellcome, London) at the optimal concentration of 1 μg/ml or LPS-B (Difco, Detroit) at the optimal concentration of 100 μg/ml were used respectively for T or B lymphocyte response. Cells were incubated for 48 hr at 37 C in humidified atmosphere of 5% CO_2 in air, and pulsed for the last 24 hr with either ^{3}H-TdR (spec. act. 21 Ci/mmole) at the concentration of 5 μCi/ml, or ^{125}I-UdR (spec. act. 5 Ci/mg) at a concentration of 5 x 10^{-1} μCi/ml. Both were purchased from the Radiochemical Centre (Amersham, England). All tests were done in triplicate. The cells were harvested on the filters of a MASH II Cell Harvester (Biological Associates) and counted for β or γ activity. The results are expressed either in CPM or as Mitogenic Index (MI) calculated as follows : CPM with mitogen/ CPM control. In control experiments the addition of mitogen was omitted.

Cytochemistry of peritoneal cells. Whole peritoneal cells were seeded in Falcon 2.5 cm diameter petri dishes and fixed for 30 min at 4 C with 1% glutaraldehyde (TAB) and 4% formaldehyde (TAB) in Cacodylate buffer 0.1 M at pH 7.2. The acid phosphatase reaction and the assessment of spreading were performed as previously described (6). The peroxidase reaction was carried out according to the Graham and Karnowsky method (4).

RESULTS

Splenomegaly induced by single i.v. or i.p. injection of glucan. Fig.1 shows that a single i.v. or i.p. injection of glucan was followed by a considerable spleen weight increase. It was already detectable on day 3 and the responses in C57BL and BDF_1 mice were similar. Fig. 2 demonstrates the reversibility of this phenomenon : after 18 days the values went down and the baseline was reached by day 34.

Evaluation of DNA metabolism in spleen and peritoneal cells after glucan administration. After glucan i.v., spleen cells (Fig. 3a) and nonadherent peritoneal cells (Fig. 3b) exhibited an intense increase of ^{3}H-TdR uptake when cultured with no mitogen. It peaked on day 6 and went back to below baseline after 14-18 days. In contrast peritoneal adherent cells, namely macrophages, did not show any significant alteration of their usual background activity.

Peritoneal macrophages. Non-elicited and glucan-elicited mouse peritoneal macrophages were recovered by a method already described (5).

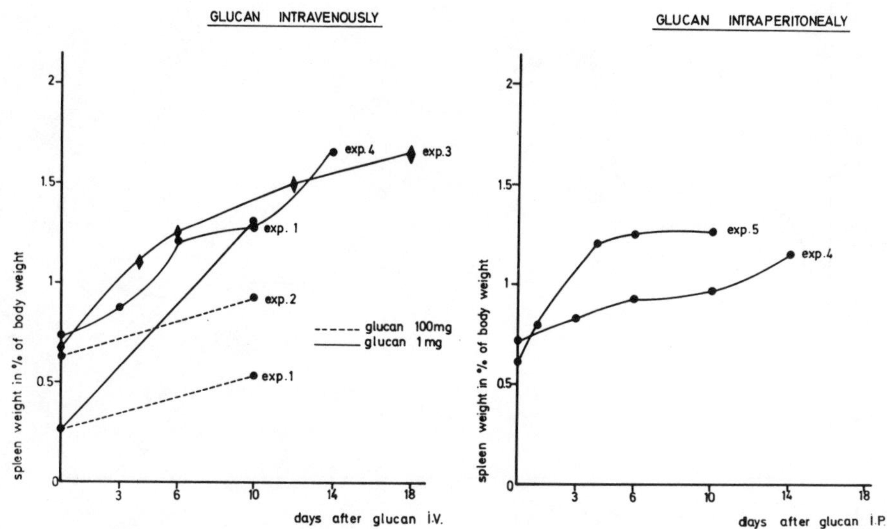

Fig. 1. Splenomegaly induced by single β 1-3 glucan injection. a. : glucan i.v. either 1 mg or 100 μg on day 0. b. : glucan i.p. 1 mg on day 0. Circle : BDF_1 mouse. Rhombus : C57BL mouse.

T and B lymphocyte response to mitogens in vitro. Spleen cells cultured with optimal concentration of LPS showed a decreased mitogenic index (MI) on day 3 after glucan. Thereafter, the values went back to and above the baseline (Fig. 4a). The PHA response was even more suppressed on days 3 and 6 and was recovered on days 12-18 (Fig. 4b). A comparison on i.v. and i.p. routes indicates a slower suppression after i.p. but the values were similar (Fig. 4c).

Mononuclear phagocyte response to glucan i.v. and i.p. The peritoneal mononuclear phagocyte populations were assessed by cytochemical and morphological criteria after glucan injection. Fig. 5 and 6 demonstrate that the changes after i.v. and i.p. injection of glucan were strikingly identical.

The percentage of acid phosphatase rich macrophages increased more than two-fold on day 3 and it was the first change. Then the percentage of spread macrophages rose after 3-6 days and decreased by day 10. An influx of peroxidase positive monocytic cells was the prominent feature on days 6 or 10. The values went back to or below baseline from days 14-18.

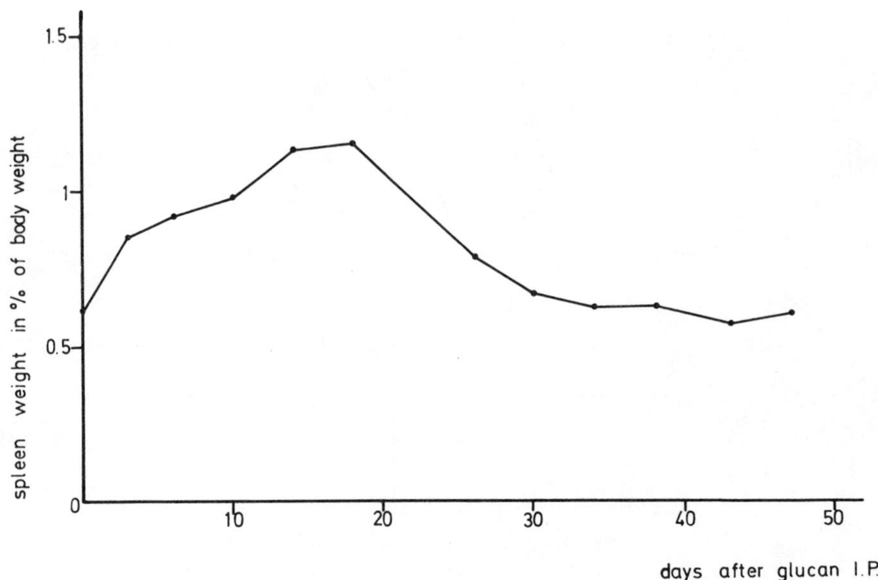

Fig. 2. Reversibility of glucan-induced splenomegaly. BDF_1 mice were injected i.p. on day 0 with 1 mg β 1-3 glucan.

Inhibition of PHA and LPS response in spleen cells by peritoneal macrophages and peritoneal macrophages secretory products. Peritoneal adherent cells containing mainly macrophages were cocultured with spleen cells at a 1:2 ratio, or the 24 hr macrophage culture supernatants (10^6 adherent cells/ml) were recovered and used as culture medium for spleen cells. Fig. 7 indicates that all macrophage preparations produced a marked inhibition of both PHA and LPS response in spleen lymphocytes. Glucan-elicited macrophages were slightly more inhibitory of PHA response than the resident macrophages but the differences were not significant. The macrophage supernatants exhibited a higher inhibition of both PHA and LPS response than the macrophages in cocultures.

DISCUSSION

Our results indicate that a single administration of β 1-3 glucan, *in vivo*, induces a sequence of various stimulative and inhibitory effects on the different cells belonging to the RE

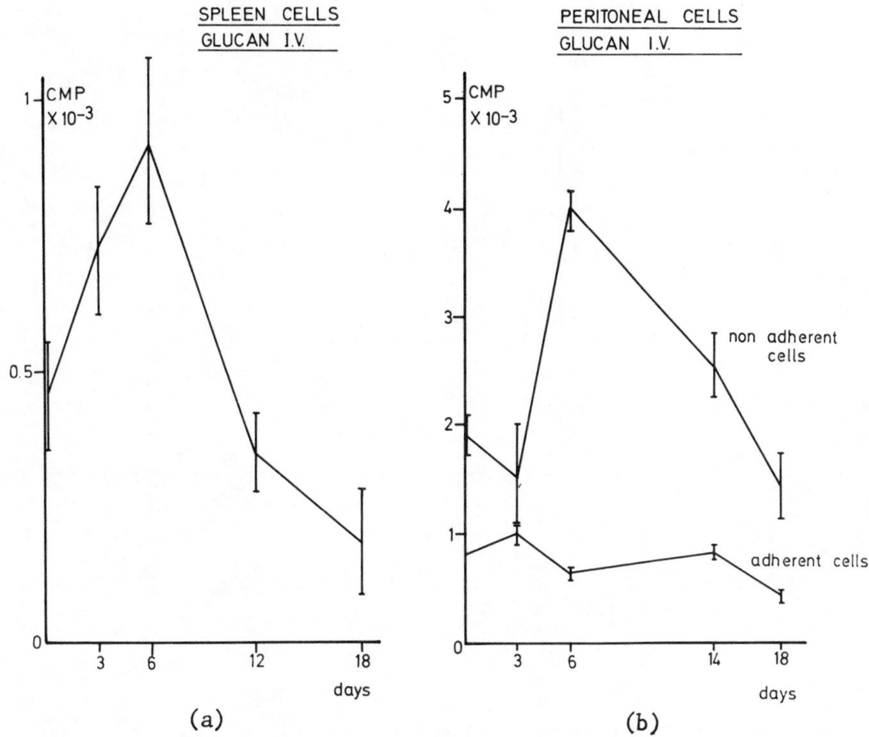

Fig. 3. Increase of *in vitro* ^{3}H-TdR uptake by spleen (a) and peritoneal lymphocytes (b) induced by glucan injected *in vivo*. BDF_1 mice received a single i.v. injection of 1 mg β 1-3 glucan on day 0.

system, and that they all are reversible. Some of the changes seem to be interrelated. Two different aspects should be separately discussed : (a) the *in vivo* and *in vitro* effects on T and B lymphocyte proliferation and (b) the mononuclear phagocyte stimulation and activation.

The reversible increase of spleen weight (Fig. 1-2) after 1 mg glucan i.v., a dose found to be optimal (8), was accompanied by an intense and also reversible proliferation of spleen lymphocytes (Fig. 3a) and of peritoneal lymphocytes (Fig. 3b). In contrast, peritoneal adherent cells did not show any significant change in DNA synthesis (Fig. 3b) but there was a marked influx of monocytes, with high peroxidase activity, in the peritoneal cavity, after glucan injection both i.v. or i.p. (Fig. 5-6). This would suggest that glucan increased the transit of blood monocytes

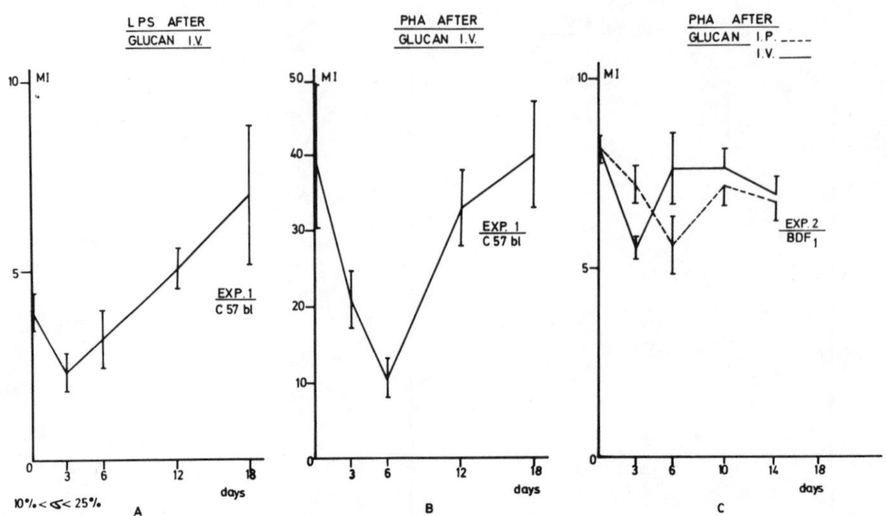

Fig. 4(a) (b) (c). Spleen lymphocyte response *in vitro* to LPS or PHA after 1 mg glucan *in vivo* on day 0.

to the peritoneal cavity, by a mechanism different from glucan chemotaxis, as it could be equally found after glucan i.v. or i.p. No detectable rise of granulocytes in the periotoneum was found. These results are in agreement with others (1) for the reported increase of macrophage colony forming cells in the bone marrow, as a phenomenon preceding the monocyte influx on days 6-10. However, they are in disagreement for the macrophage colony formation in the peritoneum as no proliferation of adherent cells was found.

Our results show that the mitogenic index of spleen cells responding *in vitro* to PHA and LPS was reversibly suppressed. This phenomenon appears to be quite different from the suppressive cells found with *C. parvum* (10). Our results indicate that the T and B lymphocyte mitogenic index was depressed and thereafter recovered in the course of splenomegaly. In contrast to the findings of others (2), an accumulation of suppressive cells in the spleen can therefore be ruled out. In addition, we report here that spleen and peritoneal lymphocytes exhibited a marked DNA synthesis 3-6 days after glucan i.v., while others did not find such an *in vivo* response neither after glucan (2) nor after *C. parvum* (10). Our finding of a simultaneous suppression of PHA and LPS response *in vitro* and stimulation of DNA synthesis *in vivo*, after a single injection of β 1-3 glucan, strongly suggests that β 1-3 glucan is a T and B mitogen *in vivo*. The reversible depression

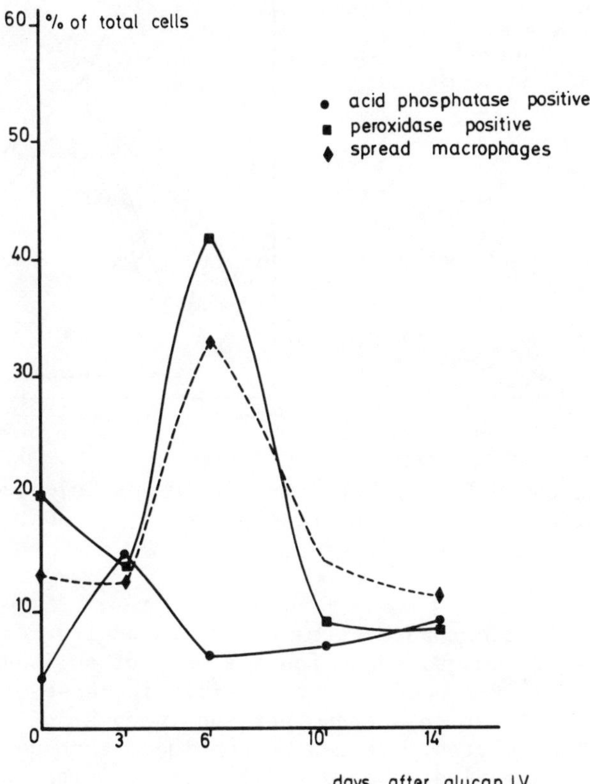

Fig. 5. Mononuclear phagocyte response to glucan. Increase of acid phosphatase positivity in peritoneal macrophages, of macrophage spreading and of peroxidase positive monocyte after 1 mg glucan i.v. on day 0 in BDF_1 mouse.

to in vitro T and B mitogens could therefore be due to a competition for the same responding cells. However, the crude CPM curves showed a trend for gradual decrease with time in PHA stimulated spleen lymphocytes cultures and not in LPS cultures (LeJeune, Vercammen, unpublished results).

In order to elucidate other mechanisms which could affect T and B lymphocytes, we studied the cytochemical and functional

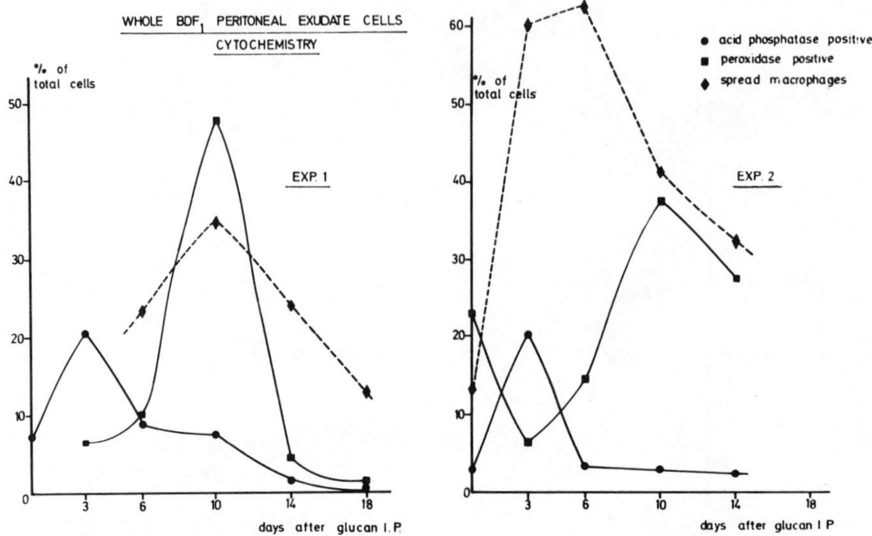

Fig. 6. Same as in Fig. 5 but 1 mg glucan was injected i.p. on day 0. Results from two separate experiments in BDF_1 mouse.

changes of mononuclear phagocytes after glucan i.v. or i.p. administration. We successively found a peak of acid phosphatase-rich macrophages, followed by a reversible increase of macrophage spreading concomitant to a transient and intense influx of peroxidase positive monocytes. It can be concluded that peritoneal macrophages were activated on day 3 : they exhibited an increase of lysosomal activity, of spreading capacity (Fig. 5-6) and became cytolytic toward tumor cells (Vercammen and LeJeune, in preparation). However, these activated macrophages did not show any significant increase of their naturally occurring cytostatic property (11) toward T and B lymphocytes.

At this stage of our studies, we can tentatively conclude that glucan is a macrophage activator and an *in vivo* mitogen. Current work is being done on the cytotoxic properties of differen RE cells on lymphocytes and tumor cells, after glucan administrati

SUMMARY

We made a sequential study of the proliferative and functiona changes occurring in RE cells after β 1-3 glucan administration in

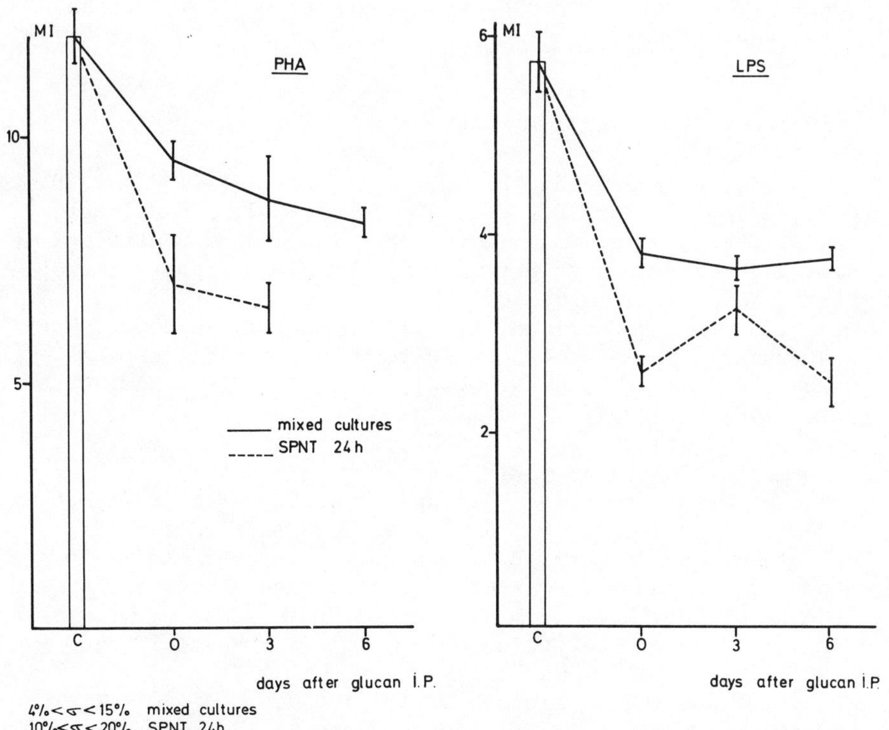

Fig. 7. Inhibition of PHA and LPS response in spleen cells by peritoneal macrophages and peritoneal macrophage secretory products. MI = Mitogenic Index. Control cells were incubated with only ^{125}I-UdR in the presence of either PHA or LPS.

BDF_1, and C57BL mouse. β 1-3 glucan was administered by single i.v. 50 mg/kg or i.p. 15 mg/kg injection. This successively induced changes in RE cells as follows : on day 3 a rise of acid phosphatase activity in peritoneal macrophages; on day 6 an increase of ^{3}H-TdR incorporation in spleen and peritoneal lymphocytes together with an intense suppression of PHA and LPS responses by spleen cells; on day 10 a 5-fold increase of the percentage of peroxidase rich monocytes in the peritoneum. Thereafter all the values went back to or below control. Our results indicate that β 1-3 glucan is an *in vivo* mitogen and a macrophage activator.

ACKNOWLEDGEMENTS

We thank Dr. N. R. Di Luzio, New Orleans, LA, for the gift of glucan. This work was supported by grant 3-4545-75 of the F.R.S.M. in Belgium.

REFERENCES

1. Burgaleta, C. and Golde, D. W., Cancer Res. 37 (1977) 1739.
2. Cook, J. A., Taylor, D., Cohen, C., Rodrique, J., Malshet, V. and Di Luzio, N. R., In: Immune Modulation and Control of Neoplasia by Adjuvant Therapy, (Ed. M. A. Chirigos), Raven Press, New York, (1978) 183.
3. Di Luzio, N. R., Hoffmann, E. O., Cook, J. A., Browder, W. and Mansell, P., Nat. Cancer Inst. Monogr. (1978) in press.
4. Graham, R. C., Jr. and Karnowsky, M. J., J. Histochem. Cytochem. 14 (1966) 291.
5. LeJeune, F. J., Beaumont, E., Garcia, Y. and Regnier, R., Biomedicine 28 (1978) 48.
6. LeJeune, F. J. and Evans, R., Europ. J. Cancer 8 (1972) 54.
7. LeJeune, F. J., Song, M., Delville, J., Stadtsbaeder, S., Gillet, J. and Jacques, P. J., Europ. J. Cancer (1978) in press.
8. Mendes da Costa, P., Defleur, V., Vercammen-Grandjean, A. and LeJeune, F. J., Europ. J. Cancer (1978) in press.
9. Riggi, S. J., and Di Luzio, N. R., Amer. J. Physiol., 200 (1961) 297.
10. Scott, M. T., Cell. Immunol. 5 (1972) 459.
11. Vercammen-Grandjean, A. F., and LeJeune, F. J., Production and mode of action of macrophage secretions that interfere with the _in vitro_ incorporation of radioactive DNA precursors by tumour cells. In: The Macrophage and Cancer. - Proc. EURES Symposium Edimburg 1977 (Eds. K. James, B. McBride, A. Stuart), (1977) 50.

THERAPEUTIC EFFECT OF INTRAVENOUSLY ADMINISTERED YEAST GLUCAN, IN MICE LOCALLY INFECTED BY *MYCOBACTERIUM LEPRAE*

J. DELVILLE and P. J. JACQUES

School of Public Health, Université Catholique de Louvain, Brussels (Belgium)

The management of leprosy is still primarily based on chemotherapy and antibiotic therapy, e.g., on directly acting substances which are simply more toxic for the parasite than for the host cells. Little efforts have been devoted thus far to the evaluation of drug candidates whose indirect antiparasitic power involves stimulation of the natural mechanism of host-defense. The dramatic problem caused by rapid spreading of resistance to sulphones prompted us to correct that situation, namely by means of immunostimulating polysaccharides whose antiparasitic efficacy had already been established against experimental tumors (19). Particulate β 1-3 glucan extracted from the cell walls of *Saccharomyces cerevisiae* was first chosen, because of its ability to act on several strategic parameters of humoral and cellular immunity (1,5,8) leading to enhancement of nonspecific resistance in a first stage (6) followed by specific immunostimulation as a second stage. Especially relevant to the case of leprosy, in which macrophages are the host-cells to the parasitic mycobacteria, is that this glucan appears as a most potent and versatile reticuloendothelial (RE) system-stimulator (5) through both activation of preexisting macrophages and overproduction of fresh mononuclear phagocytes. In the area of infectious diseases, β 1-3 glucans of fungal origin proved promising as candidates for the prevention or therapy of experimental tuberculosis (10), candidiasis (10,20), cryptococcosis (17), sporotrichosis (18), malaria (7), toxoplasmosis (11) and numerous other infections caused by extracellular bacteria (10).

Yeast glucan displayed therapeutic activity in the experimental model for leprosy when injected locally at the site of infection (2,3). Since this administration route is hardly suitable for patients because of the number of infected foci, some of which would inevitably escape detection the present study was designed to evaluate the effect of intravenously injected glucan.

MATERIAL AND METHODS

The experimental model used in this study as reported by Shepard (14) consisted of injecting human leprosy bacilli into the foot-pads of mice demonstrating its value over the last two decades for chemotherapeutic research on leprosy (13,16). Strain Tb mice were selected for their high susceptibility to tuberculosis allowing more rapid growth of *Mycobacterium leprae*. The mycobacteria, initially isolated from a human leproma (DS), were maintained by passages through the foot-pad of Tb mice. Yeast glucan (batch DL-04-P) was obtained from Dr. N. R. Di Luzio (Tulane University, New Orleans, LA) and further purified through repeated extractions on diethyl ether/water two-phase systems (P. J. Jacques, unpublished work).

Twelve mice were inoculated in one of the hind foot-pads, with a total of 4.4×10^4 acid-fast bacteria containing 15.9% of solid stained organisms. Two weeks later, treatment was initiated in five of these mice consisting of 4 weekly injections through the tail veins of glucan (40 mg. Kg^{-1}) suspended in saline for a period of 21 days. From the 12th to the 105th day after termination of treatment, the foot-pads of mice from both the control and treated groups were dissected and processed for enumeration of acid-fast bacteria (AFB; Ziehl-Neelsen method). In order to distinguish live from dead leprosy bacilli, the currently accepted criterion of granular versus solid-stained AFB (12) was retained. Granular counts were obtained by subtracting the solid-stained from the total AFB.

Statistical evaluation of the results was performed by the classical t-test variance analysis, linear regression and correlation.

RESULTS

From the individual observations gathered in Table I, it can be seen that AFB counts in control mice increased with time after infection, at rates typical of the selected mouse strain and inoculum size. Also, glucan administration seemed to decrease the three types of AFB counts.

In order to evaluate the statistical significance of the differences due to treatment, it was necessary to extract the part attributable to time after infection from the differences between

TABLE I

Effect of Glucan Treatment on Mycobacterial Counts (x 10^{-3})

Time (days) After		Control			Glucan-Treated[a]		
Infection	End of Treatment	Total AFB	Staining Solid	Staining Granular	Total AFB	Staining Solid	Staining Granular
47	12	19.5	5.86	13.6	1.72	0.00	1.72
47	12	17.2	1.92	15.3	10.3	0.00	10.3
84	49	174	38.9	135	20.2	1.55	18.7
112	77	558	208	350	47.9	16.7	31.2
112	77	163	69.0	94.0	-	-	-
140	105	1646	339	1307	104	47.9	56.1
140	105	1404	222	1182	-	-	-

[a]Glucan (40 mg.Kg^{-1}) was injected intravenously on days 14-21-28-35 after infection.

individual values. This was achieved in Table II, by expressing AFB counts of the treated mice in percent of the homologous values obtained in the corresponding control animals. It can be seen that glucan treatment significantly decreased ($p<0.1\%$) the number of granular as well as solid-stained AFB. It is therefore, not surprising to observe that their sum (total AFB) was also decreased, with a similar level of significance. In other words, should one accept literally the hypothesis put forward by Rees and Valentine (12) which considers solid-stained as live mycobacteria and granular as dead ones, it would be permitted to conclude from our results that glucan treatment reduced the number of live AFB, e.g., the source for bacterial proliferation, also the number of dead AFB. Being the most numerous, the latter can be held primarily responsible for the development of leprotic lesions which is currently attributed to the normal immune response to long lasting antigens. Moreover, glucan treatment depressed granular counts to

Table II

Statistical Significance[a] of Glucan-Treatment Effects on Mycobacterial Counts

	Mycobacterial Counts (%)		
	Total	Staining	
	AFB	Granular	Solid
Control	100 ± 0	100 ± 0	100 ± 0
Treated	10.9 ± 8.5	23.8 ± 13.0	6.64 ± 3.42
Control-treated	81.1 ± 8.5	76.2 ± 13.0	93.4 ± 3.4
P <	0.001	0.001	0.001

[a]Descriptive statistics refer to arithmetic mean ± standard error. Significance of differences between means (8 degrees of freedom) was assessed by the t-test.

a much larger extent than the solid-stained ones (Table III), at all times during the experimental period. When examined according to the theory of Rees and Valentine (12), this observation suggests that the decrease of granular AFB counts induced by glucan treatment could not only result from the decreased rate of decay of live (solid-stained) AFB which can be expected from the lowered concentration of the latter but it must involve, in addition, an increased rate of in vivo degradation of the dead (granular) leprosy bacilli.

A surprising fact also illustrated in Table III is that the intensity of all the effects of glucan treatment reported here increased as time elapsed after treatment instead of progressively vanishing.

TABLE III

Evolution of Intensity of Glucan Effect on Mycobacterial Counts[a]

Time (days) After End of Treatment	Log_e of Glucan Effect on (AFB counts x 10^{-3})			Log_e (Effect on Granular / Effect on Solid)
	Total AFB	Granular Stained	Solid Stained	
12	2.88	2.47	1.77	1.79
12	1.93	1.61	0.65	1.13
49	5.03	4.76	3.62	4.37
77	5.75	5.25	4.80	4.23
105	7.26	7.08	5.45	6.86
r[b]	0.9770	0.9757	0.9643	0.9591
b[b]	0.0518	0.0528	0.0478	0.0539
a[b]	1.928	1.5436	0.8188	0.9270
p[c]	<0.01	<0.01	<0.01	<0.01

[a]Treatment effects were expressed as differences between raw values of counts between control and treated. They were then submitted to logarithmic transformation in order to normalize their frequency distribution, as a prerequisite to applicability of linear regression and correlation analysis.

[b]Statistics: r = correlation coefficient; a and b are respectively the ordinate at origin and slope of the linear regression line : Log_e effect = a + b·time.

[c]Significance (p) of the correlation was chosen as that of the single mean b (t-test with 4 degrees of freedom).

In the exploratory conditions of dosage and drug administration schedule adopted in the present study, glucan administration had conspicuous therapeutic activity but failed to stop the infection caused by M. leprae. A significant drop of total and granular AFB in treated as compared to control animals could be observed as early as the 12th day after end of treatment. At that time, solid stained AFB were undetectable in treated animals, whereas the controls still contained an appreciable proportion of the 7,000 live AFB present in the inoculum. The bactericidal nature of glucan suggested - though not demonstrated - by these observations was rendered more than probable after applying (Table IV) a method (9,15) consisting of graphically estimating the difference in the time necessary for the AFB counts of treated mice to reach those of the controls. The fact that, in our animal model, none of the six experimental curves corresponded to a true exponential function of time, and that no parallelism could be noticed between them, prohibited us from exploiting the elegant and audacious technique of Shepard (15), and forced us to measure the delays between treated and control curves after hand-fitting the latter. Results presented in Table IV show that, for all three types of AFB counts, the delay caused by glucan treatment was longer than the 21 days

TABLE IV

Length and Evolution of Delay for Reaching Given Mycobacterial Counts, After Glucan Treatment

Bacterial Counts ($x\ 10^{-3}$)	Delays (days)		
	Total AFB	Granular AFB	Solid St. AFB
5	-	-	39
10	-	-	38
20	55	43	42
30	-	58	46
40	89	69	49
50	-	76	54
60	109	80	-
80	129	-	-
100	138	-	-

Delays were measured graphically as horizontal distances between control and treated curves obtained through handfitting on the untransformed data, for various values of bacterial counts. The latter were chosen only in the region covered by both the control and treated curves giving counts as a function of time.

representing the duration of the drug administration period. Moreover, this delay steadily increased with time throughout the experiment. The analysis was extended to total counts, for the sole purpose of facilitating comparison of present data with those from relevant literature.

DISCUSSION

Application of the current criteria would allow us to conclude that the present results unequivocally demonstrate the therapeutic value of intravenously administered glucan, and the bactericidal nature of its action in the local infection caused in the mouse foot-pad by *M. leprae*. Indeed, the number (total) of acid-fast bacteria was depressed early in treated as compared to control animals (Table I). In addition, when at a later stage, bacterial counts rose again, the delay needed for the treated foot-pads to contain the same number of AFB as the controls largely exceeded the length of the drug administration period (Table IV). However, application of the above criteria to total AFB neglects two long recognized features, especially in lepromatous lesions, that the majority of AFB are dead, and that the handling of intravacuolar microbes by lysosomal effectors involves two distinct and successive steps, e.g., bacterial killing and chemical degradation of the dead organisms. Precisely, the method of Rees and Valentine (12) offers the possibility of distinguishing between the two categories of AFB which, in addition, are thought to play distinct roles in the pathogenesis of leprosy and thus are distinct targets for drug action.

Since, and only since, the above criteria were fulfilled by solid stained counts while, in addition, the granular counts were also depressed in glucan treated mice, we claim the therapeutic effect of glucan involving bactericidal activity. Another benefit from using the more demanding technique of Rees and Valentine, was that glucan treatment also caused a considerable decrease of granular counts that largely exceeded that of the solid stained ones. This would allow us to conclude in first approximation that an acceleration of *in vivo* degradation of dead leprosy bacilli occurred, introducing a second impact point in the glucan therapeutic action after bacterial killing. Other drug models with wide antiparasitic spectrum of activity, e.g., the free radical generators (2). Triton WR-1339 and Macrocyclon (4), exhibit a similar double impact therapeutic capacity in the foot-pad model for leprosy.

Experiments are in progress in an attempt to improve the efficacy of glucan treatment after administration by systemic routes, and in order to elucidate its mechanisms.

ACKNOWLEDGEMENTS

The authors wish to express their gratitude to I. de Zurpele, W. Rayyan and F. Herman for skillful technical assistance, to Dr. N. R. Di Luzio (New Orleans, LA) for continuous supply of yeast glucan, to Drs. H. Sansarricq (WHO, Geneva) and R. J. W. Rees (London) for encouragement and stimulating discussions, and to Belgian Fonds de la Recherche Scientifique Médicale (contract 3.4580.75F), Les Amis du Père Damien and World Health Organization (Thelep Program) for financial and moral support. One of us (P. J. J.) is Maître de Recherche of Belgian Fonds National de la Recherche Scientifique.

REFERENCES

1. Browder, W., McNamee, R., Cohan, L., Taylor, D. and Di Luzio, N. R., J. Reticuloendothelial Soc., 20 (1976) 55 a.
2. Delville, J. and Jacques, P. J., Acta Leprologica, 66/67 (1977) 101.
3. Delville, J. and Jacques, P. J., Arch. Intern. Physiol. Biochim., 85 (1977) 965.
4. Delville, J. and Jacques, P. J., Biochem. Soc. Tras., 6 (1978) 395.
5. Di Luzio, N. R., The Reticuloendothelial System in Health and Disease (Eds. H. Friedman, M. R. Escobar and S. M. Reichard), Plenum Press, New York, Vol. A (1976) 412.
6. Di Luzio, N. R., Kuppfer Cells and Other Liver Sinusoidal Cells (Eds. E. Wisse and D. L. Knook), Elsevier/North Holland, Amsterdam (1977) 397.
7. Gillet, J., Jacques, P. J. and Herman, F., this volume.
8. Glovsky, M. M., Di Luzio, N. R., Alenty, A. and Ghekiere, L. R., J. Reticuloendothelial Soc., 20 (1976) 54a.
9. Holmes, I. B. and Hilson, G. R. F., Proc. Soc. Exp. Biol. Med., 145 (1974) 1395.
10. Komatsu, N., Sakai, S., Saito, G., Kikumoto, S. and Kimura, N., United States Patents, application 378054 (1976).
11. Nguyen, B. T. and Stadtsbaeder, S., this volume.
12. Rees, R. J. W. and Valentine, R. C., Intern. J. Lepr., 30 (1962) 1.
13. Sansarricq, H., Experientia, 33 (1977) 114.
14. Shepard, C. C., J. Exp. Med., 112 (1960) 445.
15. Shepard, C. C., Intern. J. Lepr., 35 (1967) 429.
16. Shepard, C. C., Ellard, G. A., Levy, L., de Araujo-Opromolla, V., Pattyn, S. R., Peters, J. H., Rees, R. J. W. and Waters, M. F. R., Bull. World Health Org., 53 (1976) 425.
17. Song, M., Demoulin-Brahy, L. and Jacques, P. J., Current Chemotherapy, Am. Soc. Microbiol., Washington (1978) 234.
18. Stevens, M. M., Stevens, P., Cook, J. A., Ichinose, H. and Di

Luzio, N. R., J. Reticuloendothelial Soc., 20 (1976) 66a.
19. Whistler, R. L., Bushway, A. A., Singh, P. P., Nakahara, W. and Tokuzen, R., Adv. Carbohydr. Chem. Biochem., 32 (1976) 235.
20. Williams, D., Cook, J. A. and Di Luzio, N. R., J. Reticuloendthelial Soc., (1977) in press.

COMPARATIVE BIOLOGICAL AND ANTITOXOPLASMIC EFFECTS OF PARTICULATE AND WATER-SOLUBLE POLYSACCHARIDES, *IN VITRO*

B. T. NGUYEN and S. STADTSBAEDER

Service Microbiologie, Cliniques Universitaires Saint Luc, Université Catholique de Louvain, Brussels (Belgium)

Toxoplasma gondii is an obligate intracellular protozoan which proliferates preferentially within reticuloendothelial mononuclear phagocytes of experimentally infected animals.

Resistance against toxoplasma infection is a form of cell-mediated immunity involving functional T cells (18,28) and macrophages specifically activated by toxoplasma-sensitized lymphocytes. These macrophages have an enhanced capacity for controlling intracellular multiplications of *T. gondii* both in immune animals (26, 27) and in cell cultures *in vitro* (10,25,26,27).

Corynebacterium parvum and BCG, which stimulate the lymphoreticular system, are usually employed as nonspecific host-resistance enhancers. More recently, however, polysaccharides have been proposed as potent stimulators of reticuloendothelial cells (7,11). Some of them are actually used in experimental bacterial (4,15), protozoal (8) and cancer (14,17,29,30) immunotherapy with promising results.

In one of our previous reports (22) β-1,3 glucan, batch n° 02, (kindly provided by Dr. N. R. Di Luzio from Tulane University School of Medicine, New Orleans, LA) showed marked toxic effect for mouse peritoneal macrophages but not for HeLa cell monolayers and was completely ineffective against infection by *T. gondii* both in experimentally infected NMRI female mice and in normal mouse peritoneal macrophages and HeLa cells in culture.

In this paper we describe experiments performed *in vitro* using five other polysaccharides with special reference to their effects on cytotoxicity,spreading, endocytosis and toxoplasma infection of normal mouse peritoneal macrophage and HeLa cell monolayers.

MATERIALS AND METHODS

Animals. Normal NMRI female mice, weighing between 20-22g were used throughout this study.

Parasites. *T. gondii* trophozoites of the virulent RH strain were collected from lethaly-infected mice and purified as previously described (27).

Culture medium. One ml volumes of normal mouse peritoneal macrophages (1×10^5 ml) and HeLa cells (5×10^4/ml) were distributed into Leighton tubes. After 24 hr of incubation of 37 C, the monolayers were washed thrice with fresh medium. Volumes of 1 ml containing varying concentrations of glucans were then added to the tubes.

Polysaccharides. Lentinan (LTN), Schizophyllan micro (SPG micro) and macromolecular forms (SPG macro) and *Coriolus versicolor* extract (PSK) were, respectively, provided by Drs. Chihara, Komatsu and Vetsuka from Tokyo (Japan). Batch n° 06 of Di Luzio insoluble particulate glucan (DL 06) and water-soluble polysaccharides were suspended or dissolved in saline as stock solutions of 5 mg/ml. All these solutions were further sterilized in the autoclave.

Cytotoxic effect. Viability of the cells after 24 hr-exposure at 37 C to varying concentrations of glucans was determined by the trypan blue exclusion method (21).

Spreading effect. Glucan-treated monolayers were rinsed once with saline and then fixed with 2% glutaraldehyde for 5 min before being examined by phase-contrast microscopy. Giemsa stain was also applied to some preparations.

Effects on endocytosis of macrophages. Phagocytic activity of macrophages treated with polysaccharides was assessed with lyophilized preparations of highest doses of polysaccharides which gave less than 10% of cytotoxicity, the cover slips were washed twice with fresh medium and 1 ml of culture medium containing 4×10^5 parasites was added to each tube. The monolayers were then incubated at 37 C for 60 min before being examined. Only pinocytic activity of PSK-treated macrophages was assessed with Pelikan drawing black ink. Macrophage monolayers were cultivated for 24 hr at 37 C in medium containing 0.2% (v/v) of the marker. Microscopic observations were performed on Giemsa-stained preparations.

Antitoxoplasmic effect. The highest doses of polysaccharides causing death of less than 10% of the cells, as judged by the trypan blue exclusion test, were added to mouse peritoneal macrophage and to HeLa cell monolayers, either 2 days before inoculation with living *T. gondii* RH (1×10^5 parasites/tube), at the time of inoculation or 2 hr later. Therefore, the percentage of infected cells and the mean number of parasites per infected cell in the presence or absence of polysaccharides were determined daily for 3 days on Giemsa-stained preparations.

RESULTS

Cytotoxic effect. Cytotoxic effect of polysaccharides for cell monolayers was assessed with the trypan blue exclusion technique. Doses of polysaccharides producing 50% of cytotoxicity (CD 50) after 24 hr of incubation at 37 C are listed in Table I. Particulate insoluble glucan showed a higher toxicity degree for macrophages than the water-soluble ones. The CD 50 for particulate 06 Di Luzio glucan was equal or greater than 40 µg/ml.

In contrast to macrophages, there was no differential cytotoxicity between either particulate or water-soluble polysaccharides for HeLa cells with doses up to 50 µg/ml.

Spreading effect. LTN and PSK induced a very marked spreading effect upon macrophage monolayers. This effect was conspicuous on more than 80% of the adherent cells as soon as 4 hr after addition of LTN or PSK to cell cultures. Spread macrophages were elongated resulting from emission of long extensions (Fig. 1-2). By 24 hr, macrophages treated with 40 µg LTN or with 500 µg PSK per ml had a mean maximal length about three times greater than that of untreated cells (Fig. 3).

Addition of LTN or PSK 2 hr instead of 24 hr after adherence of macrophages on glass cover slips delayed for about 24 hr the spreading effect.

LTN and PSK did not induce spreading of macrophages if the incubation temperature was lowered to 4 C. The macrophages had not lost their ability to spread after such a treatment since their subsequent reincubation at 37 C in the presence of LTN or PSK still produced spreading.

Spreading effect of micromolecular form of SPG was significantly lesser than that of LTN and PSK. Incubation of macrophage monolayers for 24 hr in the presence of SPG micro resulted in an increase in mean maximal length from 1.4 to 1.5, respectively, with 40 and 500 µg/ml. Macromolecular form of SPG had no demonstrable spreading effect on macrophage monolayers.

TABLE I

Effects of Polysaccharides on the Viability of Normal Mouse Peritoneal Macrophages and HeLa Cell Monolayers

Polysaccharides	CD 50[a] (μg/ml)	
	Macrophages	HeLa cells
DL 06	> 40	>50
LTN	>1,000	>50
PSK	>1,000	>50
SPG micro	>1,000	>50
SPG macro	>1,000	>50

[a]Dose of polysaccharides producing 50% of cytotoxicity after 24 hr at 37 C by the trypan blue exclusion technique.

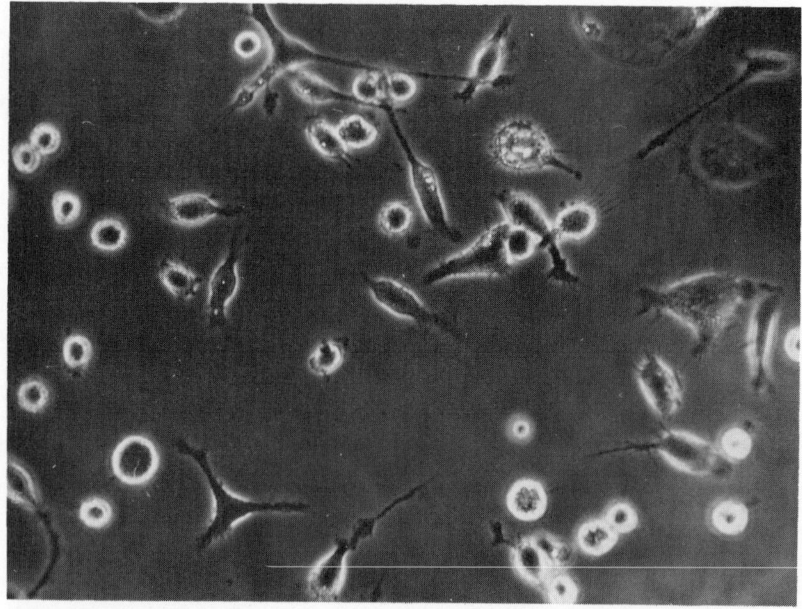

Fig. 1. Untreated control mouse peritoneal macrophage monolayer, 48 hr after cultivation at 37 C (Phase contrast. X 1,400).

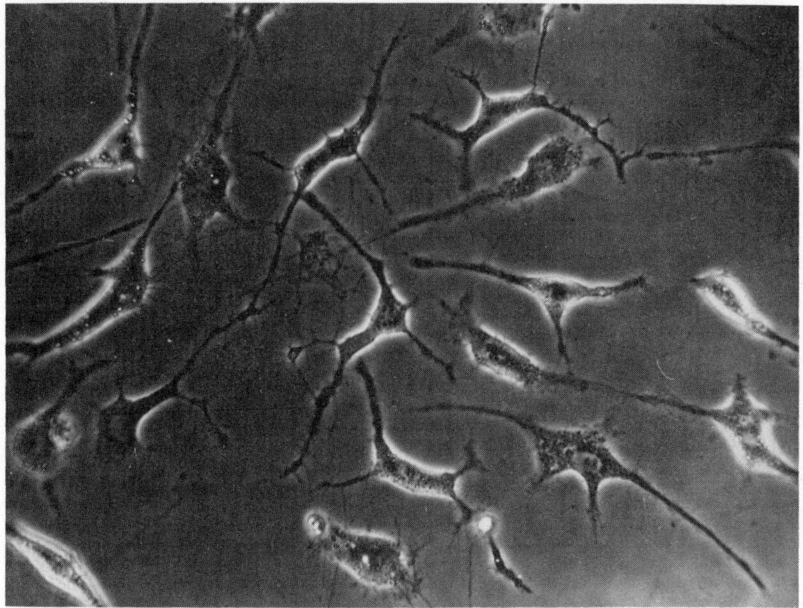

Fig. 2. 24 hr-old mouse peritoneal macrophage monolayer treated for 24 hr at 37 C with PSK (500 μg/ml) (Phase contrast. X 1,400).

Particulate Di Luzio glucan was engulfed by macrophages which rounded off and lost adherence to glass cover slips. This led to a decrease of the cell length with increasing doses.

In contrast to macrophages, none of the polysaccharides used in this study induced spreading of HeLa cells.

Effects on phagocytosis. Effects of polysaccharides on phagocytic activity of macrophages in culture are represented in Table II. Cultivation of macrophages for 2 days with nontoxic doses of both forms of SPG did not significantly alter phagocytosis by macrophages of lyophilized-preparations of killed toxoplasma. In contrast, uptake of toxoplasma by macrophages pretreated with 20 μg/ml of 06 Di Luzio glucan was markedly decreased ($p<0.001$). This dose had been chosen since it produced less than 10% of cytotoxicity. On the other hand, incubation of macrophages with LTN or with PSK prior to addition of killed toxoplasma resulted in a significant ($p<0.010$) increase uptake of the parasites;

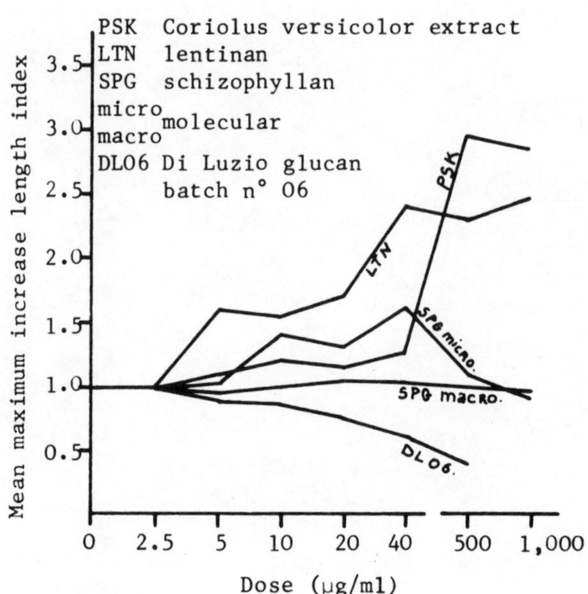

Fig. 3. Effect of polysaccharides (PLS) on macrophage spreading *in vitro*. Counts performed after 24 hr at 37 C on glutaraldehyde fixed preparations.

$$\text{Mean maximum length increase index} = \frac{\text{mean maximum length with PLS}}{\text{mean maximum length untreated}}$$

both percentages of LTN or PSK-treated macrophages containing 1 to 2 and more than 2 toxoplasma per cell were significantly higher than those of the untreated control cells for each time interval considered.

Effect of PSK on pinocytosis. Pinocytic activity was qualitatively assessed only on PSK-treated macrophages. Macrophages which had taken up China ink could be divided into three main groups as follow: cells (i) completely, (ii) moderately and (iii) slightly filled with the marker. A representative example is given in Fig. 4. These three groups represent respectively, 43, 34 and 23% in PSK-treated macrophages and 31, 33 and 36% in untreated control cells.

Antitoxoplasmic effect. The different modes of treatment (summarized in Table III) show that only treatment of macrophages prior to inoculation with living _T. gondii_ for 2 days with 500 μg/ml of PSK or LTN reduced significantly the infection of macrophage monolayers. Protection afforded by PSK or LTN significantly delayed destruction of the host cells by toxoplasma. The most consistent evidence for this protecting effect was seen on days 2 and 3 of inoculation. The evolution of untreated and PSK-treated macrophages after inoculation with living toxoplasma is illustrated in Fig. 5. Significant destruction of untreated cells by the parasites began on day 2 and reached more than 90% on day 3. Despite the presence of replicative forms of toxoplasma within PSK-treated macrophages, destruction of these cells did not exceed 60% on day 3 of inoculation.

Incubation of HeLa cells in the presence of polysaccharides for 2 days before inoculation with living _T. gondii_ did not interfere with the normal course of the infection.

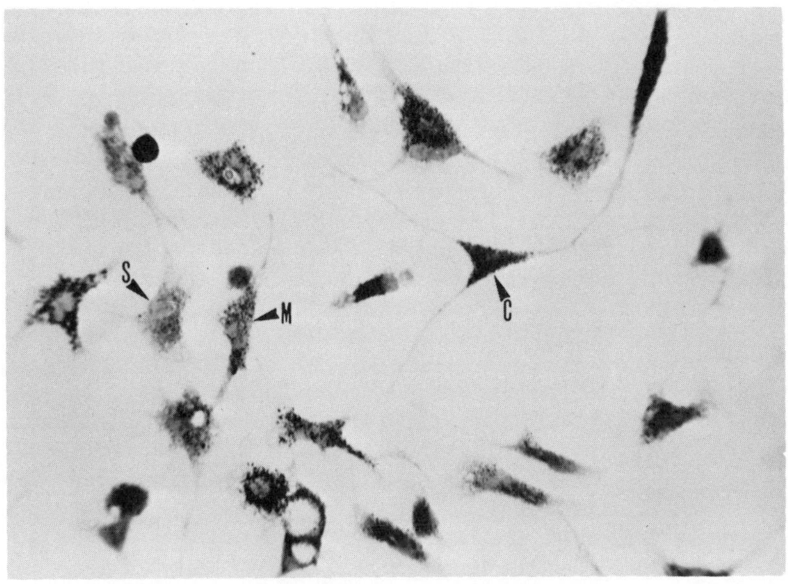

Fig. 4. Pinocytosis of China black ink by PSK-treated macrophages. Note the presence of cells completely (C), moderately (M) or slightly (S) filled with the marker (Giemsa stain. X 1,400).

TABLE II

Effect of Pretreatment with Polysaccharides for 24 Hr on Phagocytosis of Lyophilized Preparations of Killed *Toxoplasma gondii* by Mouse Peritoneal Macrophages in Culture

Polysac-charides	Dose	(%) Macrophages with		(%) Total Phagocytosis	p[b]
		1-2 parasites	>2 parasites		
DL 06	20	13,0±2,5[a]	2,9±0,5	15,9±1,8	<0.001
LTN	500	35,6±4,1	6,9±2,5	41,5±3,1	<0.025
PSK	500	40,2±4,9	8,7±1,3	48,9±2,5	<0.010
SPG micro	500	30,8±3,7	2,0±1,6	32,8±3,9	NS[c]
SPG macro	500	26,7±4,2	3,8±2,4	30,5±4,2	NS
Control	-	28,7±3,9	3,4±2,7	32,1±3,1	

[a]Mean ± standard error from six replicate experiments.
[b]Student t test.
[c]NS, not significant ($p>0.05$).

DISCUSSION

Present results indicate that insoluble particulate and water-soluble polysaccharides demonstrated differential cytotoxicity according to the cell-type employed. None of the polysaccharides used was toxic to non-phagocytic HeLa cells, whereas macrophages better tolerated water-soluble than insoluble particulate glucans. As we previously emphasized (22), phagocytosis of particulate glucans might be directly related to their cytotoxic effect since: (a) particulate glucans were observed within macrophages but not within HeLa cells; (b) macrophages which were filled with particulate glucans regularly lost their ability to exclude vital dye; and (c) the particulate Di Luzio glucan used in the present study, which was engulfed by macrophages to a lesser extent than that previously employed (22), was consequently about 8 times less toxic.

Lentinan and *Coriolus versicolor* extracts were two of the five glucans which produced the most marked spread of unelicited normal mouse peritoneal macrophages in culture. Why such an

TABLE III

Effect of Polysaccharides on Toxoplasma Infection within Mouse Peritoneal Macrophage Monolayers[a]

Time of Polysaccharide Addition to Inoculation	Days After Inoculation	Polysaccharides (μg/ml)					
		DL06(20)	LTN(500)	PSK(500)	SPG micro (500)	SPG macro (500)	Saline
2 days before	1	+	-	-	+	+	+
	2	++	+	+	++	++	++
	3	+++	++	++	+++	+++	+++
at the time	1	+	+	+	+	+	+
	2	++	++	++	++	++	++
	3	+++	+++	+++	+++	+++	+++
2 hrs after	1	+	+	+	+	+	+
	2	++	++	++	++	++	++
	3	+++	+++	+++	+++	+++	+++

[a]Each + represents 20 to 30% destruction of the monolayers by *Toxoplasma gondii*.

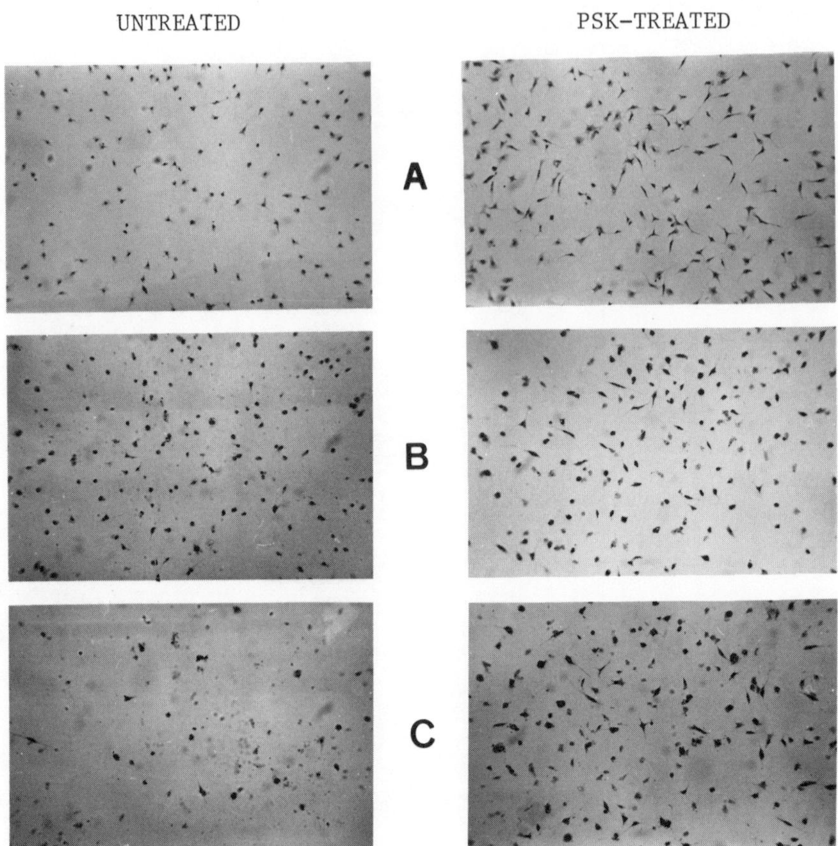

Fig. 5. Effect of PSK on mouse peritoneal macrophages infected with living *Toxoplasma gondii* RH. Macrophages were pretreated with PSK (500 μg/ml) for 2 days before inoculation. Micrographs were taken 1 (A), 2 (B) and 3 (C) days after inoculation (Giemsa stain. X 200).

effect required previous adherence of macrophages to glass-cover slips remains unclear. Furthermore, the spreading of macrophages seemed to be an active process which needed metabolic energy since low temperatures inhibited it.

Burgaleta *et al*. (2) reported that macrophages collected from peritoneal cavity of glucan-treated mice show marked spread after their adherence to cover slips. Their macrophages were morphologically identical to those we obtained after addition of LTN or PSK to cultures of macrophages collected from normal mice.

But, Di Luzio insoluble glucan was used by these authors and we did not observe any spreading effect in cultures treated with both glucans provided by Di Luzio. Again, the glucan used by Burgaleta *et al*. is different from those we recently received. Otherwise, one could postulate that LTN and PSK produced direct spreading effect upon resident peritoneal macrophages, whereas that of particulate Di Luzio glucans is merely directed towards peritoneal macrophages recruited from blood monocytes (23), most likely following chemotactic stimuli produced by glucan, with or without involvement of the host-immune system (3). Indeed, macrophages used by Burgaleta *et al*. were collected only 6 days after intraperitoneal injection of Di Luzio glucan, at a time where the total number of peritoneal macrophages was about 3 times greater than that of the untreated control animals.

Kamitsuka *et al*. (11) have demonstrated enhanced phagocytosis of *Candida tropicalis* by macrophages derived from PSK-treated mice. Similar effect can be reproduced *in vitro* with *T. gondii* after addition of LTN or PSK to culture of normal mouse peritoneal macrophages. Although comparative kinetic studies of endocytic activity between untreated and LTN or PSK-treated cells were not performed here, results obtained after the single time interval of 60 min are sufficiently representative to propose that uptake of lyophilized preparations of killed toxoplasma were significantly higher in the treated groups than in the untreated ones. Increase in size, membrane and spreading activities following exposure to LTN or PSK improve surface contact which would therefore be favorable to phagocytosis. On the other hand, engulfment of insoluble glucan during the preinoculation period likely interfered with further uptake of toxoplasma since phagocytosis was markedly reduced with Di Luzio glucan-treated macrophages.

The ability of polysaccharide-treated macrophages to delay destruction by intracellular toxoplasma infection was solely restricted to monolayers which were pretreated for 2 days with LTN or PSK. The mechanism of action of LTN and PSK in toxoplasmic resistance is not yet understood. However, it can be argued that: (a) this resistance was developed by the macrophages themselves in the absence of cooperation with any other cell types since the monolayers were extensively washed prior addition of polysaccharides to eliminate non adherent cells, mainly lymphocytes; (b) LTN and PSK had no direct action upon intracellular toxoplasma since treatment performed at the time or after inoculation had no effects as were treatments of toxoplasma-infected HeLa cells, and (c) it is clear that only cells which presented morphological features of activated macrophages at the time of inoculation were able to further prevent destruction by toxoplasma.

Activation of macrophages by LTN or PSK is different from activation by newborn calf serum (NBCS) since normal mouse peritoneal macrophages cultivated in high concentrations of NBCS also showed characteristics of activated macrophages (12,19) but failed to efficiently restrict intracellular growth of toxoplasma (24). These observations provide additional support in favor of the consideration that LTN and PSK are real immunoenhancers.

Di Luzio glucans and SPG exhibited significant protecting effects against tumors (3,14,17), bacteria (4,15,16), yeasts (13, 17) and protozoa (8) in experimental animals. This increase in resistance has been essentially attributed to activated macrophages because peritoneal macrophages collected from Di Luzio or SPG-treated mice showed enlargment in size and enhanced capacity for reducing growth of tumor cells (3) and bacteria (20) *in vitro*. Nevertheless, whether this macrophage activation occurred alone or under influence of the host-immune system remains to be determined. If such an activation did not occur alone, our failure to demonstrate macrophage activation following treatment of the macrophage monolayers with both products might be explained by the fact that our *in vitro* system deals with a single isolated resident cell population, whereas partial and/or full involvement of the immune system leading to macrophage activation by Di Luzio glucans and SPG certainly should be considered *in vivo*. In fact, it has been shown that Di Luzio glucans and SPG stimulate humoral and cellular immunity (5,6,31,32). Furthermore, Di Luzio glucans also activate complement pathways (9) and induce monocyte proliferation (1).

SUMMARY

Mouse peritoneal macrophages, but not HeLa cells, presented many characteristics of activated cells following treatment in culture with LTN or PSK. Indeed, they demonstrated increase in size, spread, endocytic and antiparasitic activities. These data lead favorably to consider that among the five polysaccharides tested under the present experimental model LTN and PSK are the most potent activators of resident mouse peritoneal macrophages *in vitro*. The mechanism of macrophage activation by LTN and PSK should be different from that of Di Luzio glucans and SPG since activated macrophages can be induced by the latter two compounds in experimental animals but not *in vitro* in cell cultures.

ACKNOWLEDGMENT

This work was supported by grant 3.4580.75 of the Belgian Fonds de la Recherche Scientifique Médicale.

REFERENCES

1. Burgaleta, C. and Golde, D. W., Cancer Res., 37 (1977) 1739.
2. Burgaleta, C., Territo, M. C., Quan, S. G. and Golde, D. W., J. Reticuloendothel. Soc., 23 (1978) 195.
3. Cook, J. A., Taylor, D., Cohen, C., Hoffman, E. O., Rodriguez, J., Malshet, V. and Di Luzio, N. R., J. Reticuloendothel. Soc. 22 (1977) 21.
4. Delville, J. and Jacques, P. J., Arch. Internat. Physiol. Biochim., (1978) in press.
5. Di Luzio, N. R., J. Reticuloendothel. Soc., 1 (1964) 160.
6. Di Luzio, N. R., Wooles, W. R. and Morrow, S. H., J. Reticuloendothel. Soc. 1 (1964) 429.
7. Di Luzio, N. R., The Reticuloendothelial System in Health and Diseases, Part A (Ed. S. M. Reichard, M. Escobar and H. Friedman), Adv. Exp. Med. Biol., Plenum Press, New York, 73 (1976) 412.
8. Gillet, J., Jacques, P. J. and Herman, F., C. R. Soc. Biol. (1978) in press.
9. Glovsky, M. M., Di Luzio, N. R. and Ghekiere, L., J. Reticuloendothel. 20 (1977) 54.
10. Jones, T. C., Len, L. and Hirsch, J. G., J. Exp. Med., 141 (1975) 466.
11. Kamitsuka, A., XXXI Ann. Meeting of the Jap. Soc. for Medical Mycology, (1977).
12. Karnovsky, M. L., Lazdins, J. and Simmons, S. R., Mononuclear Phagocytes in Immunity, Infection and Pathology, (Ed. R. van Furth), Blackwell Scientific Publ., London, (1975) 423.
13. Koike, K., Jap. J. Antibiotics, 29 (1976) 1098.
14. Komatsu, N., Okubo, S., Kikumoto, S., Kimura, K., Saito, G. and Sakai, S., GANN, 60 (1969) 137.
15. Komatsu, N., Nagumo, N., Okubo, S. and Koike, K., Jap. J. Antibiotics, 26 (1973) 277.
16. Komatsu, N., Jap. J. Antibiotics, 26 (1973) 459.
17. LeJeune, F. J., Song, M., Delville, J., Stadtsbaeder, S. and Gillet, J., Europ. J. Cancer, Special EORIC issue, (1978) in press.
18. Lindberg, R. E. and Frenkel, J. K., J. Parasitol., 63 (1977) 219.
19. Mackaness, G. B., Infectious Agents and Host Reactions, (Ed. S. Mudd), W. B. Saunders, Philadelphia, (1970) 62.
20. Nagumo, N., Jap. J. Antibiotics, 27 (1974) 101.
21. Nguyen, B. T. and Stadtsbaeder, S., Infect. Immun. 13 (1976) 884.
22. Nguyen, B. T. and Stadtsbaeder, S., Arch. Internat. Physiol. Biochim., (1977) in press.
23. Nichols, B. A. and Bainton, D. F., Mononuclear Phagocytes in Immunity, Infection and Pathology, (Ed. R. van Furth), Blackwell Scientific Publ., (1975) 17.

24. Reikvam, A., Grammeltvedt, R. and Hoiby, E. A., Acta Path. Microbiol. Scand., Sect. C., 83 (1975) 129.
25. Remington, J. S., Krahenbuhl, J. L. and Mendenhall, J. W., Infect. Immun., 6 (1972) 829.
26. Stadsbaeder, S., Piret, L. and Clotuche De Bruyn, L., Lyon Médic., 225 (1971) 175.
27. Stadtsbaeder, S., Nguyen, B. T. and Calvin-Préval, M. C., Ann. Immunol., (Inst. Pasteur), 126C (1975) 461.
28. Stadtsbaeder, S. and Nguyen, B. T., Ann. Immunol., (Inst. Pasteur), 128C (1977) 149.
29. Tsukagoshi, S., Cancer Chemother., 1 (1974) 251.
30. Tsukagoshi, S., Vth Internat. Symp. Princess Takamatsu Cancer Res. Fund, Tokyo, (1975).
31. Wooles, W. R. and Di Luzio, N. R., Science, 142 (1963) 1078.
32. Wooles, W. R. and Di Luzio, N. R., Proc. Soc. Exp. Biol. Med., 115 (1964) 756.

GLUCAN INDUCED INHIBITION OF TUMOR GROWTH AND ENHANCEMENT OF SURVIVAL IN A VARIETY OF TRANSPLANTABLE AND SPONTANEOUS MURINE TUMOR MODELS

N. R. DI LUZIO, R. B. MCNAMEE, D. L. WILLIAMS, K. M. GILBERT and M. A. SPANJERS

Department of Physiology, Tulane University School of Medicine, New Orleans, Louisiana (USA)

In recent years, attempts have been made to alter the course of neoplasia by augmenting host defense mechanisms. A number of adjuvants including bacterial vaccines and chemical compounds have been demonstrated to produce a nonspecific stimulation of the reticuloendothelial (RE) system and augment humoral and cellular immune response. The most commonly employed agents are *Bacillus Calmette-Guerin* (BCG) and *Corynebacterium parvum* (16,22). The efficacy of such nonspecific immunotherapy, however, varies depending upon the time and mode of injection (4,29,31) as well as the type of malignancy (29,33). In view of the virulent and antigeneic nature of bacterial adjuvants such as BCG, it is not surprising that complications have been observed on occasion following the intratumoral or intradermal injections of these agents (22,32). Furthermore, there is the threat of disseminated infection following inoculation with viable organisms in patients with immunodeficiency states secondary to malignancy (22) or in immunosuppressed animals (25). Indeed, Sparks, *et al*. (35) reported that rats receiving isonicotinic acid hydrazine and BCG intralesionally had better survival and smaller tumor volumes than BCG alone, possibly by inhibiting diversion of host response to the viable BCG organism.

In general, the currently employed adjuvants do not meet many of the desirable criteria developed in this laboratory (6) as well as outlined in a recent World Health Organization Technical Report (Immunological Adjuvants: WHO Technical Report, Series No. 595). Aside from bacterial adjuvants, previous studies have demonstrated that glucan, a $\beta 1 \rightarrow 3$ polyglucose derived from the cell wall of *Saccharomyces cerevisiae*, is a potent immunopotentiator (6,37-39). Administration of glucan to mice or rats is associated with the induction of a hyperphagocytic state and the hypertrophy of major RE organs due to both an increase in size and number of macrophages (1,6,39). This neutral polyglucose is effective in enhancing both humoral and cellular responses to unrelated antigens (37,38). Additionally glucan is nonantigenic (27), and nonvirulent as opposed to bacterial immunostimulants and may, therefore, be anticipated to induce fewer toxic complications. The potential of this polyglucose as an immunotherapeutic agent in treatment of malignancy remains to be fully appreciated. Studies have demonstrated that intravenous administration of glucan prior to administration of Shay acute myelogenous leukemia tumor cells resulted in significant modification of tumor growth and prolongation of survival (7). Initial clinical studies involving a variety of metastatic lesions in man, intralesional administration of glucan produced a prompt necrosis of the tumors associated with a pronounced monocytic infiltrate (26-28). Israel and Edelstein (20) studied the response of eleven patients treated with intralesional glucan. Clinical resolution of injected lesions was achieved in some but not all cases. Histological studies were conducted on two patients. In one subject, no tumor cells were observed in an injected lesion or in an uninjected nodule, which was characterized by the presence of large quantities of melanin. In the other subject, injected 4 times with 20 mg a residual metastatic nodule surrounded by inflammatory cell infiltrates containing predominantly macrophages was observed. Israel and Edelstein (20) and Mansell, *et al*. (26) observed the resolution of ulcerated lesions by the topical application of glucan possibly because of its chemotactic activity. From these previous experiments, it is apparent that glucan can markedly modify host resistance to neoplasia.

The purpose of this present study was to further evaluate glucan's ability to inhibit tumor growth in a variety of syngeneic tumor models. Four separate murine malignancies of spontaneous origin including the anaplastic mammary carcinoma 15091A, adenocarcinoma BW10232, melanoma B16, and AKR lymphocytic leukemia were selected for these studies. Both tumor weight and survival were monitored following systemic administration of glucan. The extent of metastatic involvement in experimental and control groups was ascertained by light microscopic studies employing the melanoma and AKR lymphocytic leukemia. The influence of chronic glucan administration on the development of spontaneous leukemia in aging AKR mice was also evaluated to ascertain possible immunoprophylaxis activity. Additional studies were conducted to evaluate the mechanism of glucan induced inhibition of tumor growth by an evaluation of the *in vitro* cytotoxic potential of glucan stimulated peritoneal macrophages.

MATERIALS AND METHODS

Male C57Bl/6J, AKR/J and A/J inbred mice from the Jackson Laboratory (Bar Harbor, ME) were employed as recipients for the respective syngeneic tumors listed in Table I. The mice were maintained on Purina Laboratory Chow and water ad libitum. All tumors were excised and dispersed under sterile conditions by means of a glass tissue grinder. The number of viable cells were determined by trypan blue exclusion. Established dilutions of the cells were then injected subcutaneously in the appropriate mouse strain. AKR lymphocytic leukemia cells for intravenous injection were obtained from culture. Tumor cells were maintained as suspension cultures in RPMI 1640 medium supplemented with 10% fetal calf serum, streptomycin 100 ug/ml and penicillin (100 units/ml). The cells were cultured in sterile plastic flasks (Falcon Plastics) at 37 C and 5% CO_2.

TABLE I

Origin and Source of Syngeneic and Spontaneous Mouse Tumor Models

Tumors	Origin	Host Mouse Strain
Transplantable:		
Adenocarcinoma BW 10232	Spontaneous, mammary gland	C57Bl/6J
Anaplastic carcinoma 15091A	Spontaneous, mammary gland	A/J
Melanoma B16	Spontaneous (skin at base of ear)	C57Bl/6J
Lymphocytic leukemia BW 5147	Spontaneous, spleen and nodes	AKR/J
Spontaneous:		
Lymphocytic leukemia	Spontaneous	AKR/J (aging)

Yeast glucan was isolated from *Saccharomyces cerevisiae* by a modification of the method of Hassid, *et al.* (17). The size of the particulate glucan prepared in this fashion is approximately 1 μm (27). The glucan preparation, as evaluated by the *Limulus* lysate test, was endotoxin-free. Since the dose and schedule of treatment varied for many of the experimental procedures, details as to experimental design are incorporated in each experimental phase.

In the spontaneous tumor study, 60 male AKR/J retired breeders approximately 7 months of age, were obtained from the Jackson Laboratory, (Bar Harbor, ME). They were divided equally into a saline control and glucan-treated group. The latter received 0.45 mg glucan suspended in isotonic saline intravenously every 14 days for a 5 month period. Control mice received saline intravenously. Survival was ascertained daily throughout the study.

The antitumor cytotoxic activity of peritoneal macrophages derived from control and glucan-treated mice was studied employing a modification of the cytotoxicity assay previously described by Hibbs, *et al.* (18). The experimental animals each received an intraperitoneal injection of 4 mg of glucan for 3 consecutive days while the controls received similar injections of isovolumetric 5% dextrose in water. Peritoneal cells were harvested 2 days after the last injection and suspended in RPMI 1640 solution supplemented with 10% fetal calf serum, streptomycin (100 ug/ml), penicillin (100 ug/ml), gentamicin (100 ug/ml) and amphotericin B (2.5 ug/ml). Appropriate numbers of peritoneal exudate cells were added to microtiter wells and the macrophages (4×10^5 cells) allowed to adhere for 1½ hr. The wells were washed 3 times to remove nonadherent cells at which time tumor cells were added to yield a macrophage:tumor target cell ratio of 40:1. The tumor cells were obtained from an *in vitro* culture of syngeneic melanoma B16 cells. The microcytotoxicity cultures were incubated for 72 hr and then fixed with methanol and stained with Giemsa. The relative killing ability of macrophages was ascertained by microscopic examination.

For light microscopic studies, organs were dissected from mice and tissues 0.5 cm in thickness were fixed in 4% buffered formalin. Tissues were dehydrated in a graded series of ethanol, cleared in xylene, and embedded in paraffin. Sections 6 microns in thickness were stained with hematoxylin and eosin.

Data were analyzed for statistical significance by either Student's "t" test or Chi-square test. All data were compared for statistical significance employing a confidence level of 95%.

RESULTS

Effect of glucan on tumor growth and survival of C57Bl/6J mice with melanoma B16 implants. To evaluate the effect of intravenously administered glucan on primary tumor growth, mice were injected with 1 x 10^6 melanoma cells, and glucan (0.5 mg/mouse) or saline was administered on days 3, 6, 9, 12 and 14 (Table II). When the animals were sacrificed on day 16 tumor weights were decreased by approximately 70% ($p<0.05$) in the glucan-treated group. Twelve of the twenty-three glucan-treated mice had no detectable subcutaneous tumors in contrast to only one out of 29 control animals. Associated with the reduced tumor growth in glucan-treated mice was a significant hepatomegaly and splenomegaly (Table II).

Histological examination of the liver and lung was also ascertained on day 16. None of the animals in either the glucan or control group exhibited metastatic lesion of the liver. Livers in glucan-treated mice were characterized by the presence of granuloma and a hyperplasia of Kupffer cells. Analyses of lung histology revealed metastatic tumor in eight of nine control mice in which studies were undertaken. Tumor growth was prominent throughout the lung parenchyma. In marked contrast, none of the glucan animals had detectable tumor nodules in the lung. As with the liver, however, lung tissue in mice treated with glucan exhibited hyperplasia of macrophages and granuloma formation.

TABLE II

Inhibitory Influence of Glucan on Growth of Melanoma B16[a]

Group	No.	Liver Wt (g)	Spleen Wt (g)	Tumor Wt (g)
Control	29	1.21 ± 0.006	0.18 ± 0.01	0.97 ± 0.19
Glucan	23	2.17 ± 0.09[b]	0.48 ± 0.41[b]	0.26 ± 0.08[b]

[a]Tumor cells (1 x 10^6) were injected on day 0. Glucan (0.3 mg/mouse) was administered on days 3, 6, 9, 12 and 14. Animals were sacrificed on day 16 for determinations of organ and tumor weights.

Values are expressed as means ± standard error.

[b]Significant $p<0.05$.

To further evaluate the efficacy of glucan as a post-treatment modality, mortality was evaluated following subcutaneous injection of 1 x 10^6 melanoma cells on day 0 and subsequent intravenous injections of glucan (0.3 mg/mouse) at three-day intervals over a 12 day period. Glucan was effective in prolonging survival as denoted by the marked disparity in the rate of mortality (Fig. 1). The median time of survival of saline-treated control mice was 20 days after tumor cell inoculation in contrast to 28 days in glucan-treated mice ($p<0.05$). Glucan, therefore, significantly altered the course of melanoma as reflected by reduced tumor growth, metastases and increased survival time.

Antitumor activity of glucan in C57B1/6J mice with adenocarcinoma BW 10232. Adenocarcinoma, 5 x 10^6 cells/mouse, were administered subcutaneously and followed by intravenous saline or glucan injections (0.2 mg/mouse) on days 1, 6, 10 and 15 following the administration of tumor cells. Mean tumor weights on day 21 in the control groups was 4.21 g as opposed to 0.99 g in mice treated with glucan (Table III). This inhibitory effect of glucan on neoplastic proliferation is represented by a mean 77% reduction in tumor weight. In accordance with previous experiments there was a significant hepatomegaly in the glucan-treated mice denoting hypertrophy and hyperplasia of macrophages.

To assess if a higher dosage of glucan would be even more efficacious in limiting growth of the tumor, the glucan dose was increased to 0.45 mg/mouse and administered intravenously at 2-day intervals after subcutaneous injection with the adenocarcinoma cells (Table III). The increased dose of glucan was extremely effective in retarding growth of the adenocarcinoma as denoted by a 85% decrease ($p<0.01$) in tumor weights of glucan mice relative to the control mice on day 12 post tumor cell injection.

As with the melanoma tumor, studies were initiated to evaluate the effect of glucan on survival time of the mice following the subcutaneous administration of mammary adenocarcinoma cells. Injection of glucan at 3-day intervals at a dose of 0.45 mg/mouse resulted in prolonged survival. This protective effect is denoted by the 100% survival of glucan-treated mice at day 19 as opposed to only 20% survival in control mice (Fig. 2). However, the cessation of glucan administration on day 18 appeared to be associated with rapid onset of mortality.

In contrast to the protective effect of intravenously administered glucan in prolonging mean survival time, injection of glucan intraperitoneally (1 mg/mouse) on days 1, 6, 10 and 15 after subcutaneous administration of 5 x 10^5 adenocarcinoma cells was not effective in modifying mortality patterns (Fig. 3).

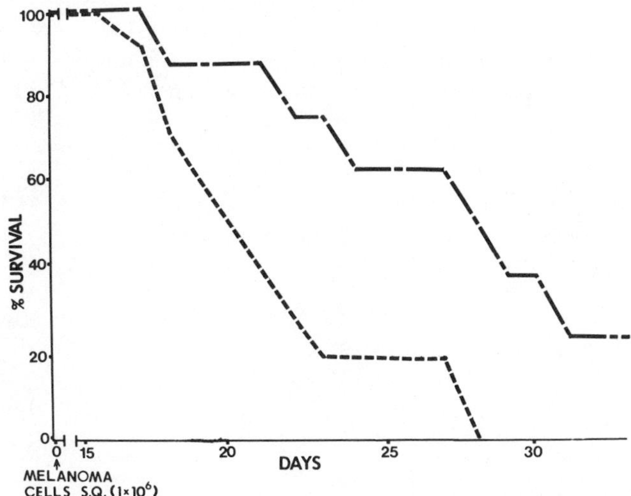

Fig. 1. Mortality of glucan and saline treated mice after subcutaneous injection of 1 x 10^6 melanoma cells, s.c. Glucan (-—-) was administered i.v. (0.3 mg/mouse) on days 0, 3, 6, 9 and 12. n = 8. Control animals received isovolumetric saline (---). n = 10.

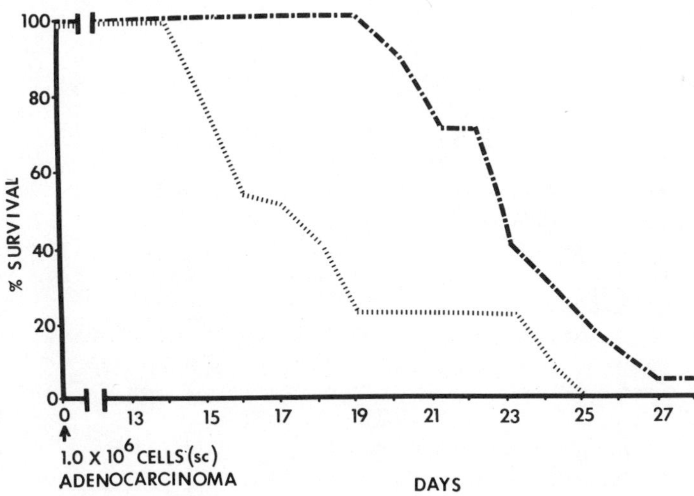

Fig. 2. Effect of intravenous glucan on survival of mice injected subcutaneously with 1 x 10^6 adenocarcinoma cells. Glucan (-—-) was injected (0.45 mg/mouse) on days 0,3,6,9,12,15 and 18. n = 14. Control (▮▮▮) groups received isovolumetric saline. n = 13

TABLE III

Inhibitory Effect of Intravenous Glucan On Subcutaneous Growth of Adenocarcinoma BW 15091A

Group	Liver Wt (g)	Spleen Wt (g)	Tumor Wt (g)
Experiment I[a]			
Control	1.56 ± 0.11	0.35 ± 0.03	4.21 ± 0.08
Glucan	1.82 ± 0.09*	0.97 ± 0.01*	0.98 ± 0.15*
Experiment II[b]			
Control	1.33 ± 0.03	0.12 ± 0.01	0.59 ± 0.17
Glucan	1.84 ± 0.13*	0.40 ± 0.02*	0.09 ± 0.01*

[a]C57Bl/6J mice were injected with 5 x 10^6 cells/mouse. Glucan (0.2 mg/mouse) or saline was administered on days 1,6,10 and 15 following tumor cell challenge. Tumors were excised on day 21.

Control n = 9; Glucan n = 6

[b]C57Bl/6J mice were injected subcutaneously with 1 x 10^6 adenocarcinoma cells. Glucan (0.45 mg/mouse) or saline was administered on days 0,2,4,6,8 and 10. Tumors were excised on day 12.

Control n = 9; Glucan n = 9

*Significant $p<0.01$

Effect of glucan on tumor growth and survival time of A/J mice with anaplastic mammary carcinoma 15091A. Subcutaneous tumors were excised and weights were determined in glucan or saline treated A/J mice 11 days after administration with 1 x 10^7 tumor cells (Table IV). Mice receiving intravenous injections of glucan (0.3 mg/mouse) at 2 day intervals up to 8 days following tumor cell challenge exhibited a significant reduction in tumor weight relative to the control group. As with the other syngeneic tumors, the antitumor action of glucan was denoted by the approximate 70% decrease of the excised tumor weights.

Of all the syngeneic tumors investigated, the employment of glucan as a post-treatment modality was most efficacious in maintaining survival of mice with the anaplastic carcinoma (Fig. 4). Mice receiving glucan intravenously on days 0,2,4,6 and 8 following subcutaneous tumor challenge exhibited only a 20% mortality after 40 days. This is in marked contrast to the 100% mortality of mice receiving isovolumetric saline during an equivalent time period.

TABLE IV

Effect of Glucan on Growth of Anaplastic Carcinoma in A/J Mice[a]

Group	No.	Tumor Wt (g)
Saline	17	1.36 ± 0.56
Glucan	19	0.71 ± 0.25[b]

[a]All mice received a subcutaneous injection of 1 x 10^7 anaplastic carcinoma cells. Glucan was administered on days 0,2,4,6 and 8 following tumor challenge at a dose of 0.3 mg/mouse. Controls received isovolumetric saline. Tumors were excised on day 11.

[b]$p<0.01$

Glucan modification of lymphocytic (AKR) leukemia. To further evaluate the effectiveness of glucan against syngeneic tumors, studies were initiated employing AKR lymphocytic leukemia cells. In contrast to our studies with solid tumors, the cultured leukemia cells were administered intravenously thus inducing highly disseminated lesions. An injected dose of 1 x 10^6 AKR leukemia cells was administered on day 0 followed by glucan injections (0.3 mg/mouse) or isovolumetric saline on days 1,2,4 and 6 (Fig. 5). These initial studies revealed that this dose of glucan was ineffective in modifying survival as denoted by the 100% mortality in both experimental and control groups by day 16. The dose of glucan was subsequently increased from 0.3 mg to 0.45 mg/mouse (Fig. 6). Administration of a higher dosage of glucan on days 1,2,5 and 7 following an intravenous challenge of 1 x 10^6 leukemia cells prolonged median survival time to approximately 18 days, compared to 13 days in the control group. In view of the relatively large tumor cell burden employed in these experiments, subsequent studies were undertaken in which the mice were challenged with a lower dose of leukemia cells (Fig. 6). The administration of glucan (0.45 mg/mouse) at 2 day intervals proved to be more effective in the reduced tumor burden mice as the glucan-treated mice manifested at 45% survival after 30 days in contrast to 10% survival in the control group.

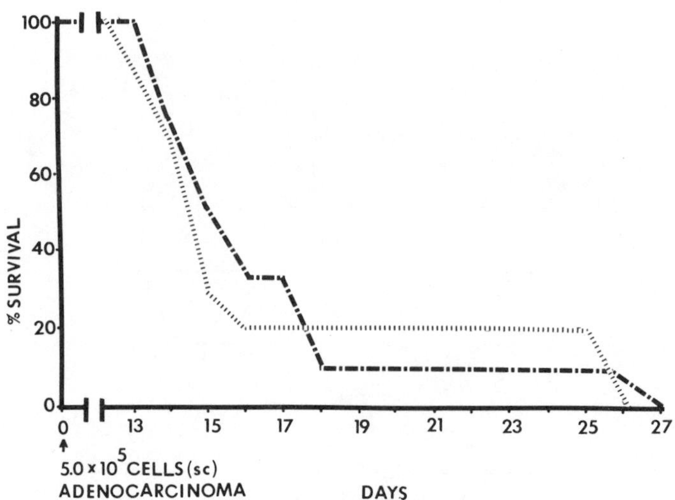

Fig. 3. Inability of intraperitoneal injections of glucan to modify survival of mice injected subcutaneously with 5 x 10^5 adenocarcinoma cells. Glucan (-—-) was administered i.p. (1 mg) on days 0,1,6,10 and 15 following tumor cell challenge. n = 12. Saline (III) was injected isovolumetrically for controls. n = 12.

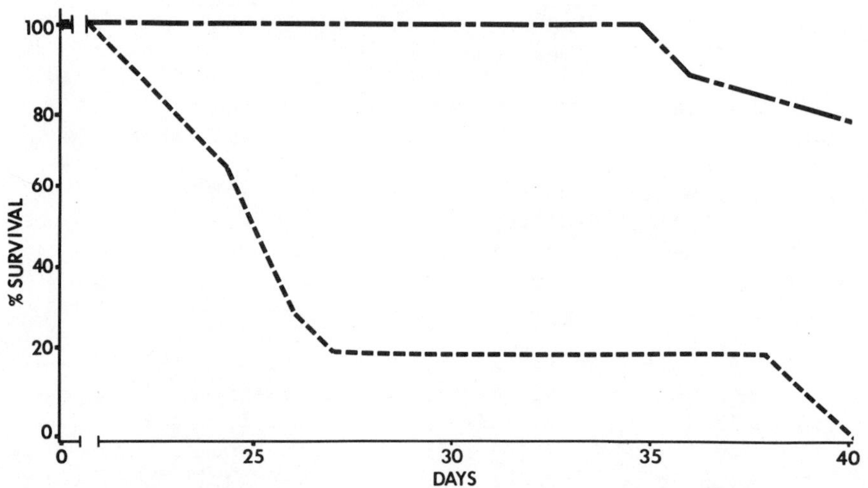

Fig. 4. Survival of A/J mice after subcutaneous administration of 1 x 10^7 anaplastic carcinoma cells. Glucan (-—-) was intravenously administered (0.3 mg/mouse) on days 0,2,4,6 and 8 following tumor challenge. Controls (---) received isovolumetric saline. n = 10/group.

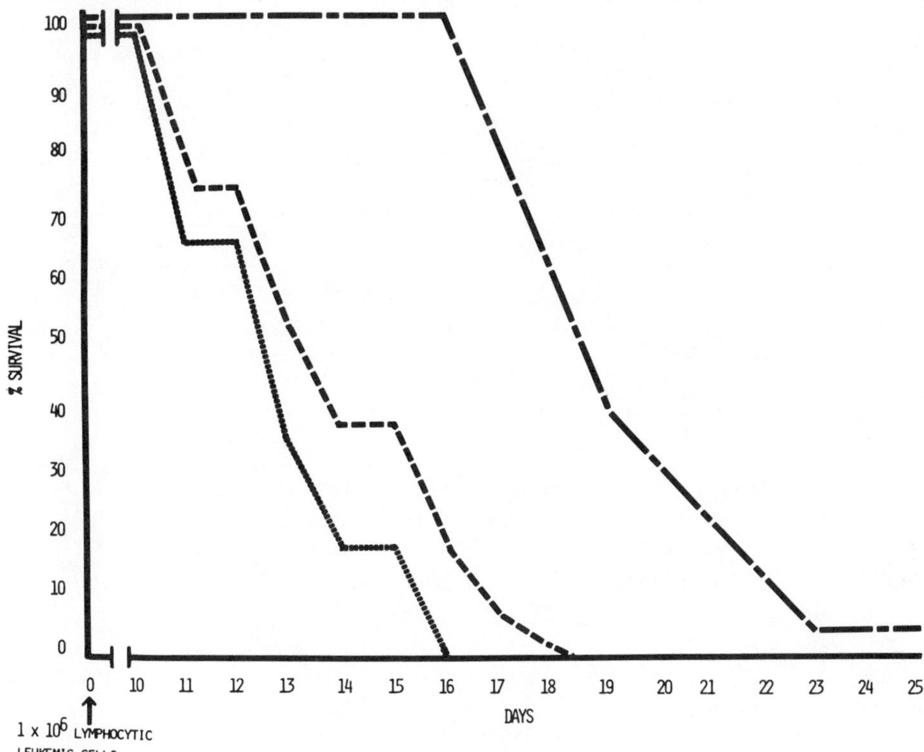

Fig. 5. Effect of glucan on survival of AKR mice which received intravenous injection of 1 x 10^6 cultured AKR lymphocytic leukemia cells. Glucan administered 0.3 mg/mouse on days 1,2,4 and 6 following tumor cell challenge (---). n = 6. Glucan also injected in dose of 0.45 mg/mouse on days 1,2,5 and 7 (-—-), n = 10. Saline controls received isovolumetric saline (▪▪▪), n = 10.

<u>Influence of chronic glucan administration on mortality of aging AKR mice developing spontaneous leukemia</u>. The chronic administration of glucan to aging AKR mice was associated with a significant modification in mortality which was observed 2½ to 3 months after the initiation of therapy (Fig. 7). At three months post-therapy, survival in the control group was 48% in contrast to 72% in the glucan group. A 24% survival manifested in the control group at 4 months was significantly different from the 68% in the glucan-treated group. At 5 months after the initiation of glucan a four-fold difference was observed as the survival rate was 12% in the control group and 48% in the glucan-treated group.

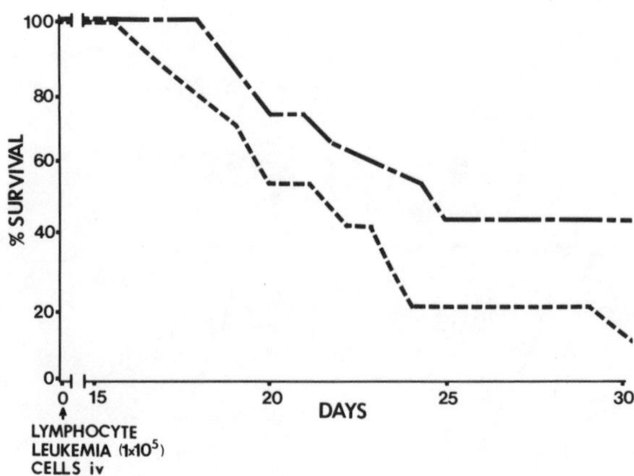

Fig. 6. Effect of glucan on survival of AKR mice with lower leukemia cell burden (1 x 10^5/mouse). Glucan (- — -) was administered intravenously (0.45 mg/mouse) on days 1,2,5 and 7 and subsequent two day intervals. Saline (---) control mice. n = 30/group.

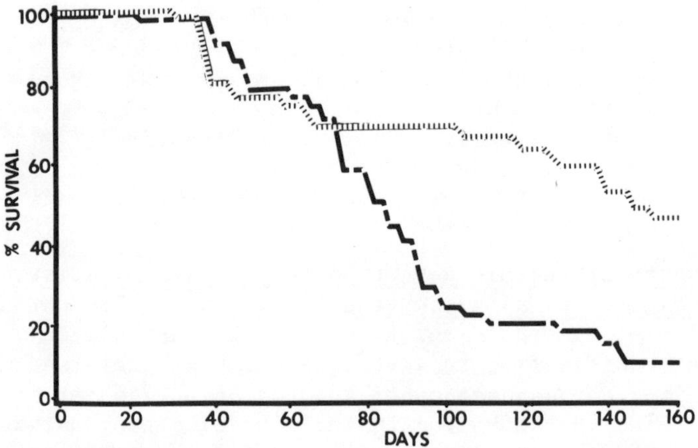

Fig. 7. Cumulative mortality of aging control (- — -) and glucan-treated (▮ ▮ ▮) AKR/J mice. Glucan (0.45 mg) was injected intravenously every 14 days, while control mice received intravenous injection of saline, the suspending medium for glucan. n = 30/group.

Evaluation of the in vitro cytoxicity of glucan stimulated peritoneal macrophages against syngeneic melanoma B16 cells. Extensive studies have been undertaken relative to *in vitro* interaction of normal and glucan peritoneal macrophages and melanoma B16 cells. Examination of the microcytoxicity assay indicated that peritoneal macrophages derived from glucan-treated mice possessed significantly greater antitumor activity against syngeneic melanoma cells than normal macrophages (Fig. 8-12). The macrophages from the glucan-treated animals appeared larger, with more vacuoles and cytoplasmic extension, characteristics usually associated with "activated" macrophages (Fig. 9).

DISCUSSION

It is evident, based upon previous preliminary clinical and experimental studies, that glucan provides a unique means to initiate enhanced host resistance to malignancy (6,9). The administration of glucan resulted in both an increase in activation and proliferation of fixed macrophage populations (1,7,37-39). The granulomatous tissue reaction induced by glucan as a result of hyperfunction and proliferation of lymphoreticular elements is of a reversible nature and will regress within approximately 2 weeks after cessation of glucan injection (39). Glucan also

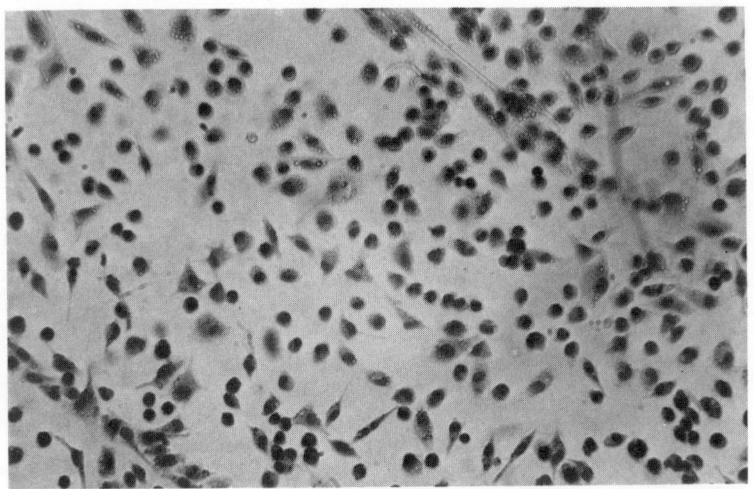

Fig. 8. Peritoneal macrophages (4×10^5/well) from control C57 mice after 72 hr in culture. These cells are relatively spherical in nature with few cytoplasmic extensions. (200 x).

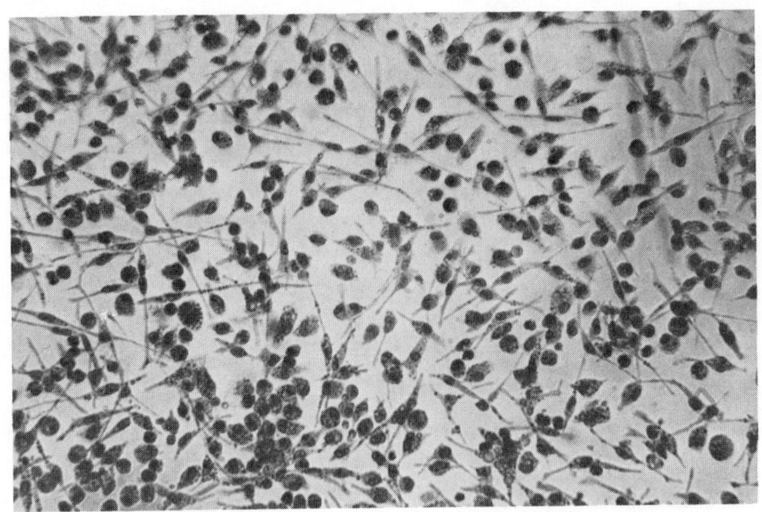

Fig. 9. Peritoneal macrophages (4 x 10^5/well) from glucan-treated C57 mice after 72 hr in culture. In contrast to Fig. 8, macrophages display extensive cytoplasmic extensions (200 x).

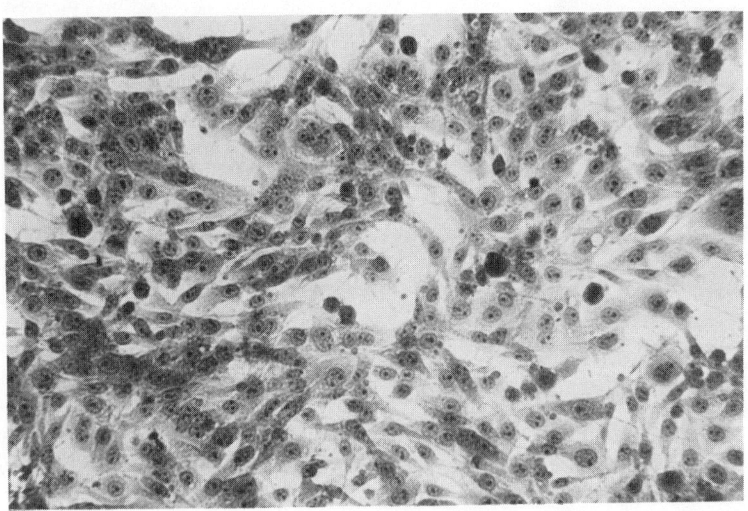

Fig. 10. Melanoma B16 cells (1 x 10^4/well) after 72 hr in culture. Cells display excellent growth and confluence (200 x).

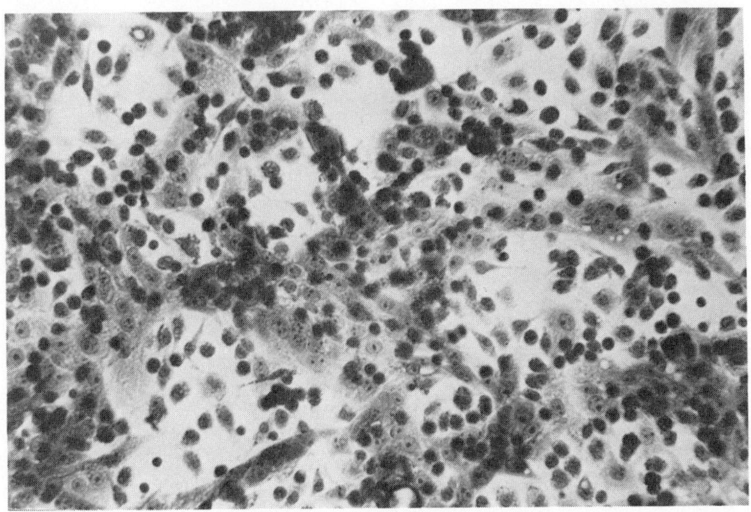

Fig. 11. Peritoneal macrophages from control mice incubated 72 hr with melanoma B16 cells. Macrophage to target cell ratio was 40:1. A slight inhibitory effect appeared to be present (200 x).

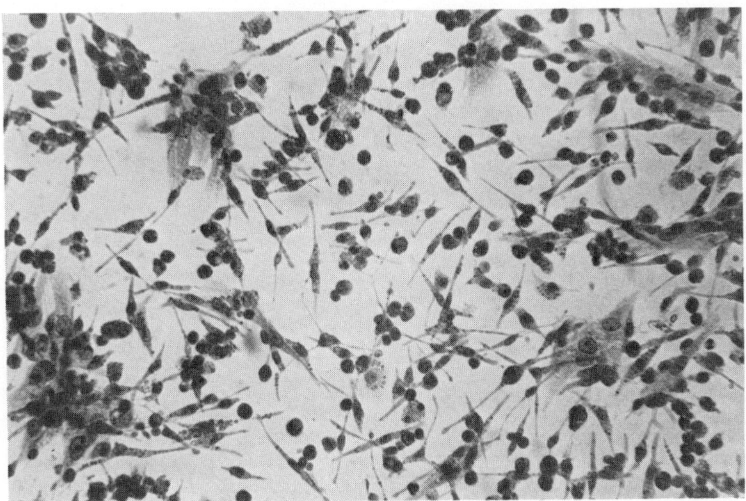

Fig. 12. Peritoneal macrophages from glucan-treated mice incubated for 72 hr with melanoma B16 cells. Macrophage to target cell ratio was 40:1. In contrast to normal macrophages, the interaction of glucan macrophages with melanoma cells produced a significant cytotoxic response (200 x).

enhances cellular (37) and humoral immunocompetence (38) as well as activates both the classical and alternate pathways of the complement cascade (14). The marked leukopoiesis and proliferation of tissue macrophage elements following glucan administration may be, in part, mediated by increased production of colony stimulatory factors (3). The ability of glucan to induce an expanded hyperfunctional macrophage population, enhance tumor macrophage content (13), and its capacity to modulate humoral and cellular immunity would be anticipated to contribute to its antineoplastic activity.

In *in vitro* interaction of peritoneal macrophages, obtained after intraperitoneal glucan administration, with syngeneic melanoma cells clearly denotes the cytotoxic potential of these cells. Melanoma cells were effectively reduced in number in the presence of glucan-activated macrophages, while relatively unaltered with control macrophages. These studies, of increased cytotoxic potential, are similar to those of Golde and Burgaleta (15) employing Friend leukemia cells and evaluated by inhibition of thymidine uptake (26 to 41%) and clonogenic ability (30 to 60%). Schultz, *et al*. (34) have also observed an enhancement in macrophage mediated cytotoxicity and cytostasis to a variety of tumor target cells. Schultz, *et al*. (34) concluded that functionally activated macrophages appear to have an important role in the enhancement of host resistance to neoplasia induced by glucan.

The present study extends the utility of glucan as a potential therapeutic agent as denoted by the significant antitumor activity in four syngeneic transplantable tumor models and one spontaneous murine leukemic model. The antitumor activity of glucan can be further appreciated when one considers the diverse characteristics and pathogenesis of the murine malignancies which were employed (Table I). Our observations however, denote a significant variation in responsiveness of the syngeneic tumor models to glucan. Glucan was most effective in maintaining survival of A/J mice with the anaplastic mammary carcinoma and least effective in prolonging survival of AKR mice with lymphocytic leukemia. Such variation in tumor responsiveness has been demonstrated with other commonly employed immunostimulants such as BCG (25) and *C. parvum*. For example, Rouminoutzeff, *et al*. (33) evaluated the efficacy of *C. parvum* in mediating antitumor activity against three tumor models: the nonsyngeneic Ehrlich's ascites, syngeneic AKR leukemia and the syngeneic YC8 ascitic tumor. Pretreatment regimen of *C. parvum* was only effective in modifying survival of AKR mice inoculated with 10^3 leukemia cells (33).

Recently, it was reported that glucan administration had no significant influence on tumor growth or mortality in a variety of syngeneic tumor models (19). Our studies employed two identical tumor models, namely B16 melanoma and adenocarcinoma 15091A and are in contrast to these observations by Hunter, *et al*. (19). However, the results of these studies are difficult to interpret in view of the two different preparations of glucan employed, one of which was prepared by this laboratory. In only one instance was it possible to identify which preparation of glucan was utilized. In none of the studies which were undertaken was it indicated that the dose of glucan and time of administration were such that macrophage activation was achieved. We have found that under certain conditions doses of glucan such as 0.2 mg/mouse had no inhibitory effect on the growth of melanoma B16 tumor, nor did it produce macrophage activation as denoted by enhanced phagocytic function or elevated serum lysozyme activity. Additionally, the effectiveness of intravenous glucan in the guinea pig hepatoma model employed by Hunter, *et al*. (19) remains to be established when appropriate dose-response studies have been undertaken. Additionally, since only one experimental mouse was killed for histology in the Hunter studies, as denoted in Table V, the validity of histopathologic studies cannot be established. Although Hunter, *et al* (19) speculatively suggest glucan will be ineffective in the treatment of human neoplasia, the conclusion is presently not supported by the observations of Mansell, *et al*. (20,26-28). Israel and Edelstein (20) reported that compared to "experience with intralesional BCG and *C. parvum*", the intralesional administration of glucan resulted in "the first documented case of resolution of a noninjected nodule". These findings do not support the concept advanced by Hunter, *et al*. (19) that tumor necrosis induced by glucan is due to "pressure necrosis". It is obvious, however, that extensive additional studies will be required to evaluate clinical efficacy of glucan or its molecular derivatives.

In contrast to the results of intralesional administration of glucan in man (20,26-28) we have found that in the acute monocytic leukemia rat model, the intralesional administration of glucan was ineffective in modifying tumor growth, while intravenous administration or the simultaneous administration of glucan with tumor cells was effective in inhibiting tumor growth. Since glucan may enhance macrophage populations by increasing CSA (3) and a delay time of several days occurs before detectable enhancement in macrophage number is apparent (7), it appears that the failure of glucan to inhibit tumor growth in mice or rats when given intralesionally may be due to a latency in macrophage proliferation and activation. Additionally, the subcutaneous injection of glucan in rats or mice produces a granulomatous pouch in contrast to an acute inflammatory response in man (26-28). The route of injection of glucan, therefore, appears to be an important factor in expression of its antitumor activity. Intraperitoneal injection was ineffective in modifying the mortality pattern of mice with adenocarcinoma. The antitumor activity of other immunostimulants such as BCG (22) and *C. parvum* also differs depending upon the route of injection and the type of malignancy. Mazurek, et al. (29) observed that a protective effect of C. parvum was obtained against lymphosarcoma when both tumor cells and C. parvum were administered intravenously. In contrast, the protection was afforded to mammary carcinoma only when both were administered intraperitoneally. In either case, the growth of subcutaneously injected tumor cells was not altered when C. parvum was injected intravenously. Since the intravenous injection of mice with C. parvum at doses approximating the dose of glucan employed in the present studies was shown to induce intravascular coagulation with consequent hepatic necrosis (23), it is possible the absence of protection may be mediated by such changes. Neither intravascular coagulation nor alterations in hepatic function were observed in glucan-treated animals. It is possible that local mechanism controlling antitumor activity may differ from the systemic antitumor activity of immunostimulants as postulated by Mazurek, et al. (29). The decreased growth of localized tumor masses, inhibition of metastases and extended survival of mice with a variety of syngeneic and spontaneous tumors following intravenous administration of glucan may reflect a nonspecific hyperfunction of the RE system.

The present study also extends the concept of employment of glucan as an immunoprophylactic agent in view of its ability to significantly modify mortality patterns of AKR mice which spontaneouly develop lymphocytic leukemia. Similar observations have been made utilizing other macrophage activating agents. Old, et al. (30) reported that BCG administration ot AKR mice produced a slight delay in the appearance of leukemia; however, a similar incidence in leukemia was observed at 290 days of age. Mortality was comparable in both the BCG-treated and control group. Lemonde (24,25) also studied the influence of BCG administration on the development of spontaneous leukemia in AKR mice. In 10 week old mice which received BCG intravenously, the incidence of spontaneous leukemia was significantly decreased. Survival was 9% in the control group at 480 days and 55% in the BCG group. When older mice were employed, a protective effect was observed in male mice but not in the female mice.

In a study somewhat similar in design to our study, Ungaro, et al. (36) evaluated the influence of biweekly intraperitoneal administration of BCG on the development of spontaneous leukemia in AKR mice. While high doses of BCG (5.4×10^6 organisms) had an adverse effect on longevity of AKR mice, lower doses ($0.2\text{-}2 \times 10^6$) had a significant effect in promoting survival. At 48 weeks of age, a time comparable to our studies, 5% of the saline group was alive while under the most optimal conditions, 35% of the BCG group was alive. Survival with other doses of BCG ranged from 10-20%. Thus, it appears that glucan is capable of promoting survival in AKR mice developing lymphocytic leukemia to a greater extent than BCG. Whether this observation is related to differences in sex of mice employed, or to the viable nature of the BCG organism and the resultant diversion of macrophages, remains to be ascertained.

It is apparent that if glucan is to be employed clinically, it must be effective as an adjunct with accepted modalities of therapy. Our previous studies have demonstrated the compatibility of glucan immunostimulation with surgery (11). Survival was enhanced in mice with melanoma following conjoint surgery and glucan administration as compared to either treatment alone. Reduction of tumor burden by the potentiation of host mediated immune response therefore, may allow more efficient elimination of residual malignancy. It is also possible that glucan will prove to be effective with other conventional types of therapy. Recent studies, for example, have demonstrated that conjoint chemotherapy with cyclophosphamide and immunostimulation with glucan is effective in inhibiting metastases and prolonging survival of rats and mice with acute leukemia (8,10).

The immunopotentiating effect of glucan is also denoted by a synergistic enhancement of survival and suppression of hepatic metastasis in leukemic rats following concurrent administration of glucan and glutaraldehyde-fixed tumor cells (2). Additionally, suppression of pulmonary metastasis has been observed in mice with melanoma B16 when glucan was injected in combination with irradiated tumor cells (32). Indeed, facilitation of metastasis was observed in this study when mice were treated with certain doses of levamisole or BCG. Such facilitation was not observed with glucan (32).

Glucan has also been observed to increase serum lysozyme, in association with enhancement in phagocytic function. In addition, glucan-treated mice showed enhanced resistance to *S. aureus* (21), denoting that glucan induces an enhanced state of host resistance against certain bacterial infections as well as neoplasia. Since infectious complications can be significant problems in patients with malignancies, the duality of therapeutic effects of glucan is a most positive feature.

The present composite studies conducted with four syngeneic transplantable tumor models and one spontaneous leukemic model, coupled with previous clinical observations, denote a potential for glucan in immunotherapy and immunoprophylaxis. Additionally, delineation of the mechanisms of antitumor activity of glucan may define the immunophysiological events which are associated with the modification of the malignant state.

SUMMARY

Extensive studies of this laboratory have demonstrated glucan, a β1→3 polyglucose derived from the cell wall of *Saccharomyces cerevisiae*, to be a potent stimulant of the RES as well as cellular and humoral immune responses. In view of the demonstrated effectiveness of intralesional glucan administration in a variety of human neoplasia and in a rat acute myelogenous leukemic model, studies were initiated to evaluate the effectiveness of glucan in mediating antitumor activity in a variety of syngeneic murine tumor models. Murine malignancies selected for these studies included the adenocarcinoma BW10232, anaplastic mammary carcinoma 15091A, melanoma B16 and the AKR lymphocytic leukemia. The ability of glucan to alter mortality of AKR mice developing leukemia was also ascertained. Administration of glucan intravenously after the subcutaneous administration of carcinoma or melanoma cells in respective host strains of mice was effective in limiting neoplastic proliferation. The decreased tumor weight generally approximated 70% in glucan-treated mice as opposed to controls. Histologic examination of mice with melanoma or leukemia also demonstrated a reduction in pulmonary and hepatic metastases, respectively. Intravenous glucan administration prolonged survival of mice with either melanoma, adenocarcinoma, anaplastic carcinoma or lymphocytic leukemia. Additionally, a four-fold increase in survival was observed in glucan-treated aging AKR mice. However, intraperitoneal administration of glucan in the adenocarcinoma model was totally ineffective in modifying survival. The assessment of the comparative *in vitro* cytotoxic effects of glucan-stimulated peritoneal macrophages revealed significant inhibition of melanoma B16 tumor growth. These composite studies suggest a therapeutic as well as a prophylactic potential for glucan which appears to be mediated, in part, by induction of cytotoxic macrophages.

ACKNOWLEDGEMENT

These studies were supported, in part, by the Cancer Research Institute of New York, MECO Cancer Research Fund, the American Cancer Society, Inc., and the National Cancer Institute.

REFERENCES

1. Ashworth, C. T., Di Luzio, N. R. and Riggi, S. J., Exp. Mol. Pathol. 1 (1963) 83.
2. Browder, W., Cohen, C., McNamee, R., Hoffmann, E. O. and Di Luzio, N. R., In: Immune Modulation and Control of Neoplasia by Adjuvant Therapy (Ed. M. A. Chirigos), Raven Press, New York, (1978) 207.
3. Burgaleta, C. and Golde, D., Can. Res. 37 (1977) 1739.

4. Chee, D. O. and Bodurtha, A. J., Int. J. Cancer 14 (1974) 137.
5. Di Luzio, N. R., McNamee, R., Miller, E. F. and Pisano, J. C., J. Reticuloendothel. Soc. 12 (1972) 314.
6. Di Luzio, N. R., Pharmacology of the reticuloendothelial system: Accent on Glucan. The Reticuloendothelial System in Health and Disease, (Eds. S. Reichard, M. Escobar and H. Friedman), Plenum Press, New York, (1976) 412.
7. Di Luzio, N. R., Influence of glucan on hepatic metastases. In: Kupffer Cells and Other Liver Sinusoidal Cells, (Eds. E. Wisse and D. L. Knook), Elsevier/N Holland Biomed. Press, Amsterdam, (1977) 397.
8. Di Luzio, N. R., Cook, J. A., Cohen, C., Rodrique, J. and Jones, E., The synergistic effect of cyclophosphamide and glucan on experimental acute myelogenous and lymphocytic leukemia. In: The Macrophage and Cancer, (Eds. K. James, B. McBride, A. Stuart), Econoprint, Scotland, (1977a) 188.
9. Di Luzio, N. R., Hoffmann, E. O., Cook, J. A., Browder, W. and Mansell, P. W. A., Glucan induced enhancement in host resistance to experimental tumors. In: Control of Neoplasia by Modulation of the Immune System, (Ed. M. Chirigos), Raven Press, New York, (1977b) 475.
10. Di Luzio, N. R., Cook, J. A., Cohen, C., Rodrique, J., Kokoshis, P. and McNamee, R., Enhancement of the inhibitory effect of cyclophosphamide on experimental acute myelogenous leukemia by glucan immunopotentiation and the response of serum lysozyme, (Ed. M. Chirigos), Raven Press, New York, (1978) 171.
11. Di Luzio, N. R., Lysozyme activity: An index of macrophage functional status. In: Lysosomes in Biology and Pathology (1978) in press.
12. Di Luzio, N. R., McNamee, R., Browder, W. and Williams, D., Cancer Tr. Resp. (1978) in press.
13. Gilbert, K., Chu, F., Jones, E. and Di Luzio, N. R., J. Reticuloendothel. Soc. 22 (1977) 319.
14. Glovsky, M. M., Di Luzio, N. R., Alenty, A. and Ghekiere, L., J. Reticuloendothel. Soc. 20 (1977) 54a.
15. Golde, D. W. and Burgaleta, C., Glucan-activated macrophages: Functional properties and cytotoxicity against syngeneic leukemia cells. In: Immune Modulation and Control of Neoplasia by Adjuvant Therapy, (Ed. M. A. Chirigos), Raven Press, New York, (1978) 201.
16. Halpern, B., Corynebacterium parvum: Applications in experimental and clinical oncology, Plenum Press, London (1975).
17. Hassid, W. Z., Joslyn, M. A., McCready, R. M., J. Am. Chem. Soc. 63 (1941) 295.
18. Hibbs, J. B., Taintor, R. R., Chapman, H. A., Jr. and Weinberg, J. B., Science 197 (1977) 279.
19. Hunter, J. T., Meltzer, M. S., Ribi, E., Fidler, I. J., Hanna, M. G., Jr. and Rapp, H. J., J. Natl. Cancer Inst. 60 (1978) 419.

20. Israel, L. and Edelstein, R., Treatment of cutaneous and subcutaneous metastatic tumors with intralesional glucan. In: Immune Modulation and Control of Neoplasia by Adjuvant Therapy, (Ed. M. A. Chirigos), Raven Press, New York, (1978) 249.
21. Kokoshis, P. L., Williams, D. L., Cook, J. A. and Di Luzio, N. R., Science 199 (1978) 1340.
22. Lemoureux, G., Turcotte, R. and Portelance, V., BCG in cancer immunotherapy, Grune and Stratton, New York, (1976).
23. Lampert, I. A., Jones, P. A., Salder, T. E. and Castro, J. E., Br. J. Cancer 36 (1977) 51.
24. Lemonde, P., Natl. Cancer Inst. Monogr. 39 (1973) 21.
25. Lemonde, P., Ambivalent effects of BCG in experimental neoplasms. In: BCG in Cancer Immunotherapy, (Eds. G. Lamoureus, R. Turcotte, V. Portelance), Grune and Stratton, New York, (1976) 155.
26. Mansell, P. W. A., Ichinose, H., Reed, R. J., Krementz, E. T., McNamee, R. and Di Luzio, N. R., J. Natl. Cancer Inst. 54 (1975) 571.
27. Mansell, P. W. A., Di Luzio, N. R., McNamee, R., Rowden, G. and Proctor, J. W., Ann. NY Acad. Sci. 277 (1976) 20.
28. Mansell, P. W. A., Roweden, G. and Hammer, D., Clinical experiences with the use of glucan. In: Immune Modulation and Control of Neoplasia by Adjuvant Therapy, (Ed. M. A. Chirigos), Raven Press, New York, (1978) 255.
29. Mazurek, C., Chaluet, H., Stiffel, C. and Giozzi, G., Br. J. Can. 17 (1976) 511.
30. Old, L. J., Benacerraf, B., Clarke, D. A., Carswell, E. A. and Stockert, E., Cancer Res. 21 (1961) 1281.
31. Pimm, M. V. and Baldwin, R. W., Int. J. Cancer 15 (1975) 260.
32. Proctor, J. W., Lewis, M. G. and Mansell, P. W. A., Ca. J. Surg. 19 (1976) 12.
33. Roumiantzell, M., Musetescu, M., Ayme, G. and Mynard, M. C., Effect of inactived Corynebacterium on different experimental tumors in mice. In: Corynebacterium parvum, (Ed. B. Halpern), Plenum Press, London, (1974) 202.
34. Schultz, R. M., Papamatheakis, J. D. and Chirigos, M. A., Tumoricidal effect in vitro of peritoneal macrophages from mice treated with glucan. In: Immune Modulation and Control of Neoplasia by Adjuvant Therapy, (Ed. M. A. Chirigos), Raven Press, New York, (1978) 241.
35. Sparks, F., Albert, N. and Breeding, J., J. Natl. Cancer Inst., 58 (1977) 367.
36. Ungargo, P. C., Drake, W. P. and Mardiney, M. R., Jr., J. Natl. Cancer Inst. 50 (1973) 125.
37. Wooles, W. R. and Di Luzio, N. R., Am. J. Physiol. 203 (1962) 404.
38. Wooles, W. R. and Di Luzio, N. R., Science 142 (1963) 1078.
39. Wooles, W. R. and Di Luzio, N. R., J. Reticuloendothel. Soc., I (1964) 160.

GLUCAN INDUCED MODIFICATION OF EXPERIMENTAL *STAPHYLOCOCCUS AUREUS* INFECTION IN NORMAL, LEUKEMIC AND IMMUNOSUPPRESSED MICE

D. L. WILLIAMS and N. R. DI LUZIO

Department of Physiology
Tulane University School of Medicine, New Orleans, Louisiana (USA)

Previous studies in our laboratory have demonstrated that glucan, a β1→ polyglucose component of the cell wall of *Saccharomyces cerevisiae*, nonspecifically activates lymphoreticular tissue (2,7,25). The intravenous administration of glucan results in a hypertrophy of the major RE organs with an intense activation and proliferation of macrophages (30-32). Glucan administration has been demonstrated to promote tumor regression and enhance survival in rats with an allogeneic Shay chloroleukemia (8) as well as in four syngeneic murine tumor models (10). Preliminary clinical investigations have demonstrated that intralesional administration of glucan results in prompt tumor necrosis with a concomitant monocytic infiltrate (23,24). Furthermore, Israel and Edelstein (19) have also reported that intratumoral administration of glucan resulted in necrosis of the lesion with a concomitant resolution of a distant nodule. Topical application of glucan resulted in disappearance of ulcerated lesions (19,23).

In view of the unique effects of glucan on various immunologic parameters and since glucan immunotherapy has been shown to enhance nonspecific host resistance, studies were undertaken in our laboratory to evaluate the effect of glucan on *Staphylococcus aureus* infection in normal, leukemic and immunosuppressed mice. This report reviews the results of these studies.

In recent years infection due to saprophytic or opportunistically pathogenic microorganisms has become a serious clinical problem (17,18). These infections are particularly prevalent in patients who are immunodeficient, due to the malignant state or immunosuppressive therapy (11,18). The gram-positive opportunistic pathogen *Staphylococcus aureus* has been implicated as a cause of secondary infection (21) and was, therefore, chosen as the infectious model for this study.

MATERIALS AND METHODS

Animals. AKR/J male mice were obtained from Jackson Laboratory (Bar Harbor, ME). The animals were housed in plastic cages and were fed Purina Laboratory Chow and water *ad libitum*.

Glucan. Glucan was prepared by a modification of the method of Hassid, *et al*. (15). Dilutions were made in sterile pyrogen-free isotonic saline.

Cyclophosphamide. Cytoxan from Mead-Johnson (Evansville, Indiana) was freshly prepared and administered intraperitoneally to mice in the dose of 30 mg/kg.

Bacteria. A clinical isolate of *Staphylococcus aureus* was obtained form the Tulane Medical Center Hospital (New Orleans, LA). The organism was subcultured in trypticase-soy broth for 18 hr at 37 C in a shaking water bath (50 rpm). Identity was verified by biochemical tests and purity by streak plating on blood agar. Isolated colonies were subcultured to trypticase-soy agar slants and maintained at 4 C. Inocula for intravenous challenge was prepared by subculturing *S. aureus* in trypticase-soy broth for 18 hr at 37 C in a shaking water bath (50 rpm). The culture was centrifuged (x 2000g) for 15 min and the cell pellet washed three times with phosphate-buffered saline (0.9% w/v). Cell numbers were determined at 24 hr in triplicate on trypticase-soy agar by standard plate count.

Leukemia. AKR/J mice with lymphocytic leukemia (BW 5147) were obtained from Jackson Laboratory (Bar Harbor, ME). The leukemic tumor was maintained by the subcutaneous injection of 1×10^6 tumor cells into 20 g AKR/J male mice. The cells for each experiment were prepared by culturing AKR/J leukemic cells. Tumor cell suspensions were subcultured into 25 cm^2 Falcon tissue culture flasks (Becton Dickinson Co. (Oxnard, CA) containing RPMI 1640 medium from Microbiological Assoc. (Walkersville, MD) with 10% (v/v) fetal calf serum from KC Biological, Inc. (Lexena, KS), 2% (v/v) penicillin-streptomycin from Micribiological Assoc. (Walkersville, MD), 0.1 mg/ml gentamicin from Schering Corp. (Kenilworth, NJ) and 1% (v/v) fungizone from Grand Island Biological Co. (Grand Island, NY). After incubation for 4 days at 37 C and 5.0% CO_2 tension, the culture was centrifuged (x 1000g) and the cell pellet washed three times with RPMI 1640, without antibiotics or antifungal agents. Cells were counted on a hemocytometer and viability determined by trypan blue exclusion. Dilutions were made in RPMI 1640 with no antibiotics or fungizone.

Experimental procedures. In the initial bacterial response study, groups of mice were injected either with glucan (1.0 mg/mouse) or isovolumetric saline on days 7 and 4 prior to challenge with $1.0 \pm 0.25 \times 10^9$ viable *S. aureus*.

In secondary infection studies, AKR lymphocytic leukemic cells (1.0×10^5) were injected intravenously to all mice on day 0. Groups of mice were given glucan (0.45 mg/mouse) or saline intravenously on day 0, 1, 2, 5 and on alternate days up to day 27. Peripheral leukocyte counts were employed to monitor the onset of lymphocytic leukemia. On day 13, one-half of the populations of each group were challenged intravenously with $1.0 \pm 0.25 \times 10^9$. *S. aureus*. All groups were monitored daily for survival.

In the immunosuppression study, groups of mice were injected either with glucan (0.45 mg/mouse), cyclophosphamide (0.6 mg/mouse), glucan (0.45 mg/mouse) and cyclophosphamide (0.6 mg/mouse), or isovolumetric saline on days 10, 7, 4 and 1 prior to intravenous challenge with $1.0 \pm 0.25 \times 10^9$ *S. aureus*. Glucan and saline were administered intravenously, while cyclophosphamide was given intraperitoneally. Differential and total leukocyte counts were performed on peripheral blood prior to each injection.

Histopathological examination. Samples of liver, lung, spleen, kidney and brain were taken on day 12 from glucan pretreated and saline control animals which were challenged with *S. aureus*. In mice pre-treated with cyclophosphamide samples of liver, lung, spleen, kidney, heart and brain were taken on day 9 following intravenous *S. aureus* challenge. All sections were fixed in 10% (v/v) formalin. The sections were stained with hematoxylin-eosin.

Statistics. Statistical comparisons between groups were performed employing Student's "t" test. A "p" value of 0.05 or less was considered significant. Statistical analyses of survival curves were based on chi-square with one degree of freedom. A chi-square value representing 95% confidence level was considered significant. All chi-square values represent a comparison between a treatment group and its appropriate control.

RESULTS

Effect of glucan on susceptibility of mice to systemic S. aureus infection. To evaluate the protective effect of glucan against systemic staphylococcal infection, glucan was administered intravenously 7 and 4 days prior to intravenous challenge with

S. aureus. At a challenge dose of 1 x 10^9 S. aureus, a 30% mortality was noted by day 1 in the saline control group (Fig. 1). In contrast, only 3% mortality was observed in the glucan pretreatment group in an equivalent time period. The median survival time for the saline control group was approximately 1.6 days as compared to 14 days in the glucan group. The glucan pretreatment group did not show a 100% mortality until day 26.

Effect of glucan on systemic staphylococcal disease in leukemic mice. Glucan administered in the dose of 0.45 mg/mouse on days 0, 1, 2, 5 and on alternate days up to day 27, resulted in a modification of mortality patterns of leukemic mice (Fig. 2) as well as leukemic mice challenged intravenously on day 13 with

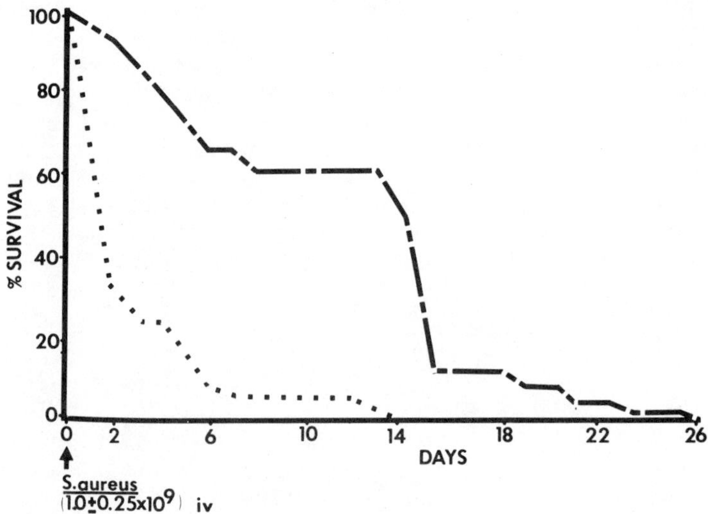

Fig. 1. Glucan (1.0 mg/mouse) induced survival of mice to intravenous challenge with 1.0 ± 0.25 x 10^9 viable S. aureus. Glucan (——) was administered intravenously 7 and 4 days prior to challenge with 1.0 ± 0.25 x 10^9 S. aureus. Isovolumetric saline (---) served as the control in S. aureus injected mice. N = 46/group.

1.0 x 10^9 S. aureus (Fig. 3). By day 20, leukemic mice which received glucan manifested an 80% survival. However, the saline control group showed a 50% survival in an equivalent time period. At day 25, the glucan group showed 70% survival as compared to 20% in the saline control group (Fig. 2).

Leukemic mice which received glucan prior to and following the administration of S. aureus, manifested a 90% survival on day 20 (Fig. 3). In contrast, the respective saline control mice showed only 10% survival in an equivalent time period. The median survival time in the control was 15 days, in contrast to 21 days in the glucan-treated group. By day 25, the glucan group showed 30% survival while all the saline control mice with lymphocytic leukemia and experimentally induced staphylococcal secondary infection had succumbed by day 23 (Fig. 3). The effectiveness of glucan in enhancing survival of mice injected with lymphocytic leukemia (Fig. 2) was significantly reduced when the mice received a subsequent injection of _S. aureus_ (Fig. 3).

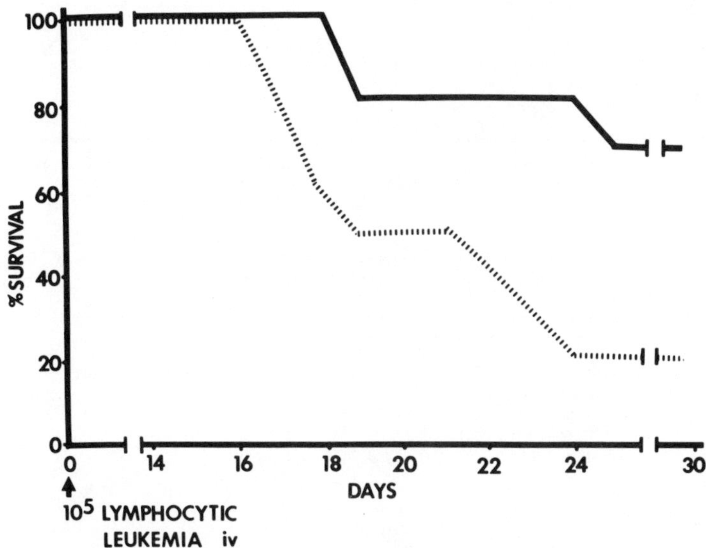

Fig. 2. Effect of glucan administration on survival of AKR/J mice following administration of 1.0×10^5 syngeneic lymphocytic leukemic cells. Glucan (——) or saline (''') was administered intravenously on days 0, 1, 2 and 5 and on alternate days up to day 27. N = 15/group.

Effect of glucan on peripheral leukocyte counts in cyclophosphamide (cytoxan) treated mice. Glucan administered in a dose of 0.45 mg/mouse resulted in a leukocyte count of 13.25×10^3/cu mm on day 6 (Fig. 4). This represents a significant ($p<0.05$) increase in peripheral leukocytes, when compared to 10×10^3/cu mm in the saline control group (Fig. 4). Cyclophosphamide treatment resulted in a significant depression in peripheral leukocytes, as reflected by a count of 4.5×10^3/cu mm on day 6 (Fig. 4). The administration of glucan significantly ($p<0.05$) increased leukocyte counts of cyclophosphamide-treated mice. By day 6, the glucan and cyclophosphamide-treated group

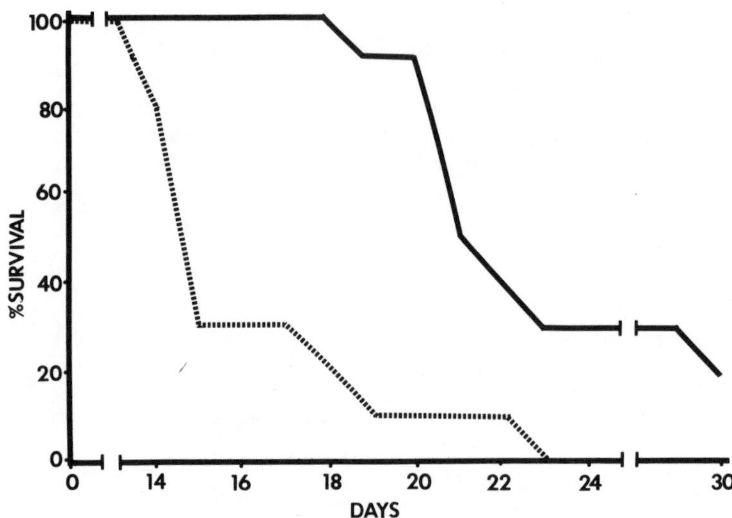

Fig. 3. Glucan-induced enhancement in survival of AKR mice injected with 1 x 10^5 lymphocytic leukemic cells on day 0 and intravenous injection of S. aureus (1 x 10^9) on day 13. Glucan (---) or saline (ııı) administered intravenously on days 0, 1, 2, 5 and on alternate days up to day 27. Increased susceptibility of leukemic mice to intravenous S. aureus is ascertained by comparison of mortality patterns of normal mice (Fig. 20. Experiments depicted in Fig. 3 and 4 were performed simultaneously. N = 15/ group.

showed a peripheral leukocyte count of 10 x 10^3/cu mm, which was equivalent to the saline control group (Fig. 4) and 122% higher than that observed in the cyclophosphamide-treated group. Differential counts of peripheral blood revealed no consistent alteration in populations of any given cell type.

Effect of glucan on survival of immunosuppressed mice with systemic staphylococcal disease. The administration of cyclophosphamide resulted in a significant decrease in survival as denoted by a median survival time of 1.4 days (Fig. 5). The mortality pattern in 17 saline injected control mice was significantly greater as denoted by a median survival time of 7.5 days. When glucan was administered conjointly with cyclophosphamide, prolongation in survival was observed with a median survival time of 9.0 days (Fig. 5). This median survival time was significantly reduced from the 12.5 days observed in the glucan-S. aureus treated group (N=17) denoting that the superimposition of cyclophosphamide reduced, to some degree, the ability of glucan

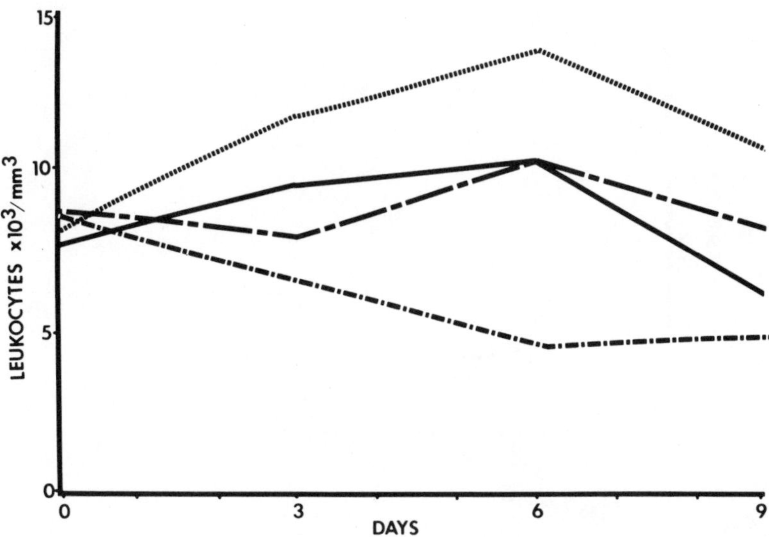

Fig. 4. Glucan-induced alterations in peripheral leukocytes of control and cyclophosphamide-treated AKR mice. Glucan (''''), cyclophosphamide (-'-'-), isovolumetric saline (——), or glucan + cyclophosphamide (-—-) were injected on days 0, 3, 6 and 9. Peripheral leukocyte counts were performed on days 0, 3, 6 and 9. N = 8/group.

to modify S. aureus sepsis.

Histopathological examination. Histological examination of glucan pre-treated and saline control animals on day 12 following intravenous injection of 1.0 x 10^9 S. aureus revealed marked pathological changes in the kidneys. There was an acute pyelonephritis in the renal cortex of saline control mice (Fig. 6). There was also a marked dilation of renal tubules which were filled with inflammatory cellular elements and necrotic debris. In contrast to the severe degenerative changes in control mice, the kidneys of glucan-treated mice exhibited relatively minimal pathological changes due to the acute septic episode (Fig. 7).

Histopathologic samples taken on day 9 from cyclophosphamide-treated mice, exhibited an acute pyelonephritis in the renal cortex with focal areas of staphylococcal colonization (Fig. 8). Extensive necrosis of renal parenchyma was observed as a consequence of abscess formation (Fig. 8). While there was some evidence of pyelonephritis and staphylococcal colonization in the glucan and cyclophosphamide-treated group, it was greatly reduced

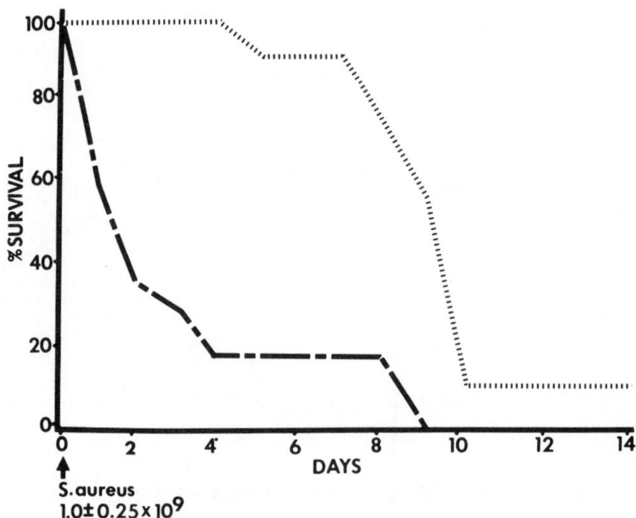

Fig. 5. Modification of the increased susceptibility of cyclophosphamide-treated mice by the conjoint administration of glucan. Glucan and cyclophosphamide (''') or cyclophosphamide (---) as a single modality were administered on days 10, 7, 4 and 1 prior to challenge with _S. aureus_. N = 17/group.

in magnitude when compared to the cyclophosphamide control (Fig. 9).

The livers of glucan and saline control mice exhibited no notable hepatic pathology. In contrast, the livers of cyclophosphamide treated mice revealed a marked lymphoid cell infiltrate with associated areas of well-defined parenchymal cell necrosis (Fig. 10). Mice pretreated with glucan and cyclophosphamide displayed the well-documented glucan-induced granuloma with mild lymphoid cell infiltrate and occasional microabscesses (Fig. 11).

DISCUSSION

The administration of glucan was effective in significantly reducing mortality due to the intravenous administration of _S. aureus_ to mice. The apparent loss of protection in the late stages of the disease may reflect the reversible nature of the glucan-induced hyperfunctional state (16,32). The present observations, demonstrating the enhanced survival of glucan-treated mice to _S. aureus_ septicemia, are in agreement with previous studies that

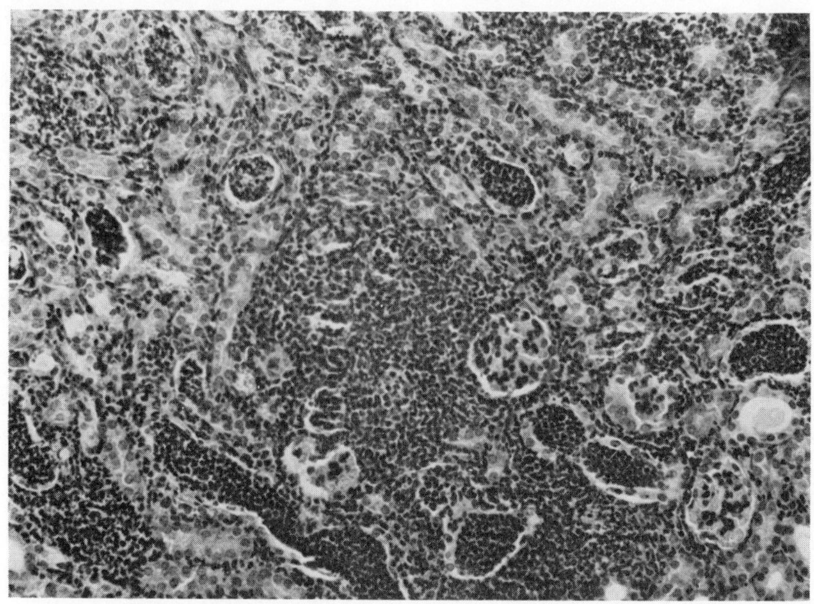

Fig. 6. Kidney of saline control mouse on day 12 showing acute pyelonephritis in renal cortex, characterized by necrosis of renal parenchyma and inflammatory cell infiltrate. Early abscess formation was observed along with a marked dilation of renal tubules filled with inflammatory elements and necrotic debris (200 x).

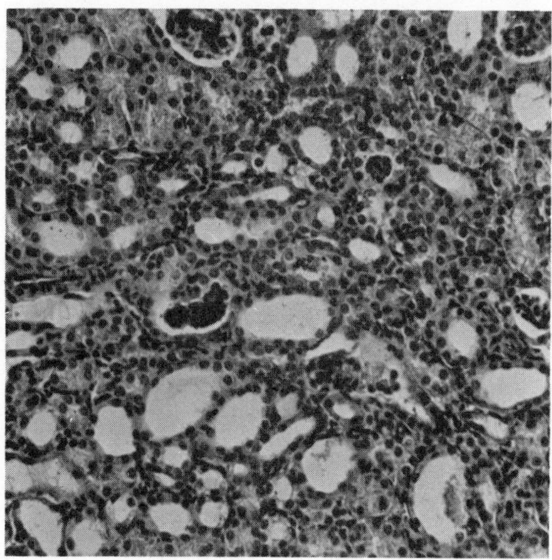

Fig. 7. Kidney of glucan pre-treated mouse on day 12 following *S. aureus* administration showing minimal dilation of renal tubules along with a maintenance of renal integrity. (200 x).

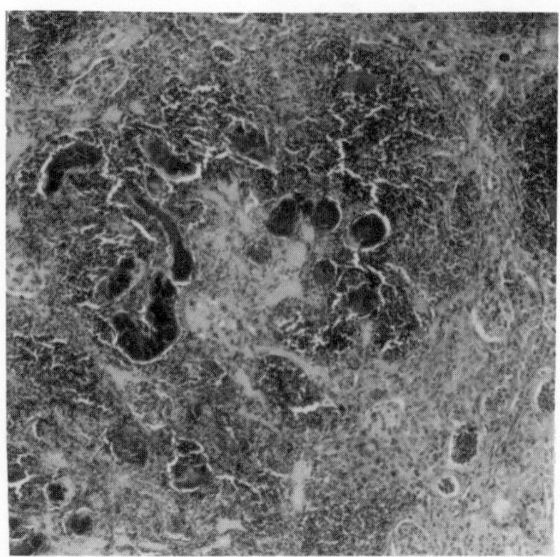

Fig. 8. Kidney of cyclophosphamide-treated mouse, day 9, showing acute pyelonephritis with focal areas of staphylococcal colonization. An inflammatory cell infiltrate along with extensive necrosis of renal parenchyma was observed in the renal cortex. (100 x).

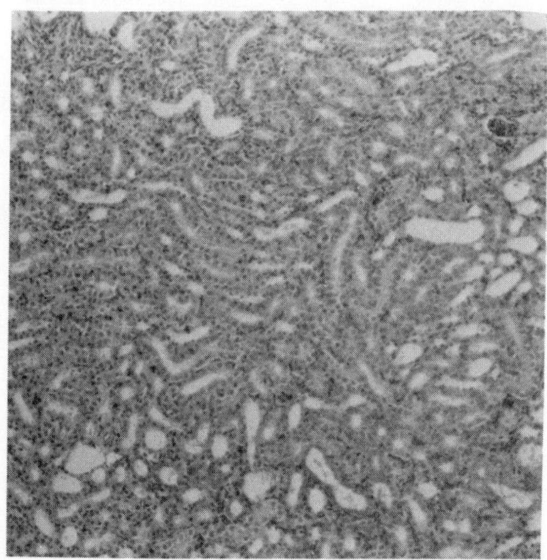

Fig. 9. Kidney of glucan and cyclophosphamide-treated mouse on day 9 showing mild pyelonephritis and dilation of renal tubules. Some evidence of staphylococcal colonization was observed along with a mild inflammatory cell infiltrate (100 x).

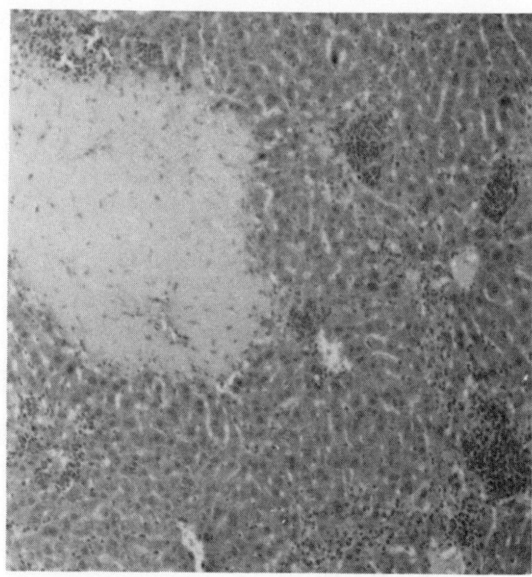

Fig. 10. Liver of a cyclophosphamide-treated mouse 9 days after staphylococcal challenge. A marked lymphoid cell infiltrate was observed with associated areas of well-defined parenchymal cell necrosis (100 x).

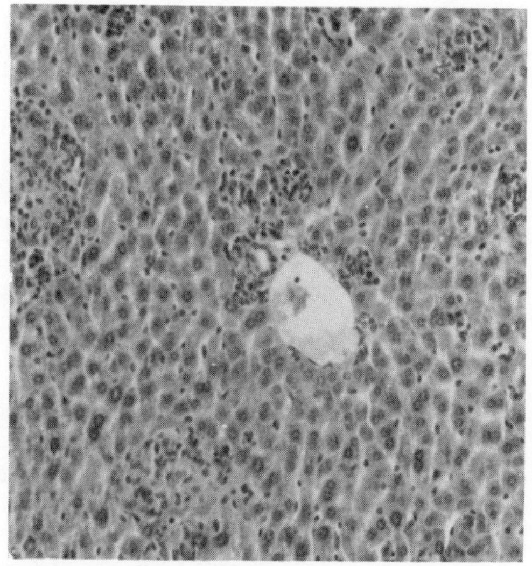

Fig. 11. Liver of a glucan and cyclophosphamide-treated mouse on day 9 after S. aureus challenge manifests the rather typical glucan-induced granuloma formation. In contrast to the cyclophosphamide-treated liver (Fig. 8) no parenchymal cell necrosis nor microabscesses were observed (100 x).

have shown glucan induced protection in a variety of murine infections such as Sporotrichum schenckii (28), Candida albicans (29), Cryptococcus neoformans and Mycobacterium leprae (22).

The precise mechanism by which glucan induces nonspecific protection against staphylococcal disease is not completely known. Previous studies in our laboratory have provided substantial evidence that glucan profoundly activates the reticuloendothelial system (7,25). Glucan-treated animals show a hypertrophy of the major reticuloendothelial organs with a concomitant increase in activation and proliferation of macrophages (30,31). Additionally, Burgaleta and Golde (6) have reported an enhanced leukopoiesis following glucan administration. Their observation is consistent with the findings reported in this investigation. Golde and Burgaleta (13) have also demonstrated that glucan-treated macrophages have enhanced function as well as altered surface morphology, generally associated with an "activated state". Other components of the immune system, such as serum lysozyme (20) and complement (C3) (12) have also been demonstrated to increase after glucan administration. These composite studies denote that glucan is capable of enhancing diverse facets of the immune system. This enhanced state of innate defenses, promoted by glucan and primarily mediated by macrophages may play a determinant role in protection of the host against systemic staphylococcal disease.

Based on earlier studies, mouse peritoneal exudate macrophages have been shown to phagocytize and destroy non-encapsulated strains of S. aureus (3). Biggar, et al. (4) have reported similar data employing rabbit alveolar macrophages against other gram-positive cocci, such as Streptocuccus faecalis and Streptococcus pneumoniae. While the role of other components of the immune system cannot be negated, the present observations in conjunction with the above cited studies, tend to support the role of macrophages in host defense against S. aureus infections.

Studies with other immunostimulants, such as BCG and C. parvum have not shown a protective effect comparable to glucan on survival of mice with experimentally induced staphylococcal septicemia. Adlam, et al. (1) reported no consistent effect with intravenous or intraperitoneal administration of C. parvum in mice that were subsequently challenged intravenously with S. aureus. In contrast, the data presented here shows that glucan provides significant protection with intravenous challenge doses of S. aureus up to an order of magnitude greater than the intraperitoneal challenge dose reported by Adlam, et al.(1). Sher, et al. (27) have reported that pretreatment with BCG will modify survival of mice challenged intravenously with 2.5×10^8 Staphylococcus aureus. Furthermore, Sher and his colleagues (27) demonstrated the effectiveness of BCG and C. parvum in cyclophosphamide-treated mice challenged with 1.68×10^5 S. aureus. In contrast, our observations demonstrate that glucan confers significant protection against intravenous challenge doses of 1.0 x 10^9 S. aureus in normal, leukemic and cyclophosphamide immunosuppressed mice.

Based upon histological examination, the kidneys appear to be the most vulnerable organ following the intravenous administration of S. aureus. This observation is in agreement with the data reported by Gorrill (14). Adlam, et al. (1) have suggested that the lack of protective efficacy of C. parvum administration against systemic S. aureus septicemia may be the result of the predilection of these microorganisms for the kidney. It was further postulated that the kidney is not affected by C. parvum induced lymphoreticular stimulation and thus the protective efficacy of C. parvum is lost following systemic infection with a nephrophilic microorganism. Our data do not support this concept since glucan stimulation of the RE system is effective in preventing the degenerative changes in the kidney. The protective efficacy of glucan administration in S. aureus-treated mice is manifested by prolonged survival as well as minimal pathological changes in the kidneys of glucan animals as compared to controls.

In cyclophosphamide-treated mice histopathological examination revealed the kidneys and liver to be the organs most vulnerable to S. aureus septicemia. When cyclophosphamide-treated mice were challenged intravenously with S. aureus a marked destruction of renal and hepatic parenchyma was observed. Sharbaugh and Grogan (26) have reported that cyclophosphamide decreased the bactericidal capacity of the kidney in rats challenged intravenously with S. aureus. This observation could, in part, account for marked renal necrosis observed in the cyclophosphamide-treated group. However, when glucan was administered conjointly with cyclophosphamide there is marked reduction in the renal and hepatic pathology of mice challenged with S. aureus.

Employing an acute monocytic leukemia rat model, Di Luzio, et al. (8) demonstrated that primary tumor growth was significantly reduced by both cyclophosphamide and glucan, with the most effective antineoplastic action being mediated by concurrent glucan and cyclophosphamide therapy. Increased survival following intravenous administration of leukemia cells was also observed in the glucan-cyclophosphamide treated rats. The degree of hepatic metastases was significantly reduced in both rats and AKR mice with acute leukemia by the conjoint use of cyclophosphamide and glucan. These studies denote that glucan can act synergistically with a conventional cancer chemotherapeutic agent, possibly since the stimulating action of glucan on macrophages is still present in cyclophosphamide treated animals.

The present data demonstrating the protective efficacy of glucan treatment against syngeneic murine lymphocytic leukemia is in accord with previous observations (9). Additionally, glucan was effective in significantly modifying staphylococcal infection in leukemic and cyclophosphamide-treated mice. Secondary infections in leukemic children are of increasing clinical concern (17,18). *Staphylococcus aureus* is commonly implicated as one of the gram-positive organisms initiating secondary infection in the leukemic or immunosuppressed host (21). In view of these observations, prophylactic treatment with glucan or other non-viable RES stimulating agents may be of potential value in combatting staphylococcal sepsis, particularly as secondary infection in malignant episodes. Furthermore, the administration of glucan may enable the patient with compromised host defense mechanisms to undergo more aggressive therapeutic measures since the induction of the immunodeficient state is significantly altered.

The current observations denote that glucan is capable of altering staphylococcal septicemia in normal, leukemic and immunosuppressed mice. These observations in conjunction with the well documented antitumor activity of glucan in both experimental animals and in man indicates that glucan may confer a unique duality of therapy by modifying neoplastic proliferation as well as enhancing host resistance to infectious disease.

SUMMARY

Glucan, a $\beta 1 \rightarrow 3$ polyglucosidic component of *Saccharomyces cerevisiae*, was evaluated for its ability to provide nonspecific resistance to *S. aureus* septicemia in AKR/J mice. Intravenous injection of glucan (0.45 mg/mouse) 7 and 4 days prior to intravenous challenge with *S. aureus* (1.0×10^9) resulted in a significantly increased survival as compared to control mice. Histological examination of the kidneys revealed that glucan decreased tissue necrosis associated with systemic staphylococcal disease. A post-treatment regimen of glucan significantly enhanced survival of AKR/J mice with lymphocytic leukemia as well as leukemic mice with experimentally induced systemic staphylococcal infection. The effect of glucan on *S. aureus* septicemia was also evaluated in cyclophosphamide-treated mice. Glucan increased peripheral leukocyte counts as well as significantly enhanced survival of cyclophosphamide-treated mice with systemic *S. aureus* infection. Histopathological examination revealed that glucan administration markedly inhibited renal and hepatic pathology in cyclophosphamide-treated mice following intravenous challenge with *S. aureus*. These data denote that glucan provides nonspecific resistance to bacterial sepsis in normal, leukemic as well as immunosuppressed mice.

ACKNOWLEDGEMENT

These studies were supported, in part, by funds from the Cancer Research Institute, Inc. (USA), American Cancer Society (USA), and the MECO Cancer Research Fund (USA).

REFERENCES

1. Adlam, C. E., Broughton, S. and Scott, M. T., Nature (London) New Biol., 235 (1972) 219.
2. Ashworth, C. T., Di Luzio, N. R. and Riggi, S. J., Exp. Mol. Pathol., 1 (1963) 83.
3. Baughn, R. E. and Bonventre, P. F., Infect. Immunol., 12(2) (1975) 346.
4. Biggar, W. D., Buran, S. and Holmes, B., Infec. Immunol., 14(1) (1976) 6.
5. Browder, W., Jones, E., McNamee, R. and Di Luzio, N. R., Surgical Forum 27 (1976) 134.
6. Burgaleta, C. and Golde, D. W., Cancer Res., 37 (1977) 1734.
7. Di Luzio, N. R., Pharmacology of the reticuloendothelial system: Accent on glucan. In: The Reticuloendothelial System in Health and Disease (Functions and Characteristics), (Eds. S. M. Reichard, M. R. Escobar and H. Friedman), Plenum Pub., N. Y., (1976) 412.
8. Di Luzio, N. R., Cook, J. A., Cohen, C., Rodrique, J and Jones, E., The synergistic effect of cyclophosphamide and glucan on experimental acute myelogenous and lymphocytic leukemia. In: The Macrophage and Cancer., (Eds. K. James, B. McBride, A. Stuart), Econoprint, Scotland, (1977a) 188.
9. Di Luzio, N. R., Hoffmann, E. O., Cook, J. A., Browder, W. and Mansell, P. W. A., Glucan-induced enhancement host resistance to experimental tumors. In: Control of Neoplasia by Modulation of the Immune System. (Ed. M. A. Chirigos), Raven Press, N. Y., (1977b) 495.
10. Di Luzio, N. R., McNamee, R., Browder, W. and Williams, D. L., Cancer Tr Rep (1978) in press.
11. Gaya, H., Tattersall, M. H., Hutchinson, R. M. and Spiers, S. S., Eur. J. Cancer, 9 (1973) 401.
12. Glovsky, M. M., Di Luzio, N. R., Alenty, A. and Ghekiere, L., J. Reticuloendothel. Soc, 20 (1976) 54a.
13. Golde, D. W. and Burgaleta, C., Glucan-activated macrophages: Functional properties and cytoxicity against syngeneic leukemic cells. In: Immune Modulation and Control and Neoplasia by Adjuvant Therapy, (Ed. M. Chirigos), Raven Press, N. Y. (1978) 201.
14. Gorrill, R. H., Br. J. Exp. Pathol., 39(2) (1958) 203.
15. Hassid, W. Z., Joslyn, M. A. and McCready, R. M., J. Am. Chem. Soc., 63 (1941) 295.
16. Hoffmann, E. O., Di Luzio, N. R., Cook, J. A., McNamee, R. B.

and Armstrong, K., Lab. Invest., 36 (1977) 340.
17. Hughes, W. T., Am. J. Dis. Child, 122 (1971) 283.
18. Hughes, W. T., Adv. Intern Med., 22 (1977) 73.
19. Israel, L. and Edelstein, R., Treatment of cutaneous and subcutaneous metastatic tumors with intralesional glucan. In: Control of Neoplasia by Modulation of the Immune System, (Ed. M. A. Chirigos), Raven Press, N. Y., (1978) 249.
20. Kokoshis, P. L., Williams, D. L., Cook, J. A. and Di Luzio, N. R., Science, 199 (1978) 1340.
21. Ladisch, S. and Pizzo, P. A., Pediatrics, 61 (1978) 231.
22. Lejeune, F. J., Delville, J., Gillet, J., Song, M., Stadtsbaeder, S. and Jacques, P., Eur. J. Cancer (1978) in press.
23. Mansell, P. W. A., Ichinose, H., Reed, R. J., Krementz, E. T., McNamee, R. and Di Luzio, N. R., J. Natl. Cancer Inst., 54 (1975) 571.
24. Mansell, P. W. A., Di Luzio, N. R., McNamee, R., Rowden, G. and Proctor, J. W., Ann. N. Y. Acad. Sci, 277 (1976) 20.
25. Riggi, S. J. and Di Luzio, N. R., Am. J. Physiol., 200 (1961) 297.
26. Sharbaugh, R. T. and Grogan, J. B., Infec. Immunol., 100 (1969) 117.
27. Sher, N. A., Chaparas, S. D., Greenburg, L. E. and Bernard, S., Infec. Immunol., 12 (1975) 1325.
28. Steven, M., Steven, P., Cook, J. A., Ichinose, H. and Di Luzio, N. T., J. Reticuloendothel. Soc., 20 (1976) 66a.
29. Williams, D. L., Cook, J. A., Hoffmann, E. O. and Di Luzio, N. R., J. Reticuloendothel. Soc., (1978) in press.
30. Wooles, W. R. and Di Luzio, N. R., Am. J. Physiol.,203 (1962) 404.
31. Wooles, W. R. and Di Luzio, N. R., Science, 142 (1963) 1078.
32. Wooles, W. R. and Di Luzio, N. R., J. Reticuloendothel. Soc., 1 (1964) 160.

PARTICULATE β 1-3 GLUCAN AND CASUAL PROPHYLAXIS OF MOUSE MALARIA (*PLASMODIUM BERGHEI*)

J. GILLET, P. J. JACQUES and F. HERMAN

School of Public Health, Université Catholique de Louvain, Brussels (Belgium)

After first contact with the erythrocytic forms of malaria parasites, the host's defense response develops in two successive steps. The first, which occurs soon after infection, is *non-specific* in nature and consists of phagocytosis of the parasites by RE-cells in the liver, spleen and bone-marrow (13,15,16). The second step, which is triggered by antigenic recognition, is characterized by specific proliferation of B and T-lymphocytes, immunoglobulin production and macrophage activation (4). In contrast, little is known about initial host defense response towards sporozoites and tissue forms of the parasite. At least, one can state that it must exist, since repeated administration of Freund's adjuvant to mice, prior to parasite inoculation, increases host resistance against infection by the sporozoites of *P. berghei* (17).

One might hope to elicit better resistance to sporozoites, by means of more potent immunostimulants or adjuvants (e.g. polysaccharides), which would first stimulate nonspecific capacity of the RES and later amplify the specific immune response. Such polysaccharides were recently classified (20) in four groups, depending on their origin : bacteria, yeasts, basidiomycetes and higher plants.

The first group of adjuvants, as represented by live or dead *Mycobacterium tuberculosis* (BCG) was already successfully used some 20 years ago in order to control experimental infections by staphylococci (8) and growth of transplantable tumors (1,18). More recently, dead *Corynebacterium pavum* was shown to exert similar inhibitory action against tumors (11). Interest in these procedures for the medical care of infections by protozoa started to develop only recently. Thus, treatment by live M.tuberculosis (BCG) or dead C.parvum was shown to protect against infections by the erythrocytic forms of plasmodia (P.yoelii, P.vinckei) and of babesia (B.microti, B.rodhaini) (5, 6); a much lighter protection was obtained with dead C.parvum and the free forms of Trypanosoma cruzi (2, 14). Ten years earlier, Nussenzweig (17) had already demonstrated protection against malaria, for 53% of the mice infected by 5000 sporozoites of P.berghei, after venous administration of dead C.parvum. The latter pioneer work namely pointed to the interest of immunoadjuvants for the causal prophylaxis of malaria, and prompted us to further explore the question, with the aid of simpler and apparently more potent adjuvants. For the present work, we chose particulate β 1-3 glucan extracted from the yeast Saccharomyces cerevisiae, which offers distinct advantages compared to BCG and causes destruction of a variety of experimental tumors (7). It appears as a potent activator of the RES (7), of complement (10) and of immunity (3). Especially important, in view of causal prophylaxis of malaria, is that glucan improves both non-specific resistance (activating property) and subsequent specific immune response (immunoapplifying property proper). Also, it leads to accumulation of inflammatory white cells (polymorphonuclear and mononuclear phagocytes) in the liver (7, 12), e.g. in the target organ for sporozoites and the growth environment for the derived tissue forms of the parasite.

MATERIALS AND METHODS

P.berghei (strain Anka) was kept highly pathogenic through cyclic passages every three weeks involving the mosquito Anopheles stephensi and mice of strain Tb. The latter which were also used for the experimental work proper, were selected on account of their high susceptibility to infection by P.berghei (19). Adult infected mosquitoes were collected by means of an automatic device (9) avoiding any manipulation and thus allowing very low insect mortality.

For each sporozoite preparation, the head and thorax from each of at least 50 mosquitoes were dissected, and crushed at 4 C in a coaxial homogenizer (Potter type) containing nutrient medium supplemented with serum. Parasite concentration was estimated in a hemocytometer and adjusted so that the inoculum volume contain 5000 to 8000 parasites. The latter was administered the intravenous route to a maximum of 12 adult Tb mice. Relative instability of the sporozoites in vitro at 0 C also required checking control mice at the end of the inoculation series.

Preparations of particulate β 1-3 glucan were kindly offered by Prof. N. R. Di Luzio (Tulane University Medical School, New

Orleans, Louisiana (USA). Suspensions in saline were administered through intravenous or intraperitoneal route, at the 3 or 4 times repeated dose of 40 or 20 mg. Kg^{-1}, prior to infection by sporozoites.

After infection, parasitemia was regularly measured until death. Animals surviving for one month without detectable parasitemia, were considered negative; subinoculation of their blood to normal untreated mice regularly confirmed lack of infection.

Two morbidity criteria were examined in all animals : (1) length of prepatent period, e.g. time interval between infection (day 0) and first appearance of parasites in blood smears, and (2) survival time, as measured in days between day 0 and that of death. In more recent experiments, two additional criteria were used, e.g. (3) frequency of parasitized red blood cells (RBC) on day 6 after infection, as expressed in number per 10,000 RBC, and (4) day on which 2% of the RBC contained parasites.

Statistical analysis of the results involved student's t-test and 2 x 2 contingency tables (X^2).

RESULTS

In an exploratory experiment, glucan (batch DL-04-P) was administered 3 times, at the maximal dosage of 40 mg. Kg^{-1}, on days 8-5-3 or 20-17-15 before inoculation of the parasites (5000 sporozoites) to 2 groups of animals differing only by the route - intravenous or intraperitoneal - used for drug administration.

As suggested in table I and validated by contingency analysis, intravenously administered glucan prevented development of malaria in about 50% of the animals ($p<2\%$), although a few of the control mice were found negative. In contrast, the animals which received the drug through the peritoneal cavity did not significantly differ from the controls ($p>95\%$); under the present circumstances, they can thus be included as controls. The striking importance of the route for drug administration becomes more significant still ($p<1\%$) when results from intravenously treated mice were directly compared to those from intraperitoneally treated ones. The results of table I also suggest a difference in the efficacy of glucan protection, depending on the period of time separating treatment from infection. Thus, both prepatent period ($p<0.1\%$) and survival time ($p<0.1\%$) were significantly increased in the three animals which developed malaria when glucan was given on days 8-5-3 before infection, whereas the same parameters remained normal when the drug was given nearly 2 weeks sooner.

TABLE I

Influence of Administration Route of Glucan on its Preventive Action Against Malaria

Glucan		Number of Animals			Morbidity in Positive Animals	
Posology 3 x 40mg.Kg^{-1}	Route	Total	Neg.	Pos.	Prepatency (days)	Survival time (days)
on days (-8),(-5),(-3)	Venous	6	3	3	7.33 % 1.33	19.00 % 3.21
	Periton.	6	0	6	4.00 ± 0.00	10.83 ± 1.28
on days (-20),(-17), (-15)	Venous	7	5	2	5.00 ± 0.00	11.00 ± 0.00
	Periton.	7	0	7	3.86 ± 0.14	10.14 ± 0.55
Control	-	16	2	14	4.39 ± 0.11	12.21 ± 0.92

All animals received 5000 sporozoites by the intravenous route, on day 0.
Statistics refer to arithmetic mean ± standard error.

TABLE II

Lower Efficacy of Glucan Treatment After Reducing Dosage and Increasing Parasites Load

Glucan Dosage	Number of Animals			Morbidity of Impaludaded Animals			
	Total	Neg.	Pos.	Prepatency (days)	Parasitemia on day 6 (c)	Day of parasitemia = 2% RBC	Survival time (days)
3 x 20 $mg.Kg^{-1}$ (a)	8	1	7	5.00 ± 0.31	24.00 ± 13.10	6.93 ± 0.17	19.43 ± 1.69
4 x 20 $mgKg^{-1}$ (b)	13	1	12	4.75 ± 0.28	38.00 ± 15.10	6.96 ± 0.16	17.58 ± 1.79
Control	13	0	13	4.46 ± 0.18	94.52 ± 19.83	6.56 ± 0.14	18.15 ± 1.46

All mice received 7500 sporozoites on day zero, by the intravenous route

a - intravenous route on days (-8), (-5), (-3).
b - intravenous route on days (-7), (-5), (-3), (-1)
c - expressed in number of infected RBC per 10,000.

Statistics refer to arithmetic mean ± standard error.

For obvious reasons, only the intravenous route was used in subsequent experiments. The latter were improved by addition of two more morbidity criteria, and through raising the number of sporozoites in the inoculum. Thus, in the experiment illustrated by table II, the inoculum contained 7,500 sporozoites and the more favorable schedule of drug administration was selected. Unfortunately, the recent preparations of glucan (DL-102777) killed Tb mice within 5 to 120 min after intravenous injection of doses higher than 20 $mg.Kg^{-1}$. If the control animals were, as expected, invariably impaludated, the protective effect of glucan dramatically decreased (table II), and the prepatent period remained normal in the unprotected though treated animals. Only parasitemia on day 6 was significantly lowered ($p<5\%$), but this did not lead to detectable prolongation of survival time.

CONCLUSIONS

Present results strongly point to yeast particulate glucan as a good candidate for medical care of malaria, provided that more reproducible and less toxic preparations can be obtained in the future. Should that hope be met, there would remain to check whether glucan acts only on the tissue phase of the plasmodium (casual etioprophylaxis) or affects subsequent forms including the merozoites of first generation. Experiments are in progress in order to solve that question, and to ascertain possible therapeutic action of that immunoamplifier on the erythrocytic stage of the disease.

ACKNOWLEDGEMENTS

The authors express their gratitude to Miss A.-M.Rona and G. Mattucilli for skillful technical assistance, to Dr. N. R. Di Luzio (New Orleans) for the supply of glucan, to Prof. P. C. C. Garnham for encouragements and stimulating discussions, and to Belgian Fonds de la Recherche Scientifique Medicale (contract 3.4580.75-F) for financial and moral support. One of us (PJJ) holds tenure of Maître de Recherche, from the Fonds National de la Recherche Scientifique.

REFERENCES

1. Biozzi, G., Stiffel, C., Halpern, B. N. and Mouton, D., C. R. Soc. Biol., 153 (1959) 987.
2. Brener, Z. and Cardoso, J. E.., J. Parasitol., 62 (1976) 645.
3. Browder, W., McNamee, R., Cohen, L., Taylor, D. and Di Luzio, N. R., J. Reticuloendothelial Soc., 20 (1976) 55a.
4. Brown, K. N., Immunology of Parasitic Infections (Eds. S. Cohen and E. Sadun), Blackwell, Oxford (1976) 268.
5. Clark, I. A., Allison, A. C. and Cox, F. E., Nature, 259 (1976) 309.
6. Clark, I. A., Cox, F. E. and Allison, A. C., Parasitology, 74 (1977) 9.
7. Di Luzio, N. R., The Reticuloendothelial System in Health and Disease (Eds. H. Friedman, M. R. Escobar and S. M. Reichard), Plenum, New York, A (1976) 412.
8. Dubos, R. J. and Schaedler, R. W., J. Exp. Med., 106 (1957) 703.
9. Gillet, J. and Herman, F., Ann. Soc. Belge Med. Trop., 56 (1976) 183.
10. Glovsky, M. M., Di Luzio, N. R., Alenty, A. and Ghekiere, L. R. J., Reticuloendothelial Soc., 20 (1976) 54a.
11. Halpern, B. N., Biozzi, G., Stiffel, C. and Mouton, D., Nature, 212 (1966) 853.
12. Hennekine, M. F., Song, M. and Jacques, P. J., Arch. Intern. Physiol. Biochim., 85 (1977) 983.
13. Hopff, B. M., Exp. Parasitol., 28 (1970) 291.
14. Kierszenbaum, F., Infect. Immun. 12 (1975) 1227.
15. Kitchen, A. G. and Di Luzio, N. R., J. Reticuloendothelial Soc., 9 (1971) 237.
16. Lucia, H. L. and Nussenzweig, R. S., Exp. Parasitol., 25 (1969) 319.
17. Nussenzweig, R. S., Exp. Parasitol., 21 (1967) 224.
18. Old, L. J., Clarke, D. A. and Benacerraf, B., Nature, 184 (1959) 291.
19. Vincke, I. and Bafort, J., Ann. Soc. Belge Med. Trop., 48 (1968) 181.
20. Whistler, R. L., Bushway, A. A., Singh, P. P., Nakahara, W. and Tokuzen, R., Adv. Carbohydr. Chem. Biochem., 32 (1976) 235.

RESTORATION OF DEPRESSED ANTIBODY RESPONSES OF LEUKEMIC SPLENOCYTES TREATED WITH LPS-INDUCED FACTORS

R. C. BUTLER, H. FRIEDMAN, and A. NOWOTNY

Depts. of Microbiology and Immunology
Albert Einstein Medical Center and University of Pennsylvania, Philadelphia, Pennsylvania and College of Medicine, University of South Florida, Tampa, Florida (USA)

Lipopolysaccharides (LPS) derived from gram negative bacteria are known to enhace antibody responses to a variety of antigens, including serum proteins and xenogeneic erythrocytes, both *in vivo* and *in vitro* (1,10,11). Recent studies in this laboratory have shown that such endotoxins may influence the immune response of splenocytes from Friend leukemia virus (FLV) infected mice which showed markedly impaired immune competence (2,3). The mechanism of action of LPS in enhancing antibody formation by leukemic splenocytes, as well as normal splenocytes, is still unclear. It is not known whether the LPS affects immunity by directly interacting with lymphocytes or by inducing intermediate immunoregulatory or immunostimulatory factors. In the present study attempts were made to determine whether pretreatment of mice with LPS causes the release of factors into·the serum which could mediate the adjuvant effect on the *in vitro* antibody response of normal or leukemia virus immunosuppressed cell cultures.

MATERIALS AND METHODS

Lipopolysaccharide derived from *Serratia marcescens* as previously described (9) was utilized for study. Twenty μg of either LPS or a detoxified PS derived from intact endotoxin by mild acid hydrolysis was injected into normal Balb/c mice (Jackson Memorial Laboratories, Bar Harbor, Maine) 6 to 8 weeks of age. In some experiments the mice were pretreated by i.p. injection of 1×10^7 viable BCG 14 days earlier. Two hr after injection of the LPS, blood was obtained from the animals and the resulting serum tested for effects on the *in vitro* antibody response of splenocytes to sheep red blood cells (SRBC). For this purpose 8 x 10^6 nucleated spleen cells from normal mice were incubated in Linbro tissue culture plates exactly as described earlier and immunized with 2 x 10^6 SRBC (7,8). The numbers of antibody plaque forming cells (PFCs) appearing in the cultures five days later were determined per culture or per 1 x 10^6 viable spleen cells by the hemolytic plaque assay according to the method of Cunningham and Szenburg (4).

In some experiments the effect of supernatants of normal spleen cells cultured with LPS was determined by an indirect method. Spleen cells were incubated with LPS and the culture supernatants harvested at various times thereafter. The supernatants were then tested for the presence of soluble immunodulating mediators by determining their effects on the antibody response of normal spleen cells immunized _in vitro_ with SRBC exactly as described above.

For some of the experiments the spleen cells treated with endotoxin were also treated with BCG _in vitro_. In all cases the PFC responses of normal spleen cells immunized with SRBC were compared with the responses of spleen cells treated with the soluble factors obtained _in vivo_ or _in vitro_. For virus infection, mice were injected i.p. with 100 ID_{50} of Friend leukemia virus (FLV). Splenocytes from these animals were harvested at various times and cultured _in vitro_ exactly as were the normal splenocytes.

RESULTS

As is evident in Table I, both LPS and PS in graded doses affected in a significant manner the antibody response of normal mouse spleen cells immunized _in vitro_ with SRBC. A concentration of 10 μg LPS resulted in maximum enhancement of the immune response _in vitro_. Ten micrograms of PS gave an enhancement similar to the intact LPS. Spleen cells from seven day FLV infected mice failed to respond normally _in vitro_ when immunized with SRBC (Table II). There was approximately a 75% reduction in the peak antibody response by infected splenocytes when compared with normal splenocytes. When LPS was added to such splenocytes a partial enhancement of the response was evident. BCG (1 x 10^5 colony forming units) had no significant effect on the suppressed response of the leukemic cells. However, when both BCG and LPS were added to such cultures, essentially normal numbers of PFCs appeared.

Muramyl dipeptide (MDP), a synthetic analogue of the cell wall moiety responsible for the adjuvanicity of mycobacteria (4), was tested in a similar manner to the LPS and PS. As can be seen in Table III, these three agents, when added to normal splenocytes, caused an immunostimulatory effect. In addition, incubation of

TABLE I

Dose Response for Stimulation of the *In Vitro* PFC Response to SRBC by Serratia LPS or PS

Treatment (μg/culture)[a]	PFC/10^6 Cells[b] ± S.E.	% Control	p
None	1281 ± 105	100	
LPS 20 μg	2324 ± 59	181	.005
10 μg	3424 ± 371	267	.005
1 μg	1780 ± 116	139	.01
0.1 μg	1345 ± 88	104	
PS 20 μg	2160 ± 65	169	.005
10 μg	2960 ± 92	231	.005
1 μg	1530 ± 84	120	.01
0.1 μg	1310 ± 64	102	

[a]Indicated dose of LPS added to cultures of 8 x 10^6 normal spleen cells immunized *in vitro* with 2 x 10^6 SRBC.

[b]Average PFC response for 8 cultures each 5 days after immunization.

TABLE II

Restoration of the Antibody Response of FLV-Infected Splenocytes by Treatment with LPS and/or BCG

Culture Treatment[a]	PFC/10^6 Cells ± S. E.	% Control	p
Normal Spleen	1429 ± 74	100	
FLV-Infected Spleen[b]	373 ± 22	26	.001
" + μg LPS	538 ± 56	38	.001
" + 10^5 BCG	354 ± 33	25	.001
" _ BCG + LPS	1507 ± 270	105	

[a]8 x 10^6 spleen cells incubated with 2 x 10^6 SRBC and treated on day of culture initiation with BCG and/or LP.S

[b]Mice were infected i.p. with 100 ID_{50} FLV 7 days before splenectomy.

TABLE III

Effects of Combinations of LPS or PS with MDP on the Antibody Responses of Normal and FLV-Suppressed Cells

Culture Treatment[a]	Normal Splenocytes		FLV-Infected Splenocytes[d]	
	PFC/10^6 Cells ± S.E.[b]	% Control[c] (p)	PFC/10^6 Cells ± S.E.	% Control (p)
None	382 ± 31	100	155 ± 10	100
20 μg LPS	1127 ± 83	295 (<.0005)	718 ± 126	470 (<.0005)
20 μg PS[e]	719 ± 61	188 (<.005)	412 ± 37	266 (<.0005)
10 μg MDP[f]	736 ± 39	193 (<.005)	368 ± 26	237 (<.0005)
20 μg LPS + μg MDP	2297 ± 171	601 (<.0005)	1331 ± 64	859 (<.0005)
20 μg PS+10 μg MDP	1061 ± 72	278 (<.0005)	664 ± 52	428 (<.0005)

[a]Cultures of 8 x 10^6 splenocytes were treated with LPS, PS and MDP and immunized *in vitro* with 2 x 10^6 SRBC.

[b]Mean numbers of PFC/1 x 10^6 viable cells from 8 cultures/group assayed on day 5.

[c]p values calculated using the Student's 't' test.

[d]0.1 ml of a cell-free homogenate of 1 x 10^6 FLV-infected cells/ml added to each culture.

[e]PS is a lipid-free, nontoxid LPS hydrolytic product.

[f]MDP is a synthetic muramyl dipeptide.

LPS or PS together with MDP resulted in an enhancement of the PFC response, with the former combination being most active. When FLV was added to normal splenocytes to induce a suppressed immune response, these materials resulted in a marked stimulation of the immune responses as compared to control cultures incubated with FLV alone. LPS appeared to have the greatest stimulatory effect when added in combination with MDP.

TABLE IV

Immunostimulatory Effects of Supernatants from LPS Stimulated Spenocyte Cultures on FLV-Induced Immunosuppression

Culture Treatment[a]	Normal		ELV[b]	
	PFC/10^6 Cells ± S.E.[c]	% (p)	PFC/10^6 Cells ± S.E.	% (p)
None	696 ± 46	100	240 ± 68	100
Normal Culture Sup'n.				
3 days	702 ± 60	101	302 ± 62	125
5 days	678 ± 36	97	324 ± 38	135
LPS-Stimulated Sup'n.				
3 days	948 ± 98	136 (.05)	592 ± 110	247 (.02)
5 days	1379 ± 82	198 (.01)	962 ± 102	401 (.01)

[a]Cultures of 8 x 10^6 normal spleen cells cultured along or with FLV and 3 or 5 day supernatants from normal or LPS stimulated splenocyte cultures.

[b]0.1 ml of a homogenate of 1 x 10^6 FLV infected cells added to cultures.

[c]Average number of PFCs for 8-24 cultures on day 5.

Supernatants from LPS stimulated spleen cell cultures were effective in reversing the immune suppression of FLV-treated splenocytes. As can be seen in Table IV, culture supernatants obtained from LPS treated splenocytes markedly enhanced the immune response of normal cells and caused a similar enhancement of PFC formation by FLV-infected splenocytes. Normal culture supernatants had no such effect. The enhancing activity of cell-free supernatants from LPS treated splenocytes was similar to that observed when post-endotoxin sera were similarly tested. As can be seen in Table V, 0.1 ml of a serum obtained from mice two hr after treatment with LPS caused a striking increase in the number of PFCs by spleen cells from FLV infected cultures. Although this effect was not as great as that induced by the LPS per se, it was significant and reproducible.

TABLE V

Restoration of FLV-Suppressed Antibody Response by Post-LPS Serum

Culture Treatment[a]	PFC/10^6 Cells ± S.E.	% Normal (p)	% FLV (p)
None	1171 ± 11	100	-
20 μg LPS	2382 ± 47	203(.0005)	-
FLV plus no addition	210 ± 17	-	100
plus 20 μg LPS	917 ± 108	-	437(.001)
plus Post-LPS Serum	586 ± 88	-	279(.005)

[a] Sera or LPS added to cell cultures with or without FLV homogenate and immunized *in vitro* with SRBC.

DISCUSSION

Various bacterial products have been shown to markedly stimulate the *in vitro* or *in vivo* antibody responses of splenocytes from normal as well as immunodepressed donors. In this regard LPS from gram negative bacteria have been studied in greatest detail in terms of adjuvanticity (1,10,11). Studies from this and other laboratories have suggested that the immunodulating effects of LPS may be mediated by soluble mediators, either similar to or identical with lymphokines (6). Other studies in this laboratory have also shown that the small molecular weight polysaccharide-rich fraction derived from LPS also has immunostimulatory properties (5). Muramyl dipeptide synthesized *in vitro* has activities similar to mycobacteria and apparently contains much of the immunostimulatory activity of the native bacterial cell wall.

In the present study the effects of these materials on the suppressed immune responsiveness of splenocytes from murine leukemia virus infected mice was studied. In addition, these materials were shown to affect the immunodepression induced by FLV on normal splenocytes *in vitro*. A combination of PS or LPS with either MDP or BCG produced a synergistic immunostimulatory effect. This effect appeared to be due to one or more soluble factors induced by these materials. For example, when supernatants from LPS stimulated spleen cells were added to normal spleen cell cultures immunized *in vitro*, an enhanced immune response occurred. The same supernatants caused a marked stimulatory response by FLV immunosuppressed cultures. The immunostimulatory effect present in the supernatants appeared similar to that found in the serum of mice pretreated with LPS or even PS. Small amounts of serum from such pretreated animals had similar immunostimulatory effects for both normal and virus-infected splenocytes. Thus it appears likely that lymphokines may mediate the adjuvant effect of LPS for both normal and FLV-infected splenocytes. Further studies are obviously necessary to define the nature of the factor(s), the cell source, and the target cell(s).

SUMMARY

Lipopolysaccharide and a nontoxic derivative, PS, from *Serratia marcescens* were studied in terms of their effects on normal and Friend leukemia virus depressed splenocytes. These materials caused a marked increase in the number of antibody producing cells by both groups of splenocytes. MDP, a synthetic analogue of myobacterial cell walls, produced a similar adjuvant response by normal and leukemic splenocytes. Combinations of PS or LPS and BCG or MDP resulted in synergistic immunostimulatory responses. A soluble factor associated with these materials appeared to mediate the response, since cell-free supernatants from LPS stimulated splenocytes or serum from LPS treated mice resulted in similar immunostimulation.

REFERENCES

1. Behling, U. H., Nowotny, A. J. Immunol 118 (1977) 1905.
2. Butler, R. C., Nowotny, A., Friedman, H. J. Res. 22 (1977) 28a.
3. Butler, R. C., Nowotny, A., and Friedman (submitted).
4. Cunningham, A. J., Szenberg, A. Immunol. 14 (1968) 599.
5. Frank, S. J., Specter, S., Nowotny, A. and Friedman, H. J. Immunol. 119 (1977) 855.
6. Hoffman, M. K., Green, S., Old, L. J., and Oettgen, H. F. Nature 263 (1976) 416.
7. Kamo, I., Pan, S. H., and Friedman, H. J. Immunol. Meth.

11 (1976) 55.
8. Nowotny, A., Behling, U. H., Chang, H. L. J. Immunol. 115 (1975) 197.
9. Nowotny, A., Cundy, K. R., Rote, N. L., Nosotny, A. M., Advuny, P. R., Thomas, S. P. and Tripodi, D. J. Ann. N. Y. Acad. Sci. 133 (1968) 586.
10. Sjoberg, O., Andersson, J. and Moller, G. Europ. J. Immunol. 2 (1972) 326.
11. Watson, J., Trenkner, E. and Cohn, M. J. Exp. Med., 138 (1973) 699.

FUNCTIONAL SIMILARITY AND DIVERSITY IN PERITONEAL MACROPHAGE POPULATIONS INDUCED *IN VIVO* BY VARIOUS STIMULI

R. GOLDMAN, Z. BAR-SHAVIT and A. RAZ

Department of Membrane Research, The Weizmann Institute of Science, Rehovot (Israel)

Intraperitoneal injection of various foreign substances results in an augmentation of the size of the population of peritoneal macrophages. Various functional differences between stimulated populations and "normal" resident macrophage populations have been documented in recent years (2,4,8,11,13,16,20-22, 24,28,29). The terminology used by different workers in the field for description of the functional differences, i.e. stimulated, elicited, activated, is not consistent and depends to a large extent on the parameter chosen for comparison. We would, therefore, use the general term "stimulation" to describe populations induced by the various stimuli. Special emphasis has been given to differences in the phagocytic capacity of normal and thioglycollate (4) or endotoxin (22) stimulated mouse macrophages, since an alteration in complement receptor function upon stimulation was implicated. Another aspect that is currently intensively studied is that of macrophage-target cell interaction and the relevance of activated macrophages in combating neoplasia (2,11, 13,21).

In this study we compared several functional parameters of macrophages stimulated by various stimuli. The results indeed show a diversity in function generated by those stimuli. Moreover, it is suggested that the notion, that stimulated macrophages are superior to resident macrophages in their phagocytic capability and especially in their ability to ingest particles attached to the phagocyte via the C3b receptor, may not be as clear-cut as posed in the literature.

MACROPHAGE STIMULATION

Various stimulating agents were injected intraperitoneally (i.p.) in order to induce peritoneal exudates. Corynebacterium parvum (CP) (heat-killed, strain CN 6137, 7 mg/ml, Burroughs Wellcome, 0.2 ml/mouse), mineral oil (Drakeol 6VI, Penerco, 0.5 ml/mouse), and glucan (prepared from Saccharomyces cerevisiae, 2 mg/mouse) were injected 5 days prior to cell harvest. Thioglycollate (2.98 gr/100 ml, 3 ml/mouse, Difco), Concanavalin A (1 mg/ 1 ml x mouse, Miles-Yeda), and Bacillus Calmette Guerin (BCG, 1 mg/1 ml x mouse, lyophilized) were injected 4 days prior to cell harvest.

MARKER ENZYMES

One of the first differences that have been noted in stimulated macrophage populations was an elevated level of lysosomal enzymes, in particular that of acid phosphatase. All of the stimulated populations listed in Table I abide to this criterion, but the extent of enzyme level elevation differs markedly within the series. The activity of the plasma membrane marker enzyme, 5'-nucleotidase, has been shown to decrease to very low levels upon macrophage stimulation (16,26). All of the stimuli compared in the present study induced exudates possessing 5-15% of the enzyme activity exhibited by normal macrophages (Table I).

PHAGOCYTOSIS MEDIATED BY THE COMPLEMENT RECEPTOR

Sheep red blood cells (SRBC) coated with IgM and C3b attach to macrophages via the complement receptor, the latter recognizing the C3b component (9). Under a certain set of experimental conditions, SRBC (IgM) C3b attach avidly to macrophages with minimal ingestion (2%). Table II represents the attachment pattern under three opsonization levels with IgM. The level of attachment and its dependence on the degree of opsonization differ for normal and stimulated macrophage populations, the most striking difference exhibited by thioglycollate-stimulated macrophages. Since in several experiments the level of ingestion of SRBC (IgM) C3b amounted to 20% of the erythrocytes attached to normal macrophages, it seemed possible that the degree of ingestion reflects the degree of opsonization and the fact that the experimental conditions allow for a limited opsonization below the threshold needed for effective ingestion. Coating with IgM is performed under sub-agglutinating conditions, and serum treatment is a delicate balance between the generation of C3b and its fixation to its cleavage to C3d that is not recognized by the macrophage receptors (14). Indeed when preformed SRBC (IgM) C3b - macrophage

TABLE I

Acid Phosphatase and 5'-Nucleotidase Activity in Normal and Stimulated Macrophages

Macrophages[a]	Acid Phosphatase Activity ± SEM (μmole Pi/mg) Protein, 2 h)	5'-Nucleotidase Activity ± SEM (μmole Pi/mg) Protein, 2 h)
Normal	1.40±0.04	3.76±0.03
Con A-stimulated	6.38±0.02	0.36±0.04
Thioglycollate-stimulated	4.32±0.04	0.26±0.02
CP-stimulated	2.46±0.03	0.31±0.03
BCG-stimulated	3.77±0.03	0.42±0.04
Mineral oil-stimulated	2.43±0.07	0.51±0.01.

[a]Macrophages were cultured for 1 hr and then washed thoroughly (x4) with saline to remove non-adherent cells and traces of Pi.

rosettes were further incubated with serum or with IgM and subsequently with serum (not shown) the percent of ingested erythrocytes out of macrophage-associated erythrocytes increased (from 20% to 41-46% for normal and to 73-78% for thioglycollate-stimulated macrophages).

The possibility that the IgM fraction contains IgG and that the ingestion stems from synergistic action of the Fc and C3b receptors (5) is not readily excluded, even though the attachment of nonserum treated IgM-coated SRBC is minimal (9-10 SRBC per 100 macrophages). In order to avoid the complications of a possible IgG contamination, we looked for a method that will relate directly the phagocytosis to the C3b component.

Zymosan induces complement activation by the alternate pathway (23) and the generated C3b becomes bound to the insoluble polysaccharide preparation (19,25). Huber and Wigzell (14) have described a simple rosette assay system for demonstration of complement receptor sites using complement-coated zymosan beads. Zymosan is a cell wall preparation of *Saccharomyces cerevisiae* and it was to be expected that the heat-killed yeast cells will be as effective as zymosan in activation of complement and fixation of C3b. Yeast cells have the advantage of being in a size

TABLE II

Interaction of Macrophages with Sheep Erythrocytes
Coated with IgM + C3b

Macrophages	No SRBC/100 Macrophages[a]					
	I IgM	A (1:30)	I IgM	A (1:75)	I IgM	A (1:150)
Normal	43	2107	24	1305	11	716
Thioglycollate-stimulated	29	123	18	116	10	56
Mineral oil-stimulated	6	1372	11	312	7	242
Glucan-stimulated	19	1477	19	450	6	361
BCG-stimulated	12	952	10	711	3	129
CP-stimulated	10	1515	9	768	4	652

[a]I - Ingested; A - Attached.

Rabbit Anti-SRBC IgM was obtained from Cordis Laboratories (Miami, Fla). SRBC (10^9/ml) were incubated for 30 min at 37 C with dilutions of IgM in medium, washed, incubated with C_5-deficient mouse serum, 10 min, 37 C, washed with cold medium. Macrophages incubated with 5 x 10^7 coated SRBC, 60 min, 37 C, fixed, stained and enumerated. SEM < 10%.

range convenient for direct microscopic enumeration (3).

The left column in Table III represents the phagocytic response to untreated yeast cells in the absence of serum. Yeast cells treated with HI-serum are phagocytosed to the same extent (2nd column from the left). Incubation of yeast cells with C_5-deficient mouse serum results in an augmentation in the phagocytic response 4-6-fold that observed with unopsonized yeast cells. The opsonizing effect depends on serum concentration and is saturable. Once opsonized, yeast cells can undergo heating (30 min, 56 C) without loss of their high affinity for macrophages. It is of interest that all the macrophage populations showed a high capacity for ingestion mediated by the C3b component, normal macrophages responded at least as the stimulated populations and thioglycollate-stimulated macrophages were inferior to the other populations in their phagocytic response. It is again possible to invoke a synergism between the C3b mediated binding and phagocytosis via nonspecific receptors as the direct effector mechanism for phagocytosis. It seems, however, that the evidence supports the notion that mouse macrophages are able to carry out phagocytosis mediated by the C3b receptors once the density of C3b on the particle is sufficient for a tight circumferential interaction prior to internalization (10). Studying lectin-mediated phagocytosis, we have clearly shown that opsonization of mouse erythrocytes with sub-agglutinating Con A concentrations leads to extensive rosette formation with no phagocytosis, and that the addition of Con A to preformed rosettes leads to ingestion of all the attached erythrocytes (7).

TABLE III

Phagocytosis[a] of C3b Coated Yeast Cells

Macrophages	-	Yeast Cells Opsonized With: H.I.C Deficient Serum (1:10)	C_5-Deficient Serum Diluted: 1:50	1:10	1:5
Normal	235	238	675	1123	1073
Thioglycollate-stimulated	97	90	216	382	309
Mineral oil-stimulated	131	152	567	846	1012
Glucan-stimulated	213	225	857	1065	1057
BCG-stimulated	144	126	713	847	687
CP-stimulated	199	129	569	1008	1018

[a] Phagocytosis: Opsonized yeast cells (10^7/ml) incubated with macrophage monolayers, 60 min, 37 C, washed, fixed, stained and enumerated. SEM < 10%.

[b] Coating: Yeast cells of *Saccharomyces cerevisiae* were boiled for 60 min, incubated (10^8/ml) in HEPES-Medium with HI or fresh C_5-deficient mouse serum of the given dilution for 30 min at 37 C.

MACROPHAGE STIMULATION AND ANTITUMOR ACTIVITY

Activation is defined as generation of strong cytostatic or cytocidal capacity in a macrophage population either *in vivo* or *in vitro*. Certain populations of stimulated macrophages, the "activated" macrophages as opposed to normal macrophages, have been shown to be involved in tumor destruction (2,6,11,13,15,21).

Nonspecific activators include chronic infection with various microorganisms, biologic immunopotentiators, such as complete Freund's adjuvant, the killed vaccines of *Corynebacterium parvum* and synthetic immunopotentiators, such as double stranded RNA and synthetic polyanions, such as pyran. In the mouse agents, such as thioglycollate glycogen and proteose peptone, do not induce activated macrophages (11,12).

We have compared the ability to inhibit target cell growth of several stimulated macrophage populations with that of normal macrophages, using two different assays, inhibition of ^{3}H-thymidine incorporation and assessment of inhibition of cell proliferation. The assessment of inhibition of target cell proliferation was based on the method described by Lagneau *et al*. (18) relating the number of cells to their quantitative staining by methylene blue. Both the KBALB (1) and N3T3.AKR(G) (27) fibroblast cell lines show a linear increase in dye eluted after staining with number of cells and the growth curve as measured by stain fixation yields the same doubling time as that assessed by direct cell count.

$$\text{Cell proliferation (\% of control)} = \frac{At{+}m - Ato - Am}{At - Ado} \times 100$$

where A - absorbance at 660 nm of 5 - targets at the end of assay, to - targets at zero time, m - macrophages, t+m - cocultures of targets and macrophages.

After 28 hr of coculture of macrophages and targets there was a reduction in the incorporation of ^{3}H-thymidine by target cells, the reduction observed in CP-stimulated macrophages exceeded that observed for any other macrophage population by orders of magnitude (Fig. 1, A-B). Using the dye fixation method an enhancement or a mild inhibition of cell proliferation was observed depending on the cell type and number of macrophages. CP-stimulated macrophages showed remarkable inhibition of cell proliferation even at 50,000 macrophages per well (Fig. 1, C-D). A longer coculture period (46 hr) led to an overall inhibition of cell proliferation differing for the different macrophage populations in its degree. Again the presence of CP-stimulated macrophages stopped totally target cell replication from very early coculture stages (Fig. 2). In 46 hr KBALB cells replicate about 2-3 times, and the percent of inhibition reflects the time of cessation of target cell replication.

Kung *et al*. (17) reported that macrophages secrete arginase to the culture medium and suggested that macrophage mediated suppression of mixed leukocyte cultures stems from depletion of arginine from the medium.

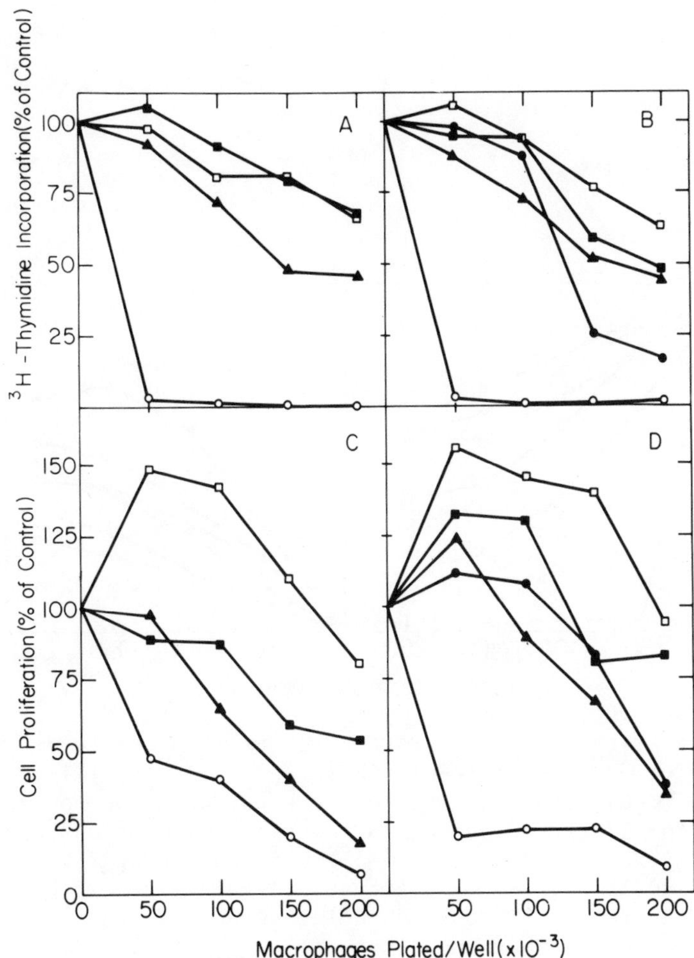

Fig. 1. ^{3}H-thymidine uptake (A-B) and inhibition of cell proliferation (C-D) of KBALB (A,C) and N3T3.AKR(G) (B,D) by: (●-●) normal, (o-o) CP, (■-■) Con A, (□-□) BCG, and (▲-▲) thioglycollate-stimulated macrophages. The specified number of macrophages were plated into triplicate wells (flat bottom, 96 wells, Linbro plates) and cultured for 22 hr. The culture medium was then aspirated and target cells (7500/well, 0.2 ml) plated for 28 hr. In A and B the medium was replaced for the last 11 hr by medium containing 0.4 μCi ^{3}H-thymidine/well. In C and D the cells were fixed after 28 hr with formaldehyde and processed according to the method of Lagneau et al. (18).

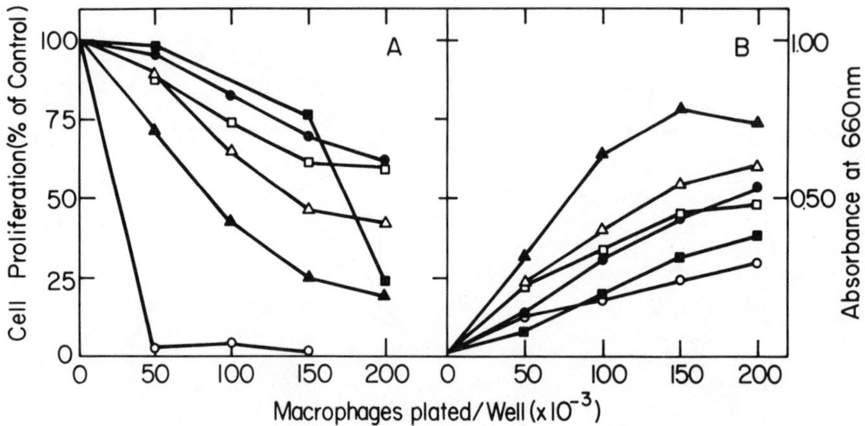

Fig. 2. A - Inhibition of KBALB proliferation by: (●-●), normal; (▲-▲), thioglycollate-; (o-o), CP-; (Δ-Δ), mineral oil-; (□-□), BCG-; and (■-■), Con A-stimulated macrophages. Macrophages were cultured for 17 hr and subsequent to aspiration of culture medium KBALB cells were plated (7500/well) and cocultured for 46 hr. Calculations as in Fig. 1. B - Amount of stain eluted from macrophage populations. The corresponding amount of stain was subtracted from each experimental point.

All the macrophage populations under study released arginase to the medium and depleted to 0-10% the arginine content in the culture medium of either the macrophages or macrophages + target cells under the conditions in which cell proliferation was assessed. KBABL proliferation depends strongly on the amount of arginine in the medium (not shown) but Dulbecco's modified Eagle's medium contains excessive amounts of arginine. Reduction of arginine content to 5% for the 46 hr of assay results in a 50% inhibition in proliferation and under the assay conditions this level of arginine would be reached only after about 18-24 hr. Addition of arginine every 12 hr during the assay abrogated the cytostatic effect to some extent but arginine depletion could not account for the effect exhibited by the different populations.

The data regarding inhibition of cell proliferation show that all the macrophage populations are endowed with a certain capacity to inhibit cell proliferation, but that the CP-stimulated macrophages must have a different or more powerful means of performing this task.

REFERENCES

1. Aaronson, S. A. and Weaver, C. A., J. Gen. Virol. 13 (1971) 245.
2. Alexander, P. and Evans, R., Nature (New Biol.) 232 (1971) 76.
3. Bar-Shavit, Z. and Goldman, R., Exp. Cell Res. 99 (1976) 221.
4. Bianco, C., Griffin, F. M., Jr. and Silverstein, S. C., J. Exp. Med. 141 (1975) 1278.
5. Ehlenberger, A. G. and Nussenzweig, V., J. Exp. Med. 145 (1977) 357.
6. Evans, R. and Alexander, P., Nature (Lond.), 228 (1970) 620.
7. Goldman, R. and Cooper, R. A., Exp. Cell Res. 95 (1975) 223.
8. Gordon, S., Unkeless, J. C. and Cohn, Z. A., J. Exp. Med. 140 (1974) 995.
9. Griffin, F. M., Jr., Bianco, C. and Silverstein, S. C., J. Exp. Med. 141 (1975) 1269.
10. Griffin, F. M., Jr., Griffin, J. A., Leider, J. E. and Silverstein, S. C., J. Exp. Med. 142 (1975) 1263.
11. Hibbs, J. B., Lambert, L. H. and Remington, J. S., Nature (New Biol.) 235 (1972) 48.
12. Hibbs, J. B.,Lambert, L. H., and Remington, J. S., Proc. Soc. Exp. Biol. (N.Y.) 139 (1972) 1049.
13. Holtermann, O. A., Lisafeld, B. A., Klein, E. and Klostergaard, J., Nature 257 (1975) 228.
14. Huber, Ch. and Wigzell, H., Eur. J. Immunol. 5 (1975) 432.
15. Kaplan, A. M., Morahan, P. S. and Regelson, W., J. Natl. Cancer Inst., 52 (1974) 1919.

16. Karnovsky, M. L., Lazdins, J., Drath, D. and Harper, A., Ann N. Y. Acad. Sci. 256 (1975) 266.
17. Kung, J. T., Brooks, S. C., Jakway, J. P., Leonard, L. L. and Talmade, D. W., J. Exp. Med.,146 (1977) 665.
18. Lagneau, A., Martin, M., Martin, F. and Michel, M. F., Compt. Ren. S. S. Biol.,171 (1977) 90.
19. Law, S. K. and Levine, R. P., Proc. Natl. Acad. Sci. USA,74 (1977) 2701.
20. Mackaness, G. B., J. Exp. Med.,120 (1964) 105.
21. Morahan, P. S. and Kaplan, A. M., Int. J. Cancer,17 (1976) 82.
22. Mørland, B. and Kaplan, G., Exp. Cell Res., 108 (1977) 279.
23. Müller-Eberhard, H. J., In: Progress in Immunology (Ed. B. Amos), Academic Press, New York, (1971).
24. Nathan, C. F., Karvousky, M. L. and David, J. R., J. Exp. Med., 133 (1971) 1356.
25. Nicholson, A., Brade, V., Lee, D. G., Shin, H. S. and Mayer, M. M., J. Immunol, 112 (1974) 1115.
26. Raz, A., Shahar, A. and Goldman, R., J. Ret. Soc., 22 (1977) 445.
27. Shellam, G. R. and Hogg, N., Int. J. Cancer, 19 (1977) 212.
28. Simon, H. B. and Seagren, J. N., J. Exp. Med., 133 (1971) 1377.
29. Unkeless, J. C., Gordon, S. and Reich, E., J. Exp. Med., 139 (1974) 834.

ACTIVATION OF PLEURAL MACROPHAGES BY INTRAPLEURAL APPLICATION OF *CORYNEBACTERIUM PARVUM*

I. BAŠIĆ, B. RODÉ, A. KAŠTELAN and L. MILAS

Department of Animal Physiology, Faculty of Natural Sci. & Math. and Central Institute for Tumors and Allied Diseases, Zagreb, (Yugoslavia)

Certain bacteria including *Corynebacterium parvum* (CP) have recently received much attention as nonspecific stimulants of the lymphoreticuloendothelial system (RES). When injected into experimental animals CP provides a chronic inflammatory stimulus leading to the extensive proliferation of lymphohistiocytic elements and activation of macrophages (9). This results in a significant enlargement of the spleen, liver, lung and lymph nodes. Induced changes in morphology are accompanied with many alterations in the functional state of the RES. Treated animals exhibit an increased phagocytic activity as evidenced by increased clearance of particulate material from the blood. They are more resistant to microbial infections and a variety of malignant tumors.

Antitumor efficacy of CP depends on many factors: dose and route of bacterial injection, size, immunogenicity and anatomical localization of investigated tumors, immune competence of the tumor host, etc. It has been established that the antitumor activity of CP is mediated mainly by activated macrophages and by the potentiated specific antitumor immunity. Which of the two mechanisms will prevail depends largely on the route of bacterial application. The former mechanism dominates following systemic application of CP and the latter requires close contact between CP and tumor cells (intratumoral injection). Our earlier studies on the role of macrophages in the CP-induced antitumor resistance have shown the following: tumors regressing in mice treated with these bacteria are heavily infiltrated with macrophages (5), CP is still effective in T-cell deficient mice (8), CP antitumor effects are resistant to the whole body irradiation (6), and peritoneal macrophages from CP-treated mice are capable of destroying tumor cells *in vitro* (1,2) and of transferring antitumor resistance to normal animals (11). Mice treated intraperitoneally (ip) with CP exhibit profound accumulation of macrophages in the peritoneal cavity (1); they are very resistant to ip injection of tumor cells (7), which indicates that accumulation of macrophages at the tumor growth site may be critical for successful tumor rejection. Similarly, intrapleural (ipl) injection of CP (12) and Bacillus-Calmette-Guerin (BCG) (13) is efficient in therapy of ipl tumor deposits in experimental animals. It has recently been demonstrated that postoperative treatment of lung cancer patients with ipl BCG markedly prolonged the disease free interval (3). These observations have stimulated our interest for studies of the effect of ipl CP on the accumulation of macrophages in the pleural cavity of mice and their antitumor activity.

MATERIALS AND METHODS

Pleural macrophages were obtained from 3-months-old CBA mice, normal or treated with CP (lot No CA 582 B generously supplied by the Wellcome Research Laboratories, Beckenham, England). Mice were given a single ipl or intravenous (iv) injection of 0.25 mg bacteria in 0.5 ml Hanks' solution. The ipl injection was performed as follows: the needle of a syringe was introduced into the pleural cavity between 5th and 6th rib near the right margin of the sternum of mice anesthesized with chloral hydrate (300 mg/kg body weight). To avoid damage of the lung a plastic tube was placed on the needle of a syringe so that the needle could penetrate only through the chest wall. Cells from the pleural cavity were harvested 1, 3, 7 and 14 days after the treatment of mice. Mice were killed, their abdomens opened and 1 ml of Medium 199 (Institute of Immunology, Zagreb, Yugoslavia) supplemented with 5% heat inactivated syngeneic serum and heparin (501U/ml medium) was injected through the diaphragm into the pleural space of each mouse. The thorax of mice was gently agitated and the fluid was withdrawn back into the syringe. The number of viable nucleated cells was determined by the trypan blue exclusion dye and was routinely 100%. Spleens were removed and weighed. Pieces of known weight were minced and passed through nylon gauze. Spleen cells were then dispersed by gentle aspiration in and out of a syringe and counted in hemocytometer.

Known number of cells obtained from the pleural cavity was plated in 35 mm plastic petri dishes and incubated for 2 hr at 37 C in a 5% CO_2 atmosphere. After incubation the plates were thoroughly washed with Hanks' solution, and the number of removed cells counted. Cells that remained attached after washing were presumed to be macrophages. The number of macrophages was also determined by their nonspecific esterase activity. Adherent cells were fixed with the phosphate buffered 4% formaldehyde and their esterase activity was determined by incubating them 10 min with 1-naphthyl phosphate and Fast Blue B diazonium salt at pH 7.4 (10).

Antitumor destructive activity of pleural macrophages was investigated against cells from a syngeneic mammary carcinoma that arose spontaneously in an old multiparous mouse. The tumor has been maintained by serial passages in syngeneic mice and it was in its 56th isotransplant generation when used in the present experiments. A primary culture of this tumor was obtained by plating 10^7 tumor cells into 60 mm plastic petri dishes containing 10 ml of Medium 199 supplemented with 10% human plasma. After 2-3 days of culture at 37 C in 5% CO_2 atmosphere nonattached cells were removed and fresh medium added. After 10 days, when cultures reached a steady growth rate, the cells were used for the experiments. We have also tested the effect of pleural macrophages on the *in vitro* growth of syngeneic and allogeneic (BALB/c) mouse embryo fibroblasts. Primary cultures of fibroblasts were prepared by a method described earlier (1). The growth of mammary carcinoma cells and mouse fibroblasts in the presence of pleural macrophages from normal mice or mice treated ipl or iv with CP 7 days earlier was monitored by plating 10,000 and 40,000 target cells, respectively, into 35 mm petri dishes containing 2 x 10^6 attached macrophages and 4 ml of medium. After 24, 48, 78 or 96 hr of growth, the medium was removed and the cells were fixed and treated with 0.05% solution of crystal violet. Target cells were counted in 10 microscope fields in each of 3 to 5 plates with the use of a x 10 ocular and x 10 objective. The counts were averaged to 1 field and the standard error was calculated (14).

Resistance of CP - treated mice to mammary carcinoma cells *in vivo* was determined by the lung colony assay. 10^4 tumor cells were suspended in 0.5 ml of Medium 199 and injected iv into normal mice. Seven days thereafter mice were divided into groups of 8 to 10 mice each and were treated ipl or iv with CP or left untreated. Seventeen days following tumor cells inoculation the mice were killed and their lungs removed. The lobes were separated and fixed in Bouin's solution. Colonies of tumor cells were seen as white, round nodules on the surface of the yellowish lung and were counted with the naked eye.

The results were statistically evaluated by Student's *t* test; differences between groups were considered significant if the P value of comparison was 0.05 or smaller.

RESULTS

Effect of CP on the number of nucleated cells in the pleural cavity. Mice were treated ipl with CP, and 1, 3, 7 or 14 days later they were killed and the number of nucleated cells in their pleural cavity determined (Table I). The number of cells increased by 2-to 5-fold; the most pronounced accumulation of cells was, however, at day 1 after treatment with CP.

TABLE I

Number of Nucleated Cells in the Pleural Cavity of CBA Mice Treated ipl with CP

Treatment of Mice	Number of Cells ($x\ 10^6$) at Days After Treatment			
	1	2	3	4
None	2.3±0.2[a]			
0.25 mg CP	11.1±0.9	5.5±0.9	6.8±0.5	6.2±0.8

[a]Mean ± S. E. This value in control mice was significantly lower from all values in CP - treated mice ($P<0.001$).

Table II shows that the majority of cells found in the pleural cavity of mice treated ipl with CP 7 days earlier were macrophages: 86% of pleural exudate cells attached to the glass surface and 98% of these attached cells were esterase positive. In contrast, 34% of pleural exudate cells from normal mice were capable of attachment; 72% of these cells were esterase positive. We included here the effect of iv injection of CP which was known to cause profound systemic stimulation of the RES (9). Iv CP did not alter the number of nucleated cells in the pleural cavity but it moderately increased the percentage of macrophages.

Systemic effects of ipl injection of CP. To investigate whether these bacteria induce systemic lymphoreticular stimulation, mice were given ipl or iv injection of CP. Seven days later the mice were killed for determination of the spleen weight and the number of nucleated cells in the spleen and peritoneal cavity (Table II). In contrast to the iv route of injection, ipl CP induced no changes in the spleen weight and cellularity. Neither routes of CP injection caused accumulation of nucleated cells in the peritoneal cavity.

TABLE II

Number of Macrophages in the Pleural Cavity of Mice Treated ipl or iv with CP

Treatment of Mice[a]	Total No. of Nucleated Cells (x 10^6)	No. of Macrophages (x 10^6)	
		Adherent Cells	Esterase Positive Adherent Cells
None	2.3±0.5	0.7±0.2(34)[b]	0.5±0.1(72)[c]
CP ipl	12.2±0.6	10.5±0.6(86)	10.2±0.5(98)
CP iv	1.7±0.2	0.7±0.1(41)	0.6±0.1(81)

[a]0.25 mg CP was given 7 days before harvesting pleural exudate cells
[b]Mean ± S. E. Numbers in parentheses are percentages
[c]Number in parentheses are the percentages of esterase positive cells in the population of adherent cells

TABLE III

Spleen Weight and the Number of Nucleated Cells in the Spleen and Peritoneal Cavity of CBA Mice Treated ipl or iv with CP

Treatment of Mice	Spleen		No. of Nucleated Cells Peritoneal Cavity (x 10^6)
	Weight (mg)	Cellularity (x 10^6)	
None	76.0±3.4[a]	101.3±8.5	6.0±1.7
CP ipl	70.8±5.3	97.6±7.5	7.0±1.3
CP iv	159.8±31.8	162.4±20.7	5.9±0.2

[a]Mean ± S. E. determined 7 days after injection of 0.25 mg CP

TABLE IV

Growth of Mammary Carcinoma (MCa) Cells on Pleural Macrophages (PM) from CBA Mice, Normal or Treated ipl or iv with CP

Cells[a]	Number of MCa Cells at Days After Plating			
	1	2	3	4
MCa	70.6 ± 3.1[b]	115.6 ± 5.2	180.0 ± 10.1	256.8 ± 19.7
Normal PM + MCa	70.4 ± 4.0	120.0 ± 7.8	189.4 ± 9.7	275.8 ± 23.5
CP[c] ipl PM + MCa	68.4 ± 3.1	15.6 ± 2.2	1.4 ± 0.9	0
CP iv PM + MCa	73.4 ± 2.5	57.8 ± 4.3	32.4 ± 7.9	29.0 ± 2.3

[a] 10^4 MCa cells were plated on 2×10^6 macrophages (1 MCa cells : 200 macrophages)
[b] Mean ± S. E.
[c] 0.25 mg CP was given 7 days before harvesting pleural exudate cells

In vitro destruction of tumor cells by CP activated pleural macrophages. Table IV presents data on the growth of 10^4 mammary carcinoma cells in petri dishes containing 2 x 10^6 pleural macrophages from either normal mice or from mice treated ipl or iv with CP 7 days earlier. Normal macrophages had no effect on the growth rate of tumor cells. However, the number of tumor cells in dishes containing CP-stimulated macrophages decreased as the incubation time was increased. Particularly effective were macrophages derived from mice injected ipl with CP; they destroyed all tumor cells within 2 days of incubation.

In vitro destructive effects of CP-activated pleural macrophages was also tested against syngeneic and allogeneic embryo fibroblasts. 4 x 10^4 target cells were plated on 2 x 10^6 macrophages obtained from mice injected ipl or iv with CP 7 days earlier. Neither normal nor activated macrophages influenced the growth rate of fibroblasts (data are not presented).

Effect of CP on the growth of tumor nodules in the lung. Our earlier studies (4) show that iv treatment of mice with CP suppresses the growth of tumor nodules generated in the lung of mice by iv injected tumor cells. The effect was found to be largely due to nonspecific activity of macrophages (1,6). In the following experiment we have investigated whether ipl CP can produce similar antitumor response. Mice were given 10^4 mammary carcinoma cells and 7 days later injected ipl or iv with 0.25 mg CP. The number of tumor nodules in the lung, determined 17 days after tumor cells inoculation, is presented in Table V. Although both treatments significantly reduced the number of tumor nodules, ipl administration of CP appeared to be more effective.

TABLE V

Effect of ipl or iv CP on the Number of Syngeneic Mammary Carcinoma Nodules in the Lung of CBA Mice

Treatment of mice[a]	Number of Tumor Nodules in the Lung		
	Mean ± S. E.	Range	P
None	36.6 ± 3.6	21 - 51	
CP ipl	24.6 ± 3.2	7 - 36	<0.001
CP iv	17.8 ± 2.8	3 - 25	<0.001

[a]0.25 mg CP given 7 days after iv inoculation of 10^4 tumor cells

DISCUSSION

Our data indicate that ipl injection of CP markedly increases the number of macrophages in the pleural cavity. Accumulation of macrophages peaks already at day 1 after treatment with CP and it persists for at least 14 days. In contrast to the iv or ip (1) route of injection, ipl treatment does not induce changes in the spleen weight and cellularity, indicating thus that the systemic effects of this route of injection may be minimal, if any. On the other hand, systemic (iv) treatment did not alter the number of nucleated cells in the pleural cavity although it slightly increased the percentage of macrophages. Pleural macrophages from mice treated ipl with CP were found to be activated. They were capable of destroying _in vitro_ cultures of cells derived from a syngeneic mammary carcinoma, but they were ineffective against normal syngeneic and allogeneic embryo fibroblasts. These cells were more effective than macrophages from mice treated iv with CP. We have previously observed that peritoneal macrophages from mice treated ip with _C. granulosum_ were nonspecifically cytotoxic for tumor cells growing _in vitro_ (1,2).

It is likely that pleural macrophages may play an important role in the prevention of tumor growth _in vivo_. It has been demonstrated (12) that ipl injection of CP suppresses the growth of tumor transplants in the pleural cavity of rats, and this effect was abolished by silica. Our results indicate that ipl CP is capable of reducing the number of metastatic tumor nodules in the lung of mice more efficiently than iv CP. It is quite possible that the pleural macrophages may have played certain role in this reduction, at least by suppressing the growth of nodules located at or near the surface of the lung. Migration of these macrophages deeper into the lung tissue can not be excluded, as well as the possibility that ipl CP also caused a strong proliferation and activation of lung macrophages. In conclusion, these data indicate that ipl administration of CP may become an efficient approach in the treatment of metastatic tumor nodules in the lung, and that this effect might be mediated to a large extent by activated macrophages.

SUMMARY

A single ipl injection of 0.25 mg CP into CBA mice led to accumulation of macrophages in the pleural cavity, but it did not influence RES as an injection given iv ipl CP caused a three-to five-fold increase in the number of nucleated cells in the pleural cavity which persisted at least 14 days. Of these cells 86% were macrophages as shown by their esterase activity. Less than 30% of cells from the pleural cavity of normal mice were esterase positive. Macrophages from the pleural cavity of CP-treated mice were capable of destroying in vitro cultures of a syngeneic mammary carcinoma, while normal pleural macrophages exerted no effect; the former were not cytotoxic for either syngeneic or allogeneic embryo fibroblasts. Ipl CP protected mice against iv injected mammary carcinoma cells; given to mice 7 days after iv inoculation of tumor cells it significantly reduced the number of tumor nodules in their lungs.

ACKNOWLEDGEMENTS

This investigation was supported by grants No 02-057-1 from USA-Yugoslav Joint board on Scientific and Technological Cooperation and IV/3 from Scientific Fund S. R. of Croatia.

REFERENCES

1. Bašić, I., Milas, L, Grdina, and Withers, R. H., J. Natl. Cancer Inst., 52 (1974) 1839.
2. Basić, I., Milas, L., Grdina, D. J. and Withers, R. H., J. Natl. Cancer Inst., 55 (1975) 589.
3. McKneally, M. F., Maver, C., and Kausel, H. W., Lancet i (1976) 377.
4. Milas, L., Gutterman, J. U., Bašić, I., Hunter, Nancy, Mavligit, G. M., Hersh, E. M., and Withers, R. H., Int. J. Cancer, 14 (1974) 493.
5. Milas, L., Hunter, Nancy, Bašić, I. and Withers, R. H., Cancer Res., 34 (1974) 2470.
6. Milas, L., Hunter, Nancy, Bašić, I. and Withers, R. H., J. Natl. Cancer Inst., 52 (1974) 1875.
7. Milas, L., Hunter, Nancy, Bašić, I., Mason, Kathy, Grdina, D. J. and Withers, R. H., J. Natl. Cancer Inst., 54 (1975) 895.
8. Milas, L., Kogelnik, H. D., Bašić, I., Mason, Kathy, Hunter, Nancy and Withers, R. H., Int. J. Cancer, 16 (1975) 738.
9. Milas, L. and Scott, M. T., Adv. Cancer Res., 26 (1977) 257.
10. Pearse, A. G. E., Histochemistry. Theoretical and Applied, 3rd Ed., Vol. 2, Churchill, Ltd., London, 1972.
11. Peters, L. J., McBride, W. H., Mason, Kathy A., Hunter, Nancy, Bašić, I. and Milas, L., J. Natl. Cancer Inst., 59 (1977) 881.
12. Pimm, M. V. and Baldwin, R. W., Int. J. Cancer, 20 (1977) 923.
13. Pimm, M. V., Hopper, D. G., and Baldwin, R. W., Br. J. Cancer, 34 (1976) 368.
14. Sinkowics, J. G., Reeves, W. J., and Cabines, J. R., J. Natl. Cancer Inst., 48 (1972) 1145.

MODULATION OF T CELLS AND MACROPHAGES BY CHOLERA TOXIN TREATMENT *IN VIVO* AND *IN VITRO*

H. FRIEDMAN and S. LYONS

College of Medicine, University of South Florida, Tampa, Florida, and Temple University Medical School, Philadelphia, Pennsylvania (USA)

Cholera toxin (CT), the enterotoxin derived from pathogenic strains of *Vibrio cholerae*, is a potent modulator of immune responses, both *in vivo* and *in vitro* (1, 2, 5, 6, 7). Mice injected with CT simultaneously with an agent such as sheep erythrocytes (SRBC) show markedly enhanced antibody responses, whereas mice pretreated with CT 2 or 3 days before challenge immunization show marked immunosuppression. These effects have been attributed to the influence of CT on the adenyl cyclase system. *In vitro* studies in this laboratory showed that CT induces only enhanced antibody responses when added to cultures of normal splenocytes, either simultaneously with antigen or 2 days earlier (3). Thus *in vivo* immunosuppression may be due to an indirect mechanism. In the present studies, spleen cells from CT pretreated mice were tested for effects on various cell classes and their responsiveness *in vitro* as compared to *in vivo*.

MATERIALS AND METHODS

Cholera toxin was obtained from the National Institutes of Health, Bethesda, Maryland and was prepared by Dr. R. Finkelstein, Southwest Medical School, Dallas, Texas. Graded quantities of CT were injected into young adult Balb/c mice, which were then challenged by intraperitoneal injection of SRBC (4×10^8 erythrocytes). The number of antibody plaque forming cells (PFC) appearing in the spleen of these animals was determined by the hemolytic plaque assay *in vitro* at various times thereafter (4). For *in vitro* studies, five million normal Balb/c splenocytes were cultured in Marbrook chambers to which were added 2×10^6 SRBC.

The spleen cells were then tested for PFCs at various times thereafter. CT was added to the cultures either at the time of culture initiation or 2 days earlier. Thymus cells, marrow cells and peritoneal cells were obtained from the mice, either normal or pretreated, and used for co-cultivational experiments with the normal splenocytes (6).

RESULTS

As is evident in Table I, pretreatment of mice with CT markedly affected the responsiveness of the spleen cells from the animals challenged *in vitro* with SRBC. Whereas splenocytes from normal control mice showed the typical rapid response to SRBC, with peak numbers of PFCs on days 4-5 after *in vitro* immunization, animals treated with CT 2-3 days before testing their spleen cells *in vitro* showed markedly depressed responses. There was a 90% or greater inhibition in the ability of the spleen cells from these animals to respond to SRBC as compared to control animals. On the other hand, when CT was injected simultaneously with antigen, the splenocytes showed an enhanced responsiveness to SRBC. Spleen cells obtained one day after injection with CT showed essentially normal responses, as did cells obtained 7 days after toxin injection.

TABLE I

Cytokinetics of Antibody Response to SRBC by Spleen Cells from Mice Injected at Varying Times with CT

Day of CT Treatment[a]	Antibody PFC Response in Day[b]				
	+2	+3	+4	+5	+6
None (controls)	358	1150	2870	3240	2100
Day 0	630	1930	3700	5250	3200
Day -1	536	1300	3100	4300	2530
-2	438	1030	1250	1870	1700
-3	98	165	283	430	210
-5	214	538	973	1630	650
-7	410	1230	2750	3000	1460

[a] 5×10^6 spleen cells from groups of mice injected i. p. at indicated time prior to sacrifice with 1.0 μg CT.
[b] Average PFC response for 3-5 cultures per group on day +5 after *in vitro* immunization with 2×10^6 SRBC.

TABLE II

Effect of Co-cultivation of Spleen Cells from Normal or CT-pretreated Mice with Different Cell Populations on *In Vitro* Antibody Formation to Sheep Erythrocytes

Cells Added to Cultures *In Vitro*[a]	Antibody Response for Spleen Cells from[b]	
	CT-treated Mice[c]	Normal mice
None (controls)	330 ± 78	3640 ± 285
Normal spleen cells		
5×10^6	3430 ± 179	4830 ± 310
1×10^6	860 ± 210	3910 ± 286
5×10^5	470 ± 120	3710 ± 197
Normal non-adherent spleen cells (1×10^6)	588 ± 97	3058 ± 280
Normal adherent spleen cells (1×10^6)	1337 ± 210	3400 ± 340
Normal PE cells		
(1×10^6)	845 ± 310	2060 ± 197
5×10^5	2830 ± 410	3430 ± 210
1×10^5	1031 ± 260	3710 ± 320

[a]Indicated cell preparations added to 5×10^6 spleen cells from normal or CT-pretreated mice; cell cultures immunized *in vitro* with 2×10^6 SRBC

[b]Average PFC response ± S. E. for 5-6 cultures per group 5 days after *in vitro* immunization

[c]Donor mice injected i. p. 3 days earlier with 1.0 μg CT

Addition of normal spleen cells to cultures of suppressed splenocytes from CT-pretreated mice had a moderate effect on the immune responsiveness of the cultures (Table II). Co-cultivation of normal splenocytes with suppressed spleen cells resulted in essentially as normal a response as would be expected when the same number of normal splenocytes were cultured alone. One million normal splenocytes partially restored the immune response, whereas half the number of such splenocytes had little effect. Nonadherent

TABLE III

Effect of T-derived Cells on *In Vitro* Restoration of Antibody Formation by CT-pretreated Spleen Cells

Cells Added to Cultures *In Vitro*[a]	Antibody Response for Spleen Cells from[b] CT-treated Mice[c]	Normal Mice
None (controls)	262 ± 32	2697 ± 311
T cells (1×10^6)	875 ± 70	3230 ± 412
PE cells (5×10^5)	795 ± 110	4150 ± 269
T cells (1×10^6) plus PE cells (5×10^5)	660 ± 148	2590 ± 141

[a]T-derived and/or PE cells added to cultures of 5×10^6 spleen cells from CT-pretreated or normal spleen cells; cell cultures immunized with 2×10^6 SRBC

[b]Average PFC response (± S. E.) of 5-6 cultures per group assayed 5 days after culture immunization

[c]Donor mice treated with 1.0 μg CT 3 days before spleen cell culture

splenocytes also had little effect. However, the adherent of splenocytes, in similar numbers, caused a significant restoration of immune responsiveness of the spleen cells in the CT pretreated mice. Five million normal PE cells had an even greater enhancing effect, whereas higher or smaller numbers of PE cells were less effective. These cell classes had little significant effect on the responsiveness of spleen cells from normal mice, except when large numbers of PE cells were used, which caused an inhibition of the response.

T-derived spleen cells from irradiated recipient mice injected with thymocytes also partially restored the immune response of spleen cells from CT pretreated mice (Table III). This effect was approximately the same as induced by PE cells and there was little, if any, additive effect when T cells and PE cells were added in combination of the suppressed splenocytes. On the other hand, when "educated" T cells were used from donor irradiated mice injected with both thymocytes and erythrocytes, a marked restoration of immune responsiveness occurred in the suppressed cultures. This response did not appear due to the

TABLE IV

Effect of "Educated" T Cells and PE Cells on Antibody Formation by Spleen Cells from CT-treated Mice Immunized *In Vitro* with SRBC

Cells Added to Cultures *In Vitro*[a]	Antibody Response for Spleen Cells from[b] CT-treated Mice[c]	Normal Mice
None (controls)	380 ± 132	3485 ± 185
"Educated" T cells (1×10^6)	4652 ± 352	3383 ± 382
PE cells (5×10^5)	1416 ± 229	3862 ± 369
"Educated" T cells (1×10^6) plus PE cells (5×10^5)	5147 ± 568	853 _ 140

[a]Cultures of 5×10^6 spleen cells from normal or CT treated mice co-cultivated with indicated cells and immunized *in vitro* with 2×10^6 SRBC; educated cells cultured from irradiated mice reconstituted with syngeneic donor T cells 8 days earlier

[b]Average number of PFC ± S. E. for 5-8 cultures 5 days *in vitro* immunization

[c]Donor mice injected i. p. with 1.0 µg CT 3 days before culture

presence of macrophages alone, since addition of PE cells to the "educated" T cell suspension had little added effect on the immune response (Table IV).

To further characterize the cell population in the educated T cell suspension, irradiation experiments were performed. When the T cell-rich preparation was heavily irradiated *in vitro*, the restorative effect of the cell suspension on the antibody responsiveness of splenocytes from CT-pretreated mice was markedly inhibited. Incubation of the T cell preparation with anti-Ig serum and complement, which removed mainly B cells, had little effect on the restorative activity of the T cell population. On the other hand, when the T cells were incubated with antiserum and complement, the restorative effect of the cells was essentially abolished (Table V). These treatments had little effect on the T cells as shown by normal responsiveness of spleen cells from untreated mice co-cultivated with either treated or untreated T cells.

TABLE V

Irradiation Reversal of Restoration of Antibody Responsiveness of Educated T cells Added to Spleen Cells from CT-pretreated Mice

Treatment of "Educated" T Cells Added to Cultures[a]	Antibody Response of Spleen Cells from[b]	
	CT-treated Mice[c]	Normal Mice
No cells added (controls)	438 ± 132	2532 ± 165
T cells - no treatment	3990 ± 120	2570 ± 195
T cells - X-irradiated	373 ± 79	2425 ± 240
T cells - incubated with anti-Ig serum + C'	3240 ± 260	2710 ± 310
T cells incubated with anti-theta serum + C'	491 ± 81	2390 ± 270

[a]Cultures of 5 x 10^6 normal spleen cells co-cultivated with 1 x 10^6 "educated" T cells, either untreated or treated with 1000 Rads irradiation or antisera and immunized with 2 x 10^6 SRBC

[b]Average PFC response ± S. E. for 5-6 cultures 5 days after *in vitro* immunizations

[c]Donor mice injected i. p. with 1.0 μg CT 3 days before use as spleen cell donors

DISCUSSION AND CONCLUSIONS

The effects of CT on the immune response of mice to SRBC has been attributed to the effect of this bacterial product on the adenyl cyclase system (5, 6). Injection of CT causes a marked increase in cAMP levels in the spleen of animals. However, the immunosuppressive effect of CT may not be directly related to an effect on immunocytes or their precursors, since adrenalectomized mice, when injected with CT, did not show altered immune responsiveness to SRBC. Thus CT, at least *in vivo*, may function through an indirect mechanism in influencing the immune response. In this regard, *in vitro* studies in this laboratory have shown that CT causes an enhanced immune response of spleen cell cultures when added either at the time of culture initiation or 2 days before challenge immunization with an antigen such as SRBC.

In the present study, spleen cells from CT pretreated mice, which evinced a marked impairment of immune responsiveness to SRBC *in vitro* were tested for immune responsiveness in the presence or absence of additional cell classes from normal mice in co-cultivation experiments. Spleen cells from CT pretreated animals, when cultured with normal splenocytes, did not inhibit the expected antibody response, indicating that suppressor cell activity was not present among splenocytes from the pretreated animals. The suppressed responses of spleen cells from CT pretreated animals could be easily reversed by addition of adherent splenocytes. However, when educated T cells obtained from donor mice injected with thymocytes and SRBC were used in similar co-cultivation experiments increases in antibody responsiveness occurred. This suggested that the defect in the splenocyte population from CT pretreated animals may be related to effects on helper T cells.

In other experiments, the helper cell activity of splenocytes from toxin pretreated animals was shown to be more depressed. Furthermore, co-cultivation of spleen cells pretreated *in vitro* with CT plus normal splenocytes indicated that the CT could induce a suppressor cell population in the spleen cell cultures. This suppressor cell activity induced *in vitro* was abrogated by incubation of CT treated cultures with anti-theta serum and complement, but not by removal of macrophages. The cells affected by the CT pretreated splenocyte cultures were antibody producing B cells. On the other hand, the results of the present studies indicate that when CT is administered *in vivo* there is a depression of helper cell activity, which can be restored by co-cultivation of the impaired splenocyte population with PE cells and/or educated T cells. These results point to complex effects of CT in modulating various classes of lymphocytes *in vivo vs in vitro*.

SUMMARY

Cholera Toxin influences the antibody response to SRBC. Enhanced responses occur *in vivo* and *in vitro* when CT is added together with antigen. However, CT depresses antibody formation when given *in vivo* before antigen but enhances *in vitro* responses under the same conditions. Modulation of antibody formation appeared due to effects of T lymphocytes as well as macrophages. Co-cultivation of immunologically impaired spleen cells from CT pretreated animals with macrophage-rich peritoneal cells or educated T cells increased the antibody response.

REFERENCES

1. Finkelstein, R. A. Crit. Rev. Microbiol. 2 (1973) 553.
2. Henney, C. S., Lichtenstein, L. M., Gillespie, E. and Rolley, T. J. Clin. Invest. 52 (1973) 2853.
3. Jerne, N. K., Nordin, A. A. and Henry, C. In: Cell bound antibodies. Wistar Press, Philadelphia, Pennsylvania (1963) 109.
4. Kateley, J. R. and Friedman, H. Ann. N. Y. Acad. Sci. 249 (1975) 404.
5. Kateley, J. R., Kasarov, L. and Friedman, H. J. Immunol. 114 (1975) 81.
6. Kateley, J. R., Kasarov, L. and Friedman, H. Proc. Soc. Exp. Biol. Med. 148 (1975) 19.
7. Lyons, S. and Friedman, H. Fed. Proc. 35 (1976) 677.

IN VIVO ACTIVATION OF MURINE PERITONEAL MACROPHAGES BY NOCARDIA WATER SOLUBLE MITOGEN (NWSM)

I. LÖWY, D. JUY, C. BONO and L. CHEDID

Inserm, Paris and Groupe de Recherche n° 31 du CNRS,
Institut Pasteur, Paris (France)

The water soluble fraction extracted from various strains of Nocardia, and hereafter referred to as NWSM (12), is a potent B-cell mitogen in several strains of mice (7) including the C3H/He Orl. mice, which are low responders to lipopolysaccharide (LPS) (10), and also in rabbits (6) and in humans (9). Bacterial lipopolysaccharides are also B-cell mitogens and adjuvants (19,14) in mice *in vivo*. However, in contrast to LPS, when NWSM was administered to mice, it failed to induce *in vivo* proliferation of splenic lymphocytes, polyclonal activation and appearance of PFC directed against syngeneic, bromelain-treated erythrocytes and thymocytes (18). These findings strongly suggest that the adjuvant activity of NWSM is not necessarily related to *in vivo* mitogenicity, and that other cells than B lymphocytes may be its primary target cell *in vivo*. During investigations of NWSM *in vivo* effects we examined the influence of this adjuvant on murine peritoneal macrophages in comparison to other water soluble adjuvants.

MATERIALS AND METHODS

Mice. CBA (6-8 weekd old), C3H/He Orl. (6-8 week old) and DBF_1 $(DBA/2xC57Bl)F_1$ hybrids) (4-5 week old) which were raised at the Centre National de la Recherche Scientifique (Orléans, France) were used.

Preparation of macrophage monolayers. Macrophages were harvested by washings of the peritoneal cavity of mice injected 4 days before with various concentrations of adjuvants in saline. After harvesting, macrophages were seeded at the concentrations of 5 x 10^5 cells in 0.2 ml of growth medium in the weels of Falcon Microtest II plates. The culture medium was RPMI 1640 (Flow Lab.) containing 25% heat-inactivated fetal calf serum (FCS) supplemented with antibiotics and glutamine. The cultures were incubated at 37 C in a 5% CO_2/95% air mixture. After the cells were allowed to adhere for 90 min at 37 C, the nonadhering cells were removed by intensive washing of monolayers with 199 medium (Pasteur Institute, France).

Inhibition of growth of mastocytoma cells. The inhibition of growth of mastocytoma cells was tested under the conditions described previously (16). Briefly, 2.5 x 10^4 P815 mastocytoma cells suspended in RPMI medium supplemented with 10% FCS, antibiotics and glutamine, were added to each macrophage-containing well (effector target ratio 20:1), and incubated for 24 hr at 37 C in 5% CO_2/95% air mixture. Four hr after adding 0.1 μCi of ^{3}H-thymidine labeled cells were collected on glass fiber filters, washed, and their radioactivity was measured in a liquid scintillation counter. The estimation of target cell damage was expressed as growth inhibition percentage and calculated according to the formula (NR-AR/NRx100) in which NR represents radioactivity of mastocytoma cells cultivated on normal macrophages and AR, radioactivity of mastocytoma cells incubated on adjuvant-activated macrophages.

Measure of phagocytosis of chicken red blood cells (CRBC). Macrophages were activated by adjuvants in vivo and monolayers were prepared as described above.

Fresh CRBC were marked with ^{51}Cr by incubation of 7.5 x 10^7 RBC with 250 μCi ^{51}Cr at 37 C during 120 min with agitation in RPMI medium supplemented with 10% FCS.

To each Falcon Microtest II well, containing a monolayer of adherent peritoneal exudate cells 3 x 10^6 ^{51}Cr marked CRBC, suspended in RPMI-FCS medium were added, and the cells were incubated together during 90 min at 37 C in 5% CO_2/95% air atmosphere. The nonphagocyted ^{51}Cr-CRBC were removed by intensive washings of monolayers with PBS; the remaining red cells were lysed by hypotonic shock, and the monolayers were washed intensively again. 0.1 ml of 1 N NaOH was added then to each well, the cells were lysed overnight and the intracellular radioactivity of lysed cells was measured in a γ-counter. The percentage of phagocytosis of ^{51}Cr-CRBC was calculated (phagocytosis % = IR/TR x 100 in which IR is intracellular radioactivity and TR total radioactivity of ^{51}Cr-CRBC added to each well).

Induction of in vivo immune response by macrophages stimulated by adjuvants. Mice were pre-injected i.p. with a solution of adjuvant in saline, 4 days later the animals were sacrificed, and their peritoneal exudate cells were suspended in RPMI medium, containing 25% FCS, antibiotics and glutamine, at the concentration of 5 x 10^6 cells/ml. 1 ml of the suspension was incubated in each of 30 mm/diameter plastic petri dishes (Nunclon) during 90 min at 37 C in 5% CO_2/95% air atmosphere. The macrophage monolayer was intensively washed, 5 x 10^7 sheep red blood cells (SRBC) suspended in 1 ml RPMI + 10% FCS were added to each dish, and the incubation continued for an additional 90 min in the same conditions. At the end of this incubation, the monolayers were again washed thoroughly with 199 medium, the remaining SRBC were lysed by hypotonic shock and the monolayers washed thoroughly a third time. The adherent cells were removed with rubber policeman, resuspended in 199 medium and injected into non-immunized syngeneic mice -3 x 10^6 cells/mouse. Controls were injected with normal, non-activated PE macrophages, incubated with SRBC under the same conditions.

The anti-SRBC plaque forming activity of macrophage-injected mice was tested 4 days later.

Adjuvant preparations tested. NWSM (Nocardia water soluble mitogen). A purified fraction of water soluble extract of *Nocardia opaca* was prepared by Dr. Ciorbaru according to the procedure described before (13).

WSA (water soluble adjuvant) which can substitute for mycobacteria in Freund's complete adjuvant, and extracted from *Mycobacterium smegmatis* as described previously (1,2).

MDP (synthetic N-acetyl-muramyl-L-alanyl-D-isoglutamine) has been shown to be the minimal structure required for adjuvant activity (20,5). MDP used was MDP-Pasteur (Institut Pasteur Production, Paris) synthetised as described previously (17).

LPS. Bacterial lipopolysaccharide extracted from *Salmonella typhimurium* by the phenol-water method (28), was obtained commercially (Difco Laboratories).

All these preparations were injected intraperitoneally in pyrogen-free saline.

RESULTS

Growth inhibition of mastocytoma target cells by activated macrophages. It has been established (3) that LPS-activated macrophages can inhibit the growth of tumor cells. We have previously reported that WSA and other mycobacterium immunostimulants could also activate macrophages *in vivo* (16). In a preliminary report we have also shown that NWSM-stimulated macrophages can inhibit the growth of L1210 lymphoma cells (8).

TABLE I

Growth Inhibition of Mastocytoma Cells by in vivo Activated Peritoneal Macrophages[a]

Experiment n°	% of Growth Inhibition of Mastocytoma Cells Cultured on Macrophages Activated In Vivo by: LPS	WSA	NWSM
1	40	71	70
2	50	96	57
3	38	79	82
4	83	ND	92
	52.75±20.84	82.00±12.77	75.25±15.13

[a] BDF_1 mice were injected intraperitoneally with 30 μg of LPS, 30 μg WSA or 30 μg NWSM 4 days before the test.

In the present study LPS, WSA and NWSM were compared by administering them at the same dosage level (30 μg) and in the same experiments. As can be seen in Table I, NWSM, like WSA, activated macrophages, and this effect was even superior to the activation by LPS.

Phagocytosis of ^{51}Cr-CRBC by adjuvant-stimulated macrophages. Peritoneal macrophages were harvested from CBA mice (LPS$^{(+)}$ responders) and from C3H/He Orl. mice, which are known to be refractory to several effects of LPS (26,10,15), 4 days after the administration of various doses of LPS and NWSM. Activation of macrophages was measured by their capacity to phagocytose ^{51}Cr-CRBC.

C3H/He Orl. macrophages in contrast to CBA macrophages were practically not activated by LPS (a very weak response was observed with 50 μg LPS/mouse (Fig. 1)). However both CBA and

C3H/He Orl. macrophages were strongly stimulated by relatively low doses of NWSM.

One μg NWSM/mouse was chosen for the following experiments, since at this dose high activation of peritoneal macrophages and optimal adjuvant effects were observed.

Comparing the ability of several adjuvants to stimulate *in vivo* the phagocytic capacity of peritoneal macrophages of CBA mice, we observed that NWSM was able to induce an important activation of the macrophages in this system (Table II). MDP had minimal activity and LPS was less efficient than NWSM.

Enhancement of the ability of antigen-treated peritoneal macrophages to induce an immune response. Peritoneal macrophages previously activated *in vivo* by different adjuvants were incubated *in vitro* with antigen (SRBC), then transferred into non-immunized syngeneic recipients. The anti-SRBC activity of the recipients was tested 4 days following the transfer of antigen-preincubated macrophages. In this system too, NWSM was able to activate significantly the peritoneal macrophages, and was found to be more active than the LPS (Table III).

Therefore, there exists a good correlation between the capacity of an adjuvant to increase both the phagocytic activity (Table II) and the ability to enhance a specific immune response of peritoneal macrophages incubated with antigen (Table III). It is thus possible that increased induction of specific antibodies is related to the amount of antigen transferred to the recipients.

DISCUSSION

In many systems, macrophages were described as target cells for adjuvant activity (25,4). In the present report, the effect of NWSM on macrophages was compared to the effects of other adjuvants: two known for their capacity to activate macrophages *in vivo*, LPS (27,23) and WSA (16); and to another adjuvant, MDP, which in certain systems does not activate macrophages *in vivo* (16). It was found that in all the systems tested, NWSM was able to stimulate murine peritoneal macrophages. Moreover, NWSM was found to be highly active as compared to the other water soluble adjuvants tested, including the bacterial lipopolysaccharide.

NWSM was also active in C3H/He Orl. mice which are congenitally low responders to LPS (26). It was demonstrated that C3H/He Orl. macrophages were poorly activated *in vitro* by LPS as measured by inhibition of tumor target cells (10). It was also reported that their peritoneal macrophages are resistant to toxic

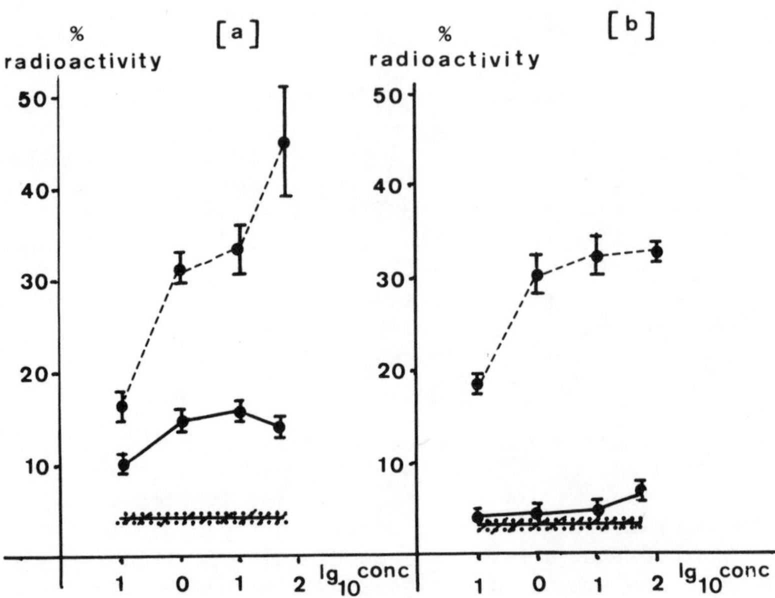

Fig. 1. The effect of adjuvant concentration on the stimulation of the phagocytic activity of peritoneal macrophages.

CBA and C3H/He Orl. mice were injected intraperitoneally with various doses of LPS and NWSM 4 days before the test. Five mice were used for each point.

{a} CBA mice {b} C3H/He Orl. mice

{ } { } { }

TABLE II

Phagocytosis of CRBC by Peritoneal Macrophages Activated *In Vivo* by Adjuvants

Activating Adjuvant	% of Phagocyted ^{51}Cr-CRBC[a]	Percent of Increase with Adjuvant
Control	7.22 ± 0.59	-
MDP	9.30 ± 0.95	23%
LPS	16.72 ± 0.51	124%
NWSM	29.12 ± 3.53	294%
WSA	21.36 ± 2.14	190%

[a]Average of 3 quadruplicate experiments.

effects of endotoxin (15). Those findings demonstrate that in C3H/He Orl. mice, not only the B lymphocytes but also their macrophage is a defective LPS-responding cell. Activation of C3H/He

TABLE III

Enhancement of Immune Response of Recipient Mice Following the Injection of Adjuvant-Treated Macrophages, Preincubated with Antigen

Activating Adjuvant	PPM Anti-SRBC[a]	Percent of Increase with Adjuvant
Control	29 ± 5[b]	-
MDP	34 ± 16	17
LPS	117 ± 26	303
NWSM	201 ± 47	593

[a]PPM: plaques per 1 x 10^6 viable cells.

[b]Average values of duplicate experiments (5 mice per each point).

CBA mice were injected intraperitoneally with aqueous solution of 30 μg MDP, 30 μg WSA, 30 μg LPS or 1 μg NWSM/mouse, and the phagocytic activity of their peritoneal macrophages was tested.

CBA mice were injected intraperitoneally with aqueous solution of 30 μg MDP, 30 μg WSA, 30 μg LPS or 1 μg NWSM/mouse. The activated peritoneal macrophages were incubated *in vitro* with Orl. macrophages by NWSM confirms that the activity of this fraction is not related to a possible endotoxin contamination.

The peak of adjuvant activity of NWSM *in vivo* was found previously to be between 0.1 and 1 μg/mouse (18). However, under the same conditions, no significant polyclonal or mitogenic activity was observed. In contrast the present findings show that the same concentrations of NWSM were able to stimulate strongly peritoneal macrophages *in vivo* (Fig. 1).

It seems that in contrast to LPS adjuvant activity which has been related to its capacity to induce proliferation of B-derived lymphocytes (11,24), the adjuvant activity of NWSM can be the consequence of its potent macrophage activating ability.

WSA, another adjuvant which in the systems tested by us, was equally able to activate the peritoneal macrophages *in vivo*, was shown to be able to enhance *in vivo* the immune response to a particulate antigen: SRBC (22). Its ability to increase the immune response to SRBC *in vitro* was mediated by the activation of macrophages (21).

Our findings do not rule out, however, the possibility of other cellular mechanisms (such as direct or indirect influence of NWSM on T cells, specific, not polyclonal activation of B cells) which could also contribute to the adjuvant activity of NWSM *in vivo*.

SUMMARY

In vitro NWSM has been shown to be a B cell mitogen and a polyclonal activator. Although NWSM has been also shown to be adjuvant active *in vivo*, motogenicity and polyclonal activation are not observed when this fraction has been administered to mice. In contrast, the experiments reported here demonstrate that after *in vivo* administration several effects of NWSM on mouse peritoneal macrophages can be observed: NWSM was able to induce an important increase in the ability of peritoneal macrophages to inhibit *in vitro* growth of tumor cells, to increase their phagocytic activity and to enhance their ability to induce an immune response, following the incubation with an antigen NWSM was able to stimulate phagocytic activity of macrophages of C3H/He Orl. mice (LPS-resistant strain). Those findings suggest that the adjuvant activity of NWSM *in vivo* can be related to its capacity to activate macrophages.

ACKNOWLEDGEMENTS

We wish to thank Dr. R. Ciorbaru and Dr. J. F. Petit for preparing NWSM used in our experiments. This work was supported by INSERM grant no. 76-59 and DGRST grant no. 77-7-1297.

REFERENCES

1. Adam, A., Ciorbaru, R., Petit, J. F. and Lederer, E., Proc. Nat. Acad. Sci. USA, 69 (1972) 851.
2. Adam, A., Ciorbaru, R., Petit, J. F., Lederer, E., Chedid, L., Lamensans, A., Parant, F., Parant, M., Rosselet, J. P. and Berger, F. M., Infect. Immunity,7 (1973) 855.
3. Alexander, P. and Evans, R., Nature New Biol., 232 (1971) 76.
4. Allison, A. C., In: Immunopotentiation, (Ed. D. W. Dresser), Elsevier Excerpta Medica, North Holland Associated Scientific Pub., (1973) 73.
5. Audibert, F., Chedid, L., Lefrancier, P. and Choay, J. Cell Immunol., 21 (1976) 243.
6. Bona, C., Chedid, L., Damais, C., Ciorbaru, R., Shek, P. N., Dubiski, S. and Cinander, B., J. Immunol., 114 (1975) 348.
7. Bona, C., Damais, C. and Chedid, L., Proc. Nat. Acad. Sci. USA, 71 (1974) 1602.
8. Bona, C., Damais, C., Juy, D. and Ciorraru, R., Abstracts of International Symposium on Bacterial Immunostimulants. Institut Pasteur, Paris, (1974) 19.
9. Brochier, J., Bona, C., Ciorbaru, R., Revillard, J. P. and Chedid, L., J. Immunol., 117 (1976) 1434.
10. Chedid, L., Parant, M., Damais, C., Parant, F., Juy, D. and Galelli, A., Infect. Immunity, 13 (1975) 722.
11. Chiller, J. M., Skidmore, B. J., Morrison, D. C. and Weigle, W. O., Proc. Nat. Acad. Sci. USA, 70 (1973) 2129.
12. Ciorbaru, R., Adams, A., Petit, J. F., Lederer, E., Bona, C., and Chedid, L., Infect. Immunity, 11 (1975) 257.
13. Ciorbaru, R., Petit, J. F., Lederer, E., Zissman, E., Bona, C. and Chedid, L., Infect. Immunity, 13 (1976) 1084.
14. Franzl, R. E. and McMaster, P. D., J. Exp. Med., 127 (1968) 1087.
15. Glode, L. M., Jacques, A., Mergenhagen, S. E. and Rosenstreich, O., J. Immunol., 119 (1977) 162.
16. Juy, D. and Chedid, L., Proc. Nat. Acad. Sci. USA, 72 (1975) 4105.
17. Lefrancier, P., Choay, J., Derrien, M. and Lederman, I., Int. J. Petp. Protein Res., 9 (1977) 249.
18. Löwy, I., Bona, C., Ciorbaru, R. and Chedid, L., Immunology, 32 (1977) 975.
19. Melchers, F., Braun, V. and Galanos, C., J. Exp. Med., 142 (1975) 473.

20. Merser, C., Sinay, P. and Adams, A., Biochem. Biophys. Res. Com., 59 (1975) 1317.
21. Modolell, M., Luckenbach, G. A., Parant, M. and Munder, P. G., J. Immunol., 113 (1974) 395.
22. Parent, M. and Chedid, L., In: Recent Results in Cancer Research, (Ed. G. Mathé), Springer Verlag, Heidelberg, 47 (1974) 190.
23. Shands, J. W., Peavy, D. L., Gormus, B. J. and McGaw, J. Infect. Immunol., 9 (1974) 106.
24. Skidmore, B. J., Chiller, J. M., Morrison, D. C. and Weigle, W. O., J. Immunity, 114 (1975) 770.
25. Unanue, E., Askonas, B. and Allison, A. C., J. Immunol., 103 (1969) 71.
26. Watson, J. and Riblet, R., J. Exp. Med., 140 (1974) 1147.
27. Weiner, E. and Levanon, D., Lab. Invest., 19 (1968) 584.
28. Westphal, O., Luderitz, O. and Bister, B., Z. Naturforsch., 7b (1952) 148.

SUPPRESSION OF IMMUNOLOGICAL RESPONSIVENESS IN AGED MICE AND ITS RELATIONSHIP WITH COENZYME Q DEFICIENCY

E. G. BLIZNAKOV

New England Institute
Ridgefield, Connecticut (USA)

In 1957, Crane and his group (13) extracted from beef heart mitochondria, a new compound-coenzyme Q- "capable of undergoing reversible oxidation and reduction." Today, coenzyme Q (Fig. 1) is accepted as a substance universally present in bacteria, plants and animals and as an essential constituent of the electron transport processes of respiration and coupled oxidative phosphorylation in mitochondria. The site of action of coenzyme Q is between NADH and succinate dehydrogenase and the cytochrome complex (reviewed in (17). Thus, coenzyme Q is indispensable for the intracellular energy metabolism and its deficiency is linked to the

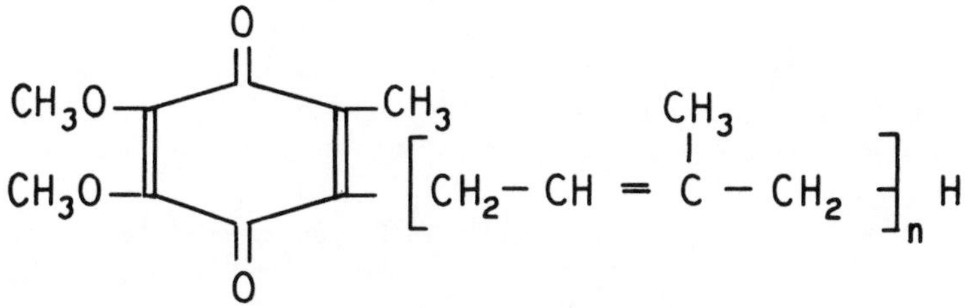

CH_3O, CH_3O, O, O, CH_3, CH_3, $[CH_2-CH=C-CH_2]_n H$

Coenzyme Q
or
Ubiquinone

Fig. 1. The host defense system, as we have broadly interpreted it, is an integrated system responsible for the defense against invasive alien particulates. "Alien" is defined as anything the body can recognize as non-self, and "particulate" ranges in size from macromolecules to cells or groups of cells.

development of many pathological processes in cardiac, gingival and distrophic tissues of humans and animals. The existing literature was reviewed recently, and the creation of a new nosologic group of diseases was proposed--diseases of bioenergetics (19).

In our extensive studies during the past ten years, we have established that coenzyme Q administration confers increased resistance in experimental animals to a variety of bacterial and protozoal infections as well as viral and chemical carcinogenesis (reviewed in 4,5). It has been postulated that this increased resistance is mediated via stimulation of various parameters of the host defense system*, a process which has high cellular energy requirements (4,5).

This presentation is a summary of our studies on the decline of one of the parameters of the host defense system in aged mice-humoral, immunological responsiveness-its relationship with coenzyme Q deficiency and the possibility of controlling this decline by administration of coenzyme Q.

DEVELOPMENT OF COENZYME Q DEFICIENCY DURING AGING

In this portion of our study, we determined the specific activities of the succinate dehydrogenase-coenzyme Q reductase in the thymus and spleen mitochondria of aged mice* (20, 22 and 24 months) as compared with young mice (10 weeks). The results shown in Fig. 2 illustrate the marked intensification of coenzyme Q deficiency in the thymus of old animals during the aging process. The slight deficiency trend in the spleen is not statistically significant.

The method of coenzyme Q-enzyme deficiency determination has been described in detail previously (7,8) and is based on the rate of reduction of 2, 6-dichlorophenol indophenol by coenzyme Q. The deficiency index was calculated per mg of protein as follows:

$$\text{Deficiency index} = \frac{\text{def. exp.-def. control}}{\text{def. experimental}} \times 100\%$$

The results of the statistical analysis are also shown in Fig. 2.

This portion of our work on aging is a joint project with Karl Folkers and his group at the Institute for Biomedical Research, University of Texas at Austin.

*The terms "aged mice" and "old mice" are used interchangeably and in accordance with the requirements established by Walford (34).

ORGAN WEIGHT CHANGES DURING AGING

We evaluated the changes in the body, liver, spleen and thymus weights in old mice (20, 22 and 24 months). For the presentation in Fig. 3, we used the ratio $\frac{\text{organ wt mg}}{\text{body wt gm}}$ in old mice, expressed as percent of control (young mice, aged 10 weeks). Clearly, the ratios of liver weight:body weight and spleen weight: body weight in old mice remain practically constant. Conversely, the thymus weight:body weight ratio decreases sharply with the advancement of the aging process.

The results of the statistical analysis are also presented in Fig. 3.

IMMUNOLOGICAL SENESCENCE IN MICE

For evaluation of the host defense system effectiveness during aging, we selected one parameter-the humoral, hemolytic, primary, immune response. Our results, shown in Fig. 4 demon-

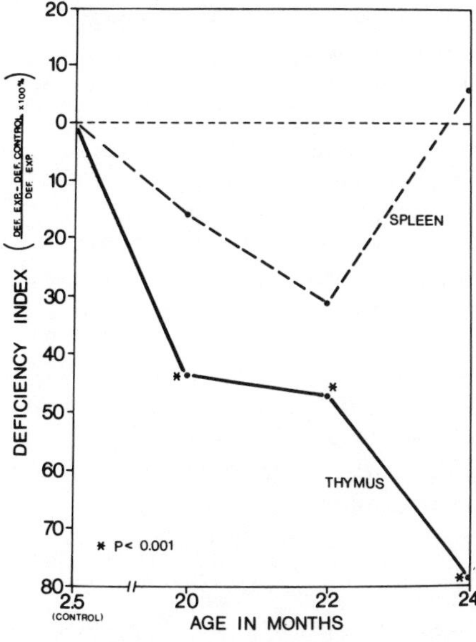

Fig. 2. Coenzyme Q deficiency index in spleen and thymus of old CF1 female mice (age 20, 22 and 24 months) as compared with control young, adult mice, age 10 weeks).

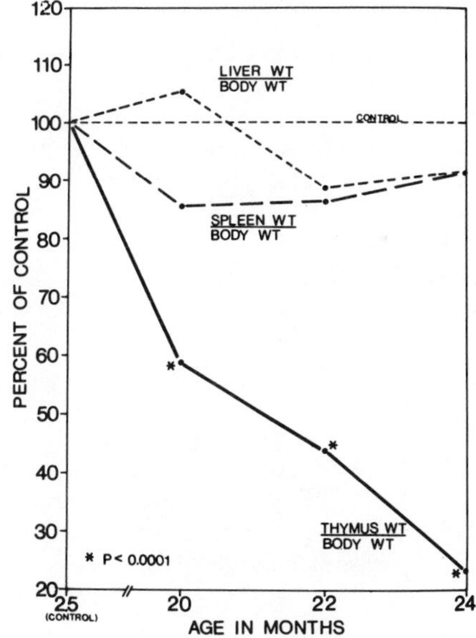

Fig. 3. Body, liver, spleen and thymus weight in old CFL female mice (age 20, 22 and 24 months) expressed as percent of control (young, adult mice, age 10 weeks).

strate the profound suppression of the humoral, hemolytic response in old mice (22 months) as compared with this response in young mice (10 weeks). As shown in Fig. 4, the age-determined suppression of the immune response can be partly reversed by a single intravenous administration of coenzyme Q (coenzyme Q_{10}) on day 4 after sheep red blood cell (FRBC) administration. The dose (coenzyme Q_{10}) response (hemolytic antibody) relationship is presented in Fig. 5.

The detailed methods used in this portion of our study were described earlier (6).

DISCUSSION AND CONCLUSIONS

There is probably no other area of biological inquiry that is so threaded by theories as is the science of gerontology. This is due in part to lack of fundamental scientific data. Another complication is the manifestation of the biological changes which, with time, affect all biological systems from the molecular level to the whole organism.

Studies in both man and experimental animals have provided solid evidence linking some diseases of adult life, such as neoplasia, autoimmune disorders and many infections, to a gradual decline in the functions of the host defense system with advancing age. Recent reviews adequately cover the existing literature (10, 26,33). In this regard, it is interesting, and probably even alarming, to cite the tremendous difference in cancer incidence rates between young and old. Data from Birmingham, U. K., shows that at age twenty-five the probability that an individual will develop cancer within the next five years is one in seven hundred. At age sixty-five, this probability is drastically increased to one in fourteen (11).

We have shown that senescent animals develop a marked deficiency of coenzyme Q-enzyme activity in the thymus. This deficiency is paralleled by gross anatomical changes in this organ, described as age-involution, and a profound suppression of the immunological responsiveness. Administration of coenzyme Q (coenzyme Q_{10}) partially restores this suppression.

The physical and chemical heterogeneity as well as functional diversity of the cells involved in the immune response is now firmly established. The discovery of the existence of two distinct pathways of differentiation of antigen-reactive cells (thymus-derived or T cells and bone marrow-derived or B cells), and the appreciation of the separate roles that each of those types of cells plays in cellular and humoral immune response have greatly enhanced our understanding of the immune system as a functional

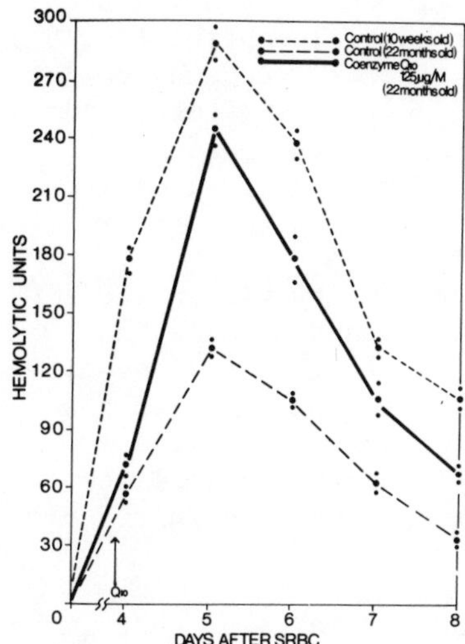

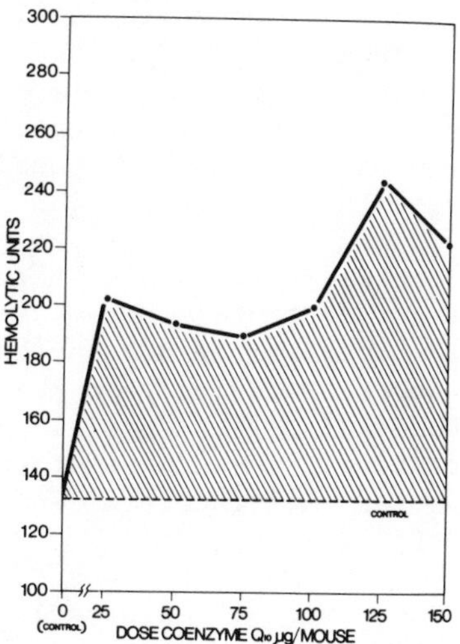

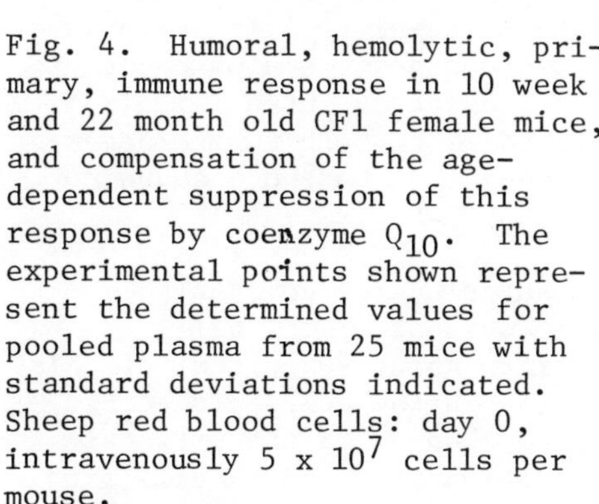
Fig. 4. Humoral, hemolytic, primary, immune response in 10 week and 22 month old CF1 female mice, and compensation of the age-dependent suppression of this response by coenzyme Q_{10}. The experimental points shown represent the determined values for pooled plasma from 25 mice with standard deviations indicated.
Sheep red blood cells: day 0, intravenously 5 x 10^7 cells per mouse.
Coenzyme Q_{10}: day 4, 125µg/mouse, intravenously as emulsion.
Antibody level evaluation: day 4-8 after SRBC.

Fig. 5. Compensation of the suppressed humoral hemolytic, primary, immune response in 22 month old CF1 female mice as a function of the dose of coenzyme Q_{10}. The experimental points shown represent the determined values for pooled plasma from 25 mice with standard deviations indicated.
Sheep red blood cells: day 0, intravenously, 5 x 10^7 cells per mouse.
Coenzyme Q_{10}: day 4, intravenously as emulsion.
Antibody level evaluation: day 5 after SRBC (peak day).

unit for the defense of the host (reviewed in 1,12).

Today, the thymus is an organ attracting considerable interest, with a cardinal role in the development and maintenance of optimal immunological responsiveness. Its integrity is essential for the full and proper development of all types of cellular immune responses and for many types of humoral responses. The general consensus is that thymus factor(s) induce T cell maturation, probably through the adenyl cyclase-cyclic AMP pathway (2). The thymus involutes by sudden or gradual depletion of its specific cellular population as a response to a wide variety of stimuli including aging and is under constant endocrine as well as neurohumoral control (14,15). Fabris *et al*. (18) suggested that thymus function depends on normal production of some hormones produced by the pituitary, and therefore thymic involution is closely related to age-dependent changes of pituitary and possibly with centrally situated hypothalamic function.

Compelling evidence suggesting heterogeneity within the two major compartments of the lymphoid system (T and B cells) has already been provided. Furthermore, it is clear that if specificity rests exclusively on the lymphocyte, macrophages also play an essential role, especially in mediation of T - B cells' cooperation. This cooperation is crucial for the optimal response to complex, multi-determined antigens, including foreign red blood cells (12,27).

The complexities of cell interactions in the senescent immune responsiveness are recognized today but not fully understood. Analysis of human blood revealed that the absolute lymphocyte count declines sharply in the first two decades, remains constant for three decades, and thereafter declines at an intensified rate (24). The production of humoral antibodies to both thymus-dependent (25) and thymus-independent antigens (20) has been shown to decline with age.

Studies in $BC3F_1$ mice indicate that old mice have only 10 percent of the humoral capacity and 25 percent of the cell-mediated capacity of young animals (21). About 90 percent of this decrease can be attributed to alteration in the cells producing an immune response and the remainder to changes in the extracellular environment. An important alteration in T and B cells with increasing age is a decrease in the ability of the cells to proliferate after mitogen (T cells) or antigen (B cells) stimulation (23). As a result of changes in the proliferative capacity of T cells and B cells in old mice, the T cell-B cell ratio is altered. Studies by Heidrick *et al*. (21) revealed that an optimal ratio T cells-B cells is required to generate a maximal response to SRBC, and that the optimal ratio is the same for cells from young or old animals.

Teasdale *et al*. (32) reported that in mammals the number of T cells decreases gradually with aging, while the absolute and percentage B cell numbers show no significant variation with age. Although B cell numbers remain stable, B cell functions are impaired with aging.

Hirokawa *et al*. (22), presented evidence that the extent of T cell maturation is determined by the degree of age involution of the thymus. It was further suggested (9) that the thymus-dependent T cells are the key factor and their exhaustion is responsible for immunological senescence in mammals. Pachciarz et al. (28) postulated that physiological thymus function(s) must continue throughout life in order to maintain the efficiency of the T cell compartment.

Segre et al. (30) reviewing the present knowledge, concluded that in mice, the first event during aging is an increase in T cell suppressor function, followed by a decrease in T cell helper function. This finally results in a loss of B cell function.

The reduction of energy metabolism during aging is now well recognized. Studies reviewed by Wilson (35) suggested an impairment of the intracellular process of respiration at the mitochondrial level. Patel (29) reported a significant reduction of the activities of several mitochondrial enzymes in tissue from aging rats, and Du et al. (16) found lower protein content in the liver mitochondria of old mice. Similarly, Siliprandi et al. (31) demonstrated that energy-linked processes are partially or completely lost during aging of mitochondria, but this is, within certain limits, a reversible phenomenon. Those functional changes are also associated with changes in the mitochondrial ultrastructure (36).

The presence of coenzyme Q in mitochondria has been known for twenty years, but its precise role as a redox carrier of the respiratory chain in mitochondria was established more recently (17). The relationship between coenzyme Q deficiency and some disease states has been postulated. Our early studies further support this postulate. In those studies (3,7) we established that a murine viral leukemogenic process is associated with a coenzyme Q deficiency state and administration of coenzyme Q reverses the clinical progression of the disease.

Indirect evidence suggests that coenzyme Q stimulates both B and T cells dependent responses (4,5). This effect is believed to be mediated via a more efficient performance by existing cells rather than by an increased number of cells. In the present study, the more efficient performance conferred by coenzyme Q compensates the decline of B cell and especially T cell functions in aged mice and probably restores the functional balance between T and B cells required, as shown by Heidrick et al. (21) for an optimal response to SRBC. A possible effect via the afferent compartment (macrophages) is not considered here because of the delayed administration of coenzyme Q (on day 4 after the antigen).

Our study strongly implies that coenzyme Q bioavailability plays an essential role in the control mechanism of immunological senescence development in mice and brings us one step closer to the possibility of restoring youthful "immunological vigor" in aging organisms.

ACKNOWLEDGEMENTS

This work was derived from research programs supported in part by grants from individuals, corporations and the following foundations: Greenaway, Griffis, Heddens-Good, International Foundation for the Fight against Cancer, Ivy Fund, Landegger, Virginia and D. K. Ludwig, J. M. McDonald, Roy R. and Marie S. Neuberger, Anne S. Richardson, Fannie E. Rippel, Rockledge, Scheider, Arnold Schwartz Fund for Health and Education Research, Ann Earle Talcott Trust, United Order True Sisters, Gilbert Verney, Wahlstrom, Wallace Genetic, Raymond J. Wean and Whitehall.

The assistance and advice of S. J. Tao for the computer program and statistical analysis is gratefully acknowledged.

We thank C. Kasche, G. Katopodis, A. Santini, A. Smith and C. Torcellini for technical assistance.

REFERENCES

1. B and T Cells in Immune Recognition (Eds. F. Loor and G. E. Roelants) John Wiley & Sons Ltd., London (1977).
2. Bach, M. A. and Beaurain, G., Ann. Immunol., 127c (1976) 967.
3. Bliznakov, E. G., Proc. Nat. Acad. Sci. (USA) 70 (1973) 390.
4. Bliznakov, E. G., The Reticuloendothelial System in Health and Disease: Functions and Characteristics (Eds. Sh. M. Reichard, M. R. Escobar and H. Friedman) Plenum Publishing Corp., New York (1976) 441.
5. Bliznakov, E. G., Biomedical and Clinical Aspects of Coenzyme Q (Eds. K. Folkers and Y. Yamamura) Elsevier/North-Holland Biomedical Press, Amsterdam (1977) 73.
6. Bliznakov, E. G., Mech. Age. Dev., 7 (1978) 189.
7. Bliznakov, E. G., Casey, A., Kishi, T., Kishi, H. and Folkers, K., J. Vit. Nutr. Res. 45 (1975) 388.
8. Bliznakov, E. G., Watanabe, T., Saji, S. and Folkers, K., (1978) submitted for publication.
9. Burnet, F. M., Lancet, II (1970) 358.
10. Burnet, F. M., Immunology, Aging, and Cancer: W. H. Freeman and Co., San Francisco, California (1976).
11. Cancer Incidence in Five Continents (Eds. R. Doll, C. Muir and J. Waterhouse), UICC (1970).
12. Claman, H. N., Ann. N. Y. Acad. Sci., 249 (1975) 27.
13. Crane, F. L., Hatefi, Y., Lester, R. L. and Widmer, C., Biochem. Biophys. Acta, 25 (1957) 220.

14. Denckla, W. D., Fed. Proc. 37 (1978) 1263.
15. Deschaux, P. and Fontanges, R., Ann. Endocrinol., 39 (1978) 23.
16. Du, J. T., Beyer, T. A. and Lang, C. A., Exp. Gerontol., 12 (1977) 181.
17. Ernster, L., Biomedical and Clinical Aspects of Coenzyme Q (Eds. K. Folkers and Y. Yamamura) Elsevier/North-Holland Biomedical Press, Amsterdam (1977) 15.
18. Fabris, N., Pierpaoli, W. and Sorkin, E., Nature, 240 (1972) 557.
19. Folkers, K., Watanabe, T., Pinphanickhakarn, V., Wan, Y., Porter, Th. Azuma, J., Yamagami, T., Kishi, T., Kishi, H., Iwamoto, Y., Nakamura, R. and Williams, R., Biomedical and Clinical Aspects of Coenzyme Q (Eds. K. Folkers and Y. Yamamura) Elsevier/North-Holland Biomedical Press, Amsterdam (1977) 299.
20. Gerbase-DeLima, M., Wilkinson, J., Smith, G. S. and Walford, R. L., J. Gerontol., 29 (1974) 261.
21. Heidrick, M. L. and Makinodan, T., Gerontologia, 18 (1972) 305.
22. Hirokawa, K. and Makinodan, T., J. Immunol., 114 (1975) 1659.
23. Kay, M. M. B., Aging and the Decline of Immune Responsiveness in Basic and Clinical Immunology (Eds. H. H. Fudenberg et al.) Lange Medical Publications, Los Altos, California (1976) 267.
24. MacKinney, A. A., Jr., J. Gerontol., 33 (1978) 213.
25. Makinodan, T. and Peterson, W. J., J. Immunol., 93 (1964) 886.
26. Makinodan, T., Wigzell, H. and Wagner, H. N., Aging and the Immune Function, MSS Information Corp., New York, New York (1974).
27. Miller, J. F. A. P., Int. Arch. Allergy Appl. Immunol., 49 (1975) 230.
28. Pachciarz, J. A. and Teague, P. O., J. Immunol., 116 (1976) 982.
29. Patel, M. S., J. Gerontol., 32 (1977) 643.
30. Segre, D. and Segre, M., Mech. Age. Dev., 6 (1977) 115.
31. Siliprandi, D., Siliprandi, N., Scutari, G. and Zoccarato, F., Biochem. Biophys. Res. Commun., 55 (1973) 563.
32. Teasdale, C., Thatcher, J., Whitehead, R. H. and Hughes, L. E., Lancet, I (1976) 1410.
33. Walford, R. L., The Immunologic Theory of Aging, Munksgaard, Copenhagen (1969).
34. Walford, R. L., J. Immunol., 117 (1976) 352.
35. Wilson, P. D., Gerontologia, 19 (1973) 79.
36. Wilson, P. D. and Franks, L. M., Gerontologia, 21 (1975) 81.

QUERCETIN, A REGULATOR OF POLYMORPHONUCLEAR LEUKOCYTE (PMNL) FUNCTIONS

C. SCHNEIDER[1], G. BERTON[2], S. SPISANI[3], S. TRANIELLO[3], and D. ROMEO[1]

Istituto di Chimica Biologica[1] and Istituto di Patologia Generale[2], Università di Trieste, Trieste, and Istituto di Chimica Biologica[3], Università di Ferrara, Ferrara (Italy)

The binding of certain small peptides, proteins or amphipathic compounds to the surface of polymorphonuclear leukocytes (PMNL) may promote a specific activation of cell functions, such as motility, endocytosis, oxidative metabolism and secretion (9, 10,12-18,20,23,25,26,31,33,35,37,39,41). The molecular mechanisms, by which this surface interaction is translated into "signals" stimulating various biochemical pathways in the PMNL, have been the subject of intense investigation for several years. The current theory is that the coordinated response of PMNL to environmental changes is triggered by a cascade of events, presumably with the utilization of some key steps for the stimulation of various cell activities. For example, an elevation of cytosol free calcium concentrations appears to be required for the enhancement of PMNL directional locomotion (38), oxidative metabolism (24,28,30) and extracellular secretion of granule enzymes (34,40).

Since the initiation of the stimulatory events occurs at the cell surface, the study of the effects of plasma membrane perturbations on the activation of PMNL functions might provide useful clues toward the understanding of the mechanism(s) of the stimulus/response coupling. With this concept in mind, we have investigated the effect of some chemically related flavonoids on several PMNL functions. The selection of these compounds was made on the basis of their known capacity of perturbing some functions of biological membranes. In fact, they inhibit transport ATPases of plasma membranes (4,36), of mitochondria (4,36), of sarcoplasmic reticulum (7,36) and of chloroplasts (3,5). Furthermore, some flavonoids have been reported to markedly reduce the antigen- or concanavalin A-induced histamine release from mast cells (6,7) and to exert an antiviral effect on enveloped viruses (2).

MATERIALS AND METHODS

PMNL were isolated from peritoneal exudates of guinea pigs or from human blood according to standard techniques (23,38,40). Cell respiration was monitored by a Clark-type oxygen electrode attached to a thermostatically controlled (37 C) plastic vessel, in which the cell suspension was stirred magnetically. Additions of the stimulant of PMNL respiration, concanavalin A (Con A) 23, 25), and of the flavonoids were made simultaneously through a narrow puncture in the lid covering the vessel.

For experiments measuring enzyme release, PMNL suspensions were incubated in disposable test tubes at 37 C in the presence of the appropriate reagents. After 30 min of incubation, the reaction mixtures were centrifuged at 400xg for 10 min at 4 C. The activity of lysozyme in the cell-free supernatants was assayed by a nephelometric method (32), and compared to the total cell activity, which was determined in the presence of 0.05% (v/v) Triton X-100 with PMNL disrupted by sonication.

The locomotion of PMNL was assayed in Gey's medium, pH 7.2, containing 1 mg human serum albumin/ml. Cells (2×10^5/0.2 ml) were placed in the upper compartment of modified Boyden chambers (38), which was separated from the lower compartment (4.5 ml) by a 3 μm pore size membrane filter. After 60 min at 37 C, PMNL migration into the filter was measured by the leading front method of Zigmond and Hirsch (42). To study chemokinetic effects the flavonoids were added to both compartments of the chamber at equal concentration, whereas chemotactic effects were evaluated with the drugs placed below the filter. The effects of flavonoids on the casein-induced chemotaxis were measured with 1 mg casein/ml in the bottom compartment and uniform concentration of the drugs throughout the chamber.

Stock solutions of the flavonoids were prepared in dimethyl sulphoxide (DMSO) and control experiments (no flavonoid) were carried out in the presence of this solvent.

RESULTS AND DISCUSSION

The effect of flavonoids on the Con A-induced stimulation of PMNL respiration is shown in Fig. 1. Of the three drugs tested, only quercetin appears to be a potent inhibitor of the stimulatory process, the inhibition being more marked in the absence than in the presence of extracellular Ca^{2+}. Several

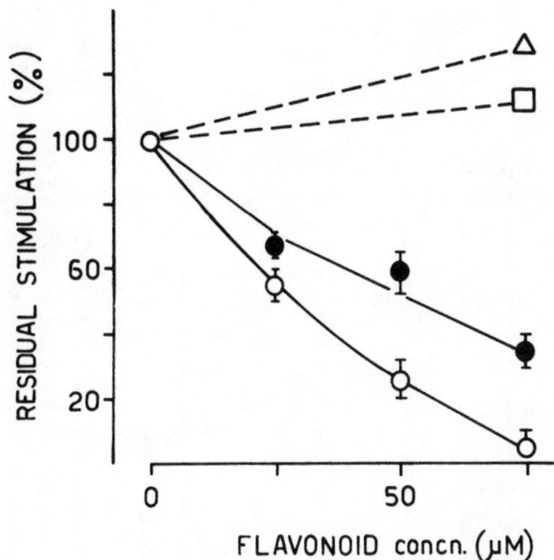

Fig. 1. Effect of flavonoids on the Con A-induced stimulation of oxygen consumption by PMNL.
Guinea pig PMNL (2 x 10^7) in 2 ml of Krebs-Ringer phosphate, pH 7.4, containing 0.2 mM glucose, with (-●-) or without (-○-, -△-, -□-) 0.5 mM $CaCl_2$, were exposed to Con A (80 μg/ml) in the presence of either dimethyl sulphoxide (100% stimulation; respiratory increment = 40.4 ± 2.7 or 50.3 ± 2.7 natoms/min, in the absence or in the presence of Ca^{2+}, respectively) or quercetin (-○-, -●-) or morin (-△-) or rutin (-□-). The data are means of at least 3 experiments ± SEM.

controls were carried out to exclude the possibility that quercetin impairs cell viability or decreases Con A binding to PMNL or inactivates the oxidase responsible for the metabolic burst (21, 29). First, in the presence of 100 μM quercetin the number of PMNL, which take up the dye trypan blue (<5%), does not increase. Second, if quercetin-treated cells are centrifuged and resuspended in fresh medium, they fully regain the sensitivity to Con A stimulation. Third, direct treatment with 75 μM quercetin of 20, 000xg subcellular fractions, isolated from either resting or previously stimulated PMNL, causes a less than 15% inhibition of the activity of particulate NADPH oxidase (21,29). Finally, as illustrated in Table I, both the glycogen-aggregating properties of Con A and the lectin binding to PMNL are unaffected by quercetin, thus ruling out the possibility that the flavonoid is inactivating the stimulant in some way before it binds to the

TABLE I

Effect of Quercetin on Con A -Induced Glycogen Aggregation and on ^{3}H-Con A Binding to PMNL

Optical Density (450 nm)[a]		μg ^{3}H-Con A Bound / 5 x 10^{6} PMNL[b]	
Glycogen + Con A	0.371	- Quercetin	0.92
" + " → α-MM	0.015	+ Quercetin	1.14
Glycogen + Quercetin + Con A	0.460		
" + " + " → α-MM	0.050		
Glycogen + Quercetin	0.035		

[a]The aggregation of glycogen was measured by a turbidimetric assay (11). 0.3 ml of Con A (1.1 mg/ml of 0.154 M NaCl) was added to 2.7 ml of calcium-free Krebs-Ringer phosphate, pH 7.4 (KRP), containing 0.8 mg of glycogen, in the absence or in the presence of quercetin. After 10 min at 37 C the optical density was recorded; at this point(α-MM) was added at the final concentration of 1 mM and 5 min thereafter the optical density was again recorded. Data are means of two experiments.

[b]5 x 10^{6} guinea pig PMNL were incubated at 37 C with 0.25 μC_i ^{3}H-Con A and 40 μg of unlabelled Con A in 1 ml of KRP, in the absence or in the presence of quercetin (50 μM). After 3 min of incubation, the suspension was diluted with 10 ml of cold KRP, the cell pellet was solubilized and the radioactivity was measured by liquid scintillation spectrometry. Specific binding was determined by the difference between total binding of Con A and binding obtained in the presence of 100 mM α-MM. Data are means of two experiments.

carbohydrate receptors.

This series of observations suggests that quercetin acts on a stage subsequent to ligand binding, very likely interacting with hydrophobic portions of the plasma membrane. The latter conclusion is consistent with the lipophilic nature of this flavonoid, which contrasts with the more hydrophilic properties of morin and rutin, the two flavonoids ineffective in inhibiting the Con A -induced metabolic stimulation.

Some evidence in favor of a cell surface-directed activity of quercetin are provided by results of experiments, in which quercetin-treated PMNL were further reacted with 1-anilino-8-naphtalene sulfonate (ANS), a compound which preferentially binds to apolar niches of the external membrane surface of cells (1,8) and competes with quercetin binding to chloroplast coupling factor 1 (3). The inhibitory effect of 50 μM quercetin on the Con A -induced stimulation of PMNL respiration is fully reversed by the subsequent addition of 500 μM ANS. Suitable controls show that ANS, at this concentration, does not modify the PMNL metabolism, either at rest or stimulated by Con A.

The flavonoids were also studied for their effects on other PMNL activities, such as exocytosis and locomotion.

Granule discharge was induced by exposing the PMNL to Con A (17,25). As shown in Table II, the release of the granule enzyme lysozyme is reduced to control levels when 30 μM quercetin is added to the reaction mixture simultaneously with Con A. Rutin and morin, up to a concentration of 100 μM, are without effect.

Quercetin also appears to modulate the motility of PMNL. From 5×10^{-8}M to 1×10^{-5}M the flavonoid exhibits both a positive chemokinetic effect and chemotactic activity (Fig. 2 a,b). Morin is much less active, showing a small positive chemokinetic effect at concentrations lower than 1×10^{-7}M, and a slight negative one at higher concentrations. Furthermore, the effect of morin on the orientation of locomotion is also much smaller than that of quercetin.

The interaction between the PMNL surface and the chemoattractants is mainly of a hydrophobic type (39). THe different activity of the two flavonoids might, therefore, again be explained on the basis of their different hydrophobicity.

Beside enhancing PMNL locomotion *per se*, quercetin, but not morin, also inhibits the chemotaxis induced by a gradient of casein (Fig. 2c). It remains to be established whether this is due to quercetin interaction with the chemoattractant or to competition for the same binding sites on the PMNL surface.

TABLE II

Effect of Flavonoids on Con A -Induced Lysozyme Secretion[a]

Additions to PMNL:	Lysozyme Release (%)	
DMSO (0.2%)	6.0 ± 0.3	$p<0.025$
DMSO + Con A (80 μg/ml)	12.7 ± 0.8	
Quercetin (30 μM)	5.0 ± 0.4	n.s.
Quercetin (30 μM) + Con A	5.7 ± 0.3	
Quercetin (10 μM)	7.7 ± 0.8	
Morin (30 μM) + Con A	13.5	
Rutin (30 μM) + Con A	13.5	

[a]Human blood PMNL (1×10^7) were incubated at 37 C for 30 min in 1 ml of calcium-free Krebs-Ringer phosphate, pH 7.4, with 0.2 mM glucose and the indicated reagents. At the end of the incubation, the cell suspensions were centrifuged and the cell-free supernatants were assayed for lysozyme activity. Data are percent of total cell enzyme activity (48.7 ± 3.3 μg/1×10^7 cells) released and are means of either three determinations ± SEM or two determinations. The difference between the means was analyzed by paired "t" statistic (n.s. = not significant).

These results indicate that we have found a novel regulator of PMNL functions. The precise mechanism by which this compound exerts its effects is at present not fully understood. As pointed out above, it is possible that quercetin interacts with hydrophobic portions of the PMNL plasma membrane. This would cause a surface perturbation, that in the absence of other extracellular ligands is translated into an activation of cell motility. Upon cell interaction with potential stimulants (secretagogues, chemoattractants, etc.), and therefore with an additional perturbation applied to the PMNL surface, quercetin would activate a reaction, which would render the PMNL less responsive to the stimuli.

One such possible reaction is the cell ejection of Ca^{2+}. In fact, according to Fewtrell and Gomperts (6,7) the inhibition of histamine release from mast cells caused by flavonoids, such as quercetin, very likely involves the regulation of cell calcium concentration. This hypothesis finds some grounds in the observations of Racker et al. (22,36) that quercetin increases the efficiency of ATP-dependent ion pumps. According to this view, ligand binding to the PMNL surface would inhibit a Ca^{2+}-dependent ATPase, normally responsible for Ca^{2+} ejection from the cells and thus for maintenance of low steady-state cytosol levels of

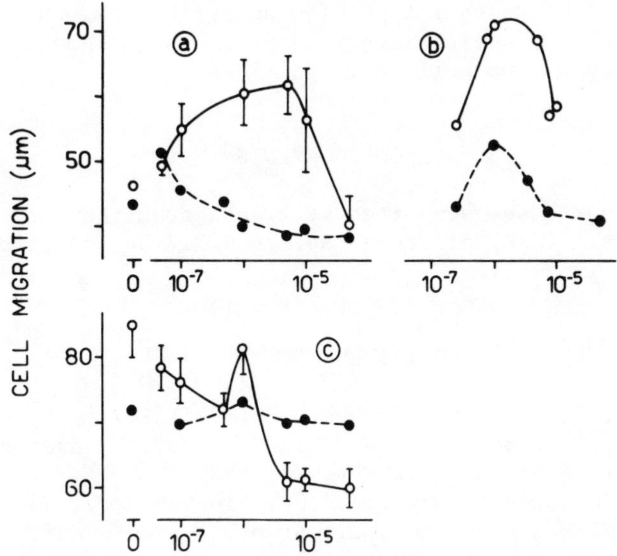

Fig. 2. Effect of quercetin (-o-) and of morin (-●-) on PMNL locomotion. Abscissas: molar concentration of the flavonoids. (a) Cells stimulated chemically but in the absence of a gradient, i.e. with uniform concentration of the flavonoids throughout the Boyden chamber (chemokinesis); (b) Cells moving towards a gradient, i.e., the flavonoids were placed below the filter (chemotaxis); (c) Cells stimulated by a gradient of casein with equal concentration of the flavonoids in the two compartments of the chambers.
The measurement of PMNL migration was taken for five fields across the filter, and duplicate chambers were always run. Data are means of either two (morin or quercetin in b) or three experiments ± SEM.

this ion (27). This inhibition would cause an increase in cytosol Ca^{2+} concentrations and stimulation of Ca^{2+}-dependent activities, such as chemotaxis, oxidative metabolism and secretion (24,28,30,34,38,40). The increase in efficiency of the Ca^{2+} pump caused by quercetin would restore low levels of Ca^{2+} and resting cell activities. This postulated mechanism finds partial support in the observation that in the presence of extracellular Ca^{2+}, which generates a steep downhill concentration gradient of this ion toward the cytoplasm (27), quercetin inhibition of Con A -induced stimulation of PMNL respiration is somewhat lower than in a calcium-free medium.

This theory would receive strong support by the demonstration of a Ca^{2+} -dependent transport ATPase at the PMNL surface. We have recently shown that such an enzyme is present in the plasma membrane of another type of phagocytic cell, the alveolar macrophage (27). Research is now in progress to show a similar enzyme activity on the surface of the PMNL.

ACKNOWLEDGEMENTS

This research was supported by grants from the National Research Council (CNR) of Italy (No. 76.01317.04) and from the University of Trieste.

REFERENCES

1. Azzi, A., Quart. Rev. Biophys., 8 (1975) 237.
2. Béládi, I., Pusztai, R., Mucsi, I., Bakay, M. and Gábor, M., Ann. N. Y. Acad. Sci., 284 (1977) 358.
3. Cantley, L. C. and Hammes, G. G., Biochemistry, 15 (1976) 1.
4. Carpenedo, F., Bortignon, C., Bruni, A. and Santi, R., Biochem. Pharm., 18 (1969) 1495.
5. Deters, D. W. and Racker, E., Nelson, N. and Nelson, H., J. Biol. Chem., 250 (1975) 1041.
6. Fewtrell, C. M. S. and Gomperts, B. D., Nature, 265 (1977) 635.
7. Fewtrell, C. M. S. and Gomperts, B. D., Biochim. Biophys. Acta, 469 (1977) 52.
8. Fortes, A. G. and Ellory, J. C., Biochim. Biophys. Acta, 413 (1975) 65.
9. Fridkin, M., Stabinsky, Y., Zakuth, V. and Spirer, Z., Biochim. Biophys. Acta, 496 (1977) 203.
10. Goetzl, E. J. and Austen, K. F., J. Clin. Invest., 53 (1974) 591.
11. Goldstein, I. J., Hollerman, C. E. and Smith, E. E., Biochemistry, 4 (1965) 876.
12. Goldstein, I. M., Hoffstein, S., Gallin, J. and Weissmann, G. Proc. Nat. Acad. Sci. USA, 70 (1973) 2916.
13. Goldstein, I. M., Cerqueira, M., Lind, S. and Kaplan, H. B., J. Clin. Invest., 59 (1977) 249.
14. Hatch, G. E., Gardner, D. E. and Menzel, D. B., J. Exp. Med., 147 (1978) 182.
15. Hawkins, D., J. Immunol., 107 (1971) 344.
16. Henson, P. M., J. Immunol., 107 (1971) 1547.
17. Hoffstein, S., Soberman, R., Goldstein, I. M. and Weissmann, G., J. Cell Biol., 68 (1976) 781.
18. Kakinuma, K., Biochim. Biophys. Acta, 348 (1974) 76.
19. Lang, D. R. and Racker, E., Biochim. Biophys. Acta, 333 (1974) 180.

20. Najjar, V. A. and Nishioka, K., Nature, 228 (1970) 672.
21. Patriarca, P., Cramer, R., Moncalvo, S., Rossi, F. and Romeo, D., Arch. Biochem. Biophys., 145 (1971) 255.
22. Racker, E., Biochem. Soc. Trans., 3 (1975) 785.
23. Romeo, D., Zabucchi, G. and Rossi, F., Nature New Biol., 243 (1973) 111.
24. Romeo, D., Zabucchi, G., Miani, N. and Rossi, F., Nature, 253, (1975) 542.
25. Romeo, D., Zabucchi, G., Jug, M., Miani, N. and Soranzo, M. R., In: Concanavalin A (Eds. T. K. Chowdhury and A. K. Weiss), Plenum Press, New York (1975) 273.
26. Romeo, D., Zabucchi, G. and Rossi, F., In: Movement, Metabolism and Bactericidal Mechanisms of Phagocytes (Eds. F. Rossi, P. Patriarca and D. Romeo), Piccin Medical Books, Padua (1977) 153.
27. Romeo, D., Schneider, C., Gennaro, R. and Mottola, C., this book.
28. Root, R. K. and Metcalf, J. A., In: Movement, Metabolism and Bactericidal Mechanisms of Phagocytes (Eds. F. Rossi, P. Patriarca and D. Romeo), Piccin Medical Books, Padua (1977) 185.
29. Rossi, F., Romeo, D. and Patriarca, P., J. Reticuloendothel. Soc., 12 (1972) 127.
30. Schell-Frederick, E., FEBS Letters, 48 (1974) 37.
31. Schiffmann, E., Corcoran, B. A. and Wahl, S. M., Proc. Nat. Acad. Sci. USA, 72 (1975) 1059.
32. Schneider, C., Gennaro, R., de Nicola, G. and Romeo, D., Exp. Cell Res., 112 (1978) 249.
33. Showell, H. J., Freer, R. J., Zogmond, S. H., Schiffmann, E., Aswanikumer, B., Corcoran, B. and Becker, E. L., J. Exp. Med., 143 (1976) 1154.
34. Smith, R. J. and Ignarro, L. J., Proc. Nat. Acad. Sci. USA, 72 (1975) 108.
35. Strauss, R. G., Mauer, A. M., Spitzer, R. E., Asbrock, T. and Stitzel, A. E., J. Immunol., 111 (1973) 313.
36. Suolinna, E. M., Buchsbaum, R. N. and Racker, E., Cancer Res., 35 (1975) 1865.
37. Tedesco, F., Trani, S., Soranzo, M. R. and Patriarca, P., FEBS Letters, 51 (1975) 232.
38. Wilkinson, P. C., Exp. Cell Res., 93 (1975) 420.
39. Wilkinson, P. C., In: Movement, Metabolism and Bactericidal Mechanisms of Phagocytes (Eds. F. Rossi, P. Patriarca and D. Romeo), Piccin Medical Books, Padua (1977) 21.
40. Zabucchi, G., Soranzo, M. R., Rossi, F. and Romeo, D., FEBS Letters, 54 (1975) 44.
41. Zatti, M. and Rossi, F., Biochim. Biophys. Acta, 148 (1967) 553.
42. Zigmond, S. H. and Hirsch, J. G., J. Exp. Med., 137 (1973)387.

THE EFFECT OF CYCLOPHOSPHAMIDE ON A SECONDARY OCULAR IMMUNE RESPONSE IN RABBITS

J. M. HALL and J. F. PRIBNOW
F. I. Proctor Foundation for Research in Ophthalmology University of California and the Naval Biosciences Laboratory, School of Public Health, University of California, San Francisco, California (USA)

Our previous experiments (7) showed that cyclophosphamide (Cytoxan) suppressed the immune response of rabbits to intravitreally injected bovine gamma globulin (BGG). Suppression of the 14 day plaque forming cell (PFC) response occurred when treatment was begun as late as 5 days after immunization. The 21 day PFC response and antibody titers were suppressed in rabbits treated from day 0 or day 2 through day 13. When treatment began later, the 21 day response was significantly depressed, but some recovery occurred. Smaller Cytoxan doses (50 mg per injection) were not as immunosuppressive as 100 mg doses. Shorter treatment (days 2 through 8) was less effective than treatment through day 13.

The present experiments were done to determine whether rabbits whose primary ocular immune response had been suppressed by Cytoxan would undergo a normal secondary response following a challenge intravitreal injection of BGG. Other experiments were done to determine whether Cytoxan would suppress a secondary response in rabbits that had undergone a primary ocular immune response to BGG.

MATERIALS AND METHODS

Effect of Cytoxan on Priming. New Zealand white rabbits weighing approximately 3 kg received intravitreal injections of BGG (Miles Laboratory, Kankakee, Ill.) into the right eyes. The methods for preparing antigen and for the intravitreal injections have been described previously (7). Cytoxan treatment began on day -3, day 0 or day 2, and was continued until day 12. These treatment regimens were chosen because they were shown to be most effective in suppressing the primary response. The Cytoxan dose was 100 mg per injection and was given intramuscularly every other day (until day 12). Cytoxan was obtained from Mead Johnson Co. (USA).

The rabbits were bled at weekly intervals and the antibody titers determined by the hemolytic antibody method described previously (6). Three months after injection we challenged the rabbits by an intravitreal injection of 1.5 mg BGG into the left eyes. The rabbits were killed 7 days after challenge. We determined the numbers of PFCs in corneas, lymph nodes, and uveal tracts, and the antibody titers in the serum, and in the aqueous and vitreous humors from both eyes.

Control rabbits were immunized intravitreally, but did not receive Cytoxan. They were challenged three months post-immunization, and the PFC assay and antibody determinations were done as described above.

Secondary Response. We injected the right eyes of New Zealand white rabbits with 1.5 mg BGG. Antibody titers were determined weekly. Three months after immunization, when serum antibody could no longer be detected, we injected the left eyes of the rabbits with 1.5 mg BGG. Cytoxan treatment was begun either 4 days, 2 days or 1 day before challenge, or on the same day as the challenge injections. The dose was 150 mg per injection. Injections were given every other day until day 6. The control rabbits were the same as those used in the priming study. We killed the rabbits on day 7 and determined the numbers of PFC in uveal tract and corneal tissue from both eyes. Hemolytic antibody titers in the serum and ocular fluids were also determined.

The rabbits in all groups were observed daily for signs of ocular inflammation. A portion of the anterior segment of the eyes of some rabbits was processed by routine histological procedures.

RESULTS

Effect of Cytoxan on Priming. Table I shows the results of the PFC assays on the tissue of control rabbits and rabbits treated with Cytoxan during the primary response. The control rabbits all developed a primary serum antibody response, but we did not detect antibody in the serum of the treated rabbits. The rabbits that had been treated from day 2 through day 12 developed ocular inflammation by the second-post challenge day, as did the controls. The PFC response of these treated rabbits was similar to that of the untreated rabbits. Fewer PFC were found in the

TABLE I

Secondary PFC Response in Tissues of Rabbits Treated with Cytoxan During Primary Response to BGG

Day CY Treatment Began	Total Cytoxan Dose	PFC per Million Cells in:	
		L. Uvea	L. Cornea
Controls	0	2160[a] (9/9)[b] (430-5250)[c]	725 (9/9) (57-3687)
+2	600 mg	1725 (5/5) (247-3846)	724 (5/5) (81-1885)
0	700 mg	100 (3/5) (0-281)	75 (4/5) (0-121)
-3	800 mg	27 (2/2) (24-30)	17 (1/2) (0-35)

[a]Numbers represent arithmetic means
[b]Number of animals with PFC/total number of animals in group
[c]Range of PFC values in group

ocular tissues of the rabbits whose treatment began before or simultaneously with immunization. As shown in Table II, some of these rabbits had normal secondary serum and aqueous humor antibody titers. There was no obvious correlation between primary antibody titers of control rabbits and the titers reached after challenge. There was no antibody in the aqueous humor or vitreous humor from the right eyes of any of the rabbits, and none in the vitreous humor of the unchallenged eyes. We detected some PFC in the right uveal tracts of 6 control rabbits, and in the right corneas of two of the rabbits, but no PFC in the right eyes of the treated rabbits. Lymph node PFC were absent or low in all rabbits.

The Effect of Cytoxan on the Secondary Response. The results during the secondary response are presented in Table III. The rabbits had shown normal primary serum antibody responses, but titers had fallen to undetectable levels before challenge. The PFC numbers in all the Cytoxan treated rabbits were much smaller than those of the controls. Only two of the 15 treated rabbits had

TABLE II

Secondary Hemolytic Antibody Titers of Rabbits Treated with Cytoxan During Primary Response to Intravitreally Injected BGG

Day CY Treatment Began	Total Cytoxan Dose	Hemolytic Antibody Titer (log2) in: L. Aqueous	Serum
Controls	0	9.4[a] (10/10)[b] (5-14)[c]	8.2 (10/10) (4-13)
+2	600 mg	8.4 (7/7) (3-14)	7.7 (7/7) (2-12)
0	700 mg	7.0 (3/5) (0-16)	6.6 (5/5) (5-8)
-3	800 mg	13.0 (2/2) (11-16)	6.0 (2/2) (4-8)

[a]Numbers represent arithmetic means
[b]Number of animals with antibody/total number of animals in group
[c]Range of antibody titers in group

uveal tract PFC, and one of these had only 5 antibody producing cells. There were no PFC in the corneal tissue of any of the rabbits. One rabbit that had received only 300 mg Cytoxan did develop a normal secondary PFC response. Lymph node PFC were low or absent in both treated and control rabbits.

Table IV shows the results of antibody titrations on the serum and ocular fluids of the rabbits. There was no antibody in the aqueous humor of any of the Cytoxan treated rabbits, but high antibody titers in the aqueous of the controls. Low serum antibody titers were found in 6 of the 17 treated rabbits.

The Cytoxan treated rabbits developed ocular inflammation by the second day after challenge. Examination of Giemsa stained smears of the uveal tract cells and of the stained sections showed that the uveal infiltrate consisted predominantly of small lymphocutes. The infiltrate in the uveal tissue of control rabbits was composed primarily of plasma cells.

TABLE III

PFC in Tissues of Rabbits Treated with Cytoxan During Secondary Response to BGG

Day CY Treatment Began	Total Average CY Dose	PFC per Million Cells in: L. Uvea	L. Cornea
Controls	0	2160[a] (9/9)[b] (430-5250)	725 (9/9)
-4 to -1	600 mg	13 (2/9) (0-108)	0
0	680 mg	60 (1/6) (0-361)	3 (1/6) (0-19)

[a]Numbers represent arithmetic means
[b]Number of animals with PFC/total number of animal in group
[c]Range of PFC values in group

DISCUSSION

Our previous experiments showed that Cytoxan suppressed the ocular inflammatory and antibody responses of rabbits that received a single intravitreal injection of BGG. The degree of suppression was related to the time treatment began and to the total Cytoxan dose given. Since uveitis is often recurrent, it seemed important to establish whether Cytoxan would prevent recurrences of ocular inflammation and antibody formation after a second exposure to the immunizing antigen.

The effects of Cytoxan on priming for a secondary response have been studied in mice and guinea pigs. Maguire and Maibach (12) suppressed anaphylactic sensitization to ovalbumin by treating guinea pigs with Cytoxan. Hoffsten and Dixon (8) challenged mice 42 days after a primary injection of keyhole limpet hemocyanin. Three hundred microgram doses of Cytoxan administered during the entire immunization period suppressed the secondary response and smaller doses were partially suppressive. Marbrook et al (13) made mice tolerant by administering large doses of SRBC. The direct PFC response of cytoxan treated mice challenged 18 days later was less than that of the control mice. Frisch and Davies (4, 5) found that Cytoxan treatment did not prevent priming

TABLE IV

Hemolytic Antibody Titers of Rabbits
Treated with Cytoxan During Secondary Response to BGG

Day CY Treatment Began	Total Average CY Dose	Hemolytic Antibody Titer (log_2) in: L. Aqueous	Serum
Controls	0	9.4[a] (10/10)[b] (5-14)[c]	8.2 (10/10) (4-13)
-4 to -1	600 mg	0	1.3 (5/11) (0-5)
0	680 mg	0	0.5 (1/6) (0-3)

[a]Numbers represent arithmetic means
[b]Number of animals with antibody/total number of animals in group
[c]Range of antibody titers in group

for a secondary response, as did Finger (3) and Kool (9). In some cases the secondary responses were depressed, but still typical secondary responses.

Our results in rabbits were similar to those of some of the other investigators. Most of the rabbits treated with immunosuppressive doses of Cytoxan during the primary response developed secondary responses following intravitreal challenge. Although the PFC numbers in the ocular tissues of the rabbits in some groups were lower than the controls, the serum and aqueous humor antibody titers were as high as those of the controls, indicating that a true secondary response had taken place. The low PFC numbers might reflect a technical problem with the plaque assay, or a partial suppression of the response. In a primary response to BGG we do not detect uveal or corneal PFC until about the 12th post-immunization day.

We can only speculate on the mechanism of action by which Cytoxan fails to prevent priming. Recent evidence indicates that the mode of action in suppressing immune responses is not as simple as first thought (10, 12). Cytoxan was thought to affect mostly B lymphocytes, and exert its humoral antibody suppression by its action on B cells. Recent experiments (2, 13, 16) suggest that Cytoxan can also affect T lymphocytes. Winkelstein (17) found that guinea pig peripheral blood and lymph node T and B cells are affected by Cytoxan, but that T cells recover faster. Ramshaw (15) suggests that Cytoxan's effect on humoral immunity is due to induction of a T cell that represses B cell activity. Kool (9) noted that Cytoxan given later than one day after immunization did not affect memory, and suggested that T cells differentiated into memory cells early in the response, and that they are not inhibited by Cytoxan. The drug seems to affect various T and B cell populations in different ways. In our experiments we found that Cytoxan-treated rabbits had some lymph node PFC even though the primary ocular immune response was completely suppressed. It would be reasonable, then, to expect a secondary response since priming for memory would have taken place. Even in the absence of early priming, it could have taken place after recovery from the immunosuppressive effects of Cytoxan, since intravitreally injected antigen remains in the vitreous for a relatively long period, and might have been available to "recovered" immunocompetent cells.

We also demonstrated in the present experiments that Cytoxan can suppress the secondary response in rabbits that had undergone a primary response to intravitreally injected BGG. The effects of Cytoxan given during secondary responses have not been extensively studied. Frisch and Davies (4, 5) were able to suppress the secondary response in mice that had undergone a primary response to human erythrocytes, even when treatment was given after challenge. We did not begin treatment after challenge, since the antibody response is detected very soon after intravitreal challenge, and it would not have been possible to give enough Cytoxan. Two hundred mg doses were toxic to our rabbits even when given intramuscularly. Again, the mechanisms of action can only be speculated upon. Cytoxan could be suppressing B cells that are stimulated to proliferate and differentiate after challenge or as shown by Ramshaw _et al._ (15) it could be activating a T cell that represses the B cell response.

SUMMARY

Treatment of rabbits with immunosuppressive doses of cyclophosphamide during the primary response to intravitreally injected bovine gamma globulin did not prevent priming for a secondary response to the same antigen. High antibody titers were found in the aqueous humor and serum of most of the treated rabbits. Ocular tissue plaque forming cell numbers were similar to those of the controls in many of the rabbits, and slightly lower in others.

Treatment with cyclophosphamide completely suppressed the ocular immune response in many rabbits that had undergone a primary response following intravitreal injection of BGG. The response in other animals was depressed but not completely inhibited. The presence of ocular inflammation and lymphocytes in the challenged eyes of the treated rabbits suggested a differential effect of cyclophosphamide on cells stimulated to divide after challenge.

REFERENCES

1. Akanese, P. W., Hayden, B. J. and Gershon, R. K. J. Exp. Med. 141 (1975) 697.
2. Balow, J. W., Parrillom, J. E. and Fauci, A. E. Immunology 32 (1977) 899.
3. Finger, H., Emmerling, P. and Bruss, E. Experentia 254 (1969) 1183.
4. Frisch, A. W. and Davies, G. H. Cancer Res 25 (1965) 745.
5. Frisch, A. W. and Davies, G. H. J. Lab. Clin. Med. 68 (1966) 103.
6. Hall, J. M. Invest. Ophthal. 10 (1971) 775.
7. Hall, J. M., Ohno, S. and Pribnow, J. F. Clin. Exp. Immunol. 30 (1977) 309.
8. Hoffsten, P. F. and Dixon, F. J. J. Immunol. 112 (1974) 564.
9. Kool, G. A. In: Microenvironmental Aspects of Immunity. Plenum Press (1973) p. 399.
10. Maguire, H. C. and Maibach, H. I. J. Allergy 32 (1961) 406.
11. Marbrook, J. and Baguley, B. G. Cell. Immunol. 25 (1976) 217.
12. Milton, J. D, Carpenter, C. B. and Addison, I. E. Cell. Immunol. 24 (1976) 308.
13. Mitsuoka, A., Baba, M. and Morikawa, S. Nature (Lond) 262 (1976) 77.
14. Otterness, I. G. and Chang, Y. H. Clin. Exp. Immunol. 26 (1976) 346.
15. Ramshaw, I. A., Bretscher, P. A. and Parish, C. R. Europ. J. Immunol. 7 (1977) 180.
16. Schwarze, G. Clin. Exp. Immunol. 27 (1977) 178.
17. Winkelstein, A. Blood 50 (1977) 81.

ACKNOWLEDGEMENT

This research was supported in part by Grants No. 01182 and EY-01597 from the National Institutes of Health (USA) and by the Office of Naval Research (USA) under a contract between the Office of Naval Research and the Regents of the University of California.

Part III
Regulatory Functions of the Reticuloendothelial System

It is quite apparent that the Reticuloendothelial (RE) System is involved in many regulatory activities. In this section, the role of the RE System in glucose homeostasis, the metabolism of metals such as iron, zinc and copper, in homopoiesis and granulopoiesis are discussed. In addition, the function of macrophage prostaglandins in phagocytosis is reviewed. The nature and mechanism of factors influencing the function of RE cell activities, especially as related to antibody formation, are also dealt with in terms of regulatory functions.

RES FUNCTION AND GLUCOSE HOMEOSTASIS

J. P. FILKINS

Stritch School of Medicine
Loyola University of Chicago
Chicago, Illinois (USA)

As well known to members of the RE Societies, the name for the collection of wandering and sessile mononuclear phagocytic cells which we so dearly love to study was coined by the German pathologist Ludwig Aschoff as the "reticuloendothelial system". Less well known, however, is that Aschoff in his original studies was so impressed by the metabolic functions of the phagocytic cells that he suggested an alternate term for the phagocyte collection - namely, the "histiocytic metabolic apparatus) (1). The studies to be presented herein deal with a novel, metabolic role for the macrophage apparatus - namely, a proposed regulatory function in glucose homeostasis which pivots around RES influences on insulin dynamics and the resultant functional insulinemic state.

DEPRESSION OF RE PHAGOCYTOSIS IN HYPOGLYCEMIA

Our interest in the connection between RES function and glucoregulation arose from a series of studies we were conducting on endotoxin shock in rats. In particular, we were impressed by data obtained on a correlation between the classic endotoxic depression of intravascular colloidal carbon clearance by the RES and the development of the characteristic progressive, profound hypoglycemia of endotoxicosis. As depicted in Table I, control male Holtzman rats had fasting plasma glucose levels of colloidal carbon of 15 ± 1.7 min. After i. v. administration of 3 mg of *Salmonella enteritis* endotoxin, plasma glucose values declined to 70 ± 4 mg/dl at 60 min, to 50 ± 3 mg/dl at 120 min, to 32 ± 3 mg/dl at 180 min, and to 10 ± mg/dl at 300 min; corresponding to the plasma glucose declines were increases in colloidal carbon clearances half-time values, i. e. RES depression, of from 22 ± 2.2, to 29 ± 3.2, to 37 ± 4.2, to 52 ± 6.1 min.

TABLE I

Effects of Endotoxin on Plasma Glucose Levels and Colloidal Carbon Clearance[a]

Experimental Group	Number of Rats	Plasma Glucose (mg/dl)	Intravascular half-time (min)
Control	28	88 ± 6	15 ± 1.7[b]
Endotoxin-3 mg:			
60 min prior	10	70 ± 4	22 ± 2.9
120 min prior	10	50 ± 3	29 ± 3.2
180 min prior	10	32 ± 3	37 ± 4.2
300 min prior	10	10 ± 1	52 ± 6.1

[a]Overnight fasted Holtzman rats (300 ± 10 gm) received either 3 mg of *S. enteritidis* endotoxin or saline i. v. and at the times specified the groups received 8 mg/100 g colloidal carbon i. v. and were sampled for plasma glucose determinations

[b]$p < .05$ as compared to all endotoxin time groups. Values are means ± SEM

In order to assess directly the effects of hypoglycemia without the host of direct and indirect complications of endotoxicosis, 2 additional groups of carbon clearance function studies were performed (4): 1, using a bevy of fed and fasted control rats with endogenously varying glucose levels (Fig. 1), and 2, using rats rendered hypoglycemic to varying levels by insulin sc (Fig. 2). In a group of 40 control rats, the correlation (r) of carbon clearance half-times *vs* blood glucose levels was -.3911 which was significant at a p value of .0126. In these 40 rats, the mean blood glucose level was 90.6 mg/dl and the mean carbon half-time was 16.8 min.

In a group of 31 insulin-treated rats with blood glucose levels as low as 10 mg/dl, the correlation (r) of carbon clearance half-times *vs* blood glucose levels was -.6423 and the p value was $< .001$ (Fig. 2). The mean blood glucose of the 31 rats was 34.8 mg/dl and the mean carbon half-time was 25.2 min. Most striking was the sub-group of 16 insulin-treated rats with blood glucose

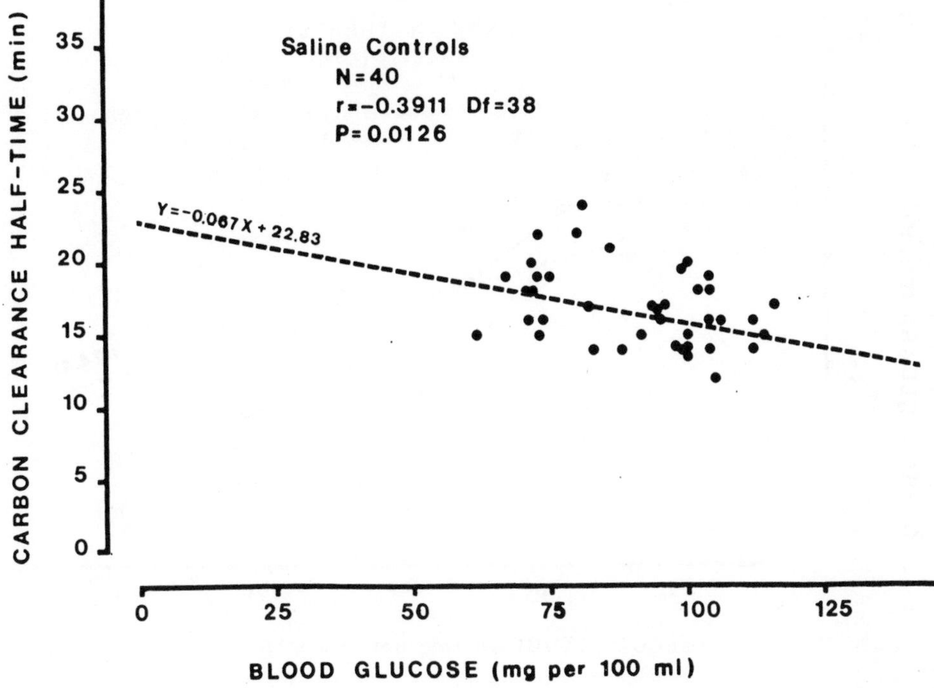

Fig. 1. Carbon clearance half-times (8 mg/100 gm) as a function of endogenous blood glucose levels in control rats. The best line through the points was computed by the method of least squares.

levels below 30 mg/dl in which marked depression of carbon clearance was manifest; i. e., a mean intravascular half-time of 30.8 min at a mean blood glucose of 21 $\pm$ 1.8 mg/dl.

In summary to this point, the phagocytic clearance data suggested that RES function was indeed influenced by the blood glucose status. This finding suggested a test of the inverse relation - namely, would the status of RES functional activity alter glucose homeostasis? The remainder of this article will be devoted to providing evidence for a definite influence of RES function on glucose homeostasis.

DEPRESSION OF RES FUNCTION AND ALTERED INSULIN SENSITIVITY

In order to alter RES function the classic colloidal carbon blockade model was employed using 32 mg/100 gm of C11/1431a Pelikan Biological Ink (2, 8). As an initial probe into the effects of RES depression on glucose homeostasis, the influence of carbon

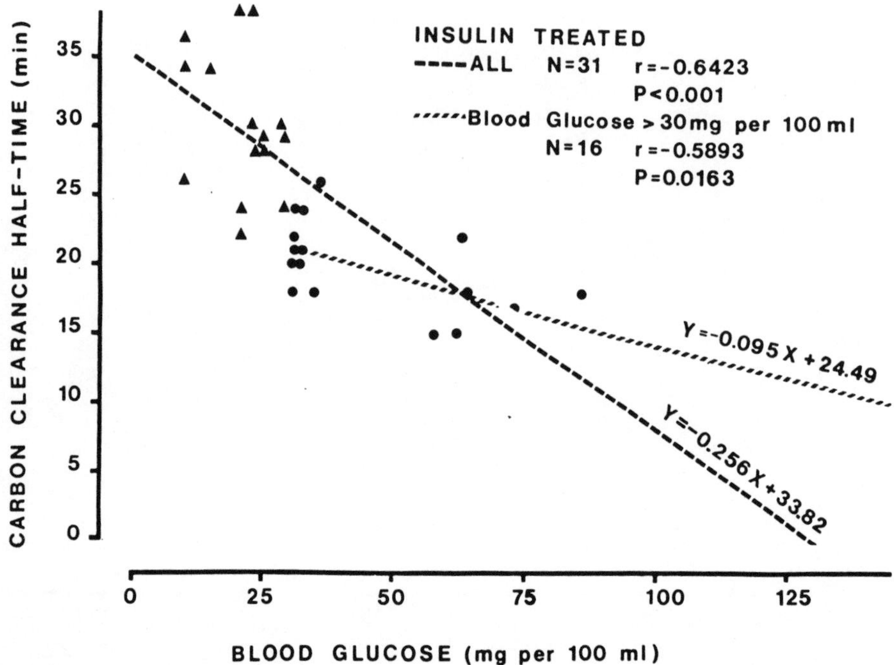

Fig. 2. Carbon clearance half-times (8 mg/100 gm) as a function of blood glucose levels in insulin hypoglycemia rats. The best lines through both the total population and the sub-group with glucose levels below 30 mg/dl were computed by the method of least squares.

blockade on sensitization to insulin lethality was evaluated (Fig. 3).

As depicted in Fig. 3, 3 groups of rats were studied: (i) control rats which were uninjected prior to insulin treatment, (ii) sham-blockade rats which received the supernatant from Pelikan ink C11/1431a as obtained by ultra-centrifugation at 25,000 x g for 60 min, and (iii) carbon-blockade rats which received 32 mg/100 gm of colloidal carbon ink at 4-6 hr prior to insulin. Crystalline insulin was administered sc at doses of 0.5 and 1.0 unit per rat; all rats were males of the Holtzman strain and were fasted overnight. Insulin induced only modest lethality in convulsive seizures in either control or sham-blockade groups, but marked increased in insulin sensitivity to lethal seizure deaths occurred after carbon-blockade.

As an additional test of insulin sensitivity after RES depression, hypoglycemia responses were evaluated (Fig. 4). The

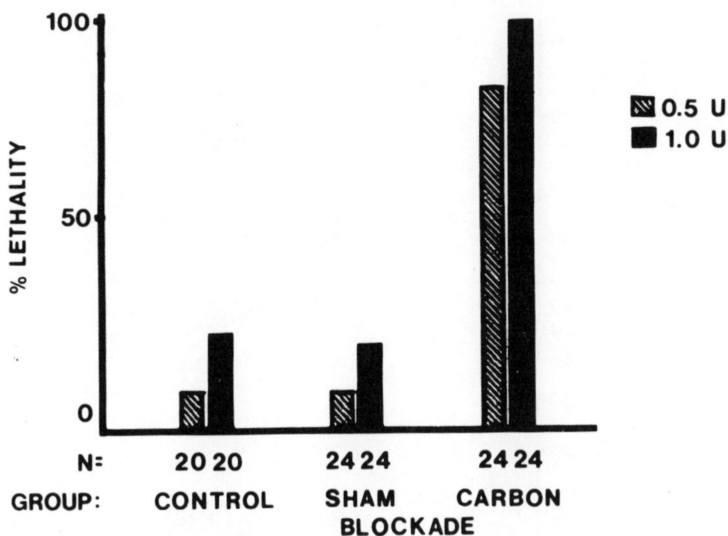

Fig. 3. Effect of RES depression on insulin lethality.

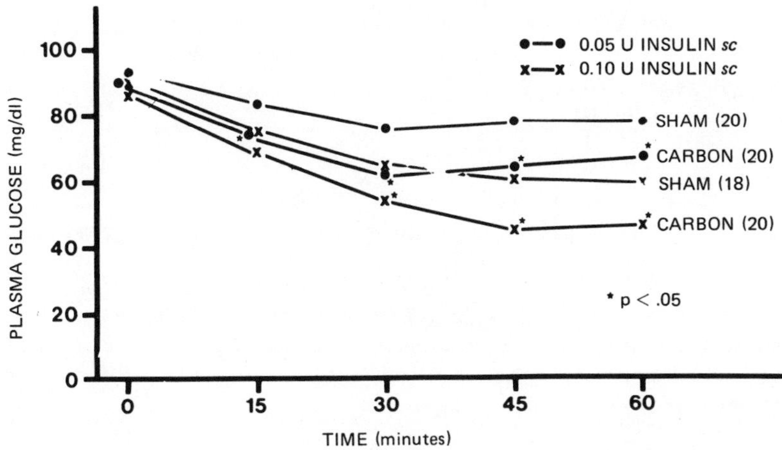

Fig. 4. Effect of RES depression on insulin hypoglycemia.

nadirs of plasma glucose were enhanced in carbon-blockade rats treated with either 0.05 or 0.10 units of insulin as compared to sham-blockade rats. Thus, RES depression also sensitized to the hypoglycemia action of insulin.

As a further index of the influence of RES depression on glu-

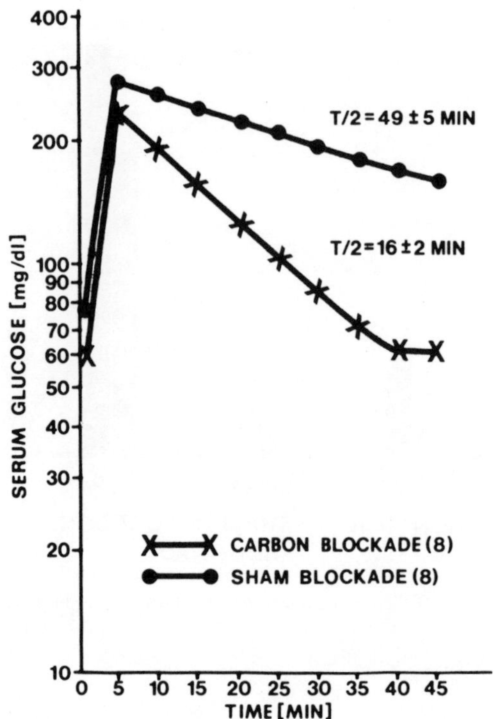

Fig. 5. Effect of RES depression of glucose tolerance. Half-time values are mean ± SEM.

cose homeostasis, glucose tolerance was evaluated in carbon-blockade *vs* sham-blockade rats (Fig. 5). In these studies rats received 400 mg D-glucose i. v. and the net glucose disappearance half-times were computed. Carbon blockade reduced the glucose half to 16 min as compared to 49 min in the sham group. This increased glucose tolerance is indicative of a functional hyperinsulinemic state in RES depression.

DEPRESSION OF RES FUNCTION AND ALTERATIONS IN HEPATIC GLUCONEOGENESIS

Based on the evidence presented above for altered glucose homeostasis and functional hyperinsulinism in a RES depressed state, the status of the 2 major glucoregulatory processes affected by insulin - (i) glucose production via gluconeogenesis and (ii) peripheral glucose utilization - were evaluated both *in vitro* and *in vivo*. In order to quantitate hepatic gluconeogenesis

TABLE II

Effect of Colloidal Carbon Depression of the RES on Gluconeogenesis in Isolated Hepatocytes[a]

Hepatocyte Donor Rats	# of Prepar- ations	Glucose Production (moles of glucose/gram protein/120 min) KRB	10mM Lactate	10mM Pyrovate	10mM Alanine
Sham-Control	6	12 ± 1.4	142 ± 12	218 ± 31	152 ± 18
Carbon Blockade	6	14 ± 1.6	91 ± 11[b]	102 ± 26[b]	74 ± 13[b]

[a]Carbon blockade was produced in overnight fasted male rats (300 ± 10 gm) with 32 mg/100 gm colloidal carbon i. v. Sham-rats received the equivalent volume of the carbon vehicle obtained by ultracentrifugation. Hepatocytes were prepared 4-6 hr after treatment.

[b]$p < .05$ values are mean ± SEM

directly, isolated hepatocyte preparations were employed (6) (Table II).

Hepatocytes isolated from carbon-blockade rats had depressed gluconeogenesis as compared to hepatocytes from sham-control rats. Thus, conversion of lactate, pyruvate, and alanine were reduced 36%, 53% and 51%, respectively, after RES depression.

In order to evaluate gluconeogenesis *in vivo*, the conversion of a 100 mg alanine load containing 4 μCi of ^{14}C-alanine to plasma glucose was evaluated (7) (Fig. 6). As indicated, both the hyperglycemic response to the alanine load and the percent conversion of alanine to glucose as computed by ^{14}C tracer analysis were depressed in carbon blockade rats as compared to sham-blockade rats.

Thus, to this point, *in vivo* and *in vitro* evidence has been presented to indicate that RES depression is associated with defects in the ability of the liver to conduct gluconeogenesis. In this fashion, input to the glucose pool is decreased. Since gluconeogenic depression is a sensitive index of hepatic insulinization, the data are suggestive of a functional hyperinsulinism incident to depression of the hepatic RES.

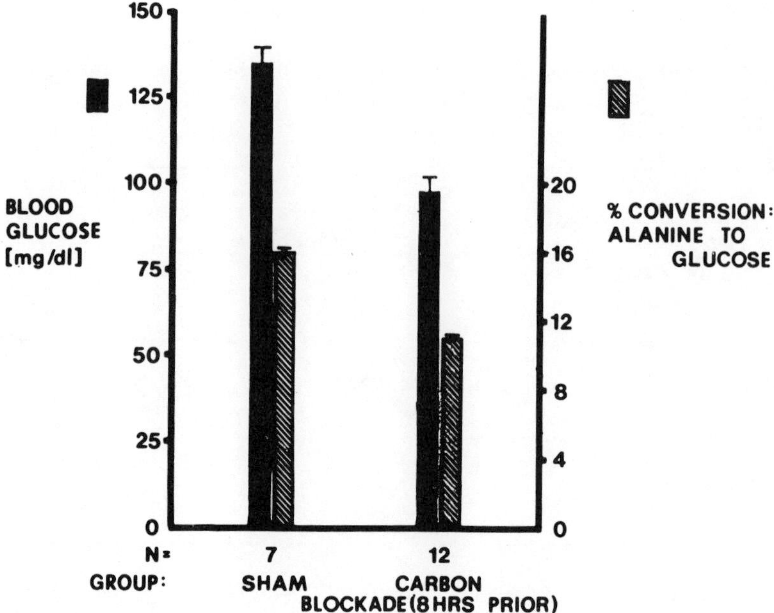

Fig. 6. Effect of RES depression of *in vivo* gluconeogenesis.

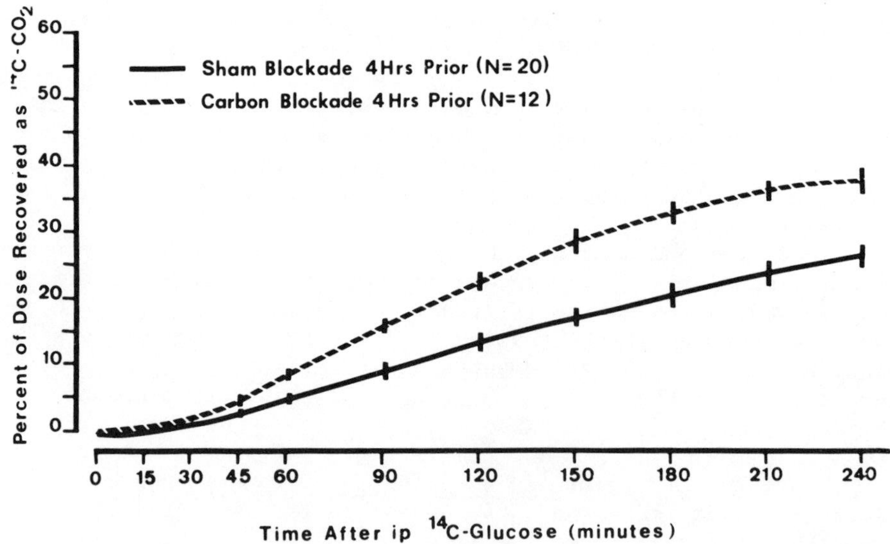

Fig. 7. Effects of RES depression on *in vivo* glucose oxidation.

TABLE III

Effect of Colloidal Carbon Depression of the RES on Glucose Oxidation in Epididymal Fat Pads[a]

Donor Group	Number of Rats	Glucose Oxidation (DPM $-^{14}CO_2$/gram/hr)
Sham-Controls	12	56,242 ± 4196
Carbon Blockade	12	74,188 ± 5211[b]

[a]Overnight fasted rats (100 ± 10 gm) received either 32 mg/100 gm of colloidal carbon or the equivalent volume of the ink supernatant i. v. All rats were sacrificed at 4 hr and epididymal fats incubated in Krebs-Ringer Bicarbonate buffer with 1 mg/dl D-glucose and 0.5 μCi-U-^{14}-C-D-glucose.

[b]$p < .05$ values are mean ± SEM

DEPRESSION OF RES FUNCTION AND ALTERATIONS IN PERIPHERAL GLUCOSE USE

In order to evaluate the effects of RES depression on glucose use *in vitro*, the isolated epididymal fat pad model was used (8). As indicated in Table III, fat pads from carbon-blockade rats manifested increased oxidation of U-^{14}C-D-glucose to $^{14}CO_2$ as compared to sham blockade controls.

In accord with the *in vitro* evidence for increased glucose oxidation after RES depression, *in vivo* studies of total body oxidation of U-^{14}C-D-glucose to expired $^{14}CO_2$ showed enhanced glucose catabolism (Fig. 7).

Thus, the studies on gluconeogenesis and glucose oxidation both *in vitro* and *in vivo* indicated that RES depression was associated with a state of functional hyperinsulinism.

DEPRESSION OF RES FUNCTION AND ALTERATIONS IN BASAL AND GLUCOSE-STIMULATED SERUM INSULIN LEVELS

Since the studies presented above indicated a state of functional hyperinsulinism after depression of the RES, a series of experiments were designed in order to measure serum insulin *per se* after carbon blockade (10). Insulin was quantitated by radio-

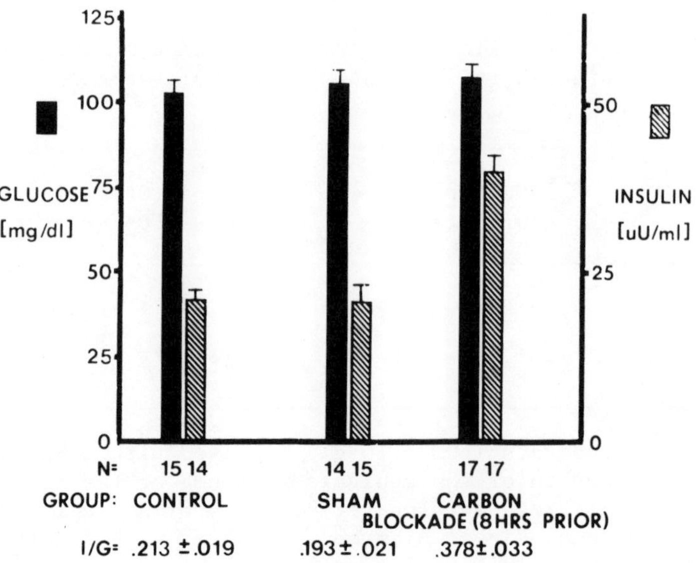

Fig. 8. Effect of RES depression on basal serum immunoreactive insulin.

immunoassay using the Phadebas method (3, 5). As depicted in Fig. 8, at 8 hr after carbon blockade an approximate doubling of basal serum immunoreactive insulin was evident. Since plasma glucose levels were not altered, the insulin to glucose ratio was also doubled after RES depression.

In order to amplify the change in insulin dynamics, insulin levels were also evaluated at 5 min after a 400 mg-D-glucose load i. p. in carbon-blockade *vs* sham-blockade rats (Fig. 9). Both the uninjected and sham-blockade controls manifested a glycemic mediated increase in insulin levels. Most striking, however, was the approximately 4-fold rise in insulin levels in the carbon-blockade rats.

SUMMARY AND CONCLUSIONS

The experiments reviewed suggest that the RES is involved in glucose homeostasis. Depression of the RES using the colloidal carbon blockade model was associated with enhanced sensitivity to insulin-induced convulsive seizure deaths and hypoglycemia, increased glucose tolerance, depressed gluconeogenesis - both *in vitro* and *in vivo*, enhanced glucose catabolism - both *in vitro* and *in vivo*, and elevation of both basal and glycemic-stimulated

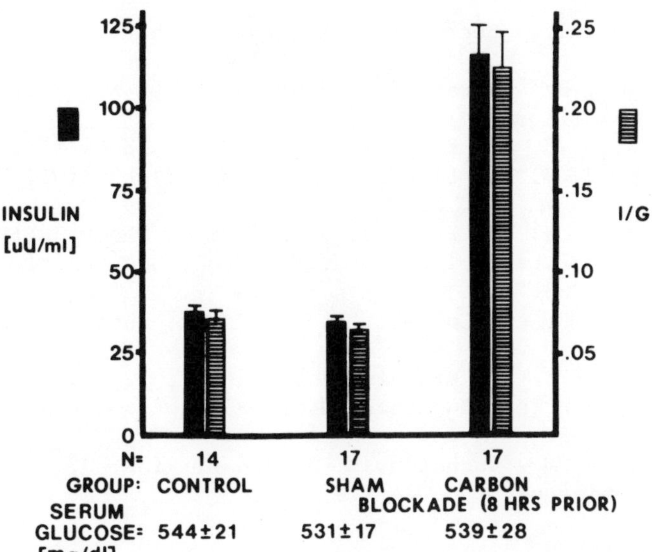

Fig. 9. Effect of RES depression on glucose-stimulated immunoreactive insulin.

serum insulin levels. It appears, therefore, that the alterations in glucose homeostasis accompanying RES depression are underwritten by a true hyperinsulinemia. Further studies are needed to elucidate the mechanism of the hyperinsulinemia, viz, is it associated with decreased insulin degradation during the transhepatic passage through depressed sinusoidal Kupffer cells, or is it due to an enhancement of pancreatic beta cell secretion?

In overview, the studies presented substantiate Aschoff's insights when he offered the expression "histiocytic metabolic apparatus" for the confederation of mononuclear phagocytes. It is our conviction that further study of the metabolic functions of the RES will unravel new insights into the regulatory function of macrophages.

ACKNOWLEDGEMENTS

The collaboration of my colleagues B. J. Buchanan and A. M. Hadbavny is gratefully recognized. These studies were supported by USPHS Grant HL 08682.

REFERENCES

1. Aschoff, L. In: Lectures in biology. Hoeber, New York (1924) 1.
2. Biozzi, G., Benacerraf, B. and Halperin, B. N. Brit. J. Exptl. Pathol. 34 (1953) 441.
3. Buchanan, B. J. and Filkins, J. P. Circ. Shock 3 (1976) 223.
4. Buchanan, B. J. and Filkins, J. P. Am. J. Physiol. 231 (1976) 265.
5. Buchanan, B. J. and Filkins, J. P. Circ. Shock 3 (1976) 267.
6. Cornell, R. P. and Filkins, J. P. Proc. Soc. Exptl. Biol. Med. 145 (1974) 203.
7. Filkins, J. P. and Cornell, R. P. Am. J. Physiol. 227 (1974) 265.
8. Filkins, J. P. J. Reticuloendothel. Soc. 22 (1977) 461.
9. Filkins, J. P. and Buchanan, J. B. J. Reticuloendothel. Soc. 21 (1977) 391.
10. Hadbavny, A. M., Buchanan, B. J. and Filkins, J. P. J. Reticuloendothel. Soc. 24 (1978) 57.

ROLE OF RES AND LEUKOCYTIC ENDOGENOUS MEDIATOR IN IRON, ZINC AND COPPER METABOLISM

R. F. KAMPSCHMIDT

Biomedical Division, The Samuel Roberts Noble Foundation

Ardmore, Oklahoma (USA)

The reticuloendothelial system (RES) influences metal metabolism in the body in many different ways. The most thoroughly studied metal is iron, and its relationship with the RES has been frequently reviewed (1, 10, 22, 24). Substantial quantities of zinc occur in phagocytic cells and there is evidence that zinc has a role in membrane stability and phagocytosis (4). During infectious diseases or other inflammatory stresses the absorption, storage and plasma levels of zinc are altered (27). The most clearly defined interaction between copper and the RES is the role of ceruloplasmin in regulating the movement of iron from the RES to transferrin (39). Iron is conserved by the body and its major use is in the formation of the hemoglobin found in erythrocytes. Aged erythrocytes are removed from the blood by the RES and the major portion of the iron is recycled to the bone marrow through the iron transport protein (transferrin). Although most of the iron is used for new hemoglobin synthesis, a small amount is stored in the RES for varying periods of time.

Infection, inflammation or neoplasia alters this normal flow of iron. During early acute phases of these disorders, reutilization of hemoglobin iron is impaired causing a decrease in transport iron (7, 21). There still is doubt about whether the restricted iron supply persists during the chronic stage (3), and some investigations indicate that impaired iron reutilization may have no role in the developing anemia (40). Erythrocyte survival time appears to be shortened for the anemias associated with arthritis (8), cancer (31) and inflammation (32); and the bone marrow fails to respond adequately to the anemia of these chronic disorders. The lack of a proper erythropoietic response is usually attributed to an inadequate increase in erythropoietin (5, 9, 37,

41); however, the limited erythropoietic response may be due to the availability of iron (5) or to the competition for the pluripotent marrow stem cell by the granulocyte and erythrocyte stimulatory factors (34). To better assess the proper role of each of these mechanisms in anemia, a search was made for an endogenous mediator responsible for the lowering of transport iron during infection, inflammation or cancer (16, 25, 26). The endogenous factor found to be responsible for lowering plasma iron (17), plasma zinc (18), and increasing plasma copper (29) is called leukocytic endogenous mediator (LEM) and has been the subject of a recent review (11). The normal cycles of metabolism for iron, zinc and copper are altered at several different points when LEM is injected (11).

Apparently all cells of the RES can produce LEM when properly activated (11). Activation occurs when the RE cells phagocytize bacteria, virus or endotoxin or it can occur through interaction with lymphokines released during delayed hypersensitivity reactions (11). Thus, the RES has not only direct effects upon metal metabolism during their transport and storage but also indirect effects by producing LEM which alters these reactions.

LEM from several different species and cell types has a molecular weight in the range of 12 to 15 thousand daltons (11, 14, 23). The LEM produced by rabbit peritoneal granulocytes has an isoelectric point at pH 7.8 (23); its activity can be destroyed by heat, trypsin or pronase (11); and free sulfhydryl groups are essential for its activity (20).

In addition to its effects upon metals LEM has been shown to increase the release and stimulate the production of neutrophils by the bone marrow (12, 19), cause fever (11), increase the flux of amino acids from muscle to liver (36), and alter the rates of synthesis of a wide variety of acute phase proteins (6, 11, 29, 36). Although much more work on purification needs to be done, the evidence thus far favors a single mediator for all these activities (2, 15, 20, 23). Some of these alterations in host metabolism are probably not direct effects of LEM but involve other mediators (11).

The effect of injections of LEM into rats on the plasma levels of copper, zinc and iron is shown in Fig. 1. LEM produced a rapid decrease in plasma zinc concentration reaching a minimum 5 to 6 hr after injection. The return to normal levels also occurred promptly. It has been suggested that LEM may be a key intermediate in altering zinc homeostasis during inflammation, since it also affects absorption and hepatic uptake (28, 30). Plasma iron reaches a minimum 8 to 12 hr after LEM injection. Plasma iron returns to normal values somewhat more slowly than zinc, but at all of the doses which have been tested it is back to nearly normal levels by 24 hr. Storage iron in the liver has been shown to increase after injection of LEM into rats (30). Plasma copper increased slowly

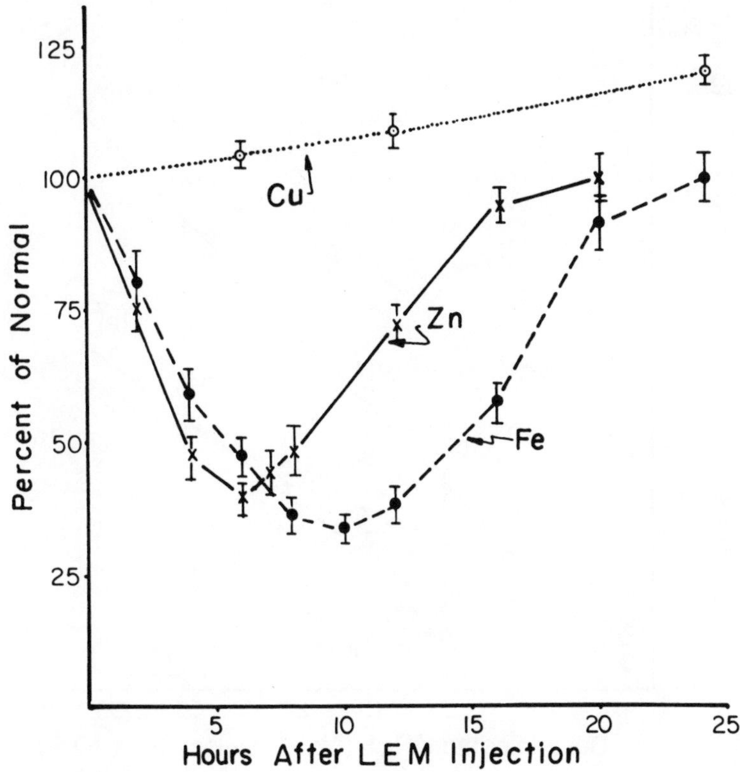

Fig. 1. Plasma copper, zinc and iron concentrations at various times after an i. p. injection of LEM. Each rat received the LEM prepared from 2 x 10^8 peritoneal granulocytes. Each point is an average value for a group of 8 to 20 rats.

and had not reached a maximum by 24 hr (29).

Effects of varying doses of LEM on the plasma levels of iron and zinc in rats are shown in Fig. 2. Increasing the dose causes a further decrease in both plasma iron and plasma zinc. If a sufficient number of animals are used the effects produced by LEM on both plasma iron and zinc give fairly reproducible log dose response curves (15).

Perhaps the most unique and useful feature of LEM is that animals will not develop a tolerance to it upon repeated injections. Rats were injected every 8 hr with crude LEM prepared from 1 x 10^8 rabbit peritoneal granulocytes per dose. The effect of these injections on the hemoglobin and hematocrit of rats is shown in Fig. 3. Each point on this figure shows the mean and standard error for groups of 14 to 60 rats. After the 13th injection of LEM both

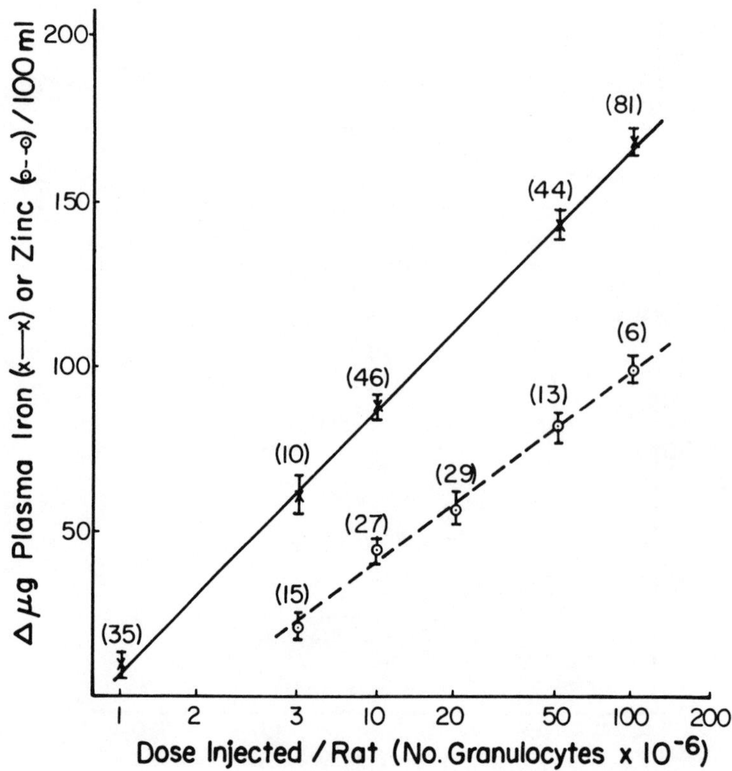

Fig. 2. The effect of varying the dose of injected LEM on plasma iron and zinc in rats. The concentration of iron or zinc in the plasma was measured 8 hr after rats received an i. p. injection of LEM. The amount of plasma iron or zinc is expressed as changes from a control group which received only the vehicle for the LEM. Each point is an average value for the number of rats indicated in the parenthesis. The brackets indicate the S. E.

the packed red cell volume and the hemoglobin concentration were significantly decreased. Under the conditions used in these initial experiments the anemia was not stabilized, as it usually is during chronic infections, but continued to decrease. It seems possible that a mild stable anemia might be produced by using a more highly purified LEM administered at lower doses and at less frequent intervals over a longer period of time. If this anemia is typical of the anemia of chronic disorders, several other alterations might reasonably be expected (3). The effects of 10, 20 or 30 injections of LEM on some of these host changes are shown in Table I. With multiple injections of LEM, plasma iron decreases rapidly and is then maintained at a lower level. Total iron stores of the liver and spleen were increased slightly by the 10th

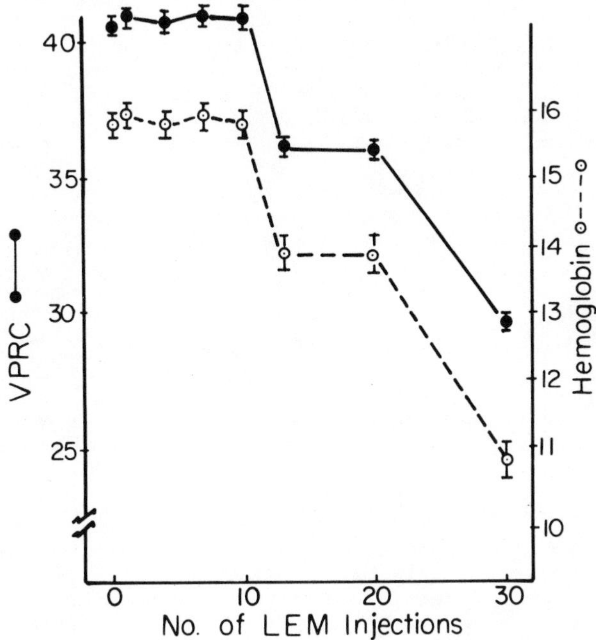

Fig. 3. The development of anemia in rats receiving multiple injections of LEM. Rats were injected every 8 hr i. p. with LEM prepared from 1 x 10^8 peritoneal granulocytes. Each point is an average value for groups of 14 to 60 rats with the brackets indicating the S. E. VPRC = volume of packed red cells.

injection and remained at this level throughout. Free protoporphin of erythrocytes was significantly increased after all three series of LEM injections. These changes are typical of those found during anemia of chronic disorders (3).

Plasma zinc decreases rapidly and after multiple LEM injections a lower level of plasma zinc is maintained (Table I). Although plasma copper increases slowly (29) through 10 injections of LEM, this higher level is then maintained through 30 injections. The total iron binding capacity, as well as the percent saturation with iron is decreased after 10, 20 and 30 injections of LEM. The number of neutrophils in the bloodstream are markedly increased with 10 or more injections. Some of this increase is due to a continued pressure for neutrophil release from the bone marrow caused by the LEM injections (12), but there is also an increase in granulopoiesis which starts after about 10 injections of LEM (19). The increase in granulopoiesis may be related to the gradual increase in colony stimulating factor found in the plasma as more LEM injections are given (19). This stimulation to leukocyte production

TABLE I

Effects of Multiple LEM Injections in Rats

Number LEM Injections[a]	0	10	20	30
Number Rats	42	20	30	10
Plasma iron µg/100 ml	267 ± 8[b]	127 ± 9[c]	104 ± 8[c]	74 ± 13[c]
Storage iron µg/liver	1356 ± 80	1555 ± 140	1614 ± 81[d]	1610 ± 146
Storage iron µg/spleen	166 ± 10	182 ± 12	196 ± 81[d]	185 ± 12
Free erythrocyte protoporphin µg/100 ml	43 ± 1	50 ± 3[d]	51 ± 2[c]	58 ± 3[c]
Plasma zinc µg/100 ml	115 ± 6	63 ± 6[c]	64 ± 5[c]	60 ± 8[c]
Plasma copper µg/100 ml	114 ± 6	151 ± 5[c]	163 ± 10[c]	155 ± 8[c]
Total iron-binding capacity µg/100 ml	386 ± 14	248 ± 10[c]	257 ± 19[c]	260 ± 23[c]
Blood neutrophils no. $mm^3 \times 10^{-2}$	12 ± 1	76 ± 15[c]	88 ± 9[c]	84 ± 13[c]

[a]Each rat received the LEM prepared from 1×10^8 granulocytes every 8 hr. The various measurements were made 5 hr after last i. p. injection.
[b]Mean ± S. E.
[c]Significantly different from normal, $P < 0.005$
[d]Significantly different from normal, $P < 0.05$

may help explain the failure of the bone marrow to respond properly to the developing anemia (34).

An area of current interest in metal metabolism involves the possibility of denying invading microbes a ready access to iron (35, 38). Hence, the hypoferremia produced by injections of LEM might be advantageous to the host during infections. It has been shown that injections of LEM 8 to 48 hr before a usually fatal dose of Salmonella typhimurium will protect rats against this bacterium (13). LEM has been shown to affect a number of different metabolic pathways and to be released from RE cells after a variety of conditions known to activate these cells (11). It is currently difficult to determine to what extent any one of these metabolic pathways might be influencing host resistance. There would seem to be little doubt that alterations in zinc (33) and iron in particular will affect host resistance (35). It appears likely, however, that some of the other metabolic host alterations that occur after LEM injections or during acute or chronic injections and inflammation have a role also (13). It probably will be necessary to investigate some of these other changes in greater detail before it is possible to thoroughly understand the role of the RES in metal metabolism or to assess the importance of metals in host resistance.

REFERENCES

1. Barry, W. E., Tallarida, R. and Rusy, B. F. J. Reticuloendothel. Soc. 5 (1968) 412.
2. Bornstein, D. L. and Walsh, E. C. J. Lab. Clin. Med. 91 (1978) 236.
3. Cartwright, G. E. Sem. Hemat. 3 (1966) 351.
4. Chvapil, M. Life Sci. 13 (1973) 1041.
5. Douglas, S. W. and Adamson, J. W. Blood 45 (1975) 55.
6. Eddington, C. L., Upchurch, H. F. and Kampschmidt, R. F. Proc. Soc. Exp. Biol. Med. 139 (1972) 565.
7. Freireich, E. J., Miller, A., Emerson, C. P. and Ross, J. F. Blood 12 (1957) 972.
8. Freireich, E. J., Ross, J. F., Bayles, T. B., Emerson, C. P. and Finch, S. C. J. Clin. Invest. 36 (1957) 1043.
9. Gutnisky, A. and Van Dyke, D. Proc. Soc. Exp. Biol. Med. 112 (1963) 75.
10. Haurani, F. L. and Meyer, A. In: The Reticuloendothelial system in health and disease (Eds. S. M. Reichard, M. R. Escobar and H. Friedman) Plenum Press, New York Vol. 73A (1976) 171.
11. Kampschmidt, R. F. J. Reticuloendothel. Soc. 23 (1978) 278.
12. Kampschmidt, R. F., Lond, R. D. and Upchurch, H. F. Proc. Soc. Exp. Biol. Med. 139 *1972) 1224.
13. Kampschmidt, R. F. and Pulliam, L. A. J. Reticuloendothel. Soc. 17 (1975) 162.
14. Kampschmidt, R. F. and Pulliam, L. A. Proc. Soc. Exp. Biol.

158 (1978) 32.
15. Kampschmidt, R. F., Pulliam, L. A. and Merriman, C. R. Am. J. Physiol. 235 (1978) in press.
16. Kampschmidt, R. F. and Upchurch, H. F. Proc. Soc. Exp. Biol. Med. 110 (1962) 191.
17. Kampschmidt, R. F. and Upchurch, H. F. Am. J. Physiol. 216 (1969) 1287.
18. Kampschmidt, R. F. and Upchurch, H. F. Proc. Soc. Exp. Biol. Med. 134 (1970) 1150.
19. Kampschmidt, R. F. and Upchurch, H. F. Proc. Soc. Exp. Biol. Med. 155 (1977) 89.
20. Kampschmidt, R. F., Upchurch, H. F., Eddington, C. L. and Pulliam, L. A. Am. J. Physiol. 224 (1973) 530.
21. Kampschmidt, R. F., Upchurch, H. F. and Johnson. H. L. Am. J. Physiol. 208 (1965) 68.
22. Lynch, S. R., Lipschitz, D. A., Bothwell, T. H. and Charlton, R. W. In: Iron in biochemistry and medicine (Eds. A. Jacobs and M. Worwood) Academic Press, New York (1974) 563.
23. Merriman, C. R., Pulliam, L. A. and Kampschmidt, R. F. Proc. Soc. Exp. Biol. Med. 154 (1977) 224.
24. Noyes, W. D., Bothwell, T. H. and Finch, C. A. Brit. J. Haemat. 6 (1960) 43.
25. Pekarek, R. S., Bostian, K. A., Bartelloni, P. J., Calia, F. M. and Beisel, W. R. Am. J. Med. Sci. 258 (1969) 14.
26. Pekarek, R. S., Burghen, G. A., Bartelloni, P. J., Calia, F. M., Bostian, K. A. and Beisel, W. R. J. Lab. Clin. Med. 76 (1970) 293.
27. Pekarek, R. S. and Evans, G. W. Proc. Soc. Exp. Biol. Med. 150 (1975) 755.
28. Pekarek, R. S. and Evans, G. W. Proc. Soc. Exp. Biol. Med. 152 (1976) 573.
29. Pekarek, R. S., Powanda, M. C. and Wannemacher, R. W., Jr. Proc. Soc. Exp. Biol. Med. 141 (1972) 1029.
30. Pekarek, R. S., Wannemacher, R. W., Jr. and Beisel, W. R. Proc. Soc. Exp. Biol. Med. 140 (1972) 685.
31. Price, V. E. and Greenfield, R. C. In: Advances in cancer research (Eds. J. P. Greenstein and A. Haddow) Academic Press, New York Vol. 5 (1958) 199.
32. Rigby, P. G., Strasser, H., Emerson, C. P., Betts, A. and Friedell, G. H. J. Lab. Clin. Med. 59 (1962) 244.
33. Sobocinski, P. Z., Canterbury, W. J., Jr. and Powanda, M. C. Proc. Soc. Exp. Biol. Med. 156 (1977) 334.
34. Steinberg, H. N., Handler, E. S. and Handler, E. E. Blood 47 (1976) 1041.
35. Sussman, M. In: Iron in biochemistry and medicine (Eds. A. Jacobs and M. Worwood) Academic Press, New York (1974) 649.
36. Wannemacher, R. W., Jr., Pekarek, R. S., Thompson, W. L., Curnow, R. T., Beall, F. A., Zenser, T. V., DuRubertis, F. R. and Beisel, W. R. Endocrinology 96 (1975) 651.
37. Ward, H. P., Kurnick, J. E. and Pisarczyk, M. J. J. Clin.

Invest. 50 (1971) 332.
38. Weinberg, E. D. Science 184 (1974) 952.
39. Williams, D. M., Lee, G. R. and Cartwright, G. E. Am. J. Physiol. 227 (1974) 1094.
40. Zarrabi, M. H., Lysik, R., Distefans, J. and Zucker, S. Brit. J. Haematol. 36 (1977) 647.
41. Zucker, S. and Lysil, R. J. Lab. Clin. Med. 84 (1974) 620.

FUNCTION OF MACROPHAGE PROSTAGLANDINS

IN THE PROCESS OF PHAGOCYTOSIS

E. RAZIN[1], U. ZOR[2] and A. GLOBERSON[1]

Departments of Cell Biology[1] and Hormone Research[2],
The Weizmann Institute of Science, Rehovot (Israel)

Prostaglandins (PGs) act as mediators in inflammation and cell-mediated immune responses (1,5,9). Since macrophages participate in the inflammatory reaction, studies were focused on the effects of PGs on macrophage functions. It has been demonstrated that addition of PGs at low doses enhances phagocytosis (8), whereas at pharmacological concentrations phagocytosis is inhibited (2,7,8,10). Furthermore, macrophages were shown to synthesize PGs (3,4), and this process is enhanced by phagocytized particles (6). We therefore attempted to find out whether synthesis of PGs by the macrophage may play a role in phagocytosis.

MATERIALS AND METHODS

Mice. Two to 4 months old (Balb/c x C37BL/6)F_1 male mice obtained from the Animal Breeding Center of the Weizmann Institute were employed throughout this study.

Prostaglandins. PGE_2, $PGF_{1\alpha}$, $PGF_{2\alpha}$ and PGA_1 (kindly donated by Dr. J. Pike, Upjohn Company, Kalamazoo, Michigan) were dissolved in ethanol and then diluted in phosphate buffer saline (PBS) so that the final concentration of ethanol did not exceed 0.1% (v.v).

Macrophage preparation and treatment. Adherent cells were separated from spleens, washed, and incubated in PBS in plastic petri dishes at 37 C in a 5% CO_2 in air atmosphere. The non-adherent cells were subsequently removed.

Phagocytosis assay. Phagocytosis by the macrophages was evaluated by incubating the cells with opsonized sheep erythro-

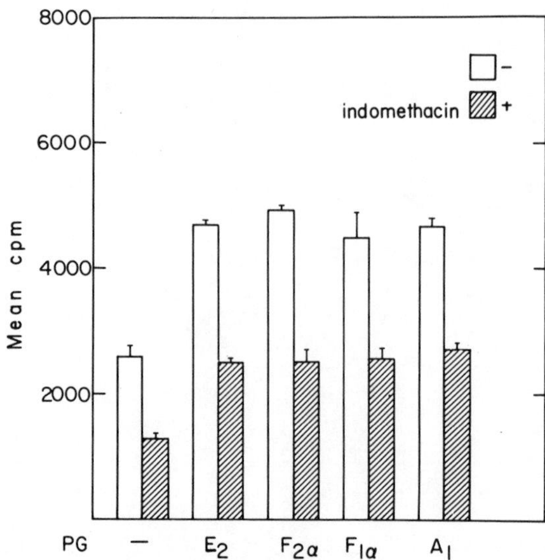

Fig. 1. Inhibition of phagocytosis of opsonized SRC by spleen macrophages treated with indomethacin. Each point represents the mean ± standard error (SE) of 3 replicates. Total cpm initially added was 157859. Results of 1 of 6 repeated experiments behaving in similar manner.

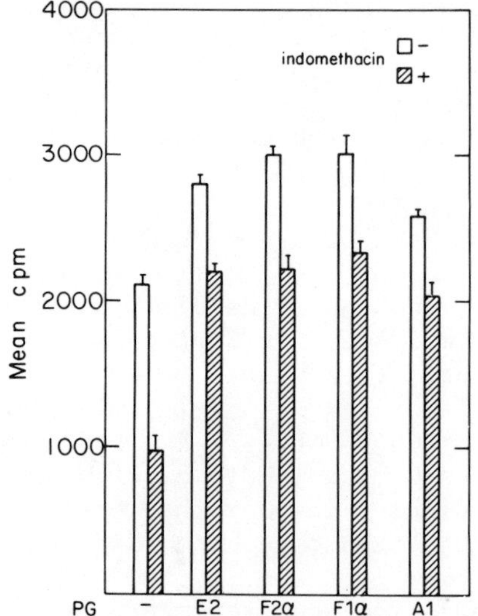

Fig. 2. Inhibition of phagocytosis of unopsonized SRC by spleen macrophages treated with indomethacin. Total cpm initially added was 400,150. Each point represents the mean ± SE of 3 replicates. Results of 1 of 6 repeated experiments behaving in a similar manner.

cytes (SRC) or with unopsonized SRC labeled with ^{51}Cr and subsequently lysing the SRC remaining attached to the cell surface (8).

RESULTS AND DISCUSSION

Our initial experiments were designed to examine the effect of Pgs at various concentrations (10^{-10} to 10^{-2} mg/ml) on phagocytosis of opsonized SRC by stimulated peritoneal macrophages. We observed that PGs (E_2, $F_{2\alpha}$, $F_{1\alpha}$ and A_1) at concentrations of 10^{-8} to 10^{-4} mg/ml, enhanced the phagocytosis significantly, whereas PGs at higher doses (10^{-2} mg/ml) had an inhibitory effect (8). The role of endogenous PGs in the process of phagocytosis was therefore examined by using indomethacin, a known inhibitor of PG synthetase.

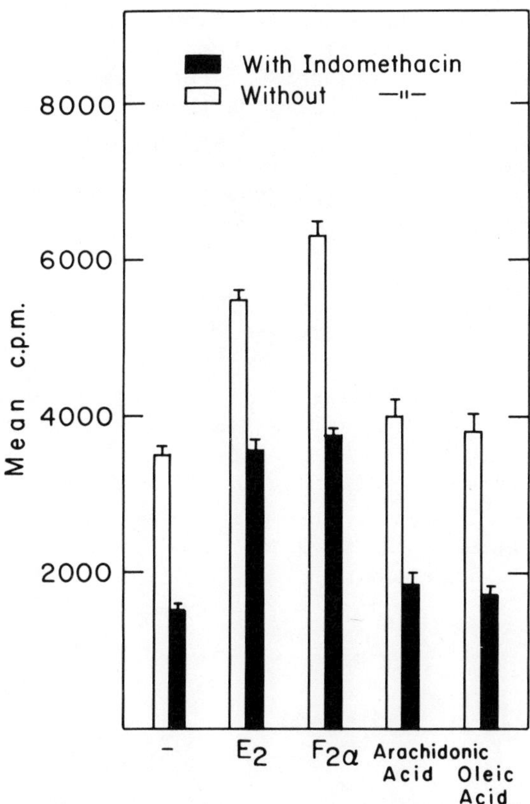

Fig. 3. Influence of arachidonic acid and oleic acid on phagocytosis of opsonized SRC by spleen macrophages, with or without indomethacin treatment. Total cpm initially added was 144,000. Each point represents the mean ± SE of 3 replicates. Results of 1 out of 2 repeated experiments behaving in similar manner.

Adherent cells were incubated at 37 C with 5 μg/ml indomethacin, with or without PGs (10^{-6} mg/ml). Control groups were treated with PBS. One hr later they were rinsed with PBS and reincubated for a further 45 min in the same solutions, except that PGs were added to the PBS control groups which were not treated with indomethacin.

A decrease of about 50% in phagocytosis of SRC was observed, employing either IgG-coated (Fig. 1) or unopsonized SRC (Fig. 2). The inhibitory effect of indomethacin was prevented in cultures in which the various PGS were added. This suggested that the effect of indomethacin was probably due to inhibition of the macrophage production of PG rather than to a nonspecific effect of the drug.

Specificity of the PG effect was further evaluated in an experiment using fatty acids. Hence, the same protocol of experiment was repeated, employing arachidonic and oleic acid instead of PGs. As shown in Fig. 3, these fatty acids did not enhance phagocytosis of opsonized SRC. Furthermore, they did not prevent the effect of indomethacin on the macrophages. Macrophages appear to be the major cell type responsible for PG production in the inflammation site (4) at which phagocytosis plays an important role in removing pathogenic bacteria and foreign particles. The exact mechanism by which PGs affect phagocytosis remains to be elucidated.

SUMMARY

The role of prostaglandins (PGs) in phagocytosis of sheep erythrocytes (SRC) by mouse spleen adherent cells was examined. A decrease of about 50% in the phagocytosis was observed when macrophages were treated with 5 μg/ml indomethacin. Concomitant addition of PGs (10^{-6} mg/ml), however, prevented the inhibitory effect of indomethacin. It is thus suggested that PGs play an important role in phagocytosis.

ACKNOWLEDGEMENT

Support for these studies was provided by the Minerva Foundation.

REFERENCES

1. Berenbaum, M. C., Purves, E. C. and Addison, I. E., Immunology,30 (1976) 815.
2. Cox, J. P. and Karnovsky, M. C., J. Cell Biol., 59 (1973) 480.
3. Flower, R. J. and Blackwell, J. G., Biochem. Pharmac., 25 (1976) 285.
4. Gordon, D., Bray, M. A. and Morley, J., Nature, 262 (1976) 401.
5. Henney, C. S., Bourne, H. R. and Lichtenstein, L. M., J. Immunol., 108 (1972) 1526.
6. Humes, J. L., Bonney, R. J., Pelus, L., Dahlger, M. E., Sadowski, S. J., Kuehl, F. A. and Davies, P., Nature, 269 (1977) 149.
7. Loose, L. D. and Di Luzio, N. R., J. Reticuloendothel. Soc., 13 (1973) 70.
8. Razin, E., Bauminger, S. and Globerson, A., J. Reticuloendothel. Soc., 23 (1978) 237.
9. Smith, J. W., Steiner, A. L. and Parker, C. W., J. Clin. Invest, 50 (1971) 442.
10. Weissman, G., Zurier, R. B. and Hoffstein, S., Am. J. Pathol., 68 (1972) 539.

THE MONONUCLEAR PHAGOCYTE SYSTEM AND HEMOPOIESIS

M. RACHMILEWITZ, B. RACHMILEWITZ, M. CHAOUAT,
H. ZLOTNIK and M. SCHLESINGER
Department of Experimental Medicine and Cancer Research
The Hebrew University-Hadassah Medical School
Jerusalem (ISRAEL)

The *in vitro* bone marrow culture technique developed in recent years and employed in extensive studies has demonstrated that mononuclear phagocytes originate in the bone marrow. The colony forming cells are the committed precursors common to the granulocytic and monocytic lines. The proliferation of the colony forming cells requires a substance or substances which possess colony stimulating activity (CSA). The principal cell in the peripheral blood responsible for the elaboration of colony stimulating activity is the monocyte (7). The close ancestral relationship between granulocytes and monocytes may explain the proliferation of both cell populations in the neoplastic process of myelomonocytic leukemia. The normal function of the monocyte is retained in cells of monocytic and myelomonocytic leukemia (9). The serum colony stimulating activity was found to correlate with the level of circulating monocytes (18). Monocyte-derived macrophages and tissue macrophages are also active producers of CSA (8). Since tissue macrophages retain their function during severe bone marrow failure, these cells may serve as a reservoir of production of CSA for restoration of granulopoiesis.

The origin of macrophages and their precursors from the bone marrow and the cell kinetics were demonstrated by *in vivo* experiments using the cell labeling with tritiated thymidine (36, 37).

The role of the monocyte-macrophage in host defense has been extensively studied and will be amply discussed in this book. The present paper will be limited to the secretory function of macrophages which has a bearing on hemopoiesis and on some clinical implications. Our interest in this field stems from our work on vitamin B_{12} binding proteins. Of the 3 vitamin B_{12} binding proteins, the transcobalamins (TC), TCII has been shown to transport vitamin B_{12} and to deliver it to the tissues (1, 25). The transport function of TCII has been demonstrated in vitro on cell systems such as Ehrlich ascites cells, reticulocytes, HeLa cells, transformed lymphocytes, fibroblasts and mouse leukemic lymphoblasts (9, 26-28). In man, the role of TCII in delivering vitamin B_{12} to tissues is evidenced by the observation that hereditary TCII deficiency leads to lack of cellular maturation of the hemopoietic system and neonatal megaloblastic anemia in spite of normal serum concentration of vitamin B_{12} (6, 12, 13).

Increased TCII levels have been found in the sera of patients suffering from different pathological conditions. These include Gaucher's disease (6, 23), systemic lupus erythematosus, rheumatoid arthritis, dermatomyositis and chronic monocytic leukemia (Table I). All these clinical conditions are characterized by the stimulation and proliferation of the reticuloendothelial system (RES). High TCII levels have also been found in the sera of patients with acute leukemia and malignant lymphoma in the active state of the disease (23, 28).

The site of TCII synthesis is not yet established. Indirect evidence from animal experiments indicates that liver and possibly other organs may be involved in the synthesis of TCII (4, 30, 34). The increased serum TCII content observed in clinical conditions in which the common denominator is the stimulation of the mononuclear-phagocyte system suggested that the cells of this system might be the site of TCII synthesis. This hypothesis was tested in an experimental model - the peritoneal exudate cells (PEC) of mice. The mouse was found to be the most suitable experimental animal for this study since mouse TCII and human TCII have similar features and analogous metabolism (33, 34). Preliminary findings of this study were reported (24).

MATERIALS AND METHODS

Animals. Male inbred mice of the BALB/c strain, kept at the animal colony of the Department of Experimental Medicine and Cancer Research, were used.

The preparation of cell suspensions. Peritoneal cells were obtained either from normal, unstimulated mice or from mice injected with a single intraperitoneal (i. p.) injection of 2.5 ml 2.98% thioglycollate. The cells were collected from the peritoneal cavity by repeated washings with saline. Bone marrow cells were obtained either from normal donors or from mice stimulated by a single i. p. injection of thioglycollate. To collect bone marrow cells the femurs of donor mice were dissected out, cut at both ends and the contents of the bone marrow cavity was

TABLE I

Serum Concentration of TCII on Healthy Individuals and in Patients with Various Disorders

	Serum TCII pg/ml (Mean ± S.D.)	Serum UBBC[b] pg/ml (Mean ± S.D.)
Normal values	886 ± 214	1200 ± 207
Acute Leukemia	3048 ± 1419	3857 ± 1483
Hodgkin and Non-Hodgkin Lymphoma	3346 ± 769	4100 ± 808
Gaucher's Disease	3195 ± 209	3797 ± 2280
Chronic Monocytic	15646	16130
Leukemia	5005	6585
Acute Immunological Diseases[a]	3244 ± 688	4090 ± 638

[a]Rheumatoid arthritis - 2 cases; Systemic Lupus erythematosis - 5 cases; Dermatomyositis - 1 case; Scleroderma - 1 case
[b]UBBC = Unsaturated vitamin B_{12} binding capacity

flushed out with saline by a syringe. Suspensions of cells from various lymphoid organs (thymus, spleen, lymph nodes) were prepared as described previously (20). All cell suspensions were exposed to 0.83% NH_4Cl according to the method of Boyle (3) to lyse red blood cells. Finally, the cells were suspended in a volume of 2 ml saline. The number of cells was determined in each sample and the cells were disintegrated by ultrasonic vibration for 2-3 min. The sonicates were centrifuged for 10 min at 12,000 rpm and the supernates were separated.

Organ homogenates. Homogenates of brain, liver and kidney were exposed to 0.83% NH_4Cl, washed and spun at 3,000 rpm for 10 min and the sediments were collected. Two ml of saline were added to the sediments, they were resuspended and exposed to ultrasonic vibration as described above. The sonicates were spun at 3,000 rpm for 10 min and the supernatant fluids were harvested. The optical density of the supernates was determined at a wavelength of 280 µm and the TCII content was assayed in each sample. In some experiments similar homogenates were prepared from cells of the peritoneal cacity, spleen and bone marrow for determination of TCII content.

Cell cultures. PEC from either normal or stimulated mice were suspended in MEM-S culture (Grand Island Biological Co., New York, New York), supplemented with 10% fetal calf serum (Grand Island Biological Co., New York, New York), penicillin (100 units/ml) and streptomycin (100 μg/ml). In a few experiments Hank's culture medium (Bio-Lab, Jerusalem) was used instead of MEM-S. The use of culture media which are supplemented with vitamin B_{12} had to be avoided to prevent interference with the assay of TCII. Two ml of cell suspensions containing 2 x 10^6 cells/ml were placed in 30 mm plastic Petri dishes (Falcon) and incubated in a humidified atmosphere containing 5% CO_2 and 95% air at 37 C. The supernatant fluid was collected at various time intervals after the cultures were set up and assayed for TCII content.

The cells grown in culture consisted of either the total population of peritoneal cells or of the adherent and nonadherent subpopulations. Separation into these subpopulations was achieved by letting the peritoneal cells attached to plastic Petri dishes for 3 hr at 37 C. The nonadherent cells were then collected with a Pasteur pipette, and kept in culture separately. Fresh culture medium was added to the cells adhering to the plastic dishes and to the nonadherent cells, and both cell types were incubated for varying time intervals. At the end of the incubation period the supernatant fluid was separated and the content of TCII was determined.

Assay of TCII. For the determination of TCII in cell sonicates a volume of sonicate containing the equivalent of 2 x 10^6 cells was used. The TCII content of tissue sonicates was assayed in volumes varying from 25 μl to 100 μg. The samples were labeled with $^{57}CoB_{12}$ using a solution containing 10,000 pg/ml $^{57}CoB_{12}$ (Radiochemical Center, Amersham, specific activity 100-130 μCi/μg). The minimal amount of radioactive vitamin B_{12} added was 100 pg $^{57}CoB_{12}$. Higher amounts of radioactive vitamin B_{12} were added whenever required to provide full saturation of the B_{12} binders. After incubation for 10 min at 37 C in a shaking bath which allowed the $^{57}CoB_{12}$ binding, the B_{12} protein binders were separated quantitatively by using the charged cellulose filter technique described by Selhub et al. (29). The principle of the technique is the following: the $^{57}CoB_{12}$ labeled solution is passed through a stack of charged cellulose filters composed of 1 negatively charged cellulose nitrate filter (Schleicher and Schull, porosity 0.45 μ, 25 mm in diameter) and 3 DEAE filters (Whatman's DE-81, 25 mm in diameter). The DEAE filters used are chemically identical with the granular Whatman's DE-52 used for chromatographic separation of the transcobalamins. TCII absorbs selectively and quantitatively to the cellulose nitrate filter. TCI and TCIII, being negatively charged molecules, pass through the negatively charged cellulose-nitrate filter and bind chemically to the DE-81 filters. The lower retention of TCIII by the DE-81 filters allows specific desorption of TCIII from a duplicate stack of filters with a low ionic strength solution. Excessive $^{57}CoB_{12}$ is removed by repeated washings of the filters with the buffer solution used in this system - borate buffer 0.1 M pH 8.5

The filters were separated after the washings and their radioactivity was determined for 1 min in a Well type scintillation counter. The results were expressed either in cpm of the radioactivity retained on the filters or as ng vitamin B_{12} bound per 2×10^6 cells. Since the molar ratio binding between the B_{12} molecule and the transcobalamins molecules is 1:1 (2), the amount of TCII was expressed as ng of vitamin B_{12} bound.

RESULTS

In vivo experiments. Sonicates of cell suspensions were prepared from lymphoid organs and assayed for TCII levels. Low concentrations of TCII were detected in sonicates of peritoneal and spleen cells from unstimulated animals (Table II). The concentration of TCII per mg protein was higher in spleen cells than in PEC. The large volume of peritoneal cells probably accounts for the higher concentration of TCII per cell found in PEC as compared with spleen cells. Considerable amounts of TCII were present in peripheral blood monocytes. The highest TCII levels were found in bone marrow cells. In contrast, no TCII was detected in cells of the mesenteric and peripheral lymph nodes nor in the thymus. In homogenates of the kidney and brain, TCII was undetectable. Liver homogenates contained low, irregular levels of TCII.

Following a single intraperitoneal injection of thioglycollate the concentration of TCII in PEC increased considerably already 4 hr after stimulation. The level of TCII continued to increase 8 hr after stimulation and reached a peak at 24 hr (Fig. 1). At that point TCII reached a concentration which was about 100-fold higher than the initial TCII concentration in the unstimulated PEC. A precipitous fall of the TCII level in PEC was observed after 48 hr. Thereafter, TCII concentration in PEC remained similar to that in unstimulated cells.

Parallel to TCII determination in PEC, the level of TCII was determined in bone marrow (BM) cells at various time intervals after thioglycollate stimulation. Prior to stimulation, BM cells contained high levels of TCII. Within 4 hr after stimulation, a slight drop in the concentration of TCII was detected in the BM (Fig. 1). At 8 hr after stimulation, the TCII level dropped markedly. At 24 hr, the level of TCII in the BM cells was almost completely recovered and continued to increase during the following 24 hr. No significant changes were found in the number of the BM cells during this period.

TABLE II

Concentration of TCII in Sonicates of Various Cells and Organ Homogenates of Unstimulated Mice

Cells and Organs Tested	Pg per 1 x 10^6 Cells	Pg per mg Protein
Bone marrow cells	32.3	459.6
Peripheral blood monocytes	6.7	N.D.
Peritoneal exudate cells	1.8	11.1
Spleen cells	1.0	32.3
Peripheral blood granulocytes	0	0
Lymph node cells	0	0
Thymus cells	0	0
Liver		0-2.1
Kidney		0
Brain		0
Serum	31.000-52.000 pg/ml	510-860

[a]Not done

TCII production in vitro. PEC from either normal of stimulated mice were cultured in vitro and TCII levels were determined in cell sonicates and in the medium. TCII concentration in the cells remained constantly low all through the incubation period, regardless of the source of the cells (less than 0.01 ng TCII/ 2 x 10^6 cells). In contrast to the constant low intracellular levels of TCII, extracellular TCII increased daily. The production and release of TCII into the medium was similar in non-stimulated PEC and in PEC harvested 24 hr after thioglycollate stimulation (Fig. 2). Both cell populations secreted considerable amounts of TCII which increased daily throughout the incubation period.

In order to identify which cell subpopulation produces TCII, peritoneal cells were separated according to their capacity to adhere to a plastic surface. Adherent cells isolated from the peritoneal cavity of either unstimulated mice or mice which were stimulated in vivo for 24 hr produced similar, high quantities of TCII throughout the incubation period (Fig. 3). The amount of

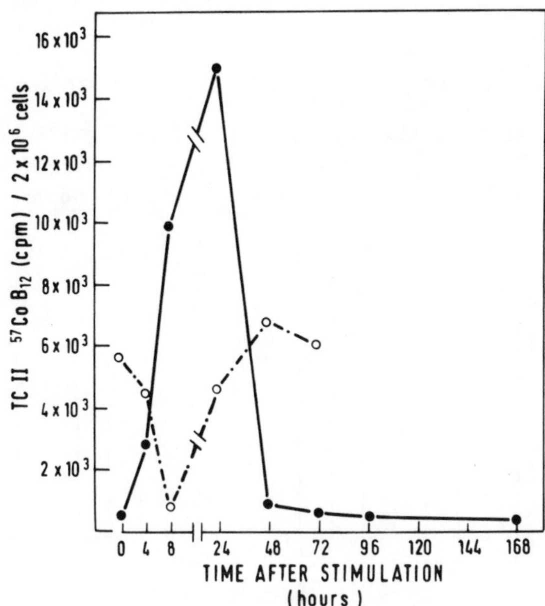

Fig. 1. The concentration of TCII in peritoneal exudate cells and in bone marrow cells at various time intervals after an intraperitoneal injection of thioglycollate. Peritoneal exudate cells (•), bone marrow cells (o).

TCII produced by the adherent cells was, in all experiments, almost as high as that produced by the total unseparated population of PEC

Nonadherent cells from either normal mice or from animals stimulated for 24 hr failed to produce significant amounts of TCII (fig. 3).

The effect of bleeding on TCII concentration in the bone marrow. Since the BM of the mouse was found to have the highest TCII concentration of all organs examined, it seemed of interest to examine the changes in TCII during increased BM activity and accelerated cell proliferation. For this purpose TCII content of the BM cells of the mouse was examined following bleeding.

Balb/c mice, 3 months old, were bled 0.25-0.3 ml of blood from the orbital vein. Four hr after bleeding the mice were killed and bone marrow cells were collected from the shaft of the femur. The cells were washed and a suspension of 3 x 10^6 cells in saline was prepared for TCII determination.

The results depicted in Table III show that within 4 hr after bleeding the hematocrit of the bled animals fell from 52 to 42

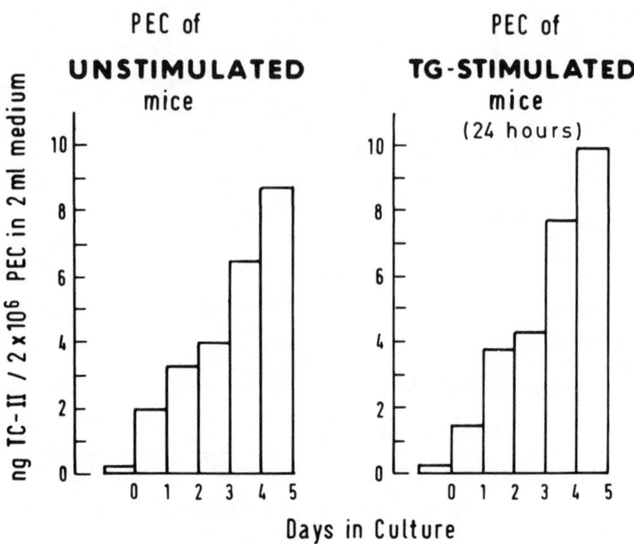

Fig. 2. In vitro secretion of TCII by peritoneal exudate cells (PEC) obtained from either unstimulated mice or from mice injected 24 hr previously with a single injection of thioglycollate (TG).

TABLE III

Effect of Bleeding on Hematocrit and TCII Concentration in Bone Marrow Cells

	Number of Determinations	Hematocrit (Mean ± S.E.)	TCII in BM[a] (Mean ± S.E.)
Normal mice	11	52 ± 1	23,700 ± 1,700
4 hr after bleeding	6	42 ± 1	15,000 ± 1,200
Percentage decrease		19.3	36.7

[a]Expressed as cpm of $^{57}CoB_{12}/3 \times 10^6$ bone marrow (BM) cells

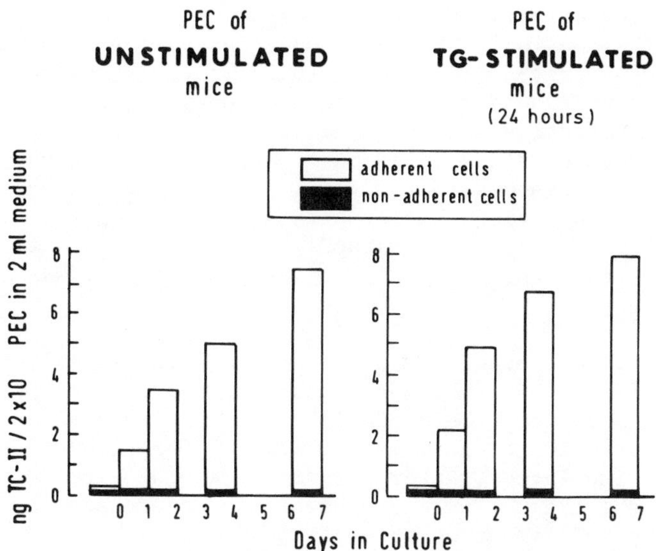

Fig. 3. _In vitro_ secretion of TCII by the adherent and nonadherent subpopulations of peritoneal exudate cells obtained from the peritoneal cavity of either unstimulated mice or from mice injected 24 hr previously with thioglycollate.

and the TCII concentration decreased by 37%, Twenty-four hr after bleeding the concentration of TCII approached normal values.

The decrease in TCII following bleeding and the consequent increased activity of the BM could be explained by release of TCII by marrow cells due to increased demands of rapidly proliferating cells for vitamin B_{12} and its carrier protein. A second possiblity is based on the concept of stem cell competition. This concept postulates that increased demands for cells of 1 line can result in depletion of stem cells required for production of another line. The increased erythropoietic activity following bleeding may thus lead to a decrease in mononuclear cell population and diminished production of TCII. This explanation is supported by the observations of Metcalf (16) that bleeding reduced the total number of _in vitro_ colony-forming cells in the BM of mice but caused a significant increase of erythropoietic cells.

DISCUSSION

Macrophages have been shown to synthesize and secrete a

number of biologically active substances (10, 11, 17, 35). These include pyrogens, lysosomal hydrolases, lysozyme, complement factors, plasminogen activators and prostaglandins. It has also been suggested that cells of the RES might possibly be involved in the synthesis of ferritin (15) and haptoglobin (19). Experimental studies on erythropoietin production in anephric rats indicate that the Kupffer cells may be the major source for erythropoietin (21). The present study based on experiments performed both *in vivo* and *in vitro* shows that TCII is produced and released by macrophages. Following thioglycollate stimulation the level of TCII in PEC was found to be markedly increased. *In vitro* experiments showed that the synthesis and release of TCII was limited to macrophages.

Of all organs examined in the unstimulated animal, the bone marrow was found to be the most active TCII producer. It is now well established that the progenitors of the mononuclear-phagocyte system situated in the bone marrow (10, 17, 35) produce blood monocytes. The latter, after a short period of circulation, migrate into the tissues as macrophages and accumulate at sites of inflammatory and immunologic reactions (31, 32).

The observation that concomitant with the rise of TCII in PEC there was a marked fall of TCII in the bone marrow indicates that TCII-producing cells from the bone marrow migrate into the peritoneal cavity. This, in turn, suggests that TCII is synthesized in the bone marrow by early stages of the mononuclear-phagocyte system.

The demonstration that macrophages actively produce and secrete TCII provides an explanation for the clinical observations which prompted studies described here. The high TCII levels found in diseases in which the marophage pools are excessively large as in chronic monocytic leukemia, seem to reflect the increased TCII production by proliferating monocytes. Lipoid storage disease, like Gaucher, is associated with proliferation of macrophages transformed into foam cells resulting in increased serum TCII in this disease (5, 23). The high serum TCII observed in the active stage of immunologic disorders and in hematological malignancies can well be explained by the reactive macrophage stimulation in these disorders. The TCII determination in the serum may provide a marker which enables the assessment of the mononuclear-phagocyte response and its extent.

The work presented demonstrates that monocytes and macrophages synthesize transcobalamin II which is essential for normal blood production. The determination of TCII in the BM which appears to be the most important site of TCII production may serve as a marker to follow the migration of TCII-producing cells to other organs.

The results of the experiments on bled mice suggest that the TCII fluctuation may reflect the response of the BM to various stimuli affecting hemopoiesis.

SUMMARY

Extensive studies on the secretory function of macrophages in recent years revealed that substances involved in blood production are synthesized by macrophages. Of these substances the production of transferrin, possibly also ferritin and haptoglobin, have been demonstrated. Experimental studies on erythropoietin production in anephric rats indicate that the Kupffer cells may be the major source of erythropoietin. This presentation is dealing with the function of macrophages in producing the primary transport protein of vitamin B_{12}, transcobalamin II (TCII), which is vital for normal blood production.

Increased TCII levels found in clinical conditions in which the common denominator is the stimulation and proliferation of the mononuclear-phagocyte system suggested the possibility that TCII may be produced by the cells of this system (macrophages, monocytes). This hypothesis was tested in peritoneal exudate cells (PEC) of mice as an experimental model.

Of all organs examined in the unstimulated mice, bone marrow (BM), peripheral blood monocytes, spleen cells and PEC contained TCII. The highest concentration of TCII was found in the BM cells. Following stimulation, TCII increased markedly in the PEC, reaching a peak after 24 hr. Concomitantly, TCII decreased in the BM cells. No change was observed in the TCII content of the other organs following stimulation. PEC of stimulated and unstimulated mice incubated _in vitro_ produced and secreted TCII into the medium. The production and secretion of TCII was found to be limited to the adherent cell population only, i. e., the macrophages.

The TCII concentration in BM cells was found to be decreased 4 hr after bleeding.

ACKNOWLEDGEMENTS

This study was supported by grants from the Israel Center Association (2/76: 7/78), the Marcia and Max Eber Fund, and the Herman Lee Fund.

REFERENCES

1. Allen, R. H. Brit. J. Haematol. 33 (1976) 161.
2. Allen, H. R. and Magerus, P. W. J. Biol. Chem. 247 (1972) 7702.
3. Boyle, W. Transplantation 6 (1968) 761.
4. England, J. M., Tavill, A. S. and Chanarin, I. Clin. Sci. Mol. Med. 45 (1973) 479.
5. Gilbert, H. S. and Weinreb, N. New Eng. J. Med. 295 (1976) 1096.
6. Gimpert, E., Jakob, M. and Hitzig, W. H. Blood 45 (1975) 71.
7. Golde, D. W. and Cline, M. J. J. Clin. Invest. 51 (1972) 2981.
8. Golde, D. W., Finley, T. N. and Cline, M. J. Lancet II (1972) 1397.
9. Golde, D. W., Rothman, B. and Cline, M. J. Blood 43 (1974) 749.
10. Gordon, S. and Cohn, Z. A. Int. Rev. Cytol. 36 (1973) 171.
11. Gordon, S., Tood, J. and Cohn, Z. A. J. Exp. Med. 139 (1974) 1228.
12. Hakami, N., Neiman, P. E., Canellos, G. P. and Lazerson, J. New Eng. J. Med. 285 (1971) 1163.
13. Hitzig, W. H., Dohmann, U., Pluss, H. J. and Vischer, D. J. Pediat. 85 (1974) 622.
14. Hoffbrand, A. V., Tripp, E. and Das, K. C. Brit. J. Haematol. 24 (1973) 147.
15. Jacob, A. and Warwood, M. New Eng. J. Med. 292 (1975) 951.
16. Metcalf, D. Brit. J. Haematol. 16 (1969) 397.
17. Meuret, G. and Hoffman, G. Brit. J. Haematol. 24 (1973) 275.
18. Moore, M. A. S., Spitzer, G., Metcalf, D., et al. Brit. J. Haematol. 27 (1974) 47.
19. Palmer, W. G. and Schuler, R. L. Biomedicine 25 (1976) 88.
20. Patinkin, D., Schlesinger, M. and Doljanski, F. Cancer Res. 30 (1970) 489.
21. Peschle, C., Mavone, G., Genovese, A., et al. Blood 47 (1976) 325.
22. Rachmilewitz, B. and Rechmilewitz, M. Isr. J. Med. Sci. 12 (1976) 583.
23. Rachmilewitz, B. and Rachmilewitz, M. New Eng. J. Med. 296 (1977) 1174.
24. Rachmilewitz, B., Rachmilewitz, M., Chaouat, M. and Schlesinger, M. Biomedicine 27 (1977) 213.
25. Rappazzo, M. E. and Hall, C. A. J. Clin. Invest. 51 (1972) 1915.
26. Retief, F. P., Gottlieb, C. W. and Herbert, V. J. Clin. Invest. 45 (1966) 1907.
27. Rosenberg, L. E., Lilljeqvist, A. and Allen, R. H. J. Clin. Invest. 52 (1973) 69a.
28. Ryel, E. M., Meyer, L. M. and Gams, R. A. Blood 44 (1974) 427.
29. Selhub, J., Rachmilewitz, M., Chaouat, M. and Schlesinger, M. Biomedicine 27 (1977) 213.
30. Sonneborn, D. W., Abouna, G. and Mendez-Picon, G. Biochim. Biophis. Acta 273 (1972) 283.

31. Spector, W. G., Walters, M. N. I. and Willoughby, D. A. J. Path. Bact. 90 (1965) 181.
32. Spector, W. G. and Willoughby, D. A. J. Path. Bact. 96 (1968) 389.
33. Tan, C. H. and Blaisdell, S. J. Biochim. Biophis. Acta 444 (1976) 416.
34. Tan, C. H. and Hansen, H. J. Proc. Soc. Exp. Biol. Med. 127 (1968) 740.
35. Van Furth, R. Sem. Hemat. 7 (1970) 125.
36. Van Furth, R. and Diessehoff-Den Dulk, M. M. C. J. Exp. Med. 132 (1970) 813.
37. Whitelaw, D. M., Bell, M. F. and Batles, H. F. J. Cell Physiol. 72 (1968) 65.
38. Zittoun, J., Zittoun, R., Marquet, J. and Sultan, C. Brit. Haematol. 31 (1975) 287.

MACROPHAGES AS REGULATORS OF GRANULOPOIESIS

R. N. APTE, E. HELLER, C. F. HERTOGS and D. H. PLUZNIK

Department of Life Sciences
Bar-Ilan University
Ramat-Gan (ISRAEL)

Much evidence is available which indicates the ability of the macrophage to elaborate factors which can either increase (5, 9, 11, 13, 16, 22) or decrease (17, 20, 21, 25) the proliferation of hemopoietic cells. The question whether committed hemopoietic stem cells proliferation can be regulated by macrophages can now be answered by using the soft agar technique. The introduction of this technique for cloning granulocyte and macrophage precursor cells by Pluznik and Sachs (27) and Bradley and Metcalf (14) provided a new approach to the evaluation of the regulation of granulopoiesis and macrophage formation. The clonal growth in soft agar cultures of such precursor cells, termed colony forming units-culture (CFU-C), is wholly dependent on the presence of a stimulatory substance designated colony stimulating factor (CSF) (28). In the mouse assay this substance is produced and/or released by cell suspensions from many organs including hemopoietic tissues, by cell lines and it is also present in the serum and urine (18, 29, 32). White blood cells are a major secretory source of CSF elaborated *in vitro*. However, the exact relationship between the various white blood cell populations in the production of CSF is unclear. Recently, different independent groups have shown that blood monocytes and tissue macrophages are the major hemopoietic source of CSF in humans and mice (12, 13, 19). It has been shown that CSF can be considered *in vivo* as granulopoietin (3). Thus, this factor plays an essential role in regulating proliferation and differentiation of committed stem cells to mature granulocytes and macrophages, not only *in vitro* but also *in vivo*.

Macrophages and granulocytes are cardinal cellular elements in host resistance and inflammation and they participate in an essential way in the elimination of various kinds of invading microorganisms. Bacterial lipopolysaccharides (LPS), products of gram-negative bacteria, cause pronounced effects on the granulopoietic system. After an injection of LPS to mice, a rise in tissue and serum CSF, as well as a rise in the number of granulocyte/macrophage progenitor cells in the marrow and spleen is observed (3). Analogous results were obtained when staphylococcal enterotoxin B (SEB), an exotoxin derived from gram-positive bacteria, *Staphylococcus aureus*, was injected into mice (14). In addition, both bacterial products are potent lymphocyte mitogens, LPS being a B cell mitogen (10), while SEB is a T cell mitogen (26). Both mitogens also induce generation of CSF when added to lymphoid cell suspensions (14, 15, 24). The mechanism of generation of CSF by macrophages and lymphocytes in lymphoid cell cultures stimulated with bacterial toxins (LPS and SEB) was studied in the present communication. Special emphasis was put on the role of the degree of activation of the macrophage on secretion of CSF, as well as on the regulatory role of macrophages and their soluble products in this secretory process.

MATERIALS AND METHODS

Mice. C3H/eB, C3H/HeJ, Balb/c and ICR, as well as C3H/eB congenitally athymic (nude) male mice were purchased from the Weizmann Institute of Science (Rehovot, Israel). CBA/N mice were generously provided by Dr. I. Scher from the Naval Medical Research Institute (Bethesda, Maryland) and were subsequently bred and raised in our facilities. All mice were used at the age of 9 to 12 weeks.

Mitogens. LPS-W from *Escherichia coli* 055:B5 was purchased from Difco Laboratories (Detroit, Michigan). Staphylococcal enterotoxin B (SEB) was kindly provided by Dr. I. Hertman of the Israel Institute for Biological Research (Ness-Ziona, Israel).

Lymphoid cell cultures. Spleen or thymus was removed aseptically from mice, dispersed through a stainless steel screen into PBS and washed twice. Nucleated viable cells (2 x 10^6/ml) were incubated in RPMI-1640 medium supplemented with 5% heat-inactivated horse serum (Bio Lab, Jerusalem, Israel) in 1 ml aliquots at 37 C in a humidified atmosphere at 5% CO_2 usually for 4 days. At the end of incubation, cells were removed by centrifugation and cell-free supernatant was stored at -20 C until used.

Enriched cell populations. (a) Peritoneal macrophages were obtained from unstimulated mice or mice which had been injected 3 days before with 1.5 ml of 10% proteose-peptone or thioglycolate solutions (Difco Laboratories, Detroit, Michigan). Mice were sacrificed and peritoneal cells were collected from the peritoneal cavity after injection of 5 ml PBS. After being aspirated from the peritoneal cavity, cells were washed and cultured under conditions similar to those described above. The cells were planted on petri dishes and incubated for 2 hr and then washed vigorously 3 times to remove nonphagocytic loosely attached cells and subsequently cultured. (b) Splenic or thymic lymphocyte suspensions were depleted of adherent cells by passage through 2 subsequent columns of pyrex wool (Pyrex Wool Owens-Corning Fiberglass Corp, Corning, New York). Adherence columns were constructed in plastic syringes and each contained 1 g pyrex wool which had previously been washed, autoclaved and equilibrated with warm PBS supplemented with 5% horse serum before use. Approximately 1 x 10^8 cells in a volume of 2 ml were loaded onto each column. The cells were incubated at first for 20 min at the upper part of the column and then washed into the lower part for an additional incubation period of 25 min. All separation procedures were performed at 37 C. At the end of the incubation time each column was washed with 30 ml of PBS and the cells were collected, washed and subsequently cultured as described above.

Assay for CSF. CSF of the culture fluids from the different cell cultures was assayed by its ability to stimulate colony formation from murine marrow cells in the soft agar system. Bone marrow (BM) cells (10^5) were cloned in soft agar medium on a harder agar base (0.5%), supplemented in experiments with LPS with 15%, or in experiments with SEB with 30% of the culture fluids and 25% of horse serum. Cultures were incubated for 7 days, and cell colonies growing in soft agar were counted microscopically.

The results shown in each figure and table are average results obtained from 5 experiments.

RESULTS

Interaction Between Macrophages and T Lymphocytes in Generation of CSF Induced by SEB

In a previous study it was shown that spleen cell suspensions, although containing less mature T cells than thymic suspensions, elaborate larger amounts of CSF when stimulated by SEB (15). These results were interpreted as indicating that a possible cooperation between macrophages and T cells is needed in generation of such type of CSF, since the spleen is richer in macrophages than the thymus. In order to test this hypothesis the experiments described below were performed.

Macrophage dependence of SEB-induced CSF generation. When thymus cell cultures (2.5 x 10^6/ml) were incubated for 4 days in an optimal dose of SEB (10 μg/ml), a large amount of CSF was generated, which supported the development of 145 $\pm$ 5 colonies/10^5

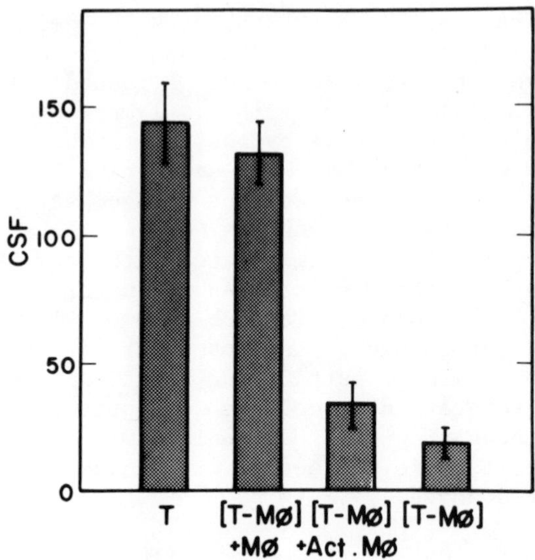

Fig. 1. Restoration of CSF generation in SEB-stimulated purified thymocytes after addition of nonactivated and activated macrophages.

bone marrow cells seeded. However, when the thymus cells were filtered through a pyrex wool adherence column, the effluent nonadherent cells (T-MØ) largely lost their ability to secrete CSF in response to SEB and could support the growth of only 18 ± 5 colonies/10^5 bone marrow cells seeded. When such SEB-stimulated nonadherent thymocytes (2 x 10^6 cells/ml) were supplemented with 5% of peritoneal macrophages from unstimulated mice, the ability to generate CSF in such cultures was reconstituted (Fig. 1). Macrophages, when cultured at the same cell concentration as added to the T lymphocyte cultures, generated only very minute amounts of CFS which could support the growth of only 9 ± 5 colonies/10^5 bone marrow cells. Activated macrophages harvested from mice stimulated with 2.93% thioglycolate (TG) augmented only slightly the secretion of CSF in cultures of nonadherent thymocytes. Thus, it seems that an interaction between macrophages and T lymphocytes leads to secretion of large amounts of CSF.

Effect of macrophage culture fluids on generation of CSF by T lymphocytes. Macrophage supernatants were prepared by incubating nonactivated macrophages (10^5/ml) for 24 hr without SEB, and the culture fluids were thereafter collected. Nonadherent thymocytes were subsequently cultured for 4 days with 10 μg/ml SEB. In culture fluids of such lymphocyte suspensions the ability to generate CSF was restored (Fig. 2). Such supernatants, when prepared from thioglycolate-activated macrophages, had only a very small restoring capacity in this system.

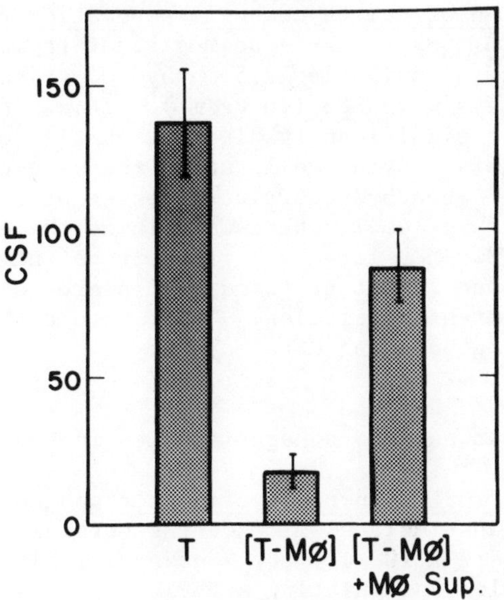

Fig. 2. Restoration of CSF generation in SEB purified thymocytes after addition of macrophage supernatants.

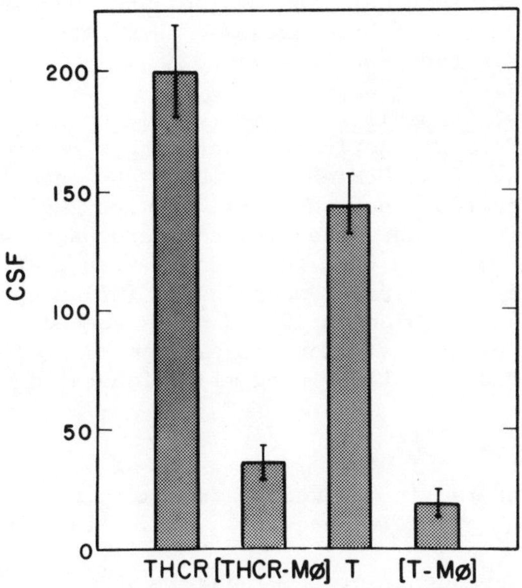

Fig. 3. Generation of CSF by SEB stimulated hydrocortisone resistant thymus cell (THCR).

Identification of the thymus cell population generating CSF in response to SEB. Hydrocortisone resistant thymus cells (THCR) (obtained 48 hr after injecting 2.5 mg hydrocortisone/mouse) were incubated for 4 days with SEB (10 μg/ml). It was found that CSF was generated in a significantly higher amount as compared to CSF obtained from regular thymus cells under the same experimental conditions (Fig. 3). When hydrocortisone resistant thymus cells were filtered through pyrex wool adherence columns the effluent non-adherent cells (THCR-MØ) largely lost their potential to generate CSF. Hydrocortisone resistant thymus cells are considered as a mature immunocompetent population. Thus, mature thymocytes can respond to SEB in generating CSF.

Interaction Between Macrophages and LPS in Generation of CSF

Generation of CSF by nonactivated macrophages. Peritoneal macrophages from unstimulated mice of the strains C3H/eB and C3H/HeJ were cultured (2×10^5/ml) for 4 days with different amounts of LPS and the colony stimulating activity was tested in the culture fluids collected. Elevated levels of CSF were detected in supernatants of macrophages from C3H/eB mice stimulated in culture by 10, 50 and 100 μg/ml LPS. Only small amounts of CSF were elaborated by macrophages obtained from C3H/HeJ (Fig. 4). Similar results were obtained when adherent spleen cells were cultured with LPS. However, such cell suspensions are unavoidably contaminated with adherent fibroblasts and therefore peritoneal macrophages were used in the present study.

Comparison of the ability of activated and nonactivated macrophages to generate CSF. Activated macrophages were obtained from the peritoneal cavity of C3H/eB mice which had been injected 3 days before with 10% proteose-peptone (PP), or with 2.93% thioglycolate broth (TG). Activated and nonactivated macrophages were cultured as described above. From Fig. 5 it can be seen that culture fluids of LPS-stimulated nonactivated macrophages (MØ) supported the development of 74 ± 8 colonies/10^5 BM cells seeded. However, culture fluids from peritoneal macrophages from PP or TG-stimulated mice, when cultured with LPS (50 μg/ml), elaborated depressed amounts of CSF.

Interaction Between Macrophages and B Lymphocytes in Generation of LPS-Induced CSF

Macrophage dependence of LPS-induced CSF generation. Spleen cell cultures (2×10^6/ml) when incubated for 4 days in the presence of an optimal dose of LPS (50 μg/ml) elaborated large amounts of CSF and supported the development of 185 ± 28 colonies/10^5 bone marrow cells seeded. However, when such cell suspensions were

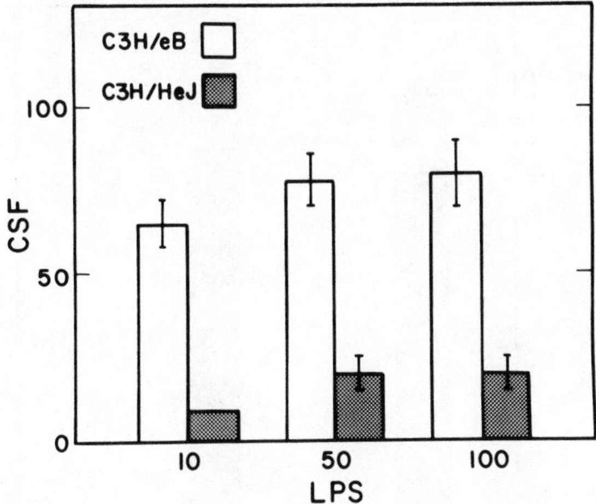

Fig. 4. Generation of CSF by peritoneal nonactivated macrophages stimulated by increasing concentrations of LPS (μg/ml).

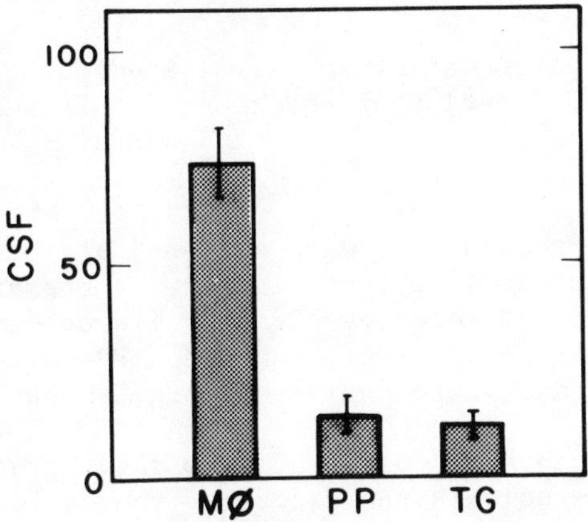

Fig. 5. Generation of CSF by LPS stimulated nonactivated proteose peptone (PP) and thioglycolate (TG) activated macrophages.

passaged through 2 successive pyrex wool adherence columns in order to deplete adherent macrophages the ability of the nonadherent effluent cells (Ly.) to secrete CSF in response to LPS decreased dramatically to about 20% of the normal secretory levels (28 $\pm$ 5 colonies/10^5 BM cells seeded) (Fig. 6). When such LPS-stimulated (50 μg/ml) nonadherent lymphocyte (Ly.) cultures (2 x 10^6 cells/ml) were supplemented with about 10% PP-induced peritoneal macrophages (2 x 10^5 cells/ml) MØ, large amounts of CSF

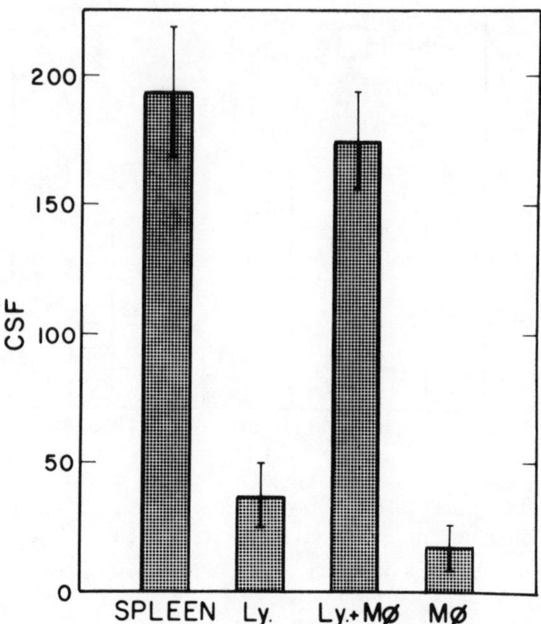

Fig. 6. Generation of CSF by LPS stimulated purified splenic lymphocytes and restoration of the response after addition of macrophages.

were generated. Macrophages, when cultured at the same cell concentration as added to lymphocyte cultures, generated only minute amounts of CSF (18 ± 3 colonies/10^5 BM cells seeded) (Fig. 6). Thus, it seems that an interaction between PP-activated macrophages and lymphocytes leads to secretion of large amounts of CSF.

Effect of macrophage culture fluids on generation of CSF by lymphocytes. To elucidate the nature of the cellular interactions between activated macrophages and lymphocytes, in the process of generation of CSF, the following experiments were undertaken. Macrophage supernatants were prepared by incubated PP-activated macrophages (2 x 10^6/ml) for 24-48 hr with or without LPS (50 μg/ml) and the culture fluids were thereafter collected and diluted 1:2 in culture medium. Nonadherent spleen lymphocytes (2 x 10^6/ml) were suspended in such macrophage supernatants and were subsequently cultured for 4 days either with or without LPS (50 μg/ml). The culture fluids of such lymphocyte suspensions were incorporated into the agar as a source of CSF at a final concentration of 15%. The results shown in Table I indicate that activate macrophage supernatants were generated when LPS was added to cultures and such supernatants could activate lymphocytes to secrete CSF even when

TABLE I

Replacing Activity of Macrophage Supernatants (Sup MØ) Obtained from LPS Stimulated Macrophage Cultures in Generation of CSF by Purified Splenic Lymphocytes

Lymphocytes \ Sup MØ	CSF - LPS	CSF + LPS
- LPS	11 ± 5	155 ± 14
+ LPS	63 ± 10	142 ± 16

the lymphocyte cultures were not stimulated by the mitogen. Supernatants prepared from macrophage cultures not stimulated by LPS manifested only a weak lymphostimulatory activity and addition of LPS to such lymphocyte cultures improved only partially the secretion of CSF. Therefore, in the following experiments which will be described macrophage cultures fluids were prepared from LPS stimulated cell cultures and lymphocytes were suspended in such supernatants diluted 1:2 in culture medium. Lymphocyte cultures were not supplemented with the mitogen. It has to be noted that macrophages were not activated to generate significant amounts of CSF by LPS-induced lymphocyte supernatants. Thus, generation of CSF in macrophage-lymphocyte mixed cultures seems to occur via a unidirectional pathway whereby LPS-stimulated macrophages secrete soluble lymphostimulatory factor(s) which, in turn, activate lymphocytes to secrete CSF.

Identification of the spleen cell population generating CSF in response to LPS. It was found that the population of lymphocytes responding to LPS-induced macrophage supernatants by generating high levels of CSF possibly consist of B lymphocytes. This was evidenced by showing that nonadherent lymphocytes from congenitally athymic nude (nu/nu) mice responded to such macrophage helper factor(s) as lymphocytes from conventional mice (Fig. 7). Further identification of the subpopulation of B lymphocytes generating LPS-induced CSF was possible by using CBA/N mice. These mice carry an x-linked defect which reduces the mitogenic and immunogenic responses to some T independent antigens including LPS (1). This defect is associated with a reduced number of splenic mature B lymphocytes (30). Spleen cells from CBA/N and the low-responder strain, C3H/HeJ, mice failed to incorporate significant amounts of ^{3}H-thymidine into DNA when stimulated by LPS. However, large amounts of CSF were generated

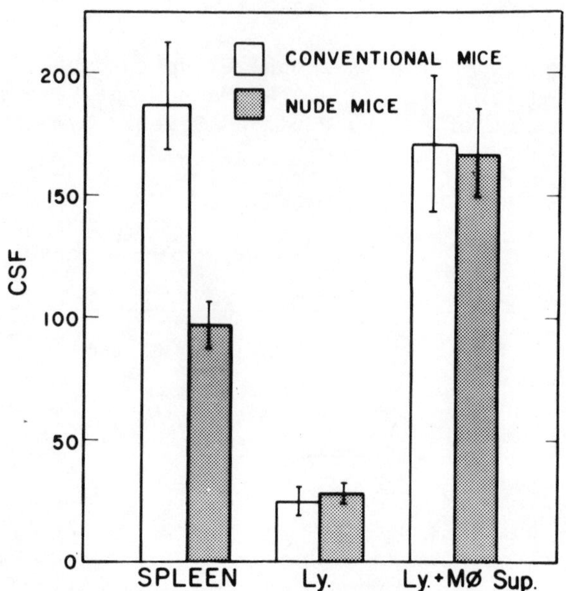

Fig. 7. Generation of CSF by purified lymphocytes from athymic nude mice induced by LPS-stimulated macrophage supernatants.

in LPS stimulated CBA/N and the high responder strain C3H/eB spleen cell cultures (Fig. 8). Thus, immature splenic B lymphocytes can respond to LPS in generating CSF.

Specificity of generation and mode of action of macrophage lymphostimulatory supernatants. The availability of LPS-low and high responder strains of mice provided us with a useful tool for further characterization of the mechanisms involved in generation of CSF in lymphoid cell cultures. C3H/HeJ mice are known to be low responders to the differential effects induced by LPS (2, 34, 37).

LPS-induced macrophage supernatants were prepared from macrophage cultures of C3H/HeJ mice as well as from such cultures of LPS-high responder mice of the inbred strain C3H/eB. The activity of each type of macrophage culture fluid was cross-tested on lymphocytes from both strains of mice. The results of these experiments are shown in Fig. 9. Macrophages obtained from C3H/HeJ mice did not elaborate any significant lymphocyte helper activity. However, such macrophage supernatants generated by macrophages from LPS-high responder mice (C3H/eB) succeeded to activate lymphocytes from C3H/HeJ mice which, in turn, secreted large amounts of CSF.

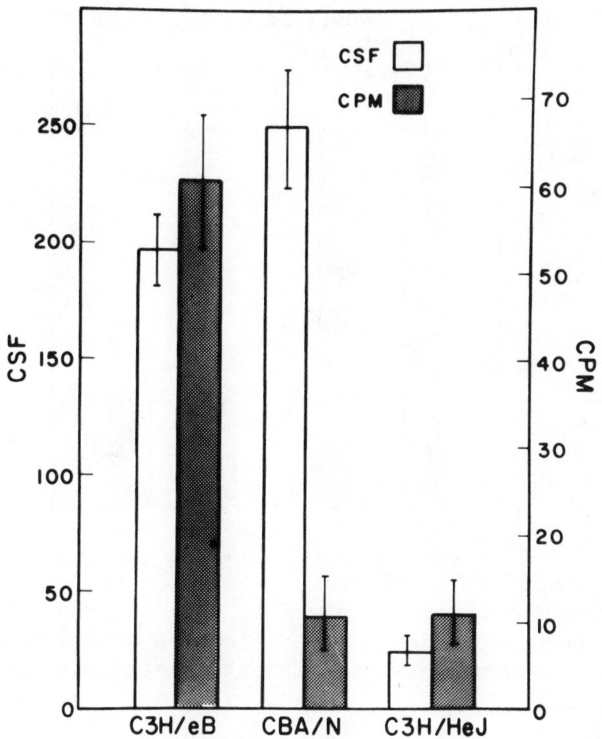

Fig. 8. Mitogenic response and generation of CSF in splenic cell cultures from different strains of mice after stimulation by LPS.

DISCUSSION

The present study indicates that secretion of CSF by B and T cells requires some type of macrophage help; nonadherent lymphocytes produce only small amounts of CSF. However, when supplemented with a small critical number of macrophages the ability to secrete CSF was restored. Macrophages when cultured at the same cell concentration as added to the lymphocytes generated themselves only small amounts of CSF. It is now widely accepted that T cell proliferation, as well as generation of lymphokines by T cells, is macrophage dependent (23). On the contrary, most studies indicate that B cell mitogens activate such lymphocytes directly without any need for auxiliary signals provided by macrophages (23). Moreover, there are even reports showing that addition of macrophages to lymphoid cultures stimulated by B cell mitogens cause suppression of the proliferative response.

The macrophage auxiliary signal needed for B lymphocyte

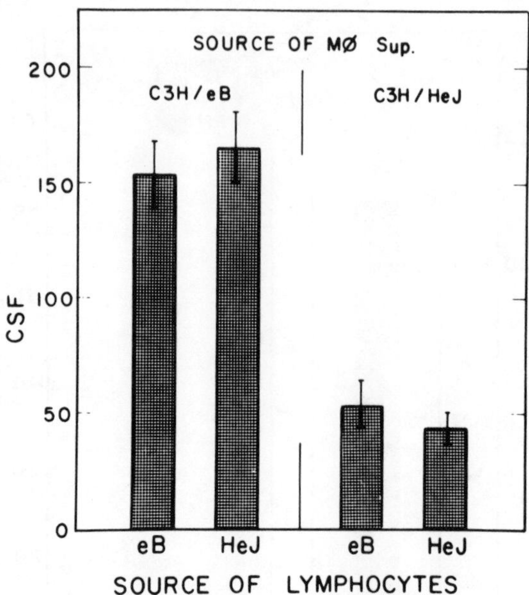

Fig. 9. Generation of CSF in purified splenic lymphocytes, from C3H/eB (high responder) and C3H/HeJ (low responder) mice, after induction with supernatants from LPS-stimulated macrophages.

activation to secrete CSF is mediated by the elaboration of 1 or more diffusible substances of macrophage origin. PP-induced macrophages, when stimulated by LPS in culture for an optimal period of 24 hr, elaborate factor(s) which subsequently stimulate B cells to secrete CSF, without need for addition of the mitogen to the lymphocyte cultures. On the other hand, macrophages are not stimulated to secrete such elevated levels of CSF when incubated with supernatants of LPS-stimulated splenic lymphocytes, thus pointing to the unidirectional specific interaction between lymphocytes and macrophages in the process of elaboration of CSF in LPS-stimulated lymphoid cell cultures.

When macrophage supernatants prepared from unstimulated peritoneal macrophages are added together with SEB to enriched non-adherent thymocytes, large amounts of CSF are generated. It seems that the mitogen binds to the T lymphocyte producing 1 activating signal, while a second activating signal is given by the macrophage soluble factor. The 2 signals are probably generated simultaneously. On the other hand, activation of B lymphocytes by LPS seems to occur via 2 subsequent signals. At first, macrophages incubated for 24 hr with LPS elaborate soluble factors which, in turn, subsequently activate B cells to secrete CSF, without any need for addition of the mitogen to lymphocytes. Only

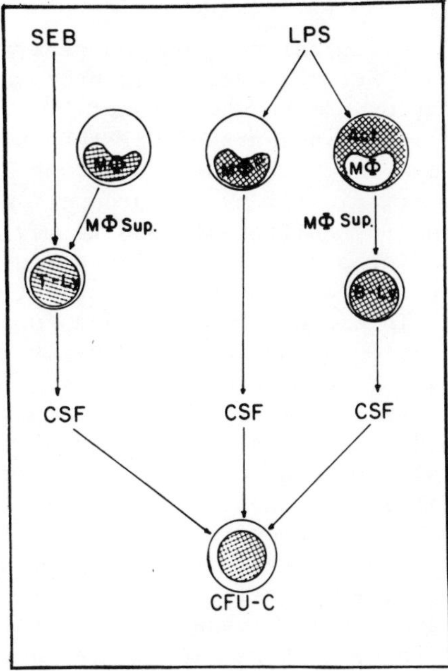

Fig. 10. Proposed mechanisms of CSF generation by SEB and LPS stimulated macrophages.

nonactivated macrophages can be directly stimulated by LPS to generate CSF. The proposed mechanisms responsible for secretion of CSF in response to LPS and SEB are schematically shown in Fig. 10.

It seems that B lymphocytes are specifically activated by LPS-induced macrophage factor(s). Such potent macrophage culture fluids stimulate lymphocytes from congenitally athymic nude (nu/nu) mice to secrete CSF, while thymocytes incubated with LPS or LPS-induced macrophage supernatants generate only minute amounts of CSF. It seems also that the B cell subpopulation, which interacts with such macrophage factors, may be distinct from that which undergoes mitogenesis and blast transformation in response to LPS. In a previous study we have shown that large amounts of CSF are present in the culture fluids of LPS-stimulated spleen cells from CBA/N mice (1). Such mice carry an x-linked inability to mount normal immune responses to thymus-independent antigens and poor _in vitro_ responsiveness to B cell mitogens (8, 37). Associated with this defect is a reduced number of splenic B cells, low serum IgM relative to putative IgD and an immature pattern of cell surface Ig-density distribution (31, 37). Quite interesting is the fact that for generation by CSF by SEB mature immunocompetent thymocytes are needed.

LPS-stimulated peritoneal macrophages generate *in vitro* significant levels of CSF. However, this process is modulated by the degree of activation of the macrophage; PP or TG-activated macrophages secrete lesser amounts of CSF than such cells from untreated mice. It is well established that such activated macrophages react characteristically by the production of large amounts of lysosomal enzymes (6). Different results may account for the reduced levels of CSF present in the culture fluids of activated macrophages. It may be that the intense activation of lysosomes causes a suppression in different macrophage functions. LPS also stimulates the production of hydrolytic enzymes in peritoneal macrophages (7, 38), however, to a lesser extent that TG or PP. Therefore, it may be that after a certain state of activation secretion of CSF is depressed in contrast to what happens with secretion of enzymes. It is also possible that the cellular composition of the activated peritoneal cavity is depleted of a subpopulation of macrophages secreting CSF. The existence of different populations of phagocytes has previously been described (33). Activation of adherent cells may increase the production of inhibitory substances which may antagonize the stimulatory effects of CSF. Macrophage culture fluids are known to contain low-molecular weight inhibitors of DNA and protein synthesis in lymphoid cell cultures, such as thymidine, prostaglandins and others, inhibitors of macromolecular nature such as interferon (36). On the other hand, macrophages when incubated in culture with SEB do not elaborate significant levels of CSF.

The availability of low and high responder strains of mice provides a useful instrument to determine mechanisms involved in the numerous humoral and cellular actions of LPS. Macrophages from LPS-low responder strains of mice, C3H/HeJ, fail to generate lympho-stimulatory factor(s) which facilitate generation of CSF by B lymphocytes. However, lymphocytes from C3H/HeJ mice respond to potent macrophage-derived culture fluids (diluted 1:2) and secrete CSF. This observation suggests that, in fact, soluble factor(s) rather than residual LPS in the macrophage supernatants activate B cells. However, it cannot be excluded that the active principle in such supernatants is LPS which has been handled and processed by macrophages, so that its recognition sites have been altered and it is able now to directly activate B cells from C3H/HeJ mice. Recently Truffa-Bachi *et al.* (35) have shown that LPS is processed by B cells from LPS-high responder mice to a low molecular weight component rendering it highly mitogenic to lymphocytes of the low responder strain, C3H/HeJ.

The present study emphasizes the regulatory role of macrophages and lymphocytes in the process of elaboration of the granulopoietic mediator-CSF by lymphocytes. Macrophages and lymphocytes are mobile, they are present in most tissues and they are in intimate contact with granuloid progenitor cells in hemopoietic tissues and may thus serve as an efficient control system which reacts to local as well as systemic granulopoietic signals.

SUMMARY

Committed progenitor cells for granulocyte and/or macrophage (MØ) differentiation proliferate in soft agar cultures to form colonies of mature granulocytes and/or MØ. Colony formation is dependent upon continuous presence of a colony stimulating factor (CSF). Murine lymphoid cells incubated with B-cell mitogen, bacterial lipopolysaccharide (LPS) or a T cell mitogen, staphylococcal enterotoxin B (SEB), elaborate CSF. Different cooperative mechanisms between MØ and lymphocytes mediate the process of generation of CSF by T and B lymphocytes (T-Ly.; B-Ly.). For T-Ly. secretion of CSF, 2 signals occurring simultaneously in culture are needed: the T-Ly. mitogen, SEB, interacts with the T-Ly., producing 1 activating signal, while the second signal is delivered by a soluble factor, released by nonactivated MØ, which is added to SEB-activated T-Ly. Thioglycolate-stimulated ("activated") MØ do not release this stimulatory factor. "Activated" or nonactivated MØ do not release CSF when incubated with SEB. Generation of CSF by LPS-induced lymphoid cells is possible by 2 different mechanisms: (a) MØ incubated with LPS generate CSF. This process is dependent on the degree of "activation" of the MØ. The more "activated" these cells are, the less CSF is generated. (b) Secretion of CSF by LPS-induced B-Ly. needs interaction between "activated" MØ and lymphocytes. In this case, 2 subsequent signals are required: first, LPS interacts directly with MØ which secrete helper factors that, in turn, stimulate lymphocytes to release CSF without direct interaction with the B-Ly.

ACKNOWLEDGEMENTS

This work was partially supported by a grant from the Hematology Research Foundation (Chicago, Illinois) and by the Bar-Ilan Research Authority (Israel).

REFERENCES

1. Amsbaugh, D. F., Hansen, C. T., Prescott, B., Stashak, P. W., Barthold, D. R. and Baker, P. J. J. Exp. Med. 136 (1972) 931.
2. Apte, R. N., Hertogs, C. F. and Pluznik, D. H. J. Immunol. 118 (1977) 1435.
3. Apte, R. N. and Pluznik, D. H. J. Cell. Physiol. 89 (1976) 313.

4. Bradley, T. R. and Metcalf, D. Aust. J. Exptl. Biol. Med. Sci. 44 (1966) 287.
5. Chervenick, P. A. and LoBuglio, A. F. Science 178 (1972) 101.
6. Cohen, Z. A. Adv. Immunol. 9 (1968) 163.
7. Cohen, Z. Z. and Morse, S. I. J. Exp. Med. 111 (1960) 689.
8. Cohen, P. L., Scher, I. and Mosier, D. E. J. Immunol. 116 (1976) 3011.
9. Eaves, A. C. and Bruce, W. R. Cell Tiss. Kinet. 7 (1970) 19.
10. Gery, I., Kruger, K. and Spiesel, S. Z. J. Immunol. 108 (1972) 1088.
11. Gery, I. and Waksman, B. H. J. Exp. Med. 136 (1972) 143.
12. Golde, D. W. and Cline, M. J. J. Clin. Invest. 51 (1972) 2981.
13. Golde, D. W., Finley, T. N. and Cline, M. J. Lancet II (1972) 1397.
14. Heller, E., Hertman, I. and Pluznik, D. H. Exp. Hematol. Suppl. 3 (1975) 12.
15. Heller, E. and Pluznik, D. H. Isr. J. Med. Sci. 13 (1977) 1041.
16. Hoffman, M. and Dutton, R. W. Science 172 (1971) 1047.
17. Ichikawa, Y., Pluznik, D. H. and Sachs, L. Proc. Natl. Acad. Sci. USA 58 (1967) 1480.
18. Iscove, N., Senn, J. S., Till, J. E. and McCulloch, E. A. Blood 37 (1971) 1.
19. Joyce, R. A. and Chervenick, P. A. J. Cell. Physiol. 89 (1976) 313.
20. Kurland, J. and Moore, M. A. S. Exp. Hematol. 5 (1977) 357.
21. Nelson, D. S. Nature (London) 246 (1973) 306.
22. Oppenheim, J. J., Levanthal, B. G. and Hersch, E. M. J. Immunol. 101 (1968) 262.
23. Oppenheim, J. J. and Rosenstreich, D. L. Prog. Allergy 20 (1976) 65.
24. Parker, J. W. and Metcalf, D. J. Immunol. 112 (1974) 502.
25. Parkhouse, R. M. E. and Dutton, R. W. J. Immunol. 97 (1966) 663.
26. Peavy, D. L., Adler, W. H. and Smith, R. T. J. Immunol. 105 (1970) 1453.
27. Pluznik, D. H. and Sachs, L. J. Cell. Comp. Physiol. 66 (1965) 319.
28. Pluznik, D. H. and Sachs, L. Exp. Cell. Res. 43 (1966) 553.
29. Robinson, W. A., Metcalf, D. and Bradley, T. R. J. Cell. Physiol. 69 (1967) 83.
30. Scher, I., Ahmed, A., Strong, D. M., Steinberg, A. D. and Paul, W. E. J. Exp. Med. 141 (1975) 788.
31. Scher, I., Sharrow, S. O. and Paul, W. E. J. Exp. Med. 144 (1976) 507.
32. Stanely, E. R. and Metcalf, D. Blood 33 (1969) 396.
33. Steinman, R. M. and Cohen, Z. A. J. Exp. Med. 139 (1974) 380.
34. Sultzer, B. M. Infect. Immunol. 5 (1972) 107.
35. Truffa-Bachi, P., Kaplan, J. G. and Bona, C. Cell. Immunol. 30 (1977) 1.

36. Unanue, E. R., Beller, D. I., et al. Am. J. Physiol. 85 (1976) 465.
37. Watson, J. and Riblet, R. J. Exp. Med. 140 (1974) 1147.
38. Wiener, E. and Levanon, D. Lab. Invest. 19 (1968) 584.

REGULATION OF ANTIGEN BINDING TO T CELLS: THE ROLE OF PRODUCTS OF ADHERENT CELLS, AND THE H-2 RESTRICTION OF THE ANTIGEN BOUND

P. LONAI, J. PURI, M. ZEICHER and L. STEINMAN

Department of Chemical Immunology, The Weizmann Institute of Science, Rehovot. (Israel)

We have described recently that antigen binding to T cells is influenced by a soluble factor of peritoneal adherent cells (MF). It was observed by microscopic autoradiography of radiolabeled antigen bound to nylon wool effluent T cells, that the number of antigen binding T cells increases several fold as a result of incubation with MF for 2 hr before antigen binding. We have shown that this effect is antigen specific and that the target cell of MF action is an Lyt-1^+, 2^-, 3^- cell. It was also observed that H-2 identity is not required between the antigen binding T cells and the adherent cells from which the MF was produced. In contrast the Ir type of the antigen binding T cell enriched population did determine whether increased antigen binding could be observed (5). In a subsequent study we have attempted to define the most important molecules involved in antigen binding to T cells. Alloantisera specific to distinct components controlled by the H-2 complex and purified antibodies against immunoglobulin V regions were used to inhibit antigen binding to T cells. It was found that antigen binding to Lyt-1^+, MF sensitive non immune T cells is inhibited by anti Ia, anti idiotype (C3H,SW anti-(T,G)-A--L) and anti-V_H antibodies. No inhibition was observed when these cells were treated with anti-H-2K, anti-H-2D and anti-V_γ antibodies (3).

Two from a number of interesting questions arising from these data were investigated in the present study:

1) If the effect of MF on antigen binding is not restricted by H-2 type, what defines the observed Ir dependence of antigens binding to MF treated T cells? 2) Are both Ia and V_H involved in the binding of antigen by T cells? The importance of these

questions is accentuated by findings of others who have demonstrated that both Lyt-1^+, 3^+ type T cells recognize antigen in conjunction with elements controlled by the major histocompatibility complex (7,11) that the expression of Ir genes can be demonstrated on adherent cells (6,8,10), and that immunoglobulin idiotypic determinants are involved in the T cell receptor (1,2).

Our approach towards the clarification of these problems originated in a series of experiments which investigated elementary conditions of antigen binding to T cells. First the temperature requirement of antigen binding was investigated. It can be seen in Table I that MF treated normal and immune T cells bind antigen only at the physiological temperature. In contraxt B cells bind equally well at all temperatures between 4 and 37 C. These findings in agreement with a number of previous findings (4,9) suggested that antigen binding to T cells is an energy dependent process in contrast to antigen binding to B cells. Indeed antigen binding to T cells was inhibited by 0.02% sodium azide (not shown here). Next the time required for antigen binding was investigated. It was found that antigen binding to T cells is a much slower process than antigen binding to B cells. From the values shown in Table II the time required to reach the half of the maximal number of antigen binding cells (ABC) for B cells is 1-2 min, while for T cells 15-25 min. These findings indicated that for optimal antigen binding by T cells an energy and time consuming process is required, which is not necessary for B cells. It was reasonable to assume that this unknown process may be required by the antigen binding cell to bind antigen more efficiently either through an effect on the receptor or on the antigen itself.

We have investigated the second possibility. We reasoned, that if this process affects the antigen, then antigen, which has been incubated with MF treated nylon wool effluent cells for 30-40 min at 37 C, should contain a moiety which will be bound to T cells with faster kinetics than regular non-treated soluble antigen. Experiments demonstrated in Table II have shown that no appreciable binding of soluble antigen to T cells occurs in the first 10 min of incubation. To test our assumption, ^{125}I-(T,G)-A--L was incubated with MF treated C3H.SW nylon wool effluent cells for 40 min. The cell free supernatant was then added for 10 min to MF treated syngeneic T cells. Table III demonstrates that antigen treated in this way bound maximally to T cells in 10 min, while the untreated antigen was not bound above the control value within this time. This finding supports our reasoning, and suggests that the time and energy required for antigen binding by T cells may be directed to a process affecting the antigen. For simplicity's sake we call this effect "processing" and the incubated, labeled antigen "processed antigen", in distinction to the non treated labeled antigen which we call "soluble" antigen. Table III thus demonstrates that T cells bind "processed antigen" with a faster kinetics than "soluble" antigen, and suggests that when "soluble" antigen is added, the time is needed for the "processing" of the "soluble" antigen. The table also shows that T cells need to be pretreated with MF to bind the processed antigen.

TABLE I

Temperature Dependence of Antigen Binding by T Cells

	ABC/10^4 cells			
	Non Immune Cells		Immune Cells	
Temperature (^oC)	T Cells + MF	B Cells	T Cells	B Cells
4	12.5	30	10	58
15	28	32,5	8	55
24	20	30	22	60
30	72	28	30	63
37	75	30	92	60

[a]T cells were incubated with or without MF for 2 hr, ^{125}I-(T,G)-A--L was added for 40 min at the stated temperature.

[b]T cells and B cells were isolated by nylon wool filtration of C3H.SW spleen cells. MF is the cell free medium of non-stimulated peritoneal adherent cells harvested after 48 hr cultivation in culture medium. As culture medium RPMI-1640, supplemented with 1% normal mouse plasma, penicillin, streptomycin, glutamin and 2-mercaptoethanol. The antigen was labeled with ^{125}I to a specific activity of 5-10 µCi/µg. The cells were processed for autoradiography after 4 washes, and exposed for two weeks. Immunized animals were injected with 10 µ (T,G)-A--L in CFA into the footpads followed by a boost after 3 weeks of 10 µ antigen in PBS i.p. and were sacrificed 7 days later. All incubations were performed in the above described culture medium. For details see (1.2).

TABLE II

Kinetics of Antigen Binding by T Cells

	ABC/10^4 cells			
	Non Immune		Immune	
Time for Binding (min)	% Cells + MF	B Cells	T Cells	B Cells
2	18	42	30	80
5	22	45	28	75
10	30	40	40	75
20	54	38	72	80
30	N.D.	N.D.	108	N.D.
40	63	40	120	82
60	65	45	115	78

[a]The cells were incubated with or without MF for 2 hr ^{125}I-(T,G) -A--L was added for the stated time interval.

TABLE III

T Cells Bind "Processed" Antigen: For Antigen Binding MF Treatment Is Necessary

Binder[a]	Antigen[b]	Time of Binding (min)	ABC/10^4
T	soluble	40	12
T+MF	"	40	62
T+MF	"	10	15
T+MF	Processed	10	58
T	Processed	10	13

[a]Binders: C3H.SW nylon wool effluent spleen cells after 2 hr incubation with or without MF (1:80) at 37 C.

[b]Antigen: ^{125}I-(T,G)-A--L 5 μg/ml. Processed antigen: ^{125}I-(T,G)-A--L (5 μg/ml) incubated for 40 min at 39 C with MF treated T cells.

Next, the nature of the processor cell was investigated. Antigen ^{125}I-(T,G)-A--L was "processed" by a suspension of immune spleen cells. Two aliquot cultures were prepared. One of them was made up from non adherent spleen cells, from which the adherent cells were removed by preincubation for 2 hr at 37 C. Table IV demonstrates that adherent cells are necessary for optimal processing. In the light of this information it was reasonable to assume that "processing" may be affected by the adherent cells remaining in the nylon wool adherent fraction used in our other experiments. It is possible that the "processed" antigen is released by adherent cells. In this case some membrane components could remain attached to the antigen. Were this be the case, oligosaccharides could be found in conjunction with the antigen, which would in turn bind to a lentil-lectin Sepharose column. Since the antigen used - (T,G)-A--L -

TABLE IV

Adherent Cells Are Necessary for "Antigen-Processing": Processed Antigen Is Bound by Lentil-Lectin.[a]

Exp.	Antigen	Processor	Lentil-Lectin Column	OA-Column	Time of Binding (min)	ADC/10^4
1	soluble	-	-	-	40	80
	"	-	-	-	10	15
	processed	immune spleen	-	-	10	72
	"	non adherent immune spleen	-	-	10	5
2	"	immune spleen	-	+	10	65
	"	"	+	-	10	7

[a] 5×10^6 immune T cells were used for processing. ^{125}I-(T,G)-A--L (See conditions as in Table III). T cells were isolated from C3H.SW spleens. Lentil-lectin (Yeda, Rehovot) or ovalbumin was bound to cyanogen bromide activated Sepharose 6MB (Pharmacia, Uppsala, Sweden). All other details according to footnote to Table I.

is not a glycoprotein, the processed antigen could be selectively retained by a lentil-lectin-Sepharose affinity column. The second experiment in Table IV, demonstrates that the component of the processed antigen, which is responsible for the fast kinetics is retained on a lentil-lectin-Sepharose column, while it goes through the control ovalbumin-Sepharose column. The amount of radioactivity retained on both columns was less than 5% of the total TCA precipitable counts applied.

Our previous experiments demonstrated that the MF induced binding of antigen is under *H-2* linked genetic control, i.e., low responder T cells did not reveal MF dependent increased antigen binding. Since the genetic origin of MF did not influence this effect, we assumed that the regulation is a property of the T cells (5). The above findings of adherent cell dependent "processing" of antigen allowed us to reinvestigate this problem. It has been demonstrated that T cell dependent immune responses can be induced by antigen-fed macrophages, and that this macrophage-T cell interaction is restricted by the H-2 type of the interacting cells (6,10). We have used the above described detection of processed antigen, to answer the hitherto directly not answerable question, whether *H-2* restriction can be demonstrated at the level of antigen binding.

^{125}I-Ovalbumin was "processed" by nylon wool effluent cells isolated from spleens of a number of mouse strains. As bindings B6 or B6-H2^k T cell enriched spleen cells were used. The "processed" antigens were allowed to bind for 10 min at 37 C. Table V demonstrates the results of this experiment. Only minimal antigen binding was observed when the processor and binder cells were totally allogeneic. Recombinants HTI and A.AL, respectively, have shown that the *D* region is not involved in this restriction, suggesting that the restriction observed with the B6 and B6-H-2^k *H-2* congeneic pair is situated in the left half of the *H-2* complex. More accurate localization could be obtained with the B10.A(4R), B10.A(5R) and B10.AKR(4N) recombinants, which mapped the restriction of antigen binding to the I-A subregion of the *H-2* complex.

MF reactive cells are of the Ly-$^+$ phenotype (3,5). These experiments demonstrate that Ly-1$^+$ T cells bind antigen which most likely was in contact with adherent cells, carriers oligosaccharide moieties which bind to lentil-lectin (α-*D*-mannose specificity), and the binding of this processed antigen requires that the processor adherent cell and the binder Ly-1$^+$ T cell should share the I-A subregion of the *H-2* complex, and that the binder should be treated by MF. The experiment suggests, but does not prove that the antigen is bound as a complex which contains glycoproteins controlled by the *I-A* subregion.

Our experiments are in good agreement with data which show that the stimulation of T cells by antigen pulsed macrophages is restricted by the *I-A* subregion of the two cells. The present

TABLE V

The Binding of Processed Antigen (^{125}I-Ovalbumin) to T Cells Is Under H-2 Restriction.

Binder[a]	Processor[b]	Difference	ABC/10^4
B6	B6	-	110
"	B6-H-2^k	whole H-2	30
"	HTI	H-2D	115
"	B10.A(5R)	I-J,I-E,I-C,S,H-2G,H-2D	90
B6-H2^k	B6-H-2^k	-	80
"	B6	whole H-2	28
"	B10.A	I-C,S,H-2G,H-2D	72
"	B10,AQR	H-2K,I-C,S,H-2G,H-2D	75
"	B10.A(4R)	I-B,I-J,I-E,I-C,S,H-2G,H-2D	90
"	B10.A(5R)	H-2K,I-A,I-B	20

[a]Binders: Nylon wool purified splenic T cells pretreated with MF for 2 hr.

[b]Processor: Nylon wool effluent spleen cells of different strains. ^{125}I ovalbumin was "processed" with these cells for 40 min as described in footnote to Table III.

data provide evidence that this restriction phenomenon is indeed involved in the binding of antigen to the T cell receptor. They suggest furthermore that the involvement of H-2 complex products seems to be a necessary condition in conjunction with the antigen but not necessary in conjunction with the T cell receptor. It is suggested, but not proved, that the processed antigen is released by adherent cells. It is however, not known whether such soluble antigenic complexes have a role in the natural immune response. Preliminary experiments have demonstrated that the "processed antigen", described here reveals 100-fold stronger immunogenicity on a molar basis when injected *in vivo* than non-treated soluble antigens (Puri and Lonai, unpublished). Whether the processed antigen described here is a naturally occurring product, or not, is not yet clear. However, it is most likely not produced by autolysis of the adherent cells, within the short time (30-50 min) used for its production. Such a product may well prove to be useful in the characterization of the complex antigenic determinants responsible for the stimulation of T cells.

These experiments reveal some interesting processes in the physiology of antigen binding by T cells. Our data suggest that T cells bind adherent cell processed antigen, but they also show that for this binding a soluble product of adherent cells is independently necessary. Thus, they imply that more than one interacting step between adherent cells and T cells are necessary for antigen binding by T cells.

Our studies presented here were based on observations concerning the effect of MF. We have described together with the effect of MF on antigen binding to Lyt-1^+ cells, similar effects caused by mouse viral interferon, and have shown that interferon acts on Ly-2^+, 3^+ T cells (3,5). It will be of considerable interest to investigate whether the interferon effect is connected also to "processed" antigen, and whether H-2 restriction is involved in this effect.

REFERENCES

1. Binz, H. and Wigzell, H. J. Exp. Med. 142 (1975) 197.
2. Eichmann, K. and Rajewsky, K. Eur. J. Immunol. 5 (1975) 661.
3. Lonai, P., Ben-Neriah, Y., Steinman, L. and Givol, D. Eur. J. Immunol. (1978) in press.
4. Lonai, P. and McDevitt, H. O. J. Exp. Med. 140 (1974) 1317.
5. Lonai, P. and Steinman, L. Proc. Nat. Acad. Sci. USA 74 (1977) 5662.
6. Rosenthal, A. L., Barcinski, M.A. and Blake, J. T. Nature 267 (1977) 747.
7. Shearer, G. M. Eur. J. Immunol. 4 (1974) 527.
8. Thomas, D. W. and Shevach, E. M. Proc. Nat. Acad. Sci. USA 74 (1977) 2104.
9. Wekerle, H., Lonai, P. and Feldman, M. Proc. Nat. Acad. Sci. USA 69 (1972) 1620.
10. Yano, a., Schwartz, R. H. and Paul, W. Z. J. Exp. Med. 146 (1977) 828.
11. Zimkernagel, R. M. and Doherty, P. C. J. Exp. Med. 141 (1975) 1427.

ALVEOLAR MACROPHAGE - INDUCED SUPPRESSION OF THE IMMUNE RESPONSE

H. B. HERSCOWITZ, R. E. CONRAD and K. J. PENNLINE

Georgetown University, Schools of Medicine and Dentistry, Washington, D. C. (USA)

Active participation of macrophages in almost every phase of the immune response is now well-accepted. There is information from both *in vivo* and *in vitro* studies to indicate that macrophages not only serve as effector cells, but also may enhance or suppress the activities of lymphocytes participating in immune responses (35).

Several experimental systems have been used to demonstrate the suppressive effects of macrophages. Kirchner *et al*. (19-20) observed that spleen cells from mice bearing Maloney sarcoma virus-induced tumors responded poorly to T cell and B cell mitogens. Ruling out the possibility that there was a lack of cells capable of responding to mitogen, they suggested that a suppressor cell was involved. This was confirmed by mixing experiments, in which spleen cells from tumor-bearing mice were cocultured with normal spleen cells in the presence of mitogen and no proliferative response was observed (20). The cell type responsible for the suppression was resistant to treatment with anti-theta serum plus complement, could be removed by treatment with iron-filings and a magnet, sensitive to carrageenan, resistant to 2500 R x-irradiation and was thought to be a macrophage (49,50). Fernback *et al*. (9) reported that spleen cells from tumor-bearing animals responded poorly to alloantigens in MCL and CML. Removal of adherent cells abrogated the suppression while thiglycollate-induced PEC reconstituted the suppressive effects (13). Folch and Waksman (10) described a subpopulation of rat splenic adherent cells which act as high doses or phytohemagglutinin or concanavalin A to suppress DNA synthesis by other cells. This cell was also capable of suppressing mixed lymphocyte cultures of allogeneic rat spleen cells (11). In spite of the fact that the cell was removed by passage through glass wool columns, these investigators interpreted their data to indicate that the suppressive cell was a thymus-derived adherent cell rather than a macrophage (10,11). In recent studies, Oehler _et al_. (34) provided further evidence that the cell responsible for inhibition of mixed lymphocyte culture and cell mediated lympholysis activity was a macrophage. This conclusion was based on the findings that the active cell in normal rat spleen was adherent, phagocytic, resistant to treatment with mitomycin C and x-irradiation and unaffected by treatment with anti-thymocyte serum plus complement. In order to reconcile the differences with the work of Folch and Waksman, it was suggested that there may be some cooperation between macrophages and T cells in order to acquire or maintain the suppressor activity. Raff and Hinrichs (40-42) reported that an adherent, phagocytic cell, presumably the macrophage, was suppressive in mitogen and antigen-stimulated rat lymphocyte cultures. Through the use of various cell separation procedures they suggested that the generation of the suppressor activity in macrophages requires an interaction with T lymphocytes. Further evidence for the existence of suppressor macrophages in normal rat spleens was recently presented by Weiss and Fitch (52). Depletion of phagocytic, adherent cells from normal rat spleen cell populations allowed the generation of the PFC response to SRBC _in vitro_. Irradiated adherent cells were capable of suppressing the PFC response of macrophage-depleted lymphoid cells.

In early work, Perkins and Makinodan (37) demonstrated that serum antibody titers were depressed in an adoptive transfer system in which primed spleen cells, RBC and PEC were implanted in diffusion chambers. Using an _in vitro_ system Hoffman (15) showed that antibody production could be inhibited by the presence of excess macrophages and suggested that the suppressive effect was mediated through an inhibition of the proliferative phase of the response. Antibody responses to SRBC have been shown to be suppressed in animals after induction of chronic graft _vs_. host (GvH) disease (31). In contrast, these animals show increased resistance to infection with _Listeria_ (3) a phenomenon which is associated with increased macrophage activation. Thus it appears that increased activation of macrophages results in the expression of immunosuppressive capabilities. That this was the case was shown by Mooler (31) in a cell transfer system. In addition to suppressed humoral responses, animals undergoing chronic GvH also have diminished cell-mediated reactions as measured by allograft survival (25). This also appears to be mediated by macrophages. In a murine plasmacytoma model, Krakauer, _et al_. (23) demonstrated that ascitic fluid from hypogammaglobulinemic mice contained a factor capable of suppressing PWM-induced Ig synthesis by normal mouse spleen cells or human peripheral blood lymphocytes. Removal of phagocytic cells from the ascites fluid resulted in loss of the suppressor factor. Similarly, Kolb _et al_. (22) found that splenic macrophages from agammaglobulinemic, myeloma-bearing mice suppressed the PFC response of normal splenic lymphocytes to SRBC when added to Mishell-Dutton cultures. These findings, taken together, indicate that macrophages can suppress Ig production by B cells from normal or tumor-bearing individuals. Further, in a recent report by Klimpel and Henney (21) it was shown that spleen cells obtained from mice infected with viable BCG organisms were unresponsive *in vitro* to both mitogenic and alloantigenic stimulation. When spleen cells from BCG infected mice were mixed with allogeneic or syngeneic cells from normal mice, the latter cells neither proliferated nor developed cytotoxic activity when cultured with mitogen or alloantigen. The suppressive activity was associated with an adherent, phagocytic cell that was unaffected by treatment with anti-Thy 1 antiserum plus complement and is thought to be a macrophage.

Lemke *et al*. (26) demonstrated that macrophages were not required for the activation of mouse B cells by LPS, indeed proliferation and polyclonal antibody synthesis were often enhanced if macrophages were depleted from spleen cell populations. Addition of peritoneal macrophages to adherent cell-depleted spleen cells resulted in suppression of these responses and suppressive activity could be demonstrated in supernatants from adherent cell cultures stimulated by LPS. Wing and Remington (53) showed that peritoneal macrophages could either enhance or suppress mitogen and antigen-stimulated lymphocyte transformation as a function of the number of macrophages present. Normal macrophages could enhance these responses at all concentrations tested while activated macrophages enhanced only at low concentrations and suppressed at high concentrations.

The mechanism involved in macrophage-mediated immunosuppression appears to be associated with inhibition of lymphocyte proliferation (18). Baird and Kaplan (1,2) suggested that suppression is the result of inhibition of blast formation rather than target cell cytotoxicity. On the other hand, Opitz *et al*. (36) have suggested that macrophage-mediated suppression of ^{3}H-thymidine incorporation is due to the release of cold thymidine or a thymidine-precursor from macrophages which competes with the labeled material. Thus, how the suppression is achieved is not clear. The suppressive effect could be ablated only by treatment of macrophages with inhibitors of protein synthesis and glycolysis (17). Suppressor activity was resistant to treatment with trypsin, neuraminidase, pronase, RNase and DNase (18). In addition, interference with phagocytosis had no effect on the suppression. In contradistinction, Ptak and Gershon (38) showed that heat-killed macrophages, but not normal spleen cells or several mouse tumor lines, suppressed the initiation of *in vitro* PFC responses by a mechanism that did not affect viability of the responding cells. Further, they showed that suppression could be accomplished with macrophage membranes and suggested that the inhibition is due to the absorption of factors which are necessary for lymphocyte cooperation.

In addition to the suppressive effects mediated by macrophages which appear to require cell contact, macrophages also elaborate soluble factors which induce suppression. Calderon _et al_. (5) have described a factor from cultures of mouse PEC which inhibited proliferation of micogen-stimulated lymphocytes and tumor cells _in vitro_. Waldman and Gottlieb (51) demonstrated that a low molecular weight factor obtained from cultures of rat PEC inhibited proliferation of antigen-stimulated lymphocytes. Recently, Elgert and Farrar (7) demonstrated that a soluble factor derived from the interaction of T cells and macrophages from tumor-bearing mice was responsible for the inhibition of mitogen-induced proliferative responses. They proposed the factor interferes with DNA polymerase resulting in an inhibition of cell proliferation (8). Rich and Pierce (44) isolated a suppressor factor from Con A-induced suppressor T cell cultures which inhibited the _in vitro_ PFC response to SRBC. This soluble immune suppressor factor (SIRS) does not act directly on T or B cells, but appears to have the macrophage as its target cell (47). The possibility that SIRS acts on macrophages to generate suppressor activity was suggested (47). It is too soon to make any definitive conclusions regarding the mechanism of action of soluble suppressor factors since the data emerging in this field indicate that the events involved in the generation of suppressor cell activity are quite complex. It is becoming apparent, however, that immunosuppression requires a collaborative interaction between macrophages and lymphocytes. Whether there are two types of suppressor cells, e.g., macrophages and lymphocytes, or one type, e.g., suppressor macrophages dependent on T cells for activation or suppressor T cells dependent on macrophages for activation, remains to be shown.

In the present study we have examined the role of alveolar macrophages, a cell type concerning which there is a paucity of information regarding its immunological function available in the literature, in the _in vitro_ immune response. Our data indicate that this cell is capable of suppressing the PFC response of rabbit lymphoid cells to RBC through a soluble factor that requires the presence of lymphocytes for its generation.

MATERIALS AND METHODS

Animals and immunization. Female New Zealand white rabbits, weighing 5 to 6 lbs., were obtained from a local dealer. For priming, the animals were injected intravenously with 1.0 ml of a 3% (v/v) suspension of washed red blood cells (RBC). In some experiments the animals were immunized as above and with 0.5 ml of a 10%

(v/v) suspension of RBC in each hind foot pad. Horse RBC (HRBC) were used in some experiments and were injected as above.

Cell suspensions. Six to ten days after *in vivo* priming, rabbits were sacrificed by air embolism and their spleen and/or thymus, popliteal and tracheo-bronchial lymph nodes were removed. Single cell suspensions were prepared by teasing with serrated forceps, the cells were washed in minimal essential medium (MEM) and resuspended to 1-2 x 10^7 cells/ml in Mishell-Dutton (29) culture medium as originally described except that fetal calf serum constituted only 5% by volume as recommended by Redelman *et al.* (43) and RPMI-1640 medium was used in place of MEM.

Removal of adherent cells. The procedure used for removal of adherent cells from lymphoid cell populations was based on the method of Mosier (1). In our hands, this procedure reduced the primary *in vitro* anti-SRBC response of nonadherent $B_6D_2F_1$ mouse spleen cells to 10% of the control response with no loss in cell viability.

Alveolar macrophages. Alveolar macrophages were obtained by lavage essentially as described by Myrvik *et al.* (32). The procedure resulted in a yield of generally 1 x 10^8 cells which were predominantly macrophages (>95%).

Culture systems. Two systems of cell culture were employed in these studies. In the first, cultures were established in 16 mm diameter wells in plastic dishes (#3524), Costar plates; Bellco Glass, Vineland, N. Y.). Each well contained 1 x 10^7 lymphoid cells and 1-10 x 10^5 RBC depending upon the experiment, except for controls (no RBC) in a total volume of 1.0 ml. When alveolar macrophages were included in these cultures, they were present in a concentration of usually 1 x 10^6/ml. Cultures were incubated with rocking in an atmosphere of 10% CO_2, 7% O_2 and 83% N_2 in gas-tight plexiglass boxes at 37 C as described previously (29). The cells were harvested by pooling the contents of two wells, centrifuging and resuspending the cells in 1.0 ml of MEM. Henceforth, these cultures will be referred to as "Mishell-Dutton" cultures.

In the second system, cells were cultured in modified Marbrook vessels (28). In some experiments, a 2 chamber system was used in which the inner chamber contained 2 x 10^6 RBC in a volume of 0.5 ml. The outer chamber contained RPMI-1640 supplemented with 10% fetal calf serum, penicillin, streptomycin and glutamine. In other experiments a 3 chamber system was used in which the inner chamber contained 2 x 10^7 lymphoid cells and 2 x 10^6 RBC in a volume of 0.5 ml, the middle chamber contained 1 x 10^6 alveolar macrophages/ml either in the presence or absence of 1 x 10^6 RBC/ml in a total volume of 2.5 to 3.0 ml and the outer chamber contained complete medium as above. The cultures were incubated undisturbed at 37 C in an atmosphere containing 5-10% CO_2. These cultures will be referred to as "Marbrook" cultures.

Culture supernatants were generated from various cells and cell combinations in the Mishell-Dutton cultures over a 4 day period as described above. Usually the contents of 6 to 12 wells were pooled. The culture supernatants were tested for biological activity in the Marbrook cultures by placing 2.5 to 3.0 ml of the cell-free culture supernatant in the middle chamber of the 3 chamber vessel. The cultures were incubated as above for 4 days.

Hemolytic plaque assay. Estimates of the number of cells secreting IgM anti-RBC antibody were based on counts of hemolytic plaques using the Cunningham-Szenberg liquid assay system (6).

RESULTS

At the initiation of our studies, an attempt was made to determine if alveolar macrophages (AM) had the capacity to reconstitute the *in vitro* immune response to SRBC of primed, nonadherent rabbit spleen cells. Spleen cells obtained from rabbits which had been immunized 6 to 10 days earlier with 4×10^8 SRBC were depleted of macrophages by adherence to plastic dishes and placed in Mishell-Dutton cultures with SRBC. In anticipation of a significant decrease in the response of nonadherent cells in culture, autologous alveolar macrophages were added to some cultures at a ratio of 1 AM: 10 nonadherent cells. Two observations should be made from the results presented in Table I. First, depletion of adherent cells had no detectable effect on the ability of the spleen cells to respond to SRBC in culture. Second, in those cultures to which AM were added, the PFC were markedly diminished. This was true for both the unseparated spleen cell population and the nonadherent cell population; the presence of alveolar macrophages resulted in greater than 90% suppression of the *in vitro* PFC response.

Studies were then initiated in connection with the observed suppression of splenic lymphocyte PFC responses by AM. A dose-response effect was tested by adding varying numbers of AM to spleen cell populations in culture. To 1×10^7 spleen cells and 1×10^5 SRBC were added the following numbers of AM: 5×10^2, 5×10^3, 5×10^4 and 5×10^5. The results are presented in Fig. 1. Suppression was greater than 95% when the number of AM added per culture was 5×10^5, a ratio of 1 AM to 20 spleen cells. When 5×10^3 or fewer AM were added, little suppression was observed (20% or less).

As the suppression was clearly a reproducible event, we

began a series of experiments designed to further characterize the system. One possible explanation for the observed AM-induced suppression was cell crowding, i.e., a supraoptimal concentration of cells in the cultures could result in a lower response by the spleen cells. To test for this possibility 1 x 10^6 cells from various sources (lymph node, thymus, spleen) were added to

TABLE I

Effect of Depletion of Adherent Cells and Addition of Alveolar Macrophages on the PFC Response of Rabbit Spleen Cells[a] to SRBC[b]

Spleen Cell Population	AM Added[c]	PFC/10^6 Cells ± S.E.M.[e] - SRBC	+ SRBC
Unseparated	-	66 ± 33	960 ± 174
	+	14 ± 16	4 ± 2
Non-adherent[d]	-	82 ± 49	922 ± 168
	+	14 ± 12	5 ± 5

[a]Rabbits immunized IV with 1 ml of a 3% SRBC suspension.

[b]Cultures contained 1 x 10^7 spleen cells, ± 1 x 10^5 SRBC, ± 1 x 10^6 alveolar macrophages

[c]AM = alveolar macrophages.

[d]Non-adherent spleen cells were prepared by incubating spleen cells on plastic culture dishes for 1 hr at 37 C under 5% CO_2. The cells were decanted to fresh plates, the incubation continued for 1 hr and the cells were harvested for culture.

[e]Results represent the mean of triplicate samples.

1 x 10^7 spleen cells in culture along with 1 x 10^5 SRBC. The added cells were obtained from both autologous SRBC-stimulated rabbits or allogeneic unstimulated rabbits. Results are presented in Fig. 2. Comparable numbers of cells obtained from lymph node, thymus or spleen had no suppressive effect on the PFC response of the spleen cells. On the contrary, autologous lymph node and spleen cells augmented the PFC response by 50 to 100% This can be readily explained by the fact that these cell populations contained antigen-primed cells. Alveolar macrophages from allogeneic unstimulated rabbits suppressed the response by 90%, of the same order of suppression observed with the autologous AM.

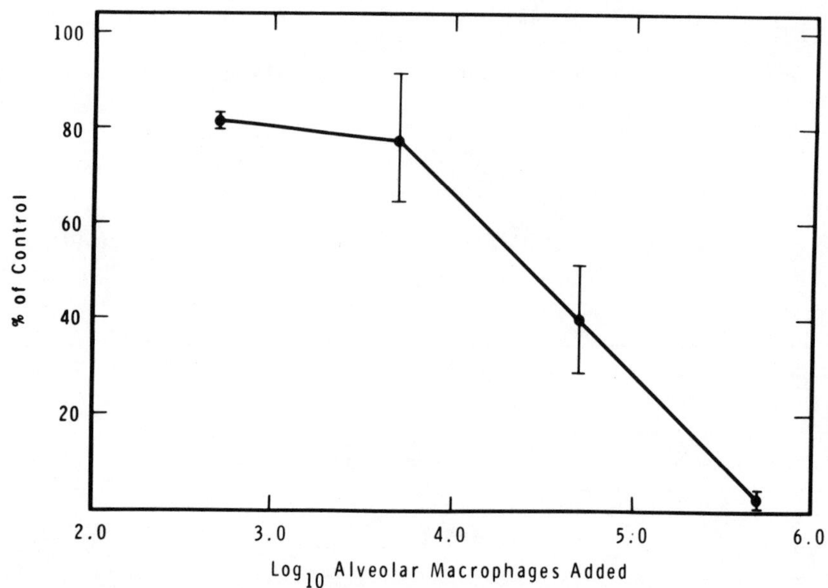

Fig. 1. Effect of the number of alveolar macrophages on the *in vitro* response of cultured spleen cells. Cultures contained 1 x 10^7 spleen cells, 1 x 10^5 SRBC and autologous alveolar macrophages at the concentrations indicated. Viabilities of cultured cells at time of harvest were equivalent (40-60%). Results are expressed as mean percent of control (no AM) ± S.E.M. for 3 experiments.

Experiments were carried out to determine the properties of the cell that mediates the suppression of the PFC response and the results are summarized in Table II.

An alternate explanation for the AM-induced suppression was that the AM removed the antigen so as to preclude stimulation of the primed lymphocytes. Two experimental designs were used to approach this possibility. In the first, excess antigen was added to the cultures, and in the second, an attempt was made to inhibit phagocytosis by saturating the AM with inert particles (latex) before adding them to the cultures. The Mishell-Dutton cultures were prepared as usual with 1 x 10^7 spleen cells and various numbers of autologous AM. SRBC were added to the cultures at 1 x 10^5, 1 x 10^6 and 1 x 10^7 cells/culture. Controls consisted of cultures without AM and/or without SRBC. The results are presented in Fig. 3. Data for each concentration of SRBC are compared to the

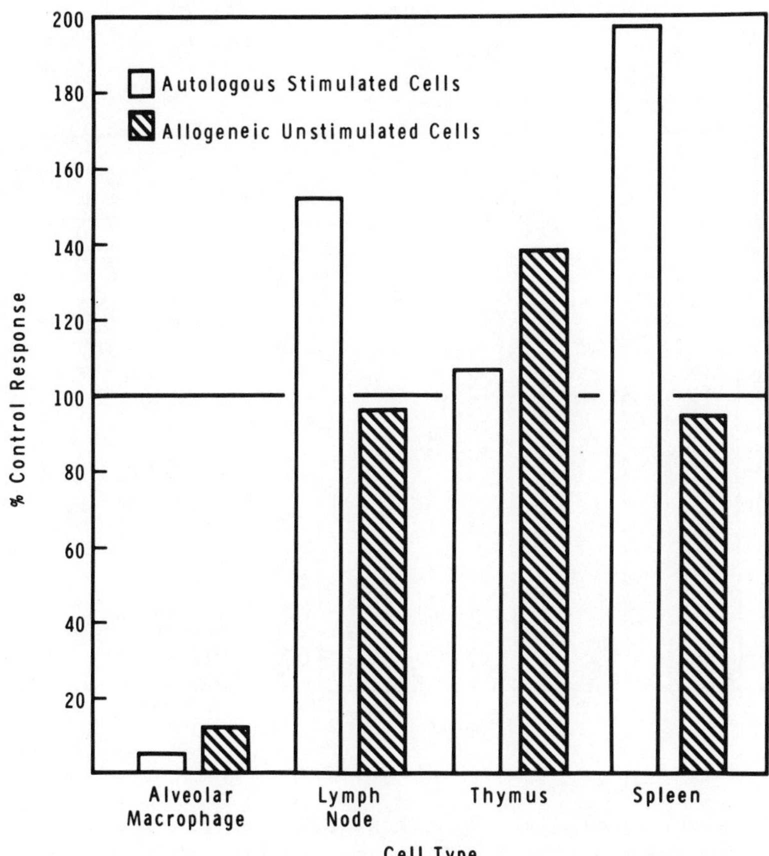

Fig. 2. Effect of addition of various cell types on the *in vitro* PFC response of rabbit spleen cells to SRBC. Cultures contained 1 x 10^7 spleen cells, 1 x 10^5 SRBC and 1 x 10^6 cells from the indicated sources. Results are expressed as percent of control and represent 4 experiments.

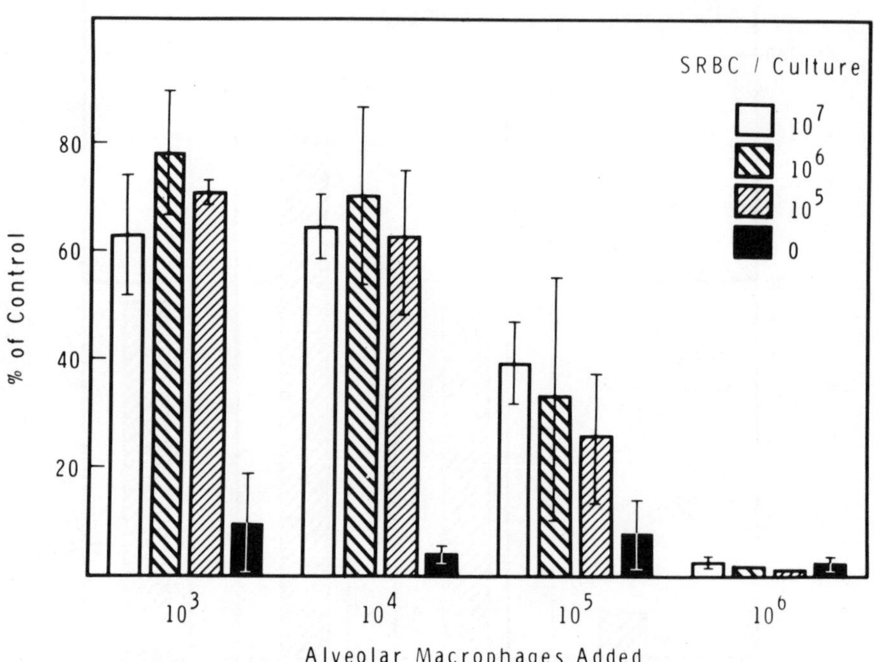

Fig. 3. Effect of addition of excess SRBC on inhibition of the *in vitro* PFC response by AM. Cultures contained 1 x 10^7 spleen cells, RBC and Am as indicated. Results are expressed as mean percent of control (no AM) ± S.E.M. for 4 experiments.

TABLE II

Properties of the Suppressor Cell

- resemble macrophages morphologically
- esterase positive
- phagocytic
- adherent to plastic dishes
- resistant to 2000 R irradiation
- resistant to anti-thymus serum plus complement

respective control for that dose. It is apparent that addition of antigen in amounts up to 100 times the optimal dose (1×10^5 SRBC) had no significant effect on the level of suppression observed at any ratio of AM to spleen cells tested. An attempt was made to impair phagocytosis in AM by preincubating them with 0.8 μm diameter polystyrene latex beads at a multiplicity of 500 beads per AM followed by washing the AM free of beads. Although not shown, the results of these experiments indicated that interference with phagocytosis had no effect on the suppression induced by AM.

The possibility also existed that the observed suppression could be attributed to a trivial phenomenon which was associated with the interaction between spleen cells and alveolar macrophages and which was restricted to the response to SRBC. To test this, rabbits were immunized intravenously, as well as in the hindfoot pads, and spleen, tracheo-bronchial and popliteal lymph nodes were collected. The cells were established in Mishell-Dutton cultures and were stimulated with SRBC either in the absence or presence of normally suppressive concentrations of AM. The results shown in Table III indicate that the suppressive effect of AM is not restricted to an interaction with spleen cells, but also occurs in cultures of popliteal and tracheo-bronchial lymph node cells. Table IV shows that the suppression mediated by AM is not restricted to the *in vitro* response to SRBC since the presence of AM in cultures of spleen cells or popliteal lymph nodes

TABLE III

Effect of Alveolar Macrophages on the PFC Response of Rabbit[a] Lymphocytes to SRBC

Culture Conditions[b]	PFC Response/10^6 Cells[c]		
	Tracheo-bronchial Lymphocytes	Spleen Cells	Popliteal Lymphocytes
-	135 ± 19	145 ± 20	491 ± 85
SRBC	2586 ± 71	2777 ± 48	5233 ± 101
SRBC + AM	126 ± 34	157 ± 14	156 ± 28

[a]Rabbits immunized IV with 1 ml of a 3% SRBC suspension and 0.5 ml of a 10% SRBC suspension in each hind foot pad.
[b]Conditions: 1 x 10^7 lymphocytes, 1 x 10^6 SRBC and 1 x 10^6 AM. Incubated 4 days at 37 C and 5% CO_2.
[c]Results represent mean ± SE for triplicate samples.

TABLE IV

Effect of Alveolar Macrophages on the PFC Response of Rabbit[a] Lymphocytes to Horse Red Blood Cells (HRBC)

Culture Conditions[b]	PFC Response/10^6 Cells[c]	
	Spleen Cells	Popliteal Lymphocytes
-	150 ± 28	1582 ± 87
HRBC	2457 ± 34	9203 ± 98
HRBC + AM	569 ± 48	2274 ± 97

[a]Rabbits immunized IV with 1 ml of a 3% HRBC suspension and 0.5 ml of a 10% HRBC suspension in each hind foot pad.
[b]Conditions: 1 x 10^7 lymphocytes, 1 x 10^6 HRBC and 1 x 10^6 AM. Incubated for 4 days at 37 C and 5% CO_2.
[c]Results represent the mean ± SE for triplicate samples.

obtained from animals immunized with horse red blood cells and challenged *in vitro* with the same antigen were also suppressed.

Experiments were designed using Marbrook vessels to determine if cell contact was a requirement for the observed suppression. Primed spleen cells were placed in the inner chamber of the vessel along with the normal challenge dose of SRBC. The AM were either added to the inner chamber (within) of the vessel in contact with the spleen cells or to the middle chamber (outside) of the vessel which made the possibility of cell contact unlikely. Fig. 4 shows the results of these experiments. Suppression was observed both when the AM were in direct contact with the spleen cells (AM within) or separated from the spleen cells by a 0.4 μm Nucleopore membrane (AM outside). The latter observation suggests that the suppression is mediated by a soluble factor(s). In order to determine the relative size of the soluble factor the spleen cells were separated from the AM by a standard dialysis membrane in place of the Nucleopore membrane. Suppression of the PFC response was not observed in these cultures (data not shown). The results can be interpreted in several ways. First, it may be that the dialysis membrane prevented cell contact which was necessary for the generation of the suppressive effect and which possibly could have occurred via cell extensions through a 0.4 μm Nucleopore membrane. This seems unlikely due to the physical arrangement of the Marbrook vessel. Second and more likely, the suppressive factor, whatever its cellular origin may be, has a molecular weight greater than 10,000 to 12,000 daltons, since a molecule of this size would be restricted from passage through a dialysis membrane.

In order to determine if the AM required the presence of antigen for the generation of the suppressor factor, the following experiment was carried out. Spleen cells were placed in the inner chamber of the vessel along with SRBC. The AM were placed in the middle chamber either in the presence or absence of SRBC. It can be seen from the data presented in Table V that AM did not have to interact with the SRBC to generate the suppressive effect. It should be recalled, however, that both the AM and spleen cells were obtained from previously immunized animals.

The next series of experiments were designed to obtain information on the temporal events involved in the suppression. The AM were added to the middle chamber of the Marbrook vessel at various times after culture initiation and allowed to remain until day 4 when the spleen cells were assayed for PFC. Fig. 5 shows that significant suppression was achieved only if the AM were added during the initial 24 hr of culture. The addition of AM at 48 hr after culture initiation resulted in partial suppression, while the addition of AM at 72 hr was virtually without

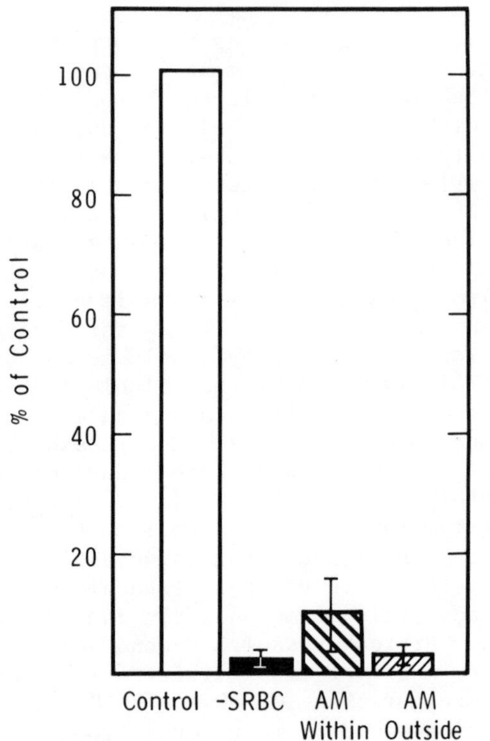

Fig. 4. Inhibition of the *in vitro* PFC response to SRBC by AM in Marbrook culture vessels. Inner chamber contained 2 x 10^7 spleen cells and 2 x 10^6 SRBC. AM were placed either in the inner chamber or middle chamber at a concentration of 2 x 10^6 cells. The inner chamber was separated from the middle chamber by either a 0.45 μm Nucleopore membrane or a piece of standard dialysis tubing. Results are expressed as mean percent of control (no AM) ± S.E.M. for 5 experiments.

effect. In other experiments, the AM were added to the middle chamber of the Marbrook vessel at the time of culture initiation and were then removed at various time intervals thereafter. The results presented in Fig. 6 show that a brief exposure of the spleen cells to the AM (up to 10 hr) did not result in suppression of the PFC response. However, if the AM were present at the time of culture initiation and remained for 24 hr then maximal suppression was observed. These results taken together, demonstrate that the suppressive effect is manifest early in the

TABLE V

Lack of Requirement for Exposure of Alveolar Macrophages to SRBC for Suppression of the PFC Response of Rabbit[a] Spleen Cells

Culture Conditions[b]			PFC ± S.E./10^6 Spleen Cells[c]	
Spleen Cells	SRBC	Alveolar MØ	Experiment 1	Experiment 2
+	-	-	7 ± 2	9 ± 1.5
+	+	-	597 ± 68	307 ± 41
+	+	Inner	9 ± 0.9	11 ± 1.8
+	+	Middle (+SRBC)	7 ± 1.3	16 ± 2
+	+	Middle (-SRBC)	3 ± 0.3	25 ± 5

[a]Rabbits immunized IV with 1 ml of a 3% SRBC suspension.

[b]Autologous alveolar lavage cells were added to the inner chamber or to the middle chamber of Marbrook vessels either in the presence or absence of additional SRBC. Cultures were harvested on day 4.

[c]Results are expressed as mean ± S.E. for 3 cultures.

response and that macrophages must be present for a definite period to be effective suggesting that suppression requires an active process.

The data from the preceeding studies suggested that the suppression is mediated by a soluble factor. To test this directly, cell-free culture supernatants were used in further experiments. Supernatant fluids were generated from the following cell combinations: (a) spleen cells, (b) spleen cells + SRBC, (c) spleen cells + SRBC + AM, (d) spleen cells + AM, (e) AM + SRBC, and (f) AM alone. This series of cultures is referred to as the "supernatant generating system" (see top portion of Table VI). Before testing the supernatants, the PFC response of each culture was determined to establish the functional capabilities of the system. Most important were the observations that culture (b) was stimulated approximately 10-fold greater than culture (a) and that there was substantial suppression in culture (c). Our experience has indicated that an active suppressing culture supernatant can be obtained from Mischell-Dutton cultures in which the AM have suppressed the PFC response by 70 to 95%. The supernatants from each of the cultures were tested in a 3 chamber Marbrook culture vessel in which the cells were placed in the inner chamber separated from the supernatant fluids in the middle vessel by a Nucleopore membrane. Control cultures, in

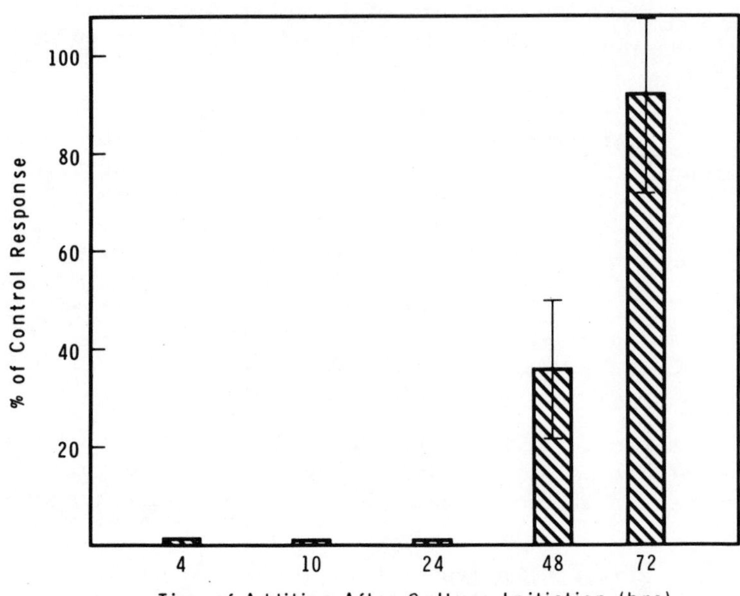

Fig. 5. Effect of time of addition of AM to spleen cells on the *in vitro* PFC response. Primed spleen cells (2 x 10^7) were placed in the inner chamber of the Marbrook vessel along with SRBC (2 x 10^6). AM (2 x 10^6). AM (2 x 10^6) were added to the middle chamber at various times after culture initiation as indicated. Results are expressed as man ± S.E.M. for 5 experiments.

which various cell combinations were incubated in the absence of culture supernatants showed the generation of a significant PFC response in SRBC-stimulated spleen cells, while cultures incubated with AM displayed a diminished PFC response (middle portion of Table VI - controls for detecting system). Several observations were made when the effects of the various culture supernatants on the PFC response were evaluated. These can be seen in the lower portion of Table VI. First, supernatants from cultures of spleen cells along (a), AM + SRBC (e) or AM alone (f) had no detectable effect on the generation of the PFC response. Second, was the observation that supernatants obtained from cultures of spleen cells + AM, with or without SRBC (cultures (c) and (d)), contained a soluble factor that significantly suppressed the PFC response at a magnitude equal to that of the AM in the control cultures. An unexpected observation was made when the

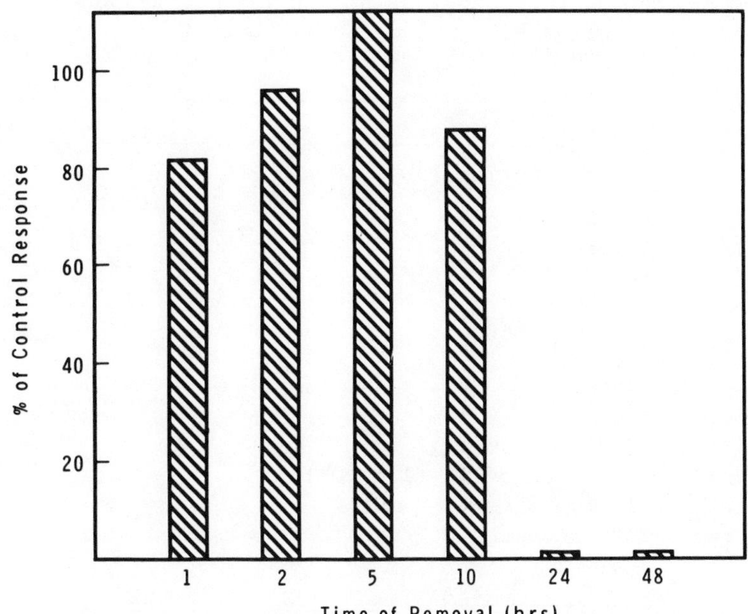

Fig. 6. Effect of removal of AM at various times after culture initiation on the *in vitro* PFC response. Primed spleen cells (2×10^7) were added to the inner chamber of Marbrook vessels along with the SRBC (2×10^6). AM (2×10^6) were placed in the middle chamber at time 0 and were then removed at the indicated time. Results are expressed as the mean ± S.E.M. for 3 experiments.

supernatant from spleen cells + SRBC (b) enhanced the response some 2-fold over the untreated control (e.g., 3773 PFC in cultures treated with supernatant (b) vs. 1855 PFC in untreated control cultures). The last line of Table VI shows the results of an experiment in which the normally suppressing cell combination, that is, spleen cells + AM + SRBC was incubated in the presence of the "enhancing" culture supernatant (b). The results indicate that the presence of the pre-formed enhancing factor prevented the AM-induced suppression. This provides further evidence that the generation of the suppressing factor is an active process occurring over a definitive time period in culture.

An attempt was then made to determine how rapidly suppression would occur if primed spleen cells were exposed to a pre-

TABLE VI

Effect of Culture Supernatants on the PFC Response of Rabbit[a] Spleen Cells to SRBC

A. Supernatant Generating System

Cell Combinations	PFC ± S. E./10^6 Cells[e]
(a) SC[b]	194 ± 22
(b) SC + SRBC[c]	1955 ± 235
(c) SC + SRBC + AM[d]	168 ± 18
(d) SC + AM	134 ± 14
(e) AM + SRBC	-
(f) AM	-

[a]Rabbits immunized IV with 1 ml of a 3% SRBC suspension.
[b]SC = spleen cells (1 x 10^7).
[c]SRBC = sheep red blood cells (1 x 10^6).
[d]AM = alveolar macrophages (1 x 10^6).
[e]Result represents the mean of triplicate samples.

B. Detecting System

Inner Chamber Cell Combinations	Middle Chamber Supernatant Source[d]	PFC ± S.E./10^6 Cells[e]	Observed Effect
1. Control			
SC[a]	-	425 ± 99	-
SC + SRBC[b]	-	1855 ± 305	Stimulation
SC - SRBC - AM[c]	-	409 ± 46	Suppression
2. Test System			
SC + SRBC	SC[a] (a)	1609 ± 113	None
SC + SRBC	SC + SRBC (b)	3773 ± 295	Enhancement
SC + SRBC	SC + SRBC + AM (c)	469 ± 55	Suppression
SC + SRBC	SC + AM (d)	501 ± 42	Suppression
SC + SRBC	AM - SRBC (e)	1769 ± 97	None
SC + SRBC	AM (f)	1873 ± 125	None
SC + SRBC + AM	SC + SRBC (b)	2896 ± 172	Suppression inhibited

[a]SC = spleen cells (2 x 10^7).
[b]SRBC = sheep red blood cells (2 x 10^6).
[c]AM = alveolar macrophages (2 x 10^6).
[d]Supernatant in 3.3 ml.
[e]Results represent the mean of triplicate samples.

formed suppressor factor prior to culture initiation. Spleen cells were incubated with various culture supernatants for 30 min at 37 C, washed and established in Mishell-Dutton cultures with added SRBC. Fig. 7 indicates that this relatively short exposure to supernatants from cultures of spleen cells + AM either in the presence or absence of antigen was sufficient to significantly suppress the PFC response whereas supernatants from spleen cells along or spleen cells + SRBC had no detectable effect.

Experiments were then carried out in an attempt to elucidate the mechanism of the AM-induced suppression. Since previous reports have suggested that macrophages suppress by interfering with cell proliferation coupled with our finding that suppression occurs early in the response, an experiment was carried out to evaluate the effect of AM on antigen-induced lymphocyte proliferation. Various cell combinations were established in Mishell-Dutton cultures. At 24 hr intervals, replicate samples were removed, harvested, washed, placed in microtiter plates at a concentration of 2×10^5 cells/well and pulsed with 1 μCi of ^{3}H-thymidine for 18 hr. Fig. 8 shows that incorporation was maximal in SRBC-stimulated spleen cell cultures pulsed at 48 hr (an approximate 4.5 fold increase over unstimulated cells) whereas cultures of spleen cells incubated with AM were inhibited in their ability to incorporate ^{3}H-thymidine into acid-precipitable counts suggesting that AM suppress PFC responses by inhibiting antigen-induced lymphoproliferation.

While the precise mechanism has not as of yet been clarified, the results summarized in Table VII preclude several possibilities that have been previously associated with macrophage-induced suppression.

TABLE VII

Characteristics of Alveolar Macrophage-induced Suppression

- heat killed AM (56 C, 45 min) do not suppress the PFC response directly or participate in the generation of suppressing supernatants
- freeze-thawed AM fail to suppress
- pre-treatment of AM with iodoacetamide (10^{-1} to 10^{-4}M) abolishes the suppressive capacity
- suppression by AM is not attributed to the release of:
    - a factor cytotoxic for lymphocytes
    - prostaglandin
    - thymidine
    - arginase

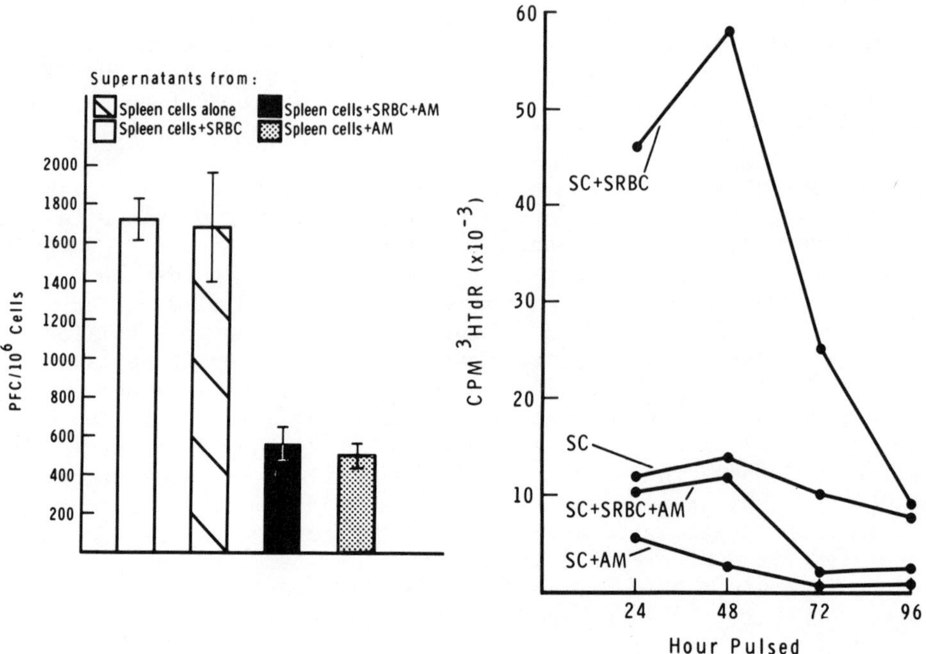

Fig. 7. (left) Effect of time of exposure to culture supernatants on the PFC response of rabbit spleen cells. Primed spleen cells (1×10^7) were exposed to the various supernatants for 30 min, washed 3 times and placed in Mishell-Dutton cultures with SRBC (1×10^6). Results represent the mean ± SE for duplicate cultures.

Fig. 8. (right) Effect of alveolar macrophages (AM) on the lymphoproliferative response of rabbit spleen cells (SC) to SRBC. Aliquots of cells were removed from Mishell-Dutton cultures, washed, placed in microtiter plates at 2×10^5 spleen cells per well, and pulsed for 18 hr with 1 μCi of ^{3}H-thymidine at the time intervals indicated. Results represent the mean of triplicate samples. SE was less than 10% at all points.

DISCUSSION

There is an impressive body of evidence accumulating which suggests that macrophages are capable of modulating immune responses (35). In this communication we have described a potential immunoregulatory role for the alveolar macrophage.

It was our intention at the initiation of these experiments to establish a role for alveolar macrophages in the induction of immune responses. The experimental design utilized the Mishell-Dutton in vitro culture system as a means of manipulating the cellular components of the system. Based on studies in the mouse system, we initially anticipated a reduced response of the adherent cell-depleted rabbit spleen population, therefore, AM were added to several cultures in an effort to effect reconstitution of the response. Those cultures to which AM were added demonstrated markedly reduced responses compared to the respective controls of either unseparated or adherent cell-depleted spleen cell populations (Table I). The experiments to be discussed herein concern our efforts to elucidate the nature of this suppression.

When varying numbers of autologous AM were added to spleen cells (either adherent cell-depleted or unseparated), the suppression of the response was found to be dependent on the concentration of AM in the cultures (Fig. 1). At ratios of 1:1000 (AM:spleen cells) only minimal suppression was observed, while at 1:10 the response was suppressed by 90%. The dose-response curve observed for AM suppression of the in vitro PFC response of rabbit spleen cells was similar to that seen in previously published studies which showed peritoneal exudate macrophage suppression of lymphocyte function as determined by PFC responses (4,26) and antibody production (27).

Several explanations were considered as possible mechanisms of the observed suppression. Certainly cell crowding in the cultures could result in a diminution in the response of antigen-stimulated splenocytes. This seems unlikely from the results of experiments in which a variety of cell types were added to the spleen cell cultures (Fig. 2). At equivalent cell concentrations, only macrophages were suppressive, while lymph node cells, spleen cells or thymocytes either augmented the response or were without effect. The finding that allogeneic unstimulated AM, but no other allogeneic cell types suppress the response deserves further comment. First, it adds credibility to the argument that suppression is not due to cell crowding and supports the concept that a macrophage-like cell is responsible for the suppression. Second, it suggests that a sharing of antigens in the major histocompatibility complex (MHC) is not required to achieve suppression, whereas it has been suggested for other macrophage-lymphocyte interactions (45). The lack of a requirement for shared MHC is not required to achieve suppression, whereas it has been suggested for other macrophage-lymphocyte interactions (45). The lack of a requirement for shared MHC antigens in suppression has been reported (12,21). Finally, it suggests that an interaction between the AM and antigen is not required for the suppressive effect. However, it should be kept in mind that the AM from unstimulated rabbits were incubated with SRBC-primed lymphocytes in the presence of additional SRBC and therefore, we cannot rule out the possibility that antigen is not required.

That the cell type responsible for the immunosuppression was a macrophage was suggested from the results presented in Table II. Giemsa stained preparations revealed that about 95% of the cells obtained by lavage had the morphological properties of macrophages. These cells were uniformly esterase positive, were capable of phagocytizing latex particles and sensitized SRBC and were adherent to plastic surfaces. The suppressive effect was not inhibited by pre-treatment of the cells with up to 2000 R of γ-irradiation or anti-thymus serum plus complement. Using similar criteria, others have suggested that the macrophage was the responsible cell type (7,21,22,52).

Macrophages as phagocytic cells may sequester antigen and therefore compete for it with lymphocytes (4). If sequestration of antigen was responsible for the loss of responsiveness in the spleen cell population, one would expect a possible shift in the macrophage-dose suppression curve when additional antigen was added so that a higher number of macrophages would be required to achieve a similar level of suppression. This did not appear to be the case (Fig. 3).

That the observed immunosuppressive effect mediated by AM was due to some culture artifact that was restricted to the interaction among spleen cells, AM and SRBC was considered unlikely based on the observations that the AM suppressed the response of both popliteal lymph node cells and tracheo-bronchial lymphocytes stimulated with SRBC (Table III) as well as the response of both spleen cells and popliteal lymph node cells stimulated with horse RBC (Table IV).

There have been several reports (2,5,7,23,26,33,36,51) which demonstrate that macrophages exert their suppressive effect by the elaboration of soluble factors. A similar observation was made herein (FIg. 4) whereby it was shown that AM separated from spleen cells by a membrane which purportedly restricted cell contact but allowed for the passage of macromolecules, resulted in suppression of the *in vitro* PFC response. The observed suppression did not require a further interaction between AM and antigen (Table V) and suggests the possibility that suppression was due to a nonspecific mechanism involving an interaction between macrophages and lymphocytes. The finding that AM had to be present at the time of culture initiation (Fig. 5) in order to achieve suppression suggests that an early event is involved. This is in contrast to the report of Tadakuma and Pierce (47) who demonstrated that SIRS-treated macrophages suppressed PFC development by a mechanism that appeared to involve a premature termination rather than a failure at the level of induction of the response. The finding that the AM had to be present in the cultures for at least 24 hr (Fig. 6) suggests that an active process is involved in the generation of the suppressor factor(s). Further support for an active process was provided by experiments in which it was shown that freeze-thawed, heat-killed and iodoacetamide-treated macrophages were incapable of inducing a suppressive effect. These results suggest that a viable, metabolically active macrophage is required. This is in contrast to reports (38,39) which showed that heat-killed macrophages or membrane preparations from macrophages could suppress *in vitro* PFC responses. They attributed the suppression to the absorption of T cell factors by macrophage surfaces thereby interfering with cooperative events.

The generation of biologically active culture supernatants (Table VI) provided some indication of potential mechanisms involved in the suppression of PFC responses. The finding that active suppressing supernatants were generated only by cultures containing spleen cells and viable AM suggests that a macrophage-lymphocyte interaction is involved. Similar conclusions were reached by others (42,46,47). At least two such interactions should be considered. First, it is possible that macrophages produce a product that acts directly on T lymphocytes to induce suppressor activity. Such a mechanism has been proposed by Stobo (46) in the macrophage-induced suppression observed in patients with disseminated fungal disease. A second mechanism, which is consistent with the work of Tadakuma and Pierce (48), suggests that activated suppressor T cells produce a mediator that directs macrophages to produce a factor which in turn suppresses lymphocyte responses. The observation that culture supernatants generated by alveolar macrophages alone did not suppress the PFC response would tend to support the latter as a possible mechanism to explain the suppression occurring in our system. Further, the finding that supernatants derived from cultures containing spleen cells plus antigen enhanced *in vitro* PFC responses provides additional evidence that several factors may be produced in this system. Whether these factors are similar to other factors produced by cells involved in the immune response or whether they are unique, as well as the relationship among these factors required for suppression of the immune response, necessitates additional investigation.

Several factors released by macrophages have been shown to inhibit lymphocyte activity. Kung *et al.* (24) reported that suppression of *in vitro* cytotoxic responses was attributable to the release of arginase from activated macrophages. In our studies, the addition of arginase to cultures of spleen cells stimulated by SRBC did not result in suppression nor was the suppression observed in cultures of spleen cells, SRBC and AM reversed upon the addition of excess arginine. There have been reports (16,36) which suggest that thymidine and thymidine monophosphate released from macrophages were responsible for inhibition of lymphoproliferative responses. In our system addition of thymidine, even at concentrations greater than 100 μg/culture, did not suppress the PFC response of SRBC-stimulated rabbit spleen cells while it did inhibit the incorporation of ^{3}H-thymidine if added at the time of pulse. Additional factors released from macrophages, namely prostaglandins, have been associated with the suppression of immune responses (14). We observed that addition of supraphysiological concentrations (10^{-4} to 10^{-7}M) of PGE_1 and PGE_2 did not affect the PFC response of _in vitro_ stimulated splenocytes nor did the addition of indomethacin, an inhibitor of prostaglandin synthetase, reverse the suppression by alveolar macrophages. Finally, we can not attribute the suppression to the release of a cytotoxic factor from the alveolar macrophages since viability was equivalent in AM-treated and control cultures.

There are numerous reports to indicate that the ultimate mechanism by which macrophages inhibit immune response is associated with the inhibition of lymphocyte proliferation (1,5,12, 26,48,51,53). The results presented in Fig. 8, in which it was shown that antigen-induced proliferation was suppressed by AM, supports this conclusion.

SUMMARY

Alveolar macrophages were shown to suppress the _in vitro_ immune response of rabbit lymphoid cells stimulated with heterologous erythrocytes. Suppression was associated with an adherent, phagocytic cell that was resistant to the effects of irradiation and treatment with anti-thymus serum. Suppression was mediated by a soluble factor whose production was independent of antigen and required an interaction of viable alveolar macrophages and lymphocytes. Suppression was associated with an early event in the induction of the PFC response and appeared to affect lymphocyte proliferation. Suppression could not be attributed to cytotoxicity, sequestration of antigen, depletion of nutrients or release of prostaglandins, arginase or thymidine. These results, taken together, provide additional information regarding immunological function of alveolar macrophages and suggest that they play a regulatory role in the immune response.

ACKNOWLEDGEMENTS

This investigation was supported gy Grant No. HLAI 16748, from the National Institutes of Health (Bethesda, MD). We gratefully acknowledge the technical assistance of Ms. Harriet Gerber. We thank Ms. Janet Phoenix Dixon for secretarial assistance in preparation of this manuscript. We are grateful to Dr. A. B. Stavitsky for his gift of the anti-thymus serum.

REFERENCES

1. Baird, L. G. and Kaplan, A. M., Cell. Immunol., 28 (1977) 22.
2. Baird, L. G. and Kaplan, A. M., Cell. Immunol., 28 (1977) 36.
3. Blanden, R. V., TRansplantation, 7 (1969) 484.
4. Broder, S., Humphrey, R., Durn, M., Blackman, M., Meade, B., Goldman, B., Strober, W. and Waldmann, T., New Engl. J. Med., 293 (1975) 887.
5. Calderon, J., Williams, R. T. and Unanue, E. R., Proc. Natl. Acad. Sci., 71 (1974) 4273.
6. Cunningham, A. and Szenberg, A., Immunol., 14 (1968) 599.
7. Elgert, K. D. and Farrar, W. L., J. Immunol., 120 (1978) 1345.
8. Farrar, W. L. and Elgert, K. D., J. Immunol., 120 (1978) 1354.
9. Fernbach, B. R., Kirchner, H., Bernard, G. D. and Herberman, R. B., Transplantation, 21 (1976) 381.
10. Folch, H. and Waksman, B. H., J. Immunol., 113 (1974) 127.
11. Folch, H. and Waksman, B. H., J. Immunol., 113 (1974) 140.
12. Gillette, R. W., Cell. Immunol., 33 (1977) 309.
13. Glaser, M., Kirchner, H., Holden, H. T. and Herberman, R. B., J. Natl. Cancer Inst., 56 (1976) 865.
14. Goodwin, J. S., Bankhurst, A. D. and Messner, R. P., J. Exp. Med., 146 (1977) 1719.
15. Hoffman, M., Immunology, 18 (1970) 791.
16. Kasahara, T. and Nakano, K. S., J. Immunol., 116 (1976) 1251.
17. Keller, R., Immunology, 27 (1974) 285.
18. Keller, R., Cell. Immunol., 17 (1975) 542.
19. Kirchner, H., Chused, T. M., Herberman, R. B., Holden, H. T. and Lavrin, D. H., J. Exp. Med., 139 (1974) 1473.
20. Kirchner, H., Herberman, R.B., Glaser, M. and Lavrin, D. H., Cell. Immunol. 13 (1974) 32.
21. Klimpel, G. R. and Henney, C. S., J. Immunol., 120 (1978) 563.
22. Kolb, J. P., Arrian, S. and Zolla-Pazner, S., J. Immunol., 118 (1977) 702.
23. Krakauer, R. S., Strober, W. S. and Waldmann, T., Clin. Res., 24 (1976) 377.
24. Kung, J. T., Brooks, S. B., Jakway, J. P., Leonard, L. L. and Talmage, D. W., J. Exp. Med., 146 (1977) 665.
25. Lapp, W. S. and Mooler, G., Immunology, 17 (1969) 339.
26. Lemke, H., Coutinko, A., Opitz, H. G. and Gronowicz, E., Scand. J. Immunol., 4 (1975) 707.
27. Luzzati, A. L. and LaFleur, L., Eur. J. Immunol., 6 (1976) 125.
28. Marbrook, J., Lancet, 2 (1967) 1279.
29. Mishell, R. I. and Dutton, R. W., J. Exp. Med., 126 (1967) 423.
30. Moller, G., Immunology, 20 (1971) 597.

31. Mosier, D. E., Science, 158 (1967) 1575.
32. Myrvik, Q. N., Leake, E. S. and Farris, B., J. Immunol. 86 (1961) 128.
33. Nelson, D., Nature, 246 (1973) 306.
34. Oehler, J. R., Herberman, R. B., Campbell, D. A. and Djeur, J. Y., Cell Immunol. 29 (1977) 238.
35. Oehler, J. R., Herberman, R. B. and Holden, H. T., J. Pharmacol. Exper. Therap., 2 (1978) 551.
36. Opitz, H. G., Niethammer, D., Lemke, H., Flad, H. D. and Huget, R., Cell. Immunol., 16 (1975) 379.
37. Perkins, E. H. and Makinodan, T., J. Immunol., 94 (1965) 765.
38. Ptak, W. and Gershon, R. K., J. Immunol., 115 (1975) 1346.
39. Ptak, W., Naidorf, K. F. and Gershon, R. K., J. Immunol., 119 (1977) 444.
40. Raff, H. V. and Hinricks, D. J., Cell Immunol., 29 (1977) 96.
41. Raff, H. V. and Hinricks, D. J., Cell Immunol., 29 (1977) 109.
42. Raff, H. V. and Hinricks, D. J., Cell Immunol., 29 (1977) 118.
43. Redelman, D., Scott, C. B. and Sell, S., Cell Immunol., 19 (1975) 230.
44. Rich, R. R. and Pierce, C. W., J. Immunol., 112 (1974) 1360.
45. Rosenthal, A. S. and Shevack, E. M., J. Exp. Med., 138 (1973) 1194.
46. Stobo, J. D., J. Immunol., 119 (1977) 918.
47. Tadakuma, T. and Pierce, C. W., J. Immunol., 117 (1976) 967.
48. Tadakuma, T. and Pierce, C. W., J. Immunol., 120 (1978) 481.
49. Viet, B. C. and Feldman, J. D., J. Immunol., 117 (1976) 646.
50. Veit, B. C. and Feldman, J. D., J. Immunol., 117 (1976) 655.
51. Waldman, S. R. and Gottlieb, A. A., Cell Immunol., 9 (1973)142.
52. Weiss, A. and Fitch, F. W., J. Immunol., 120 (1978) 357.
53. Wing, E. J. and Remington, J. S., Cell. Immunol., 30 (1977) 108.

SUPPRESSION OF ANTIBODY FORMING CELLS BY RAT SPLEEN MACROPHAGES

S. M. REICHARD

Medical College of Georgia
Augusta, Georgia (USA)

In tumor-bearing or stressed hosts, immunologic functions are impaired (2,10,27,28). We have shown that antibody synthesis was altered in traumatic shock (22). The reticuloendothelial system (RES) plays a central role in the physiologic adaptation to this severe stress. Stimulation of RE function protects against the consequences of this stress whereas RE impairment causes a deterioration of the body's defense against trauma (20).

Paradoxically it was found that these procedures appeared to have the opposite effect on the hemolysin plaque forming capacity in the spleens of rats. Impairment of the RES increased the number of antibody plaque forming cells (PFC) cultured from rat spleens *in vitro* (23). Rat spleens were shown to contain suppressor cells which inhibit the proliferative and cytotoxic responses of lymphocytes to alloantigen *in vitro* (3,5,9,17,29,31). The activated macrophage was implicated to act as a suppressor cell in many of the systems (14,19,31). Macrophages have also been observed to inhibit the PFC responses by mouse (19) and rat (32) spleen cells to heterologous erythrocytes. The current study was designed to determine whether macrophages present in normal spleen cells were, in fact, suppressing the generation of PFC. It was demonstrated that the depletion of macrophages stimulates the development of antibody producing cells and the addition of spleen or peritoneal macrophages inhibits the primary *in vitro* immune response.

MATERIALS AND METHODS

Impairment of the phagocytic activity of the RES was produced by blockading the reticuloendothelial elements with colloidal agents, which physically overload the phagocytic cells of the liver and spleen so that no further uptake occurs during a distinct time interval. Animals were injected via the jugular vein with 24 mg (1.2 ml volume) of Proferrin, a saccharated iron oxide, or 77 mg (0.3 ml) of Thorotrast, a stabilized colloidal suspension of thorium dioxide. Control animals received equal volumes of physiological saline by the same route. Two hours after receiving this colloidal agent, rats were subjected to trauma or received an intravenous injection of sheep erythrocytes.

The effectiveness of RES-blocking agents has been shown to be both dose and time-dependent, and within 4-5 hr after a single blocking injection, phagocytic activity returns to normal. Several colloidal agents were shown to stimulate phagocytic activity after an initial depression (4). An effective stimulating procedure included the intravenous administration of 2 mg saccharated iron oxide (Proferrin) daily for 3 days.

Antibody plaque forming cells (PFC) were determined in the spleens of experimental and control rats using the Jerne hemolytic plaque assay (13). Cells were prepared by gently teasing apart the spleens of normal, unimmunized or immunized rats in cold Hanks balanced salt solution. Cell suspensions were washed three times by serial centrifugation and used for the plaque assay. Suspensions of 1-5 x 10^6 of these cells and 2 x 10^8 sheep red blood cells (SRBC) were added to 2 ml of 0.6% agar solution at 45 C. The mixture was then poured onto a supporting layer of 1.2% Agarose in a small (50 x 15 mm) plastic Petri dish. After 90 min incubation at 32 C, 0.5 ml complement (1:2 dil) was added. Within 30 min, single visible hemolytic plaques about 0.25 mm diameter were found.

For immunization _in vivo_, rats were injected intravenously with 0.5 ml of 10% SRBC. Optimal numbers of PFC appeared 4 days after intravenous administration. For immunization _in vitro_, the Mishell and Dutton culture system was used (15) in which spleen cells or peritoneal cells were stimulated with 1 x 10^5 SRBC for 6 days in culture.

One milliliter cultures containing 5 x 10^6 spleen cells or 1 x 10^6 peritoneal macrophages in Hanks solution supplemented with nonessential amino acids, glutamine, pyruvate, 10% fetal bovine serum and 5 x 10^{-5} M 2-mercaptoethanol, plus 100 units penicillin and 100 mg of streptomycin were prepared. They were placed in 35 mm plastic culture dishes and incubated with gentle rotation in a humidified atmosphere of 5% CO_2. Nutritional mixtures and fetal calf serum were added daily.

Macrophage depleted spleen cells (MDSC) were prepared by incubating mixed spleen cells (1 x 10^8) in 10 ml of medium with

200 mg of carbonyl iron powder in 35 mm plastic culture dishes for 1 hr at 37 C. The phagocytic cells and remaining unphagocytized iron was removed with a powerful magnet. There was approximately 70% recovery of macrophages with this method.

Adherent spleen cells (ASC) were harvested after incubation for 1 hr at 37 C in culture medium. The nonadhering cells were carefully removed and the procedure was repeated. The adherent cells were removed with a rubber policeman or by elution with 10 mM lidocaine (31). Viability as determined by trypan blue exclusion was about 60-70%, and contained approximately 85-90% macrophages by morphological criteria.

Peritoneal exudate cells (PFC) were harvested from rats injected 4 days previously with 2 ml of 10% thioglycollate medium, by flusing out the peritoneal cavity with sterile Hanks balanced salt solution (BSS). Cells were washed twice and incubated on glass Petri dishes for 90 min at 37 C. The nonadhering cells were carefully removed and the procedure was repeated. The adherent cells were removed with a rubber policeman or by elution with 10 mM lidocaine. Viability as determined by trypan blue exclusion was about 60-70% and contained approximately 85-90% macrophages by morphological criteria.

RESULTS

Listed in Table I are the number of PFC found 4 days after an injection of 0.5 ml of 10% sheep erythrocytes. Low numbers are seen in rats compared to the larger numbers ordinarily observed in mice. There were no significant changes in plaque forming capacity in rats receiving an LD_{50}dose of trauma, i.e. 500 turns in a Noble-Collip apparatus 24 hr before or after SRBC.

As seen in Table II there was a significant decrease in PFC in animals made resistant to this trauma by prior repeated sublethal exposures, Trauma Resistant (TR) rats were given intravenous injections of SRBC 4 days before the hemolysin agar test. TR rats also received an LD_{50} dose of trauma 24 hr before or after SRBC. Trauma received before SRBC in TR rats further decreased the number of PFC.

Since this state of resistance is also produced by RES stimulation, it appears that whereas stimulation may increase survival to traumatic shock it suppresses PFC generation.

The effect of RES impairment of PFC is shown in Table III. The intravenous administration of colloidal agents, Proferrin or Thorotrast, 2 hr before the injection of SRBC enhanced the numbers of PFC in both normal and Trauma Resistant rats.

TABLE I

PFC Response of Rats Injected with SRBC[a]

Treatment	Number of Rats	PFC/10^6 Spleen Cells
SRBC	16	155
SRBC + Trauma	20	133
Trauma + SRBC	20	171

[a]Plaque forming cells (PFC) 4 days after iv injection of 0.5 ml of 10% sheep erythrocytes (SRBC). Rats received 500 turns in Noble-Collip apparatus 24 hr before or after SRBC.

TABLE II

PFC Response of Trauma Resistant (TR) Rats Injected with SRBC[a]

Treatment	Number of Rats	PFC/10^6 Spleen Cells
SRBC only	12	188
TR - SRBC	16	96[b]
TR: SRBC + Trauma	16	100[b]
TR: Trauma + SRBC	16	57[b]

[a]Plaque forming cells (PFC) 4 days after iv injection of 0.5 ml of 10% sheep erythrocytes (SRBC). Rats received 500 turns in Noble-Collip apparatus 24 hr before or after SRBC.

[b]P = 0.05.

TABLE III

RES Suppression and Plaque-Forming Cells[a]

Treatment	PFC/10^6 Spleen Cells
SRBC only	154
Proferrin + SRBC	266[b]
ThO_2 + SRBC	250[b]
Saline + SRBC	148
TR: SRBC	76
TR: Proferrin + SRBC	220[b]
TR: ThO_2 + SRBC	165[b]
TR: Saline = SRBC	76

[a]Proferrin and Thorotrast (ThO_2) given 2 hr prior to injection of SRBC in normal and TR rats. Plaques at 4 days.

[b]P = <.05.

The data in Table IV demonstrate the potentiation of the lowering of PFC in TR rats with additional trauma 24 hr prior to SRBC administration. They also show the abrogation of this effect by impairing RES phagocytic function before exposure to trauma. Proferrin given after trauma but before SRBC injection overcame the added effect of trauma but the lowered effect of TR was still evident.

These results again point out the fact that macrophages may be suppressing the PFC response *in vivo*. Impairing their function increases the number of PFC observed *in vitro*. To test this hypothesis the following experiments were carried out.

Mixed Spleen Cells were obtained from normal, traumatized and trauma resistant animals. Mixed Spleen Cells (MSC) were stimulated *in vitro* with SRBC for 6 days and the PFC were developed. Again a decreased number of PFC were evident in spleens of TR rats (Table V).

TABLE IV

Effect of RES Suppression on Antibody Response to Trauma in TR Rats[a]

Treatment	PFC/10^6 Spleen Cells
SRBC only	168
Trauma Resistant:	
Saline + SRBC	96[b]
Trauma + SRBC	57[b]
Trauma-Prof + SRBC	112
Prof + Trauma-SRBC	154

[a]Proferrin given 2 hr prior to SRBC or 500 turns. Plaques at 4 days.

[b]$P = <.05$.

In other cultures, cells in which the adherent or phagocytic cells were removed by incubation with carbonyl iron powder for 1 hr (MDSC), a greatly enhanced number of PFC was seen. This indicates that the presence of macrophages suppresses this generation of PFC.

The effect of the addition of Mixed Spleen Cells or adherent macrophages obtained by elution with 10 mM lidocaine is shown in Table VI. Both procedures lowered the antibody producing cells again to levels seen with MSC alone from levels of MDSC of about 2000 PFC. The lowered number of cells for TR rats is still evident.

The addition of Peritoneal Macrophages (Table VII) obtained from normal, traumatized and TR rats had similar results to macrophages obtained from the spleen. Levels of MDSC of about 2000 PFC were reduced to 22 in normal rats, 2 in TR rats.

Macrophages were added to the culture at various times after the initiation of incubation. It was found that macrophages could be added anytime during the first day in order to be suppressive (Table VIII). Thereafter, there was no suppressive effect.

TABLE V

PFC Response to SRBC of Mixed Spleen Cells (MSC) and Macrophage Depleted Spleen Cells (MDSC)[a]

Treatment	PFC/5 x 10^6 Spleen Cells MSC	MDSC
None	40	2018
Trauma	55	2110
TR	10	625

[a]Plaque forming cells (PFC) present in unimmunized rats stimulated with 1 x 10^5 SRBC for 6 days in culture.

TABLE VI

Suppression on Immune Response by Addition of Adherent Spleen Macrophages[a]

	MDSC plus	
Treatment	MSC (PFC/culture)	ASC (PFC/culture
None	58	11
Trauma	70	12
TR	10	0

[a]Plaque forming cells (PFC) present in unimminized rats stimulated with 1 x 10^5 SRBC for 6 days in culture. 5 x 10^6 Mixed Spleen Cells (MSC) or 5 x 10^6 Adherent Spleen Cells (ASC) added to 5 x 10^6 Macrophage Depleted Spleen Cells (MDSC).

TABLE VII

Suppression of Immune Response by Addition of Peritoneal Macrophages[a]

	MDSC Plus	
Treatment	MSC (PFC/Culture)	PEC (PFC/Culture)
None	60	22
Trauma	74	15
TR	12	2

[a]Plaque forming cells (PFC) present in unimmunized rats stimulated with 1 x 10^5 SRBC for 6 days in culture. 5 x 10^6 Mixed Spleen Cells (MSC) or 10^6 Peritoneal Exudate Cells (PEC) added to 5 x 10^6 Macrophage Depleted Spleen Cells (MDSC).

TABLE VIII

Effect of Macrophages Added at Various Times[a]

Addition	PFC/Culture
MDSC alone	2050
0 hr	22
+8	35
+16	27
+24	2100
+48	1990

[a]Plaque forming cells (PFC) present in unimmunized rats stimulated with 1 x 10^5 SRBC for 6 days in culture. 5 x 10^6 Adherent Spleen Cells (ASC) added at various times after culture initiation to 5 x 10^6 Macrophage Depleted Spleen Cells (MDSC).

DISCUSSION

The data demonstrate that macrophages act to suppress the generation of antibody forming cells in the spleens of rats. In previous studies, the state of resistance against traumatic shock was found to be associated with an increased RES activity. This induced resistance was correlated with an inhibition of the number of plaque forming cells in the spleen (20). It appeared that heightened RES activity which increases survival at the same time suppresses the PFC capacity in the rat. Experiments in which the RES phagocytic function was impaired _in vivo_ were also supportive of the idea that enhanced RES activity inhibits PFC generation. As seen in Table III, the intravenous administration of colloidal agents, a procedure known to curtail RES function, clearly stimulated the numbers of PFC in both normal and TR rats.

On the assumption that phagocytic or adherent cells from mixed spleen cells were suppressing the PFC response, these cells were removed _in vitro_ with a magnet after incubating with carbonyl iron powder. The remaining macrophage depleted spleen cells (MDSC) showed a greatly increased PFC response. As seen in Table V, a dramatic increase in the number of antibody forming cells occurred in cultures depleted of macrophages as compared to cultures of mixed spleen cells alone (from 40 PFC per 10^6MSC to 2018 per 10^6 MDSC). A similar enhancement was seen with MDSC derived from TR rats even though the lowered effect of trauma resistance on rat cells was still evident.

Finally, the addition of an equal number of mixed spleen cells (Table VI) to cultures of macrophage depleted cells returned this increased level of PFC down to those seen with MSC alone (from about 2000 PFC per culture for MDSC to 58). The addition of viable rat spleen macrophages reduced the levels nearly 200 fold for cells from normal rats, and 2000 fold for cells from TR rats (see Table VII).

Macrophages are known to play an important role in the immune process. Fishman and Adler (8) suggested that antibody synthesis results from the interaction of two functionally different cell types, one which phagocytizes and "processes" the antigen, and provides the stimulus for lymphoid cells to synthesize specific antibody. Mosier (16) showed that both adherent phagocytic and nonadherent mouse spleen cells were essential for the development of plaque forming cells _in vitro_. The importance of macrophages in the generation of PFC in the mouse has since been confirmed by many investigators (6,25,32). Macrophages have also been shown to be required in other aspects of cell-mediated immunity, including the production of cytolytic lymphocytes in mixed lymphocyte cultures in mice (1,11,30) and in man (26) and and the response to T cell mitogens (24).

In some instances, macrophages were found to suppress the immune response in mice. The PFC response to heterologous erythrocytes was suppressed by macrophages (19), mitogen induced activation of T lymphocytes *in vitro* was inhibited in normal (7,18) and tumor-bearing mice (14).

Lymphoproliferative responses and responses dependent upon them have been more difficult to demonstrate in spleens of rats (3,33). Folch and Waksman (9) described a thymus-dependent adherent spleen cell in the rat that suppressed proliferative responses to mitogenic stimuli, and Bernstein and Wright (3) were able to obtain the generation of a primary cytotoxic response to alloantigen *in vitro* using nonadherent spleen cells. In tumor-bearing rats, spleens were shown to contain phagocytic adherent cells that suppressed lymphocyte response to mitogens (10,14,17,28,31) as well as rapidly proliferating tumor cells growing *in vitro* (17). Macrophages were also observed to inhibit the formation of plaque forming cells by spleen cells (12,21,32).

It seems apparent that the action of suppressor macrophages in spleens accounts for the difficulty in demonstrating *in vitro* lymphoproliferative responses in the rat as compared to the mouse. This difference is vividly seen *in vivo* by RES blockade which results in an increased PFC response in spleens of rats, whereas in mice this procedure was reported to cause a marked suppression of PFC (25).

In summary, impairment of the phagocytic activity of RE elements produced by the intravenous injection of colloidal iron was found to cause of 2 fold increase in the number of plaque forming cells. On the assumption that phagocytic or adherent cells from rat spleen cell preparations were suppressing the PFC response, these cells were removed by incubation with carbonyl iron powder. Cultures were prepared with mixed spleen cells (MSC), macrophage depleted spleen cells (MDSC) and MDSC supplemented with spleen or peritoneal macrophages. The hemolytic plaque forming capacity increased nearly 50-fold in MDSC as compared to MSC. This increase was prevented by the addition of an equal number of macrophages. These results suggest that macrophages present in the spleen cell preparations are suppressive and may be responsible for the low *in vitro* PFC response with rat cells.

REFERENCES

1. Alter, B. J., Bach, F. H., J. Exp. Med., 140 (1974) 1410.
2. Asherson, G. L. and Zembala, M., Eur. J. Immunol., 4 (1974) 804.
3. Bernstein, I. D. and Wright, P. W., Transplantation, 21

(1976) 173.
4. Biozzi, G., Halpern, B. N., Bennacerraf, B. and Stiffel, C., Physiopathology of the Reticuloendothelial System (Ed. B. N. Halpern), Thomas Springfield (1957) 204.
5. Bruce, J., Goldstein, P. and Mitchison, N. A., Transplantation, 20 (1975) 88.
6. Chen, C. and Hirsch, J. G., J. Exp. Med., 136 (1972) 604.
7. Fernbach, B. R., Kirchner, H. and Herberman, R. B., Cell Immunol., 22 (1976) 399.
8. Fishman, M. and Adler, F. C., J. Exp. Med., 117 (1963) 595.
9. Folch, H. and Waksman, B. H., J. Immunol., 113 (1974) 127.
10. Gorczynski, R. M., J. Immunol., 112 (1974) 1826.
11. Hayry, P. and Defendi, V., Science, 168 (1970) 133.
12. Hellering, I. and Stern, K., Eur. J. Immunol., 5 (1975) 705.
13. Jerne, N. K. and Nordin, A. A., Science, 140 (1963) 405.
14. Kirchner, H., Muchmore, A. V., Chused, T. M., Holden, H. T. and Herberman, R. B., J. Immunol., 114 (1975) 206.
15. Mishell, R. I. and Dutton, R. W., Science, 153 (1966) 1004.
16. Mosier, D. E., Science, 158 (1967) 1573.
17. Oehler, J. R., Herberman, R. B., Campbell, D. A., Jr. and Djeu, J. Y., Cell. Immunol., 29 (1977) 238.
18. Parkhouse, R. M. E. and Dutton, R. W., J. Immunol., 97 (1966) 663.
19. Ptak, W. and Gershon, R. K., J. Immunol., 115 (1975) 1346.
20. Reichard, S. M., J. Reticuloendothel. Soc., 12 (1972) 604.
21. Reichard, S. M., J. Reticuloendothel. Soc., 23 (1978) 61.
22. Reichard, S. M., Russell, B. and Lefkowitz, S. S., 6th Internatl. Meeting RES Society, Freiburg (1970) 119.
23. Reichard, S. M., Russell, B. and Lefkowitz, S. S., J. Reticuloendothel. Soc., 9 (1971) 638.
24. Rosenstreich, D. L., Farrar, J. J. and Dougherty, S., J. Immunol., 116 (1976) 131.
25. Sabet, T., Newlin, C. and Friedman, H., Proc. Soc. Exp. Biol. Med., 128 (1968) 274.
26. Soliday, S. and Bach, F. H., Science, 170 (1970) 1456.
27. Sucii-Foca, N., Buda, J., McManus, J., Thiem, J. and Reemtsma, K., Cancer Res., 33 (1973) 3474.
28. Veit, B. C. and Feldman, J. D., J. Immunol., 117 (1976) 646.
29. Veit, B. C. and Feldman, J. D., J. Immunol., 117 (1976) 655.
30. Wagner, H. and Feldman, H., Cell. Immunol., 3 (1972) 405.
31. Weiss, A. and Fitch, F. W., J. Immunol., 119 (1977) 510.
32. Weiss, A. and Fitch, F. W., J. Immunol., 120 (1978) 357.
33. Wilson, D. B., J. Exp. Med., 126 (1967) 625.

Part IV
Environmental Factors Influencing the Reticuloendothelial System

It is quite evident that environmental factors and agents can influence the host responses of living organisms. We are well aware of the effects that "pollution" and environmental toxins can exert on mankind so that the interest in this area is at its peak. In this section the influence of a wide variety of substances often present in the environment on RE function and activity is discussed. It is noteworthy that many environmental chemicals can modify both cell-mediated and humoral immune responses. The immunodepressive effect of phenols are of special concern in experimental medicine and immunology since phenolic disinfectants are widely used, especially in animal quarters. Asbestos, tobacco smoke, pesticides, etc. are all known to have detrimental effects on individuals. The effects of these agents on phagocytic cells and lymphocytes, and on immune functions per se are treated in great detail. In addition, substances from natural sources, such as those isolated from marine organisms, are also shown to influence immune responses. A chapter on the role of UV-radiation in carcinogenesis and immunity is included in this section. Protein-calorie malnutrition, though not an environmental factor per se, is certainly important in immunomodulation and within the general areas dealing with effects of the environment on the RE System. In this connection, qualitative and quantitative aspects of one's diet are worthy of consideration since both undernutrition and overnutrition can affect host responses to various stimuli. Further studies dealing with the influence of these and other factors on the immune system, in general, and on the RE System, in particular, certainly seem warranted.

ENVIRONMENTAL CHEMICAL-INDUCED MODIFICATION OF CELL-MEDIATED IMMUNE RESPONSES

J. B. SILKWORTH and L. D. LOOSE

Institute of Comparative and Human Toxicology
Albany Medical College
Albany, New York (USA)

Technological advancement is accompanied by the development of many new chemical compounds followed by their dispersion, both intentional and accidental, throughout the biosphere. Although originally found in the environment at low, possibly harmless levels, many compounds are concentrated by biomagnification resulting in the exposure of mammals to potentially deleterious levels of the chemical compounds (26). In addition, certain mammalian tissues including primary lymphoid organs can concentrate dietary chemicals to levels well above those ingested (22), thereby resulting in exposure to concentrations above established maximal safety limits.

Although the influence of many environmental chemicals such as the aliphatic hydrocarbons, organochlorines, oranophosphates and heavy metals on biochemical, physiological and morphological aspects of cell behavior has received much attention, evaluation of host defense status and the immune system has received scant attention.

Recent evidence has indicated that host resistance, antibody-mediated immunity and cell-mediated immunity may be altered by environmental chemicals. Chemical-induced alteration of host resistance to viral, bacterial and protozoan infections has been reported. Friend and Trainer (5) demonstrated an increased mortality of ducklings fed polychlorinated biphenyl (PCB) and infected with duck hepatitis virus as compared to infected ducklings fed a control diet. Gainer (6) reported an increased mortality of encephalomyocarditis virus-infected mice exposed to cobalt sulfate. Thigpen (36) reported an increased susceptibility of mice to infection with Salmonella bern following exposure to 2,3,7,8-tetrachlorodibenzo-p-dioxin (TCDD) although altered resistance to pseudorabies virus was not detected. Loose and Silkworth (19) demonstrated enhanced sensitivity of mice to gram-negative bacterial lipopolysaccharide (endotoxin) and a decreased mean survival time of Plasmodium berghei-infected mice following short-term exposure to 167 ppm PCB or hexachlorobenzene (HCB). In a later study by Loose et al. (20), the exposure of mice to 5 ppm PCB 1016, PCB 1242 or HCB also resulted in the increase in endotoxin sensitivity. Since endotoxin detoxification is primarily mediated by macrophages, it was suggested that the increased sensitivity to endotoxin may be due to macrophage dysfunction resulting from exposure to PCB or HCB and thus an impairment of host defense mechanisms.

Chemical-induced alterations of humoral immunity have also been demonstrated in several species. Rabbits fed PCB produced significantly lower serum-neutralizing antibody titers to pseudorabies virus than did control animals (16). Vos and DeRoij (37) reported that guinea pigs fed PCB 1260 for 8 weeks had fewer gamma-globulin concentrations following injections of tetanus toxoid than control diet animals, thereby indirectly measuring an alteration in antibody-mediated immunity since the parameter measured was not specific for the antigen used. Loose et al. (19) demonstrated a greater than 50% reduction in the peak primary splenic antibody direct plaque forming cell responses to SRBC antigen in mice fed 167 ppm PCB 1242 or HCB for 6 weeks. In addition, a concomitant reduction of serum IgG_1, IgA, and IgM levels was also noted. Although a centrilobular and pericentral hepatocyte hypertrophy was observed, the lung, spleen, thymus and mesenteric lymph nodes did not reveal any histopathologic alterations. These results suggest that evaluation of immunological status may be a very sensitive and perhaps early assessment of environmental chemical toxicity.

The influence of environmental chemicals on cell-mediated immunity has been almost entirely neglected. Vos (39) reported that (TCDD)-treated guinea pigs displayed a significantly reduced tuberculin delayed hypersensitivity reaction, as compared to control animals; a similar effect was not observed in rats. In the same study, Vos reported a decreased graft-versus-host response (GVHR), as compared to controls, when (TCDD)-treated parental strain spleen cells were injected into adult F_1 hybrid recipients. In a later study, Vos (38) reported a decrease from control values in the phytohemagglutinin (PHA) responsiveness of spleen cells from 25-day-old male rats following postnatal maternal exposure to TCDD. Since thymic atrophy was present in pre- and post-natally treated rats, a thymo-toxic mechanism was proposed to explain the observations.

The involvement of the immune system in the expression of

environmental chemical toxicity is proposed. It is appropriate, then, to delineate the mechanism of functional alteration of the immune system by environmental chemicals and simultaneously develop a test system for the early assessment of the potential toxicity of new chemicals. The sensitivity of the immune system to modification by environmental chemicals can be conveniently evaluated.

The development of an immune response depends upon the proper function of three basic phases: (a) initial recognition of the foreign substance, (b) activation, which includes proliferation and differentiation of reactive clones, and (c) the expression of immunity. This concept can be applied to the assessment of environmental chemical toxicity on cell mediated immune responses.

Depending on the nature of the foreign substance, initial recognition of the antigen may occur through a combination of direct or indirect interactions. T-lymphocyte recognition of the antigen may be by means of a non-immunoglobulin receptor with an immunoglobulin receptor; however, the nature of the T-cell receptor has not been resolved. There is also evidence to support the concept that antigen recognition and processing may be one of the most critical functions of the macrophage (8). It has been suggested that the macrophage-bound antigen is recognized by the T-lymphocyte resulting in activation of the T-lymphocyte. The activated T-lympohcyte may then, depending on the nature of the antigen, activate other T-cell clones such as suppressor, helper, or cytotoxic T-cells, or may modify B-cell reaction to the antigen. Since surface membrane components of the immunocompetent cells play such an integral role in the recognition phase, the importance of the integrity of cell surface structures and their possible alteration by xenobiotics can be understood. The specificity of the final response will depend on the specificity of the initial recognition.

Lymphocyte activation results in proliferation and differentiation of responding clones of lymphocytes and many events of activation have been investigated following stimulation with mitogens such as PHA, pokeweed mitogen or concanavalin A. Increased turnover and synthesis of phospholipids occurs with the first hr following exposure to PHA (4, 29). An increased turnover of the fatty acid moiety of lecithin is also observed within this time interval (31). An increase in the level of cAMP is noted within 2 min of PHA exposure and is followed by a gradual decline to below control levels by 6 hr (33). Nuclear changes include the increased phosphorylation of nuclear proteins (15). PHA stimulates RNA synthesis within 30 min and protein synthesis within 4 hr followed by DNA synthesis within 24 hr which reaches a peak between 48 and 72 hr (11). Enzymes which display increased activity following activation include acid phosphatase, glucose-6-phosphate dehydrogenase, lactate dehydrogenase, DNA polymerase and DNAase (12, 18, 25, 28, 30). Lymphokine activity increased within 2 days (17, 27). Morphological and cytochemical changes also occur following activation and include lymphocyte enlargement, basophilia, and pyroninophilia (9).

The final effector stage of cell-mediated immunity includes T-cell cytotoxicity and lymphokine production. Direct cytotoxicity is primarily mediated by the T-lymphocyte (7). Brief contact of T-lymphocytes with target cells results in target cell death within 3 to 24 hr (40). This response can be inhibited by a millipore barrier between the target cells or trypsinization of the cytotoxic lymphocyte. T-cell recognition and contact with the target cell surface appears to be necessary for target cell destruction (23, 41). However, macrophages, once armed by a specific arming factor produced by the T-lymphocyte, can kill specifically. Once the armed macrophage reacts with the specific antigen, it becomes activated. The activated macrophage will then continue to kill nonspecifically (3). Antibody-mediated B-lymphocyte specific cytotoxicity requiring lymphocyte-target cell contact has also been demonstrated (24) and the production of soluble factors by lymphocytes, such as lymphotoxin, has been described (10).

Available in vivo and in vitro techniques allow the examination of the developing immune response and perhaps clarification of the mechanisms of environmental chemical toxicity (Fig. 1).

Injection of immunocompetent cells into an immunoincompetent animal expressing histoincompatible antigens results in a graft-versus-host response (GVHR). It has been firmly established that the GVHR is an expression of cell-mediated immunity (1). The GVHR has three prerequisites. First, the recipient must be unable to react against the donor cells. Experimentally this may be accomplished with the use of irradiated recipients or the use of immunocompetent parental strain cells injected into young F_1 hybrids. Second, the donor and recipient cells must be histoincompatible. Use of allogeneic mice or the injection of parental strain cells into F_1 hybrid recipients satisfies this requirement. Third, the donor cells must be immunocompetent. The severity of the graft-versus-host response is an assessment of the functional status of the recognition, activation and expression phases of the immune response as indicated by the development of a completed response. However, compensation among the three phases may occur and may not be detected by the assay.

The use of the GVHR as an assessment of immune status of environmental chemical-exposed animals is unique in that the stimulating cells of the host differ from the responding cells of the donor only in the expression of histocompatibility antigens and therefore requires an operable, specific recognition system

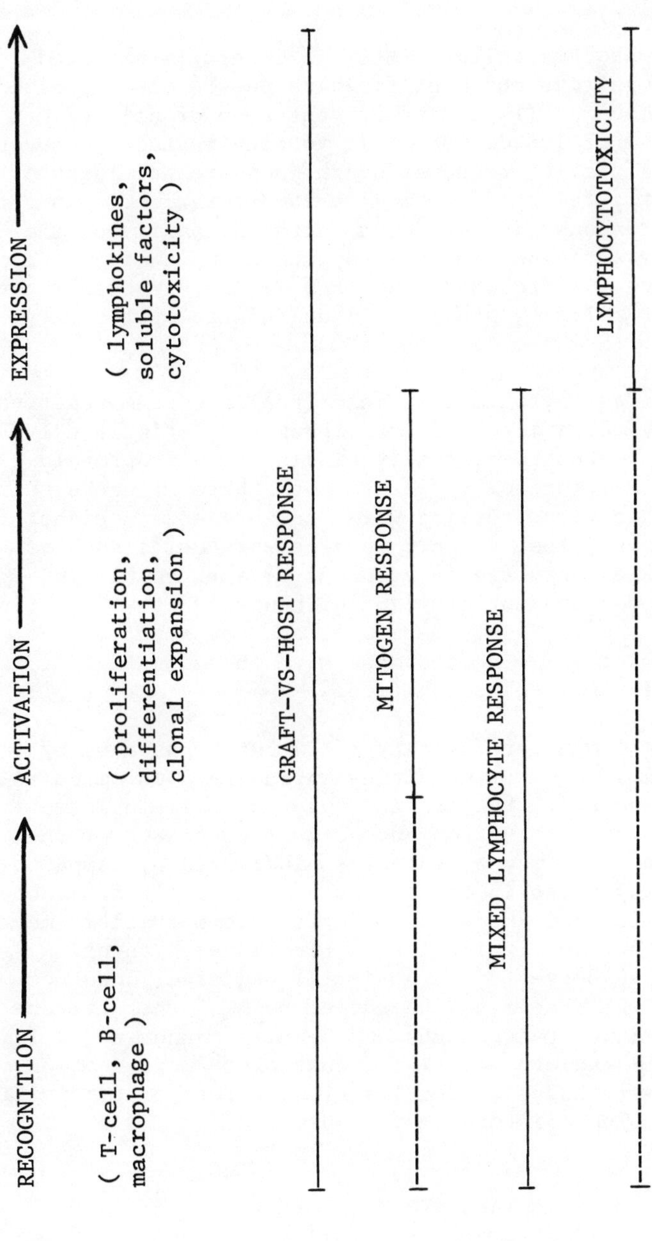

Fig. 1. Developmental phases of a cell-mediated immune response and assays which can be used for the functional assessment of each phase.

and an equally specific effector system. This experimental design contrasts with the use of erythrocytes, bacteria and viruses as antigens which present the host with numerous foreign antigenic determinants and does not require sensitive self, non-self distinction.

The mixed lymphocyte culture (MLC) is generally accepted to represent the recognitive and proliferative phases of the cell-mediated immune reaction (14). The presentation of alloantigen of mitomycin-C-treated or irradiated cells to non-treated lymphocytes results in a proliferative response by the non-treated lymphocytes which can be quantitated by ^{3}H-thymidine incorporation. Since the intensity of the response is dependent on the disparity of the histocompatibility antigens expressed by the stimulator and responder cell populations, Balb/c (H-2^d) and $B_6D_2F_1$ (H-2^{b,d}) cells can be used as stimulator cells to provide unequal histocompatibility stimuli to C57Bl/5 (H-2^b) mice.

Mitogens such as phytohemagglutinin (PHA) and gram-negative bacterial lipopolysaccharide (LPS) are thought to stimulate lymphocyte activation by nonspecifically binding to glycoprotein receptors on the cell surface (2). Although these mitogens seem to bind only certain glycoproteins which are present on either T-lymphocytes, B-lymphocytes, or only on accessory cells such as macrophages, their effects are independent of antigen binding specificity. The measurement of mitogen induced ^{3}H-thymidine incorporation in lymphocytes is, therefore, an assessment of the activation phase of the immune response with the advantage of by-passing specific antigen recognition.

Cell-mediated lymphocytotoxicity (CML) can be assayed by several _in vitro_ and _in vivo_ techniques including ^{51}chromium release and is a measure of the effector phase of cell-mediated immunity. Although the recognition and activation phases of the response to alloantigens may be intact as indicated by comparable values in MLC ^{3}H-thymidine incorporation between cells from control and chemical-treated animals, the cytotoxic mechanisms may nevertheless be functionally impaired. Functional cytotoxic impairment, although suggested to be T-cell mediated, does not clearly implicate the T-cell as the target cell of the environmental chemical. Since macrophages and B-cells cannot be excluded from cultures with absolute certainty, control or modification of the response by macrophages or B-cells (in the form of cytophilic antibodies or soluble mediators) may occur.

MATERIALS AND METHODS

Animals. Male C57Bl/6 Tex (H-2^b) and $B_6D_2F_1$ (H-2^{b,d}) weighing 18-20 gm and pregnant C57Bl/6 Tex mated with D_6B_2A (H-2^d) were supplied by Timco, Texas. Male Balb/c mice weighing 18-20 grams were supplied by Charles River, Massachusetts. Mice were housed individually. Control animals were fed Wayne Mash. Experimental animals were fed a diet containing either 167 ppm Aroclor 1016 (PCB) or 167 ppm hexachlorobenzene (HCB) in Wayne Mash. Diet analyses assured proper concentration of test chemicals. Food and water were provided *ad libitum* to all animals. Body and organ weights were followed throughout the study.

Chemicals. The test chemicals used were polychlorinated biphenyl (PCB) Aroclor 1016 (Monsanto) and hexachlorobenzene (HCB) (Eastman practical grade), which was purified by being passed through activated charcoal and then 2x crystallized from boiling benzene.

Cell isolation procedure. Spleens were removed aseptically from ether anesthetized animals, minced with a fine scissors and teased across #60 mesh stainless steel into cold Hanks Balanced Salt Solution (HBSS), Grand Island Biological Company, Grand Island, New York. Cells which remained in suspension after a 5 min settling period were used, thereby discarding unwanted debris and cell aggregates. Cell yield and viability was assessed immediately using Trypan Blue. The cells were then washed three times in cold HBSS and spun at 180 x g before being suspended to appropriate concentrations with RPMI 1640 media (GIBCO). Cell suspensions were counted just before use to assure proper concentrations. The concentration of PCB 1016 and HCB per 10^6 isolated cells was determined by electron capture gas chromatography as previously described (19).

Graft-versus-host response (GVHR). A GVHR was induced in neonatal (< 24 hr) $B_6D_2F_1$ mice by the intraperitoneal injection of 1×10^7 spleen cells isolated from control or chemical-treated C57Bl/6 mice following 3, 6, 13 or 37 weeks of dietary administration of the test chemical. The inoculum was administered in a volume of 0.05 cc RPMI 1640. Injection of spleen cells isolated from control $B_6D_2F_1$ mice (isogeneic) served as a control for the GVHR. The split litter procedure (21) was used to obviate experimental error due to variation between litters and to allow comparison of test chemicals within litters. Spleen and body weights of neonates were determined on the ninth day of maternal rearing following inoculation with spleen cells. Results were expressed as the spleen index calculated by dividing the relative spleen weights of neonates inoculated with cells from control or chemical-treated donors by the mean relative spleen weight of non-injected littermates. A spleen index of greater than 1.3 was considered to be a positive GVHR (34). The Student's t-Test was used to determine statistical significance between positive GVH responses.

Mixed lymphocyte response (MLR). Responder lymphocytes from chemical-treated or control adult C57Bl/6 mice were co-cultured with equal numbers (5×10^5 cells) of stimulator lymphocytes from control isogeneic (C57Bl/6) or allogeneic (Balb/c, $B_6D_2F_1$) lymphocytes in a final volume of 0.2 ml RPMI 1640 supplemented with 10% fetal calf serum and 50-100 units penicillin and 50-100 μg streptomycin per ml in flat bottom microtiter plates (Falcon 3040 Micro Test II with lids) at 37 C with 5% CO_2 for 1-6 days. The stimulator cells were treated with 50 μg/ml mitomycin-C (Sigma Chemical Co., St. Louis, Missouri) at a cell concentration of 2×10^7 cells per ml for 30 min at 37 C and washed three times prior to culturing. DNA synthesis of the responder cells was assayed by the addition to each culture of 1.0 μCi tritiated thymidine (Spec. Act. 6.7 Ci/mM, New England Nuclear Corp., Boston, Mass.) for the last 18 hr of culture. Cells were lysed with a water wash and the DNA collected by aspiration onto glass fiber filter strips using an automated sample harvester (Skatron, Flow Laboratories, Rockville Maryland). The filter discs were dried and the radioactivity of triplicate cultures was measured in a universal LSC cocktail (Aquasol-2, New England Nuclear Corp., Boston, Mass.) using an automatic scintillation counter (Packard). Data are presented as the stimulation index (SI) calculated by dividing the counts per min (cpm) of responder cells cultured with allogeneic cells by the cpm of the responder cells cultured with syngeneic cells. The ratio

$$\frac{\text{SI of MLR using C57Bl/6 responder cells from mice fed an experimental diet}}{\text{SI of MLR using C57Bl/6 responder cells from mice fed a control diet}}$$

was calculated. Thus a ratio of less than 1,1 or greater than 1 represents inhibition, no effect, or stimulation of the mixed lymphocyte response, respectively, of the responding C57Bl/6 spleen cells by the dietary chemicals. A ratio $\pm$ its standard error was considered to be statistically significant if less than .07 or greater than 1.30 (34).

Mitogen-induced blast transformation. Mitogen responsiveness assays were conducted using the same method as employed in mixed-lymphocyte cultures, however, 40 μg/ml phytohemagglutinin (PHA-M, B grade, Calbiochem, La Jolla, California) or gram—negative bacterial lipopolysaccharide (LPS, *Salmonella typhosa*, Westphal, Difco, Detroit, Michigan) was added to the appropriate cultures when initiated in place of isogeneic or allogeneic spleen cells.

RESULTS

There were no consistent differences from control values in body weight, spleen weight, liver weight, thymus weight, or spleen

TABLE I

Body, Spleen and Relative Spleen Weights of Mice Fed Aroclor 1016 or HCB[a,b]

	DIET	WEEKS ON DIET 3	6	13	19	24	37	41
BODY WEIGHT (g)	CON	22.6 ±0.8	26.7 ±0.5	28.9 ±0.7	29.8 ±1.3	30.0 ±1.5	33.2 ±0.6	36.8 ±3.8
	PCB	21.7 ±1.1	24.2 ±0.6[c]	28.6 ±0.7	33.6 ±2.1	30.2 ±2.8	40.5 ±2.6[c]	38.7 ±2.6
	HCB	21.8 ±0.8	25.1 ±0.5[c]	27.2 ±0.7	22.5 ±0.6[c]	22.7 ±0.7[c]	25.2 ±0.9[c]	27.8 ±0.3
SPLEEN WEIGHT (mg)	CON	101.9±9.6	94.9 ±5.4	69.6 ±4.9	67.9 ±6.0	68.5 ±8.5	68.7 ±1.6	83.7 ±8.7
	PCB	75.3 ±6.6[c]	71.3 ±2.7[c]	70.1 ±2.5	57.2 ±3.2	57.9 ±1.0	70.4 ±5.1	77.0 ±11.3
	HCB	84.0 ±2.8	91.7 ±2.3	82.9 ±3.9	111.8±21.7	174.9±13.9[c]	150.4±53.1[c]	73.0 ±2.4
REL. SPLEEN WEIGHT (%)	CON	.522 ±.07	.357 ±.03	.242 ±.02	.230 ±.03	.227 ±.02	.208 ±.01	.216 ±.03
	PCB	.352 ±.03[c]	.295 ±.01[c]	.245 ±.01	.174 ±.02	.194 ±.02	.173 ±.01[c]	.200 ±.02
	HCB	.389 ±.02	.368 ±.02	.305 ±.01[c]	.492 ±.08[c]	.773 ±.09[c]	.608 ±.23	.263 ±.01

a Male C57B1/6 mice were fed a diet containing 167 ppm Aroclor 1016 (PCB) or hexachlorobenzene (HCB) for up to 41 weeks.

b Data are presented as mean weight or relative weight (%) ± standard error; n=2-10 in all groups.

c Significantly different from control values at $p<0.05$ as determined by the Student's t-Test.

TABLE II

Liver and Thymus Weights of Mice Fed Aroclor 1016 or HCB[a,b]

	DIET	WEEKS ON DIET 13	19	41
LIVER	CON	1.5060 ±.0759	1.4711 ±.0735	1.8218 ±.1667
WEIGHT	PCB	1.4110 ±.0573	1.7779 ±.1220	1.8748 ±.1221
(g)	HCB	2.7674 ±.3188[c]	2.8533 ±.2493[c]	1.7604 ±.1010
REL.	CON	5.25 ±.11	4.94 ±.09	4.62 ±.28
LIVER	PCB	5.13 ±.20	5.30 ±.17	4.88 ±.23
WEIGHT (%)	HCB	9.96 ±1.0[c]	12.66±.79[c]	6.34 ±.31[c]
THYMUS	CON	50.5 ±2.6	31.3 ±1.6	30.6 ±1.6
WEIGHT	PCB	37.1 ±3.1[c]	41.3 ±4.0	25.8 ±2.0
(mg)	HCB	29.9 ±8.9	20.1 ±3.0[c]	27.8 ±3.7
REL.	CON	.178 ±.015	.109 ±.011	.078 ±.003
THYMUS	PCB	.135 ±.011	.123 ±.010	.070 ±.005
WEIGHT (%)	HCB	.105 ±.029	.090 ±.014	.099 ±.012[c]

[a] Male C57Bl/6 mice were fed a diet containing 167 ppm Aroclor 1016 (PCB) or hexachlorobenzene (HCB) for up to 41 weeks.

[b] Data are presented as mean weight or relative weight (%) ± standard error; n=2-10 in all groups.

[c] Significantly different from control values at $p<0.05$ as determined by the Student's t-Test.

cell yield in mice fed a diet containing 167 ppm Aroclor 1016 (PCB) for up to 41 weeks (Tables I and II) hereafter referred to as PCB-treated mice.

Mice fed a diet containing 167 ppm HCB for 19 weeks and longer consistently weighed 24% less than control mice. The liver weights were 84 and 94% greater, respectively, than control values. In addition, the absolute spleen weights of these mice were increased 74-155% above control values following 19 to 24 weeks, respectively, of dietary exposure to HCB. The relative spleen weights of HCB-treated mice also increased with continued dietary exposure of up to 24 weeks when they began to decrease. Associated with this increase in spleen size was a 25 to 86% increase in viable spleen cell yield over control values. In contrast to the increased spleen and liver weights, the thymus weights of mice which received HCB for 13 and 19 weeks were decreased 41 and 36%, respectively, from control values. After dietary exposure to HCB for 41 weeks, the liver, spleen and thymus weights were comparable to control values; however, the relative liver and thymus weights were significantly increased.

Analysis of spleen cells by gas chromatography revealed the presence of 0.437 ng PCB 1016 per 10^6 cells from mice fed 167 ppm PCB 1016 for 13 weeks and 22.1 ng HCB per 10^6 cells from mice fed 167 ppm HCB for 13 weeks.

Graft-versus-host response. The inoculation of neonatal $B_6D_2F_1$ (BDF_1) mice with spleen cells from C57Bl/6 mice fed a control diet or a diet containing 167 ppm HCB for 3, 6, or 13 weeks resulted in a positive graft-versus-host response in all groups. No significant effect of chemical exposure of the donors on the GVH response was demonstrated (Table III). However, exposure to HCB for 37 weeks resulted in a statistically significant reduction of 20% in the graft-versus-host activity of HCB-treated cells. Spleen cells from normal BDF_1 mice did not produce a GVHR in neonatal BDF_1 mice.

Mixed lymphocyte culture. Spleen cells isolated from control C57Bl/6 mice or from mice fed 167 ppm PCB or HCB for 19-24 weeks all elicited a transient increase in DNA synthesis when stimulated in a one-way mixed lymphocyte culture with mitomycin-D-treated spleen cells from Balb/c or BDF_1 mice (Table IV). The peak response occurred on the fourth or fifth day after initiation of the culture in control and HCB-treated cultures; however, cultures containing PCB-treated responder cells generally peaked on day 3.

The stimulation index (SI) during days 3, 4 and 5 of the cultures in which spleen cells from mice fed a control diet were mixed in a one-way culture with mitomycin-C-treated Balb/c stimulator cells was greater than when cultured with BDF_1 cells as the stimulator cells in 10 out of 10 cultures. However, the SI of cultures

TABLE III

Graft-Versus-Host Activity[a,b]

DONOR CELL STRAIN	DIET	WEEKS ON DIET			
		3	6	13	37
C57Bl/6	CON	2.78 ±.21 (5,5)	2.07 ±.28 (5,5)	2.21 ±.12 (6,18)	2.24 ±.12 (6,8)
C57Bl/6	PCB	2.77 ±.25 (7,7)	2.57 ±.34 (7,7)	2.13 ±.11 (6,15)	2.63 ±.20 (6,8)
C57Bl/6	HCB	2.38 ±.28 (5,5)	2.26 ±.24 (5,5)	2.25 ±.12 (6,18)	1.80 ±.09[c] (4,9)
$B_6D_2F_1$	CON	1.10 ±.10 (5,5)	0.91 ±.02 (4,4)	0.93 ±.04 (5,10)	———

a A graft-versus-host response was induced in neonatal $B_6D_2F_1$ mice by the intraperitoneal inoculation of $1x10^7$ spleen cells from C57Bl/6 mice fed a control diet or a diet containing 167 ppm Aroclor 1016 (PCB) or hexachlorobenzene (HCB). The spleen index was calculated nine days after inoculation. Inoculation with $B_6D_2F_1$ spleen cells served as a control.

b Data are presented as mean spleen index ± standard error; numbers in parentheses indicate the number of donor and recipient mice, respectively.

c Significantly different from the spleen index of control mice at $p < 0.01$ as determined by the Student's t-Test.

TABLE IV
Stimulation Indices of Mixed Lymphocyte Cultures[a,b]

TRIAL	DIET	DAY OF CULTURE 1		2		3		4		5	
		Stimulator Strain									
		Balb/c	BDF_1	Balb/c	BDF_1	Balb/c	BDF_1	Balb/c	BDF_1	Balb/c	BDF_1
1	CON	----	----	7.34	5.43	16.61	12.75	19.08	17.93	12.34	11.90
	PCB	----	----	----	----	12.31	14.22	18.43	20.29	15.35	13.72
	HCB	----	----	5.21	4.53	6.88	9.17	9.23	11.27	7.69	7.61
2	CON	3.38	1.31	7.18	4.45	12.94	8.41	----	16.44	----	----
	PCB	3.03	1.41	4.69	3.18	16.85	17.03	----	11.20	----	----
	HCB	1.26	1.01	5.15	3.84	8.04	5.10	----	6.85	----	----
3	CON	1.51	1.26	3.06	2.59	4.08	3.31	4.39	3.66	8.03	6.66
	PCB	2.96	2.19	2.62	2.26	7.19	5.06	5.65	4.34	7.31	4.78
	HCB	1.24	1.31	1.60	2.17	2.35	2.23	2.59	2.66	6.96	6.39
4	CON	1.73	1.57	3.51	3.04	5.28	3.88	7.02	5.70	7.30	6.84
	PCB	1.78	1.49	2.15	1.83	3.94	3.13	3.58	2.98	2.74	2.43
	HCB	1.15	1.14	2.90	2.64	3.40	2.53	5.11	3.31	4.94	3.62

[a] Spleen cells, $5x10^5$, from C57B1/6 mice fed a control diet or a diet containing 167 ppm Aroclor 1016 (PCB) or hexachlorobenzene (HCB) were co-cultured in a one-way mixed lymphocyte culture with $5x10^5$ mitomycin-C-treated Balb/c or B_6D_2F1 spleen cells and pulsed with 1 μCi ^{3}H-TdR/culture 18 hr prior to culture.
[b] Data are presented as the stimulation index of one mouse per diet per trial.

of spleen cells from mice fed PCB or HCB mixed in one-way cultures with mitomycin-C-treated Balb/c stimulator spleen cells was greater than when cultured with BDF_1 cells as the stimulator cells in only 7 out of 10 cultures.

The SI of cultures containing cells from PCB-treated mice were not significantly different from the SI of cultures containing cells from control mice when Balb/c cells were the stimulator cells; however, it was significantly greater than the SI of control cultures on day 3 of cultures in which BDF_1 cells were the stimulator cells (Table V).

In contrast, the SI of cultures containing HCB-treated cells was consistently below control values on days 1-5 of the culture period when either Balb/c or BDF_1 spleen cells are the stimulator cells and is significantly below (34-44%) control values on days 3 and 4 of the response.

Mitogen responsiveness. Tables VI and VII show the stimulation indices from mitogen-induced blast transformation of cultured spleen cells from C57Bl/6 mice fed a control diet or a diet containing 167 ppm PCB 1016 or HCB for 13, 24 and 41 weeks. A transient increase in tritiated thymidine (^{3}H-TdR) incorporation following addition of 40 μg/ml PHA-M (a T-cell mitogen), which peaked on days 2 or 3, was noted in control and experimental cultures (Table VI). Cultures which contained PCB-treated spleen cells demonstrated a ^{3}H-TdR incorporation rate above control levels on day 4 in cultures containing cells from mice fed PCB for 13, 24 and 41 weeks. An increase in DNA synthesis over control values was present as early as day 2 of cultures of spleen cells from mice fed PCB for 41 weeks. PHA-M-induced DNA synthesis by spleen cells from mice fed HCB for 13 and 24 weeks was significantly reduced below control values on day 2 of the response. However, by 41 weeks PHA-M-induced DNA synthesis had returned to control values.

The addition of 40 μg LPS/ml (a B-cell mitogen) to cultures of spleen cells from control mice or mice fed PCB for 13, 24 or 41 weeks resulted in an increase in ^{3}H-TdR incorporation rate which peaked on the third or fourth day of culture (Table VII). The SI of LPS-stimulated spleen cells from mice fed PCB for 13 weeks was significantly greater than control values only on the first day of culture. LPS-induced DNA synthesis by spleen cells from mice fed HCB for 13 and 24 weeks was consistently below control values in the 13 week group; the reduction was even more pronounced in animals which received HCB for 24 weeks. Although peak ^{3}H-TdR incorporation in control spleen cells was manifest on day 3-4 in control animals, the spleen cells from the mice which received HCB for 13 or 24 weeks demonstrated a peak incorporation rate on the second day of culture. Although significantly lower

TABLE V

Ratio of Stimulation Indices of Experimental Mixed Lymphocyte Cultures to Control Mixed Lymphocyte Cultures[a,b]

C57Bl/6 Responder cell treatment	Stimulator cell	DAY OF CULTURE				
		1	2	3	4	5
PCB	Balb/c	1.30 ±.34	.71 ±.07	1.14 ±.25	.92 ±.23	.84 ±.25
PCB	BDF_1	1.25 ±.25	.73 ±.08	1.56 ±.23[b]	.88 ±.17	.74 ±.23
HCB	Balb/c	.62 ±.13	.70 ±.08	.56 ±.05[b]	.60 ±.08[b]	.73 ±.08
HCB	BDF_1	.85 ±.10	.85 ±.01	.66 ±.02[b]	.59 ±.07[b]	.71 ±.13

[a] Data are presented as the ratio of stimulation indices of mixed lymphocyte cultures containing spleen cells from chemical-treated mice to the stimulation indices of cultures containing spleen cells from normal mice ± standard error; n=3-4 trials in all groups.
[b] Significantly different from control values (see materials and methods section).

TABLE VI

Stimulation Indices of PHA-M-Induced ^{3}H-TdR Incorporation of Spleen Cells from Mice Fed Aroclor 1016 or HCB for 13, 24 and 41 Weeks[a,b]

	13 WEEKS				24 WEEKS				41 WEEKS			
	DAY OF RESPONSE											
DIET	1	2	3	4	1	2	3	4	1	2	3	4
CON	2.20 ±.23	19.66 ±1.77	10.96 ±2.23	7.17 ±.99	1.53 ±.24	10.97 ±.13	9.74 ±.63	7.92 ±2.84	2.56 ±.37	9.56 ±.98	10.13 ±1.23	4.89 ±.81
PCB	2.79 ±.16	19.64 ±2.83	8.67 ±1.48	11.43 ±1.32[c]	2.21 ±.13	8.23 ±1.41	13.52 ±5.29	10.12 ±3.47	2.44 ±.16	15.72 ±1.72[c]	12.67 ±.50	10.17 ±2.02[c]
HCB	1.71 ±.17	9.63 ±1.53[c]	7.34 ±2.12	4.74 ±.73	1.08 ±.02	3.19 ±1.19[c]	7.32 ±3.95	5.18 ±3.02	1.94 ±.04	11.08 ±1.21	8.49 ±.30	8.07 ±2.42

[a] Spleen cells, 5×10^{5}, isolated from C57B1/6 mice fed a diet containing 167 ppm Aroclor 1016 (PCB) or hexachlorobenzene (HCB) for up to 41 weeks were cultured with 40 µg/ml phytohemagglutinin (PHA-M) for up to 4 days. Cultures were pulsed 18 hr prior to harvest with 1 µCi ^{3}H-TdR per culture. Stimulation indices were then determined.

[b] Data are presented as mean stimulation index ± standard error; n=2-5 in all groups.

[c] Significantly different from control values at $p < 0.05$ as determined by the Student's t-Test.

TABLE VII

Stimulation Indices of LPS-Induced ^{3}H-TdR Incorporation of Spleen Cells from Mice Fed Aroclor 1016 or HCB for 13, 24 and 41 Weeks[a,b]

	13 WEEKS				24 WEEKS				41 WEEKS			
	DAY OF RESPONSE											
DIET	1	2	3	4	1	2	3	4	1	2	3	4
CON	2.97 ±.22	10.73 ±.85	11.50 ±2.48	11.48 ±4.11	2.34 ±.46	9.39 ±.91	11.36 ±3.04	9.74 ±5.17	4.21 ±.54	8.24 ±.92	8.84 ±1.32	7.12 ±2.54
PCB	3.97 ±.14[c]	10.88 ±1.43	9.01 ±1.82	13.00 ±2.92	3.00 ±.20	6.99 ±1.91	17.23 ±8.45	11.60 ±1.28	3.82 ±.25	10.95 ±1.20	11.73 ±1.21	13.53 ±2.98
HCB	2.48 ±.26	8.43 ±1.62	6.50 ±.79	6.94 ±2.70	1.25 ±.01	3.60 ±.66[c]	2.67 ±.90	1.96 ±.64	2.64 ±.02[c]	6.40 ±.72	7.98 ±1.26	8.50 ±.38

a Spleen cells, 5×10^5, isolated from C57B1/6 mice fed a diet containing 167 ppm Aroclor 1016 (PCB) or hexachlorobenzene (HCB) for up to 41 weeks were cultured with 40 µg/ml gram-negative bacterial lipopolysaccharide (LPS) for up to 4 days. Cultures were pulsed 18 hr prior to harvest with 1 µCi ^{3}H-TdR per culture. Stimulation indices were then determined.

b Data are presented as mean stimulation index ± standard error; n=2-5 in all groups.

c Significantly different from control values at $p < 0.05$ as determined by the Student's t-Test.

than control values on the first day of culture in spleen cells of mice fed HCB for 41 weeks, the SI approached control values on days 2-4 of the response.

Spleen cells isolated from mice fed HCB for 13 weeks and cultured alone in media demonstrated an elevated background ^{3}H-TdR incorporation rate which was 5 times greater than the background ^{3}H-TdR incorporation rate of either control or PCB-treated cells (Table VIII). The increased ^{3}H-TdR incorporation rate was observed on the first day of culture and returned to control values by the fourth day of culture. After 24 weeks of dietary exposure to HCB, a 13-fold increase in the ^{3}H-TdR incorporation rate over control values was observed but this effect was seen only on the first day of culture. This elevated ^{3}H-TdR incorporation rate by HCB-treated spleen cells could be further enhanced by the addition to the culture of alloantigen (Balb/c or BDF$_1$) or mitogen (PHA or LPS) (Tables IV, VI, VII). There were no alterations from control values of ^{3}H-TdR incorporation in spleen cells from mice fed HCB or PCB for 41 weeks.

DISCUSSION

The influence of the dietary administration of two common environmental contaminants (PCB and HCB) on cell-mediated immune responses has been investigated. PCB, at the levels used in this study, had no profound influence on the graft-versus-host activity or the mixed lymphocyte responsiveness of spleen cells isolated from the experimental animals. The peak activity of spleen cells from PCB-treated mice, although occurring one day before control cells, was comparable in magnitude to the peak control response in a mixed lymphocyte culture. An enhancement of PHA- and LPS-induced activation of lymphocytes from PCB-treated mice which became more pronounced with continued exposure to PCB was demonstrated. This is the first demonstration that PCBs may stimulate lymphoid activity. There were no consistently significant alterations in body weight or the weights of spleen, liver, or thymus during the period of observation.

These findings extend those reported by Loose *et al.*(19) that a 6 week dietary exposure of mice to 167 ppm of Aroclor 1242, a form of polychlorinated biphenyls having a greater diversity in the isomer content of chlorine by weight than Aroclor 1016, resulted in a greater than 2-fold reduction in the peak primary splenic antibody response to sheep erythrocytes. These results suggest that environmental chemicals, such as PCBs, can express selective toxicity on different portions of the immune system. They also indicate that the target site of PCB causing the depression of antibody-mediated immunity is a mechanism or cell type which is not shared by the components of cell-mediated immunity.

TABLE VIII

Background ^{3}H-TdR Incorporation in CPM of Cultures of Spleen Cells from C57BL/6 Mice Fed Aroclor 1016 or HCB for 13, 24 and 41 Weeks[a]

WEEKS ON DIET	DIET	DAY OF CULTURE 1	2	3	4
13	CON	1314 ± 89 (10)	4728 ± 501 (10)	3707 ± 782 (10)	3792 ± 698 (10)
	PCB	1907 ± 554 (9)	4936 ± 454 (9)	4396 ± 622 (10)	3666 ± 483 (10)
	HCB	6566 ±1768[b] (9)	8302 ± 873[b] (9)	6922 ±1052[b] (9)	5980 ± 775 (9)
24	CON	2849 ± 992 (4)	3278 ±1033 (4)	1721 ± 590 (4)	1150 ± 508 (4)
	PCB	1786 ± 405 (4)	5077 ±1942 (4)	1790 ± 908 (4)	1291 ± 669 (4)
	HCB	37682 ±8241[b] (4)	4050 ± 681 (4)	2528 ± 584 (4)	1950 ± 665 (4)
41	CON	2879 ± 513 (4)	9683 ±1056 (5)	8332 ± 990 (5)	7009 ±1011 (5)
	PCB	2597 ± 942 (4)	7181 ±1166 (5)	7208 ± 886 (5)	4905 ± 951 (5)
	HCB	2826 ± 176 (2)	10169 ± 522 (2)	8653 ± 640 (2)	4325 ± 832 (2)

[a] Data are presented as the mean ± standard error of mean counts per minute (CPM) of triplicate cultures of 5×10^{5} spleen cells isolated from C57B1/6 mice fed a diet containing 167 ppm Aroclor 1016 (PCB) or hexachlorobenzene (HCB) for up to 41 weeks and cultured alone in media. Cultures were pulsed 18 hr prior to harvest with 1 μCi ^{3}H-TdR per culture. The number in parentheses represents the number of trials.

[b] Significantly different from control values at $p < 0.05$ as determined by the Student's t-Test.

It is possible, however, that a regulatory cell which normally acts to balance both the cell-mediated and the humoral-mediated arms of the immune system is functionally impaired by PCBs and allows an imbalanced response to occur.

Dietary exposure to hexachlorobenzene (HCB) resulted in an approximate 20% supression of spleen cell activity in the graft-versus-host response, a 44% reduction from control values in a mixed lymphocyte culture and an approximate 68% reduction from the peak response of control cells to mitogen stimulation using either PHA or LPS. Similar results which demonstrate the immunosuppressive activity of chlorinated hydrocarbons have been reported in animals using 2,3,7,8—tetrachlorodibenzo-p-dioxin (TCDD) (38) and DDT (24).

A reduction in GVH activity was not observed until after 37 weeks dietary exposure to HCB. Although this observation may indicate a lack of sensitivity of the GVH assay, a reduction in LPS-induced blast transformation was demonstrated following only 13 weeks exposure and was further reduced after 24 weeks exposure. Such increased functional impairment of the immune system with continued chemical exposure is similar to the observations reported by Loose _et_ _al_.(22), who demonstrated an impairment of host resistance to endotoxin and malaria in mice fed HCB after 3 weeks which was further impaired after 6 weeks. Furthermore, the functional impairment was suggested to be correlated with the concentration of the chemical in the primary lymphoid organs, spleen and thymus, which more than doubled during the 3 week period. The present observations in which there were no detectable chemical induced alterations in GVH activity until after 37 weeks exposure whereas mitogen induced responsiveness was noted as early as 13 weeks exposure could, therefore, be explained if component parts of the immune system are not influenced by chemical compounds until certain threshold tissue concentrations are reached.

The influence of HCB administration on cell-mediated immune functions, in contrast to those seen with PCB, could reflect the different patterns of absorption of these chemicals. In rats, Iatropoulos (13) demonstrated that 48 hr after oral administration of a single dose of either ^{14}C-labeled dichlorobiphenyl (DCB) or HCB, that DCB is rapidly absorbed from the upper gastrointestinal tract and is transported to the liver by the venous portal system. In contrast, HCB is primarily absorbed by the lymphatic system. This pattern of absorption of HCB results in the direct exposure of thoracic duct lymphocytes to high concentrations of chemical before any detoxification by the liver or dilution in the blood is possible. Thoracic duct lymphocyte adsorption or absorption of HCB may help to explain the high concentrations of HCB found in lymphoid tissue.

Although the reduced mitogen responsiveness observed in the present study following 13 weeks dietary exposure to HCB was further reduced after 24 weeks exposure, a response comparable to control values was demonstrated after 41 weeks exposure to the chemical. This suggests that in addition to a dose response relationship between chemical concentrations in lymphoid tissue and impairment of the immune response, environmental chemicals can transiently suppress parts of the immune system while having no effect on other functions of the system. Also, the return to control values in mitogen response to LPS and PHA of spleen cells from mice fed HCB for 41 weeks indicates either the development of more appropriate bio-handling, e. g., absorption, distribution, metabolism, or excretion of this compound after long term exposure, or a metabolic or functional compensation by either lymphoid or non-lymphoid tissue.

The HCB-induced transient functional impairment of lymphocyte function observed in this study was coincident with the transient changes in liver, spleen and thymus weights. The greatest increase in absolute and relative spleen weights occurred when mitogen responsiveness was most impaired. During this period thymus weight was significantly decreased whereas liver weight was significantly increased. When mitogen responsiveness had returned to control values, the absolute spleen, thymus and liver weights were comparable to control weights whereas the relative weights of spleen and liver had decreased somewhat but still remained above control values. The relative thymus weight of these mice had also increased.

The mechanism of impairment of cell-mediated immune function caused by HCB may be related to that induced by another chlorinated hydrocarbon (TCDD) reported by Vos and Moore (38). Following pre- and post-natal maternal exposure of rats to 25 g/kg of TCDD, allograft rejection times were prolonged, GVH activity was reduced, and responsiveness of spleen cells to PHA were reduced. In addition, a dose-dependent cortical atrophy was observed along with a decrease in thymus and spleen weights. Since the exposure of month-old rats to the same concentration of TCDD for 6 weeks did not result in comparable effects, a thymus dependent age related mechanism of toxicity was proposed.

In the present study, the transient dysfunction of cell-mediated immunological parameters associated with thymus weight reduction and spleen weight increase may again reflect a thymus-dependent age or, more correctly, a developmental phenomenon. That is, the thymo-tropic properties of hexachlorobenzene result in high tissue concentrations of hexachlorobenzene in mature thymus tissue where it exerts thymo-toxic effects. The immature thymus may be more susceptible to permanent damage than the mature organ. Reduction in thymus weight may be due to a reduction of thymocyte development and since non-primed T-lymphocytes are short-lived cells (35), splenic T-lymphocytes may not be replaced and, therefore, T-lymphocyte-mediated splenocyte function may be impaired.

The increased background tritiated thymidine incorporation rate present in cultures of spleen cells from HCB-treated mice has also been demonstrated with mouse lymphocytes following exposure to vinyl chloride (32). However, in the present study this effect, which became most pronounced after 24 weeks exposure and disappeared with continued exposure, was coincident with transient impairment in lymphocyte function and changes in organ weights.

The reduced stimulation index of HCB-treated cells activated in mixed lymphocyte cultures or following mitogen stimulation can not be due to the increased background incorporation levels since the ^{3}H-TdR incorporation rate by HCB-treated cells could be further elevated above the high background incorporation rate by stimulation with alloantigen or mitogen. Thus, a stimulation index comparable to control values was attained on the first day of culture of cells from mice which received HCB for 24 weeks when the background incorporation rate was 13 times greater than in control cultures.

The high ^{3}H-TdR incorporation rate which took four days to fall to control levels in cultures of cells treated with HCB for 13 weeks fell from an even higher rate in cultures containing cells treated with HCB for 24 weeks to control levels by the second day of culture. This suggests either the gradual depletion in the culture of a population of cells which have a stimulated rate of DNA synthesis or the gradual dilution during the culture period of a factor or factors which could stimulate DNA synthesis such as HCB, a metabolite of HCB, or a factor, the production of which is induced by the presence of a certain level of HCB. It is possible that HCB could be acting in a manner similar to concanavalin A, i. e., as a stimulator of nonspecific, suppressor T-cell proliferation and activity (32) thereby explaining the elevated ^{3}H-TdR incorporation rate of HCB-treated cell cultures in combination with the suppressed mixed lymphocyte activity and mitogen responsiveness.

To delineate the mechanism of action causing the functional suppression mediated by HCB in the development of an immune response, the data of the present study suggest that the lesion is not due to an impaired ability to recognize specific cell surface antigens for the following reasons: 1) HCB-treated cells can distinguish between the antigen diversity present on Balb/c versus BDF$_1$ cells, and 2) mitogen responsiveness, which is thought to bypass initial specific recognition, is impaired. Therefore, the HCB-induced lesion probably occurs beyond antigen recognition and exists either in the activation phase, due to the metabolic dysfunction of the cells involved; or, later in the response, due to a disorder in the regulation of the immune response.

SUMMARY

It is therefore proposed that: 1) environmental chemicals can have specific mechanisms of toxicity and can influence antibody-mediated immunity while having no detectable effect on cell-mediated immunity, 2) immune dysfunction is related to exposure time to a chemical and the tissue concentration of that chemical, 3) recovery of immune function may occur even though chemical exposure continues, and 4) a single assay of immune function may not be appropriate to detect chemical induced immune dysfunction.

ACKNOWLEDGEMENTS

J. B. Silkworth is a Monsanto Fund Fellow. This work was also supported in part by a joint program between the Gesellschaft F. Strahlen-und Umweltforschung mbH, Munich, Germany and the Institute of Comparative and Human Toxicology, Albany Medical College, Albany, New York (USA).

REFERENCES

1. Cohen, S., Ward, P. A. and Bigazzi, P. E. In: Mechanisms of cell-mediated immunity. (Eds. R. T. McCluskey and S. Cohn) John Wiley & Sons, New York (1974) 338.
2. Edelman, G. M. Science 180 (1973) 830.
3. Evans, R. and Alexander, P. Nature 236 (1972) 168.
4. Fisher, D. B. and Mueller, B. C. Biochem. Biophys. Acta 248 (1971) 434.
5. Friend, M. and Trainer, D. O. Science 170 (1970) 1314.
6. Gainer, J. H. Am. J. Bet. Res. 33 (1972) 2067.
7. Good, R. A., Dalmasso, A. P., Martinez, C., Archer, O. K., Pierce, J. C. and Papermaster, B. W. J. Exp. Med. 116 (1962) 773.
8. Gottlieb, A. A. Biochemistry 8 (1969) 2111.
9. Gowans, J. L. and McGregor, D. D. Prog. Allergy 9 (1965) 1.
10. Granger, G. A. and Williams, T. W. Nature 218 (1968) 1253.
11. Hirschorn, K. and Hirschorn, R. In: Mechanisms of cell-mediated immunity (Eds. R. T. McCluskey and S. Cohn) John Wiley & Sons, New York (1974) 115.
12. Hirschorn, R., Hirschorn, K. and Weissmann, G. Blood 30 (1967) 84.
13. Iatropoulos, J. J., Milling, A., Mueller, W. F., Nohynek, G., Rozman, K., Coulston, F. and Koret, F. Environ. Res. 10 (1975) 384.

14. Klein, J. In: Biology of the mouse histocompatibility-2 complex. Springer-Verlag, New York (1975) 472.
15. Kleinsmith, L. J., Allfrey, V. G. and Mirsky, A. Science 154 (1966) 780.
16. Koller, L. D. and Thigpen, J. E. Am. J. Vet. Res. 34 (1973) 1605.
17. Lawrence, H. G. Adv. Immunol. 11 (1969) 195.
18. Loeb, L. A. and Agaruwal, S. S. Exp. Cell Res. 66 (1971) 299.
19. Loose, L. D., Pittman, K. A., Benitz, K.-F. and Silkworth, J. B. J. Reticuloendothel. Soc. 22 (1977) 253.
20. Loose, L. D., Pittman, K. A., Benitz, K.-F., Silkworth, J. B., Mueller, W. and Coulston, F. Ecotox, Environ. Safety 2 (1978) in press.
21. Loose, L. D., Silkworth, J. B., Pittman, K. A., Benitz, K. -F. and Mueller, W. Inf. Imm. 20 (1978) 30.
22. Michie, D. In: Handbook of experimental immunology (Ed. D. M. Weir) Blackwell Scientific Publications, Oxford (1973) 30.1.
23. Mauel, J., Rudolph, H., Chapius, B. and Brunner, K. T. Immunology 18 (1970) 517.
24. Moller, G. and Svehag, S. -E. Cell. Immunol. 4 (1972) 1.
25. Nadler, H. L., Dowben, R. M. and Hsia, D. Y. Y. Blood 34 (1969) 52.
26. Nelson, N. Environ. Res. 5 (1972) 249.
27. Papageorgiou, P. S. and Glade, P. R. Lymphology 5 (1972) 80.
28. Pedrini, A. M., Nuzzo, F., Carrocchi, G., Dalpra, L. and Falaschi, A. Biochem. Biophys. Res. Com. 47 (1972) 1221.
29. Pasternak, C. A. and Friedericks, B. Biochem. J. 119 (1970) 481.
30. Rabinowitz, Y. and Dietz, A. A. Biochem. Biophys. Acta 139 (1967) 254.
31. Resch, K., Ferber, E. and Gelfand, E. W. 7th Leukocyte Culture Conference (1972).
32. Sharma, R. P. and Gehring, P. J. Fed. Proc. 37 (1978) 502.
33. Smith, J. W., Steiner, A. L., Newberry, W. M., Jr. and Parker, C. W. J. Clin. Invest. 50 (1971) 432.
34. Simonsen, M., Jensen, E. In: Biological problems of grafting. (Ed. F. Albert) Blackwell Scientific Publications, Oxford (1959) 214.
35. Sprent, J. In: The lymphocyte structure and function. Marcel Dekker, Inc., New York (1975).
36. Thigpen, J. E., Faith, R. E., McConnel, E. E. and Moore, J. A. Inf. Imm. 12 (1975) 1319.
37. Vos, J. G. and DeRoij, T. Toxicol. Appl. Pharmacol. 21 (1978) in press.
38. Vos, J. G. and Moore, J. A. Int. Arch. Allergy 47 (1974) 777.
39. Vos, J. G., Moore, J. A. and Zinkl, J. G. Environ. Hlth. Persp. 5 (1973) 149.
40. Waksman, B. H. In: Mechanisms of cell-mediated immunity. (Eds. R. T. McCluskey and S. Cohn), John Wiley & Sons, New York (1974) 135.
41. Wilson, D. B. J. Exp. Med. 122 (1965) 143.

THE IMMUNODEPRESSIVE EFFECT OF PHENOL DERIVATIVES

M. F. LA VIA[1], L. D. LOOSE[2], D. S. LA VIA[1], and M. S. SILBERMAN[1]

[1]Department of Pathology, Emory University School of Medicine, Atlanta, Georgia and
[2]Institute of Comparative and Human Toxicology, Albany Medical College, Albany, New York (USA)

The potentially damaging impact of manmade environmental contaminants on biological systems was first brought to our attention by the astute observations of Sir Percival Potts over 200 years ago. With impressive scientific acumen, he related the high incidence of scrotal neoplasia in chimney sweeps to their continued exposure to soot. The full significance of these observations remained hidden for more than 100 years until Japanese workers developed experimental models to study chemical carcinogenesis. As we look back at this series of events, it is regrettable to realize that greater scientific awareness might have contributed to shortening the time between Potts' original observation and further research on the phenomenon of chemical carcinogenesis. Great concern has existed since that first observation about possible noxious effects of the many new chemicals which are introduced in the environment daily.

At the FASEB meeting in April 1978, Dr. Donald Kennedy, Commissioner of the Food and Drug Administration of the United States, spoke emphatically of these dangers and pointed out that they are of particular concern because organisms are exposed to agents for which they have no prior evolutionary experience. That this is a problem of great importance is underscored by the institution, after appropriate investigation, of mandated screening tests for toxicity, carcinogenicity and teratogenicity.

Unfortunately little concern has existed for possible noxious effects at the level of host-parasite interactions and of individual manifestations of these interactions such as inflammatory, phagocytic or immune responses. This is particularly disturbing because of the mounting body of evidence which strongly indicates that disturbances of the balance of host-parasite interactions may be important in the etiology and/or pathogenesis of numerous disease states. The work on the role of macrophages in the pathogenesis of neoplastic disorders presented in an accompanying Symposium in this volume, leaves little doubt concerning the significant role of defense mechanisms in at least one very prominent pathologic condition: neoplasia. It is encouraging therefore that several laboratories are turning their efforts to studies which will hopefully become useful in screening programs to detect possible noxious effects of environmental chemicals on host-parasite interactions.

A fairly recent review by Vos (9) summarizes well the status of research in this area up to the end of 1976. In the last year and a half, however, a number of reports have appeared which are of interest in pointing out the exquisite sensitivity of immune responses to environmental chemicals.

In a study of immunodepressive effects in humans, Bekesy and coworkers (2) (Table I) investigated the mitogenic response, the number of T and B lymphocytes and the response in mixed lymphocyte cultures in Michigan dairy farmers exposed to polybrominated biphenyls (PBB) in a now famous accident. They reported that in over one-third of these individuals, when compared to non-exposed Wisconsin dairy farmers or New York residents, there was a significant decrease in all three parameters examined and concluded that this indicated an impairment of the function of lymphocytes, an important measure of their immune potential.

Fidler (3) (Table II) reported that mice given hyperchlorinated water, when compared to mice receiving tap water, show a decrease in cytotoxic effect of peritoneal macrophages on tumor cells, which progresses with time of chlorine exposure.

Loose and coworkers (4) examined the effect of polychlorinated biphenyls and of hexachlorbenzene on the immunological responsiveness of mice. They were able to show that doses which are well within the dose range of our present environment resulted in significant immunosuppression of the response to sheep erythrocytes and inability to mount a defense response to _Plasmodium berghei_.

These few examples point out in clear terms the need to start evaluating the safety of environmental agents in terms of possible effects on the immune response.

TABLE I

Response to Mitogenic and Antigenic Challenge of Lymphocytes from PBB-exposed and nonexposed individuals

Subjects	N	Phytohemagglutinin		Pokeweed Mitogen		Mixed Leukocyte Culture	
		Maximum Stimulation (count/min)	SI	Maximum Stimulation (count/min)	SI	Maximum Stimulation (count/min)	SI
Normal subjects (New York)	79	102,226±8,720	257	95,130±6,369	194		
Wisconsin dairy farm residents	46	97,662±2,693	292	90,636±3,406	190	38,172±1,209	66
PBB-Exposed Michigan dairy farm residents							
Demonstrating normal lymphoblastogenesis	27	92,272±2,241	281	93,199±7,412	186	28,248±2,072[a]	49
With abnormal lymphoblastogenesis	18	28,457±3,406[a]	71	39,159±3,537[a]	77	10,147± 317[a]	20

[a]Statistical significance (Student's t-test) between maximum blastogenesis of Wisconsin farm residents and that of Michigan farm residents ($P<.00001$).

From Bekesi *et al.* (2); copyright 1978 by the American Association for the Advancement of Science.

TABLE II

Changes in Macrophage-Mediated Cytoxicity After Hyperchlorinated Water Administration[a]

Week of Treatment	Drinking Water	% Macrophage-Mediated Cytotoxicity †Against B16 Melanoma	UV-112 Fibrosarcoma
1	Tap	55	76
	Hyperchlorinated	28	48
2	Tap	68	70
	Hyperchlorinated	31	24
3	Tap	43	62
	Hyperchlorinated	0	0
4	Tap	48	72
	Hyperchlorinated	0	0

[a]From Fidler (3).

Our interest in this area was stimulated by a laboratory accident which indicated that mice housed in cages washed with a disinfectant containing 3 phenol derivatives, developed a marked depression of the immune response to T dependent antigens in 4 to 6 weeks. The composition of this disinfectant is illustrated in Table III. One or more of the phenol derivatives contained in this compound are present in a number of disinfectants, insecticides and fungicides which are widely used throughout the world.

The toxicity of this compound and of one of its components, orthophenylphenol (OPP), has been studied extensively by Oehme (7 and personal communication) finding that the compound as well as OPP do not differ in their respective behavior in the dog and in the cat, although they are handled quite differently by these two species. The plasma concentration of OPP after administration of 1 gm/kg body weight, as shown in Fig. 1, is sharply different in the two species used. In cats it builds up to high levels and shows no decline, whereas in dogs it rapidly increases and disappears within 12 hr. Reflecting the plasma concentration, urinary excretion is marked in the dog but negligible in the cat over a 72 hr period (Fig. 2). These very different patterns of plasma accumulation and of urinary excretion are reflected in the survival times of both species illustrated in Fig. 3. Cats are clearly much more sensitive to the toxic effects of phenol derivatives as indicated by a survival time of only 14 hr at the lower dose of

TABLE III

Composition of Polyphenolic Disinfectant Examined in Our Studies

o-phenylphenol	5.0 %	
o-benzyl-p-chlorophenol	4.5 %	
p-tert-amylphenol	1.0 %	in water
sodium EDTA	3.04%	
isopropyl alcohol	1.5 %	

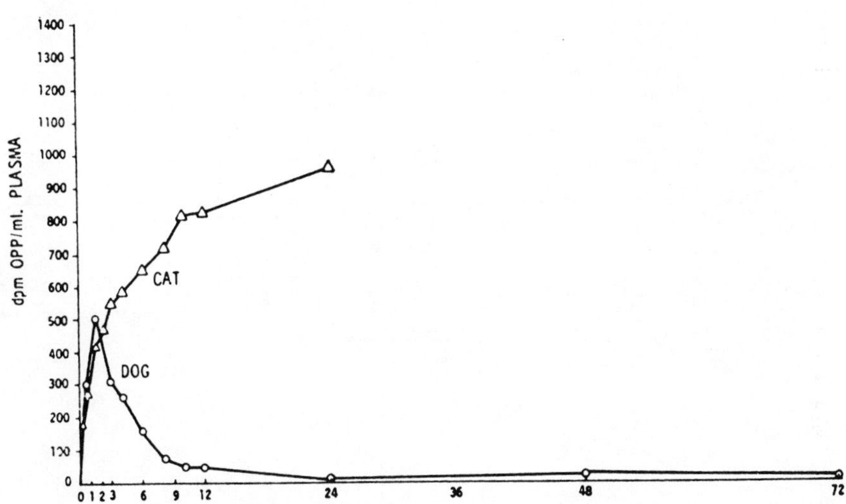

Fig. 1. Concentration of OPP in the plasma of dogs and cats given a single 1 gm dose of this chemical. From Oehme (7).

1 gm/kg body weight. Of particular interest in the context of our work, are the data presented by Oehme on tissue concentration of OPP (Fig. 4). The gastrointestinal tract, liver, bile and feces, are highest in OPP content as one would expect because of their role in detoxification and excretion. What is worthy of note, however, is the high concentration of OPP in the spleen, an organ very important to immune competence.

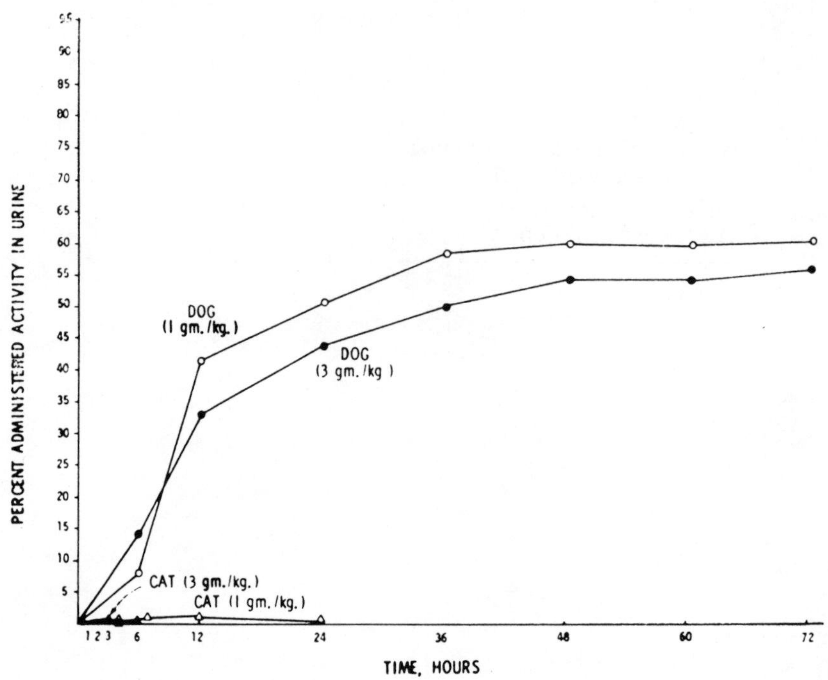

Fig. 2. Urinary excretion of OPP in dogs and cats given a single 1 gm dose of this chemical. From Oehme (7).

In pursuing our original observations, we first sought to establish whether very small amounts of phenol derivatives can be administered in the drinking water, in order to achieve a controlled exposure to known doses. If this were feasible, we then wanted to examine various tissues and organs for possible lesions induced by these compounds, to study their effects on the immune response to various antigens, and to investigate mechanism(s) of immunodepression caused by these compounds.

Three to six month old BALB/c female mice were used in the experiments reported below. Mice were housed in experimental groups of three per cage and were given measured amounts of water. By daily examination of drinking bottles, water intake was monitored and found to be constant (2.6 ml/mouse/day) over a period of three

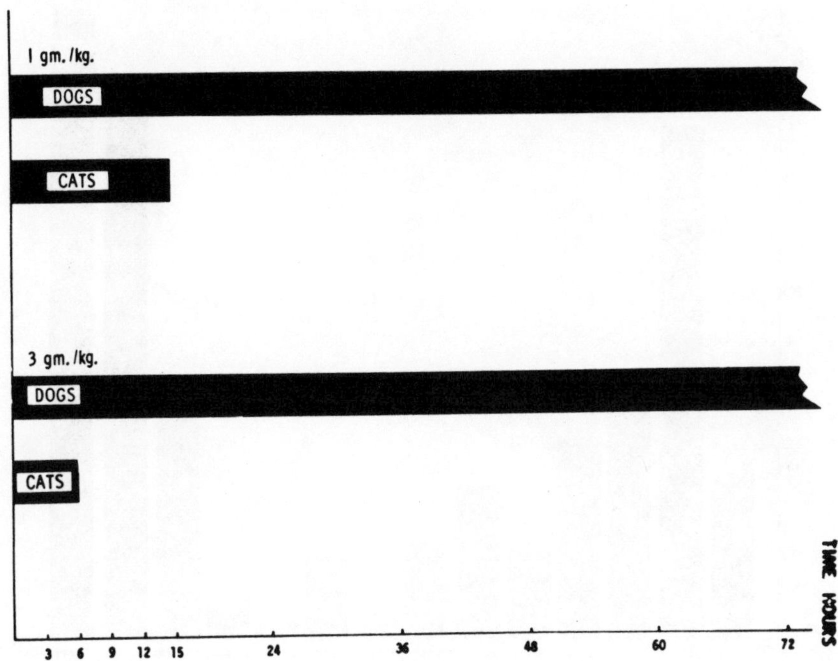

Fig. 3. Survival time of dogs and cats following a single dose of OPP of 1 or 3 gm. From Oehme (7).

weeks. These water consumption figures were used to calculate amounts of compound to be added in order to administer a known daily dose. This, however, represents more than the dose ingested, because of some water leakage into the cages which cannot be precisely measured but can be assumed to be constant. In all experiments, water consumption was also monitored daily to calculate actual consumption of the compound under study in each experiment. When phenol derivatives were added to the drinking water, there was no change in water consumption. This series of experiments demonstrated that phenol derivatives can be administered to mice in the drinking water thus assuring that a repro-

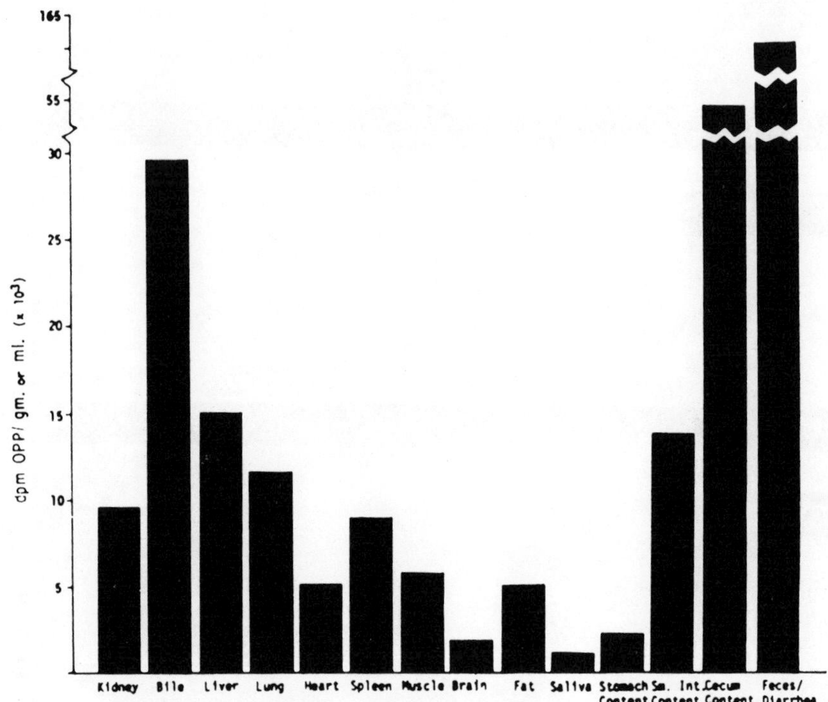

Fig. 4. Tissue concentration of OPP in dogs and cats given a single dose of radioactive chemical. From Oehme (7).

ducible and constant dose can be given. We then exposed mice to the whole disinfectant in the drinking water to establish whether this route of administration would induce the same degree of immunodepression observed by housing in treated cages. Groups of 3 mice each were given water containing (in mg/kg/day) 0.46 OPP, 0.41 OBpCP and 0.09 pTAP (see Table I for full names of derivatives). At weekly intervals 3 mice were immunized intraperitoneally with 1 x 10^8 sheep erythrocytes (SRBC) and at 4 days post immunization the number of IgM plaque forming cells (DPFC) was determined. All techniques for DPFC determination have been described previously (6). Table IV presents the results of these experiments. A significant immunodepression (45%) is already present by the end of the second week of exposure and is even more severe by the end of the fourth week (77%) at which time the experiment was terminated. In these and all other ex-

TABLE IV

Immunodepressive Effect in Mice of a Phenol Derivative Containing Disinfectant Administered in the Drinking Water[a]

Length of Exposure	"Phenol"	PFC/10^6 Cells			Average	Percent Depression
		1	2	3		
2 weeks	-	927	928	1094	983	
	+	626	586	322	511	48
	-	822	984	917	908	
	+	211	210	190	207	77

[a]No difference was found in spleen cell yields between control and treated mice. "Phenol" consumption in mg/kg/day was 0.46 OPP, 0.41 OBpCP and 0.09 pTAP. BALB/c mice were used in these experiments.

periments, cell counts were routinely performed to determine number of cells to be plated for DPFC assay. The total number of spleen cells was always the same in the exposed and control animals. In view of Oehme's data on phenol derivative concentration in the spleen, these data suggest that there is no direct cytotoxic effect on spleen cells in situ, dependent on the concentration of phenol derivatives in this organ. Clearly, because of the small dose effective in inducing immunodepression, the levels of phenol derivatives in the spleen can be assumed to be very low. The next series of experiments was directed to an examination of the effect of administering OPP in the drinking water and comparing it to the whole disinfectant. These experiments followed the same plan as in the previous series. Table V presents data showing that OPP is an effective in depressing the immune response as the entire mixture at comparable doses. OPP was selected as the first phenol derivative to study because of the demonstration by Oehme that it has a toxicity similar to the whole mixture of derivatives. Groups of mice were also set up and exposed to the whole disinfectant in the drinking water in order to enumerate T and B lymphocytes in the spleen. To accomplish this, single cell suspensions were prepared by teasing this organ in cold Veronal buffer (supplemented with Ca^{++} and Mg^{++}) containing 5% fetal calf serum (FCS). Cells were washed twice by centrifugation at 200 x g for 10 min and resuspended in RPMI with 10% FCS. The final cell concentration was adjusted to 1×10^7/ml. To detect B lymphocytes a 50 µl aliquot of the cell suspension was incubated with µl of fluorescein-tagged, goat anti-mouse Ig

TABLE V

Immunodepressive Effect in Mice of o-Phenylphenol as Compared to a Polyphenolic Disinfectant[a]

Length of Exposure	Treatment	PFC/10^6 Cells			Average	Percent Depression
		1	2	3		
3 weeks	"Phenol"	219	252	327	266	78
3 weeks	OPP	221	210	190	207	83
	Control	1294	1127	1232	1218	

[a]No difference was found in spleen cell yields between control and treated mice. OPP consumption was 0.7 mg/kg/day. "Phenol" consumption in mg/kg/day was 0.6 OPP, 0.54 OBpCP and 0.12 pTAP.

(Hyland Lab) for 45 min at 0 C. The cell suspension was then centrifuged for 5 sec in a Beckman microfuge and washed three times. The cells were resuspended in RPMI 1640 + 10% fetal calf serum in a 50 µl volume and 1 drop was placed on a glass microscope slide under a coverslip. A Zeiss microscope with an HBO 200 mercury arc (OSRAM) light source was used. At least 300 cells per preparation were examined. Cells were examined with darkfield illumination using a Zeiss 1.2/1.4 NA oil immersion darkfield condenser and a Zeiss 100x oil immersion planachromat objective with an iris diaphragm. A combination of a Zeiss PIL 546 nm excitation filter and 2 layers of Kodak Wratten 23A gelatin barrier filter were used to detect fluorescence. All cells were first examined under white light darkfield conditions and those with intact plasma membranes which under u.v. illumination exhibited speckled, ringed (peripheral) or crescent (polar, capping) fluorescence were noted. T lymphocytes were identified as spleen cells killed by anti-serum and complement as measured by trypan blue exlusion. Anti-θ serum was prepared by injecting rabbits subcutaneously with Sprague-Dawley rat brain emulsified in complete Freund's adjuvant. Inoculations were done once a week for 3 consecutive weeks and serum was collected one week after the last injection. This serum killed 95% of BALB/c thymocytes and 30-35% of spleen cells at dilutions of up to 1:16.

Phagocytic spleen cell macrophages were identified by a modification (5) of an *in vitro* yeast phagocytosis assay initially described by Schmid and Bruen (8). Briefly, a phagocyte:yeast (*Saccharomyces cerevisiae*) ratio of 1:3 was utilized. To sterile 12 x 75 mm capped plastic test tubes were added 0.20 ml of methylene blue (25.6×10^{-3} gm/100 ml in Hanks Balanced Salt Solution), 0.25 ml of the cell suspension, 0.25 ml of yeast in fetal calf serum and 0.10 ml of saline. Tubes were incubated at 37 C in a Dubnoff shaking water bath for 30 min. Following a 30 min incubation period, the tubes were removed and centrifuged at 315 g for 6 min at 4 C. The supernatant was discarded and the cell pellet resuspended in 20 = 1 HBSS. A wet mount was prepared for microscopic examination and 200 cells were counted and assessed for cells containing yeast particles.

The results of these determinations are presented in Table VI. Clearly no differences exist between T or B lymphocyte numbers in control and OPP exposed mice. However, the percent of macrophages capable of phagocytosing yeast particles is significantly reduced in treated mice as compared to controls. It must be noted again that the total number of spleen cells does not differ significantly between control and treated mice, confirming the possibility that no direct cytotoxic effect resulting in cell killing accounts for the changes induced by OPP.

The data presented also suggest that there is no change in the ability of surface receptors for the ligands used to study B lymphocytes (anti-IgG), to bind this ligand effectively as no changes were observed in the binding pattern of treated as compared to control mice. We cannot, however, exclude the possibility that antigen receptors were unable to bind antigen and this point will be examined in future experiments.

We may conclude from these results that one possible reason for the immunodepression caused by OPP could be the lowered ability of macrophages to phagocytose antigen (SRBC) or a decrease in macrophage number. One may further hypothesize that part of the impairment of immune responsiveness to a T dependent antigen may result from the lowered phagocytic ability or the decreased number of macrophages which may prevent macrophages from carrying out fully their needed function in the cell cooperative interactions necessary to activate B lymphocytes. Experiments by Archer (1) summarized below seem to support a macrophage defect as an important causative factor in immunodepression by phenol derivatives.

Mice exposed to either the disinfectant or to OPP developed very superficial lesions around the nostrils and these were examined histologically. Fig. 5 a and b illustrates the microscopic appearance of these lesions. There are focal areas of thickening of the stratified squamous epithelium and an increase in the amount of keratin over the epithelium. Several hair shafts appear fractured at the exit from the hair follicles. These lesions were diagnosed as hyperkeratosis, a condition known to be caused by exposure to phenol and its derivatives, and may have resulted from

TABLE VI

Influence of a Phenol Derivative-Containing Disinfectant on Splenic Lymphocyte and Macrophage Numbers

	O-Bearing Lymphocytes	Ig-Bearing Lymphocytes	Macrophages
Control	32 ± 3.4 (7)	54 ± 7.0 (7)	12 ± 0.9 (7)
OPP	34 ± 3.1 (8)	51 ± 6.6 (7)	2 ± 0.1 (7)*

Lymphocyte and macrophage numbers are expressed as a percent of the total spleen cell number. The data presented as the mean ± standard error with the number in parentheses representing the group size. Asterisk denotes significance at p less than 0.05. Spleen cell numbers in treated and control groups approximated 2.4 x 10^8 without any significant intergroup differences. "Phenol" consumption in mg/kg/day was 0.5 OPP, 0.45 OBpCP and 0.1 pTAP.

the constant exposure, during drinking, of the nose area. No other gross lesions were noted in several mice which were carefully examined by complete autopsy. However, we cannot exclude that microscopic lesions may have been present in the gastrointestinal tract or in other tissues and this point will be examined in future experiments.

Before discussing further the data presented here, we would like to review briefly some recently published results of Archer (1) which indicate that gallic acid, a phenol derivative widely present as a natural component of some foods and used as a food additive, is immunodepressive by a direct action at the level of immunocompetent cells.

In his work, this author showed that gallic acid added to mouse spleen cell cultures immunized with SRBC is capable of depressing markedly the immune response and that this depression can be reversed by addition to the cultures of either 2 mercaptoethanol (Table VII or adherent cell supernatant (Table VIII). Archer's results (1) suggest that a direct effect of phenol derivatives may occur at the level of macrophages and may be responsible for the immunodepression.

Our results indicate clearly that phenol derivatives, in particular OPP, are capable of interacting with mouse immunocompetent cells, most likely macrophages, and to induce profound immunode-

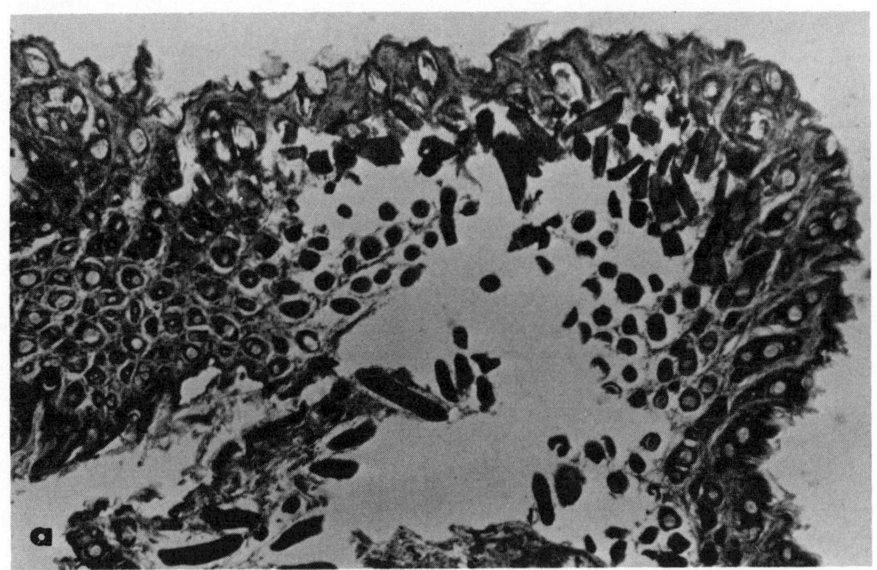

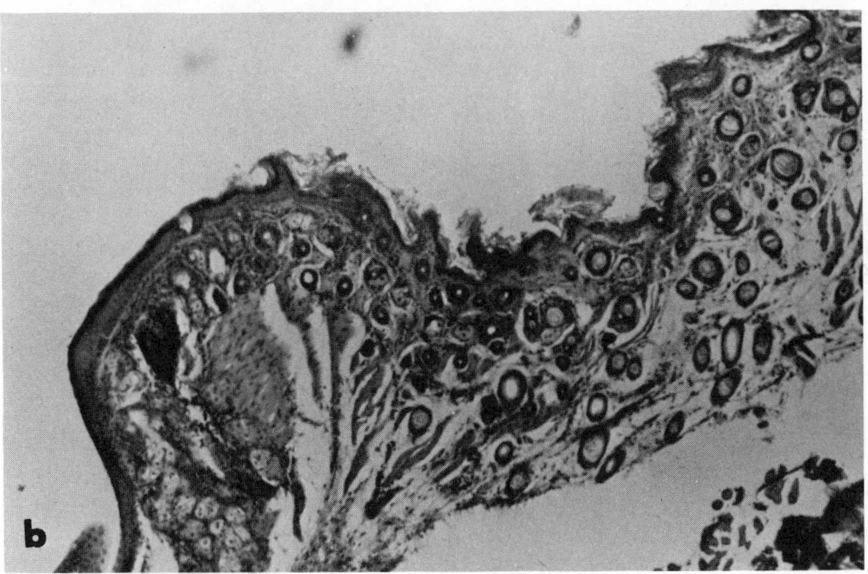

Fig. 5. Sections of the nose area of a mouse exposed to phenol derivative containing disinfectant for 4 weeks.

A. Hair shafts are seen to be fractured as they exit from the follicles.

B. A diffuse increase in the amount of keratin overlaying an extensive area of the epithelium is apparent.

TABLE VII

Effect of 2 Mercaptoethanol on the Immunodepression Produced by Gallic Acid in Culture

Culture Content	Direct Anti-SRBC PFC/Culture	PFC/10^6 Viable Cells
Control (SRBC stimulated)	22,533 ± 1,671[a] (400)[b]	2,448 ± 182
2 ME added at same time as antigen	19,200 ± 1,973	2,462 ± 253
10 μg of GA added at same time as antigen	<50	<5
10 μg of GA + 2-ME added at same time as antigen	1,467 ± 2,794	2,094 ± 273

[a]Means ± SEM of triplicate determinations; background corrected.

[b]Background PFC/culture.

From Archer et al. (1)

pression at low doses given for a relatively short time. This effect does not appear to be due to a direct cytotoxic effect, since cell numbers in the spleen are similar in control and treated mice. It appears, however, that macrophage phagocytic function or macrophage numbers are affected significantly and it may well be that the immunodepression derives from interference with macrophage-dependent events which are needed for B lymphocyte activation. Clearly this cannot yet be taken as a definite conclusion, since our studies have not excluded effects at the level of other systems (i.e. endocrine) which are intimately involved in the regulation of immune responses. It must also be determined whether macrophages are decreased in numbers, by means other than measuring phagocytic ability which may reflect a functional defect. One interesting aspect of experiments of this nature is the indication, apparent from work in different laboratories, that immune functions are exquisitely sensitive to environmental agents and thus may provide a very useful indicator of toxicity at toxicant doses much lower than those needed to induce morphologic changes or DNA damage. This sensitivity in turn points out the need for continuing to study the effect of environmental agents

TABLE VIII

Effect of Adherent Cell Supernatant on the Immunodepression Produced by Gallic Acid in Culture[a]

Culture Content	Direct Anti-SRBC PFC/Culture
Control (SRBC stimulated), washed at 24 hr	2700 ± 173[b]
10 μg of GA, washed at 24 hr	<50
10 μg of GA, washed at 24 hr, ACS added after wash	1167 ± 83
Control, washed at 24 hr, ACS added after wash	2333 ± 213
10 μg of GA, washed at 24 hr, ACS plus 10 μg of GA added at 24 hr	<50

[a]Prepared as described in text; 100 μl of final ACS added to designated cultures.

[b]Mean ± SEM of triplicate determinations.

From Archer *et al*. (1).

on the immune response in view of the major role which this response plays in a number of biological functions and disease states. While the results of our experiments are based on data obtained in a few dozen animals, they are highly reproducible and statistically significant and suggest that they should form the basis for further investigation of this problem. In particular, future work should be directed to an examination of effect in other animal species, of other antigens and of other aspects of the immune response. They should also elucidate the nature of target cells, the site(s) of action at the cell level, the effect of metabolic products of phenol derivatives, the effect of dose, length of exposure and the recovery time after exposure is discontinued.

A vast store of knowledge has been set up concerning immunologic phenomena and we are fully aware of their considerable importance in defense mechanisms and in disease phathogenesis. Thus it would be desirable to continue to investigate the possibility suggested by our studies, and those of others, that some environmental agents may have deleterious effects on immune function.

Only by furthering our understanding of these phenomena will we be able to evaluate the possible dangers posed by our environment and to learn to control them.

ACKNOWLEDGEMENT

This work was supported in part by NIH Grant AG 00132.

REFERENCES

1. Archer, D. L., Bukovic-Wess, J. A. and Smith, B. G., Proc. Soc. Exper. Biol. Med. 156 (1977) 465.
2. Bekesi, J. G., Holland, J. F., Anderson, H. A., Fischbein, A. S., Rom, W., Wolff, M. S. and Selikoff, T. J., Science 199 (1978) 1207.
3. Fidler, T. J., Nature 270 (1977) 735.
4. Loose, L. D., Pittman, K. A., Benitz, K. F. and Silkworth, J. B., J. Reticuloend. Soc. 22 (1977) 253.
5. Loose, L. D., Silkworth, J. B. and Warrington, D., Infect. Immun. (1978) in press.
6. McIntyre, J. A., La Via, M. F., Prater, R. F. K. and Niblack, G. D., Lab. Invest. 29 (1973) 703.
7. Oehme, F. W., Proc. 21st Gaines Vet. Symp., Gaines Dog Research Center, White Plains, N. Y. (1972) 8.
8. Schmid, L. and Brune, K., Infect. Immun. 10 (1974) 1120.
9. Vos, J. G., CRC Crit. Rev. Toxicol. 12 (1977) 67.

ALVEOLAR MACROPHAGE - SPLENIC LYMPHOCYTE INTERACTIONS FOLLOWING CHRONIC ASBESTOS INHALATION IN THE RAT

E. KAGAN[1] and K. MILLER[2]

Georgetown University Medical Center[1], Washington, D. C. (USA) and National Research Institute for Occupational Diseases[2], Johannesburg (South Africa)

While the alveolar macrophage undoubtedly plays a crucial role in the early stages of asbestosis (3,24) little is known about the possible contribution of the immune system to the pathogenesis of this disorder. There is evidence, from a number of clinical studies, which suggests that some disturbance of immunoregulation may be operative in patients with asbestosis. Impaired expression of several parameters of cell-mediated immunity has been demonstrated both *in vivo* (8,10) and *in* vitro (7,8,10), in such patients. In contrast, these patients manifest hyperactivity of the humoral immune response, as evidenced by their increased production of serum immunoglobulins (9,11), secretory IgA (9) and a variety of autoantibodies (9,11,30).

The reason for these immunologic abnormalities in patients with asbestosis is not clear, but the experimental induction of asbestosis in laboratory animals has provided a suitable model for studying the phenomenology of asbestos-related disease. In an earlier study we showed that alveolar macrophages obtained from rats chronically exposed to inhaled crocidolite asbestos dust (dusted rats) displayed striking alterations in surface morphology and an increased number of surface Fc receptors, compared with resident alveolar macrophages obtained from control (non-dusted) animals (15). It was postulated that these surface-related morphologic changes in macrophages obtained from dusted rats may be paralleled by changes in surface antigenicity. This hypothesis was reinforced when, in a subsequent study, we demonstrated the *in vivo* membrane deposition of complement components on alveolar macrophages from dusted, but not from control, rats (16). This finding indicates that prolonged inhalation of asbestos dust may initiate a humoral immune response directed against surface membrane determinants of alveolar macrophages.

The present study was designed to investigate the possible contribution of cell-mediated immunologic mechanisms to the pathogenesis of asbestosis. Attention was focused on the physical interactions between alveolar macrophages and enriched T cell populations from rats chronically exposed to crocidolite asbestos. Although regional thoracic lymph nodes would be the ideal source of lymphocytes for studying cellular interactions with alveolar macrophages, insufficient numbers of such lymphocytes are procurable in the rat. Instead the spleen was used as a lymphocyte source.

MATERIALS AND METHODS

Animals and exposure and conditions. Adult male rats, BD-IX strain (Freiburg, Germany) or AGUS strain (MRC Laboratory Animal Center, England), were used for all experiments. Dusted animals were exposed at 3 month of age to U.I.C.C. crocidolite asbestos (National Research Institute for Occupational Diseases, Johannesburg, South Africa) at a concentration of 1350 fibers/cc. Exposures were maintained for 8 hr a day, 5 days a week, over 5-8 months. Control (non-dusted) rats, matched for age and weight, were maintained under conventional animal house conditions.

Alveolar macrophages. Dusted and control rats were sacrificed and the alveolar macrophages obtained, as previously described (15). The macrophage concentration was adjusted to 1×10^6 cells/ml in Hepes-buffered RPMI 1640 and 1 ml aliquots were applied to Lab-Tek Tissue Culture Chamber/Slides (Miles) for 45 min at 37 C, after which non-adherent cells were removed by vigorous washing. The macrophages were then cultured for a further 4 hr at 37 C in RPMI 1640, containing 10% fetal calf serum (RPMI-FCS). Cell viability in all instances exceeded 94%.

In some experiments, 1×10^6 alveolar macrophages from dusted animals were applied to Lab-Tek slide chambers in RPMI 1640, containing 0.8 mM L-cysteine (BDH), incubated for 45 min at 37 C, washed 6 times with RPMI 1640 (to remove all traces of cysteine) and incubated for a further 4 hr as above. In other experiments $5\text{-}10 \times 10^6$ alveolar macrophages from control animals were pretreated with 1 ml of 2 mM sodium metaperiodate ($NaIO_4$, BDH) for 10 min at ambient temperature (6). After 3 washes, the macrophages were resuspended at 1×10^6 cells/ml, transferred to Lab-Tek slide chambers and cultured as above.

Spleen lymphocytes. Splenic fragments were gently homogenized in Joklik medium and the resulting cell suspensions were washed and resuspended in RPMI-FCS at a concentration of $1\text{-}1.5 \times 10^8$

cells/ml. The cell suspensions were then carefully layered onto Leukopak Leukocyte Filter (Fenwal) nylon wool columns (5). The spleen cell population was eluted with 40 ml of warmed RPMI 1640, resuspended and incubated over a second nylon column for 30 min at 37 C. A second eluate was obtained, centrifuged and the contaminant erythrocytes hemolysed with 0.83% NH_4Cl. After washing, the lymphocytes were resuspended in RPMI-FCS, at a concentration of 1×10^7 cells/ml. The final suspensions comprised 81-87% T cells and 5-11% B cells, as demonstrated by rosetting techniques and surface Ig immunofluorescence. Lymphocyte viability always exceeded 95%.

Lymphocyte-macrophage co-culture experiments. Various combinations of alveolar macrophages and enriched splenic T cell populations were incubated for 1 hr or 22 hr on Lab-Tek slide chambers (26) at an optimal lymphocyte: macrophage ratio of 10:1. Macrophages from control animals (control macrophages) were incubated with either autochthonous lymphocytes or syngeneic lymphocytes from dusted animals (dusted lymphocytes), while macrophages from dusted rats (dusted macrophages) were incubated with either autochthonous lymphocytes or syngeneic lymphocytes from control animals (control lymphocytes). In some experiments, dusted BD-IX macrophages were co-cultured with dusted AGUS lymphocytes and *vice versa*. In other experiments, dusted BD-IX macrophages were pre-treated with L-cysteine, prior to incubation with dusted AGUS lymphocytes, dusted BD-IX lymphocytes or syngeneic lymphocytes from control macrophages (with and without subsequent L-cysteine treatment) were co-cultured with autochthonous lymphocytes. The cultures were all subsequently fixed with Bouin's fixative, stained with hematoxylin and eosin, an examined morphologically. The results were expressed as the number of lymphocytes bound per 100 macrophages. The percentage of macrophages with 1 or more attached lymphocytes was also noted in each instance.

Lymphocyte blastogenic assay. Parallel lymphoproliferative assays were also performed, using the identical cross-combinations of syngeneic macrophages and lymphocytes employed in the morphologic co-culture experiments. The proliferative assays were performed in microtiter wells (26) which each contained 5×10^4 alveolar macrophages and 2.5×10^5 T cell-enriched spleen cells in RPMI-FCS with 2.5×10^{-5}M 2-mercatoethanol. Maximal uptake of ^{3}H-thymidine (^{3}H-TdR) occurred after 72 or 96 hr in syngeneic cultures.

Scanning electron microscopy. Specimens were prepared for scanning electron microscopy, as previously described (15).

RESULTS

Binding of lymphocytes to control macrophages. After 1

hr of incubation, alveolar macrophages from control rats bound comparable numbers of autochthonous lymphocytes and syngeneic dusted lymphocytes (Fig. 1). Similarly, no significant differences were noted in the proportion of control macrophages binding one or more lymphocytes, when co-cultures were performed with either autochthonous lymphocytes or syngeneic dusted splenic lymphocytes (Fig. 2). Most of the macrophage-associated lymphocytes adhered directly to the macrophage surface membrane and, in general, only one or two lymphocytes were bound to a single macrophage (Fig. 3a). After 22 hr of incubation, however, the numbers of lymphocytes adherent to control macrophages had, in both instances, decreased strikingly (Fig. 1). The percentage of the control macrophage population which was capable of sustained lymphocyte binding had also decreased with time, since only 3-14% of such macrophages had at least one lymphocyte attached after 22 hr.

Binding of lymphocytes to dusted macrophages. Striking differences were, however, observed with respect to the interaction of dusted macrophages with control or dusted splenic lymphocytes. After 1 hr of culture, more than 60% of the dusted macrophages had one or more adherent autochthonous lymphocytes (Fig. 2). Since a comparable percentage of the dusted macrophage population also bound syngeneic control lymphocytes in a like fashion, the proportion of alveolar macrophages capable of binding splenic lymphocytes non-specifically to their surface at 1 hr had increased by about 70% after asbestos inhalation. Large clusters of lymphocytes had formed around individual alveolar macrophages (Fig. 3b) and significantly greater numbers of autochthonous lymphocytes were attached to dusted macrophages ($p<0.001$), compared with control macrophages, at 1 hr (Fig. 1). Little decrease in binding of dusted lymphocytes was observed after 22 hr in autochthonous cultures (Fig. 1) and, in some instances, the size of the lymphocyte cluster had actually increased. A number of dusted macrophages contained 7 or more adherent lymphocytes, which were generally attached to surface ruffles and pseudopod extensions of the alveolar macrophages (Fig. 3b). However, some of the lymphocytes appeared to form secondary clusters around other macrophage-bound lymphocytes, in a manner similar to that described by Nielsen et al. (20) in a guinea pig PPD model.

When dusted alveolar macrophages were co-cultured with syngeneic lymphocytes from control rats, the numbers of lymphocytes bound per 100 macrophages at 1 hr were essentially similar to the values recorded for autochthonous cultures from dusted rats (Fig. 1). After 22 hr, however, a sharp drop was recorded in the numbers of adherent control lymphocytes, compared with the sustained clustering effect noted with dusted

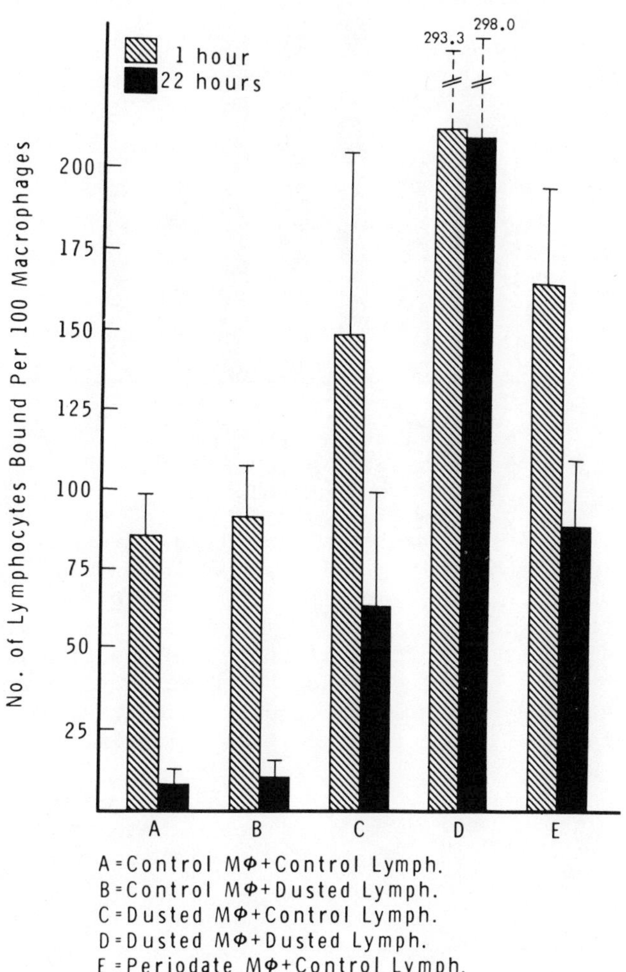

Fig. 1. Binding at 1 hr and 22 hr of T cell-enriched spleen suspensions to untreated control alveolar macrophages, dusted alveolar macrophages and $NaIO_4$ - treated control alveolar macrophages. Each result expressed as mean + S. D.

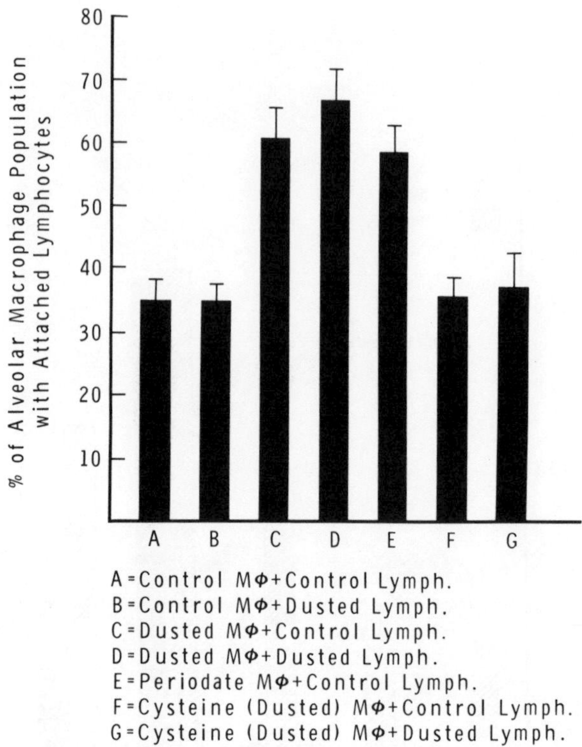

Fig. 2. Percentages of various alveolar macrophage populations binding one or more splenic lymphocytes after co-culture for 1 hr. Cysteine (dusted) M = alveolar macrophage pre-treated with L-cysteine, prior to lymphocyte co-culture. Each result expressed as mean + S. D.

lymphocytes (Fig. 1). The contrasting effects of incubating control and dusted splenic lymphocytes with dusted alveolar macrophages for 1 hr and 22 hr suggested that the effects of asbestos on macrophage-lymphocyte interactions were complex, involving a non-specific clustering effect (optimal at 1 hr) as well as an immunologically specific effect (optimal at 22 hr). A series of additional experiments were then designed, to test this assumption further.

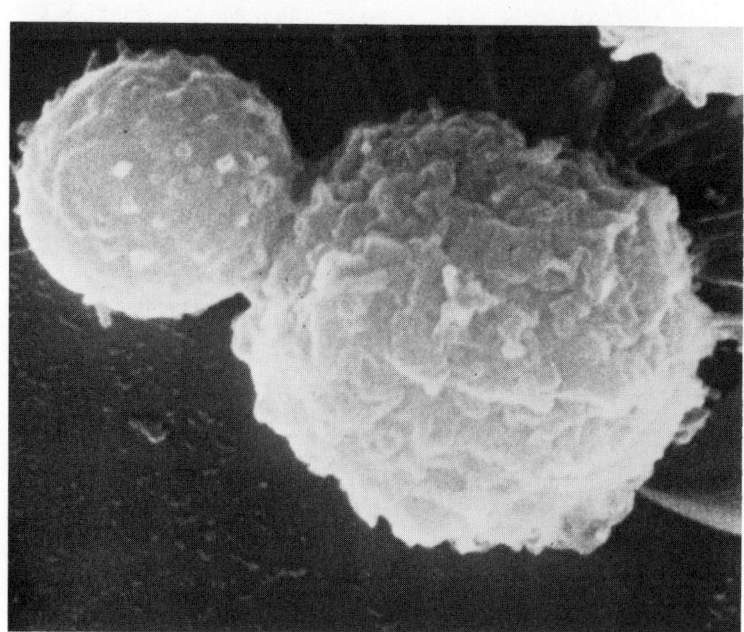

(a)

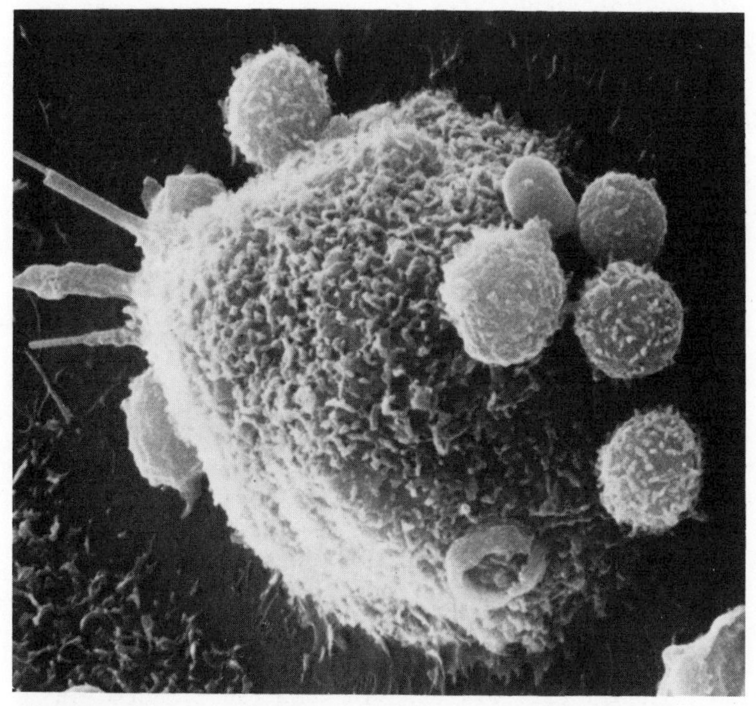

(b)

Fig. 3. Scanning electron photomicrographs showing (a) a solitary splenic lymphocyte attached to an autochthonous control alveolar macrophage, after incubation for 1 hr and (b) numerous splenic lymphocytes attached to an autochthonous dusted alveolar macrophage, after incubation for 1 hr (several ingested crocidolite fibers are protruding from one pole of the macrophage).

Binding of control lymphocytes to periodate-treated macrophages. Comparisons were made between the foregoing experiments and the interactions of control lymphocytes with autochthonous macrophages pre-treated with $NaIO_4$, a nonspecific inducer of macrophage-dependent lymphocyte blastogenesis (6). After 1 hr of incubation, $NaIO_4$-treated alveolar macrophages bound a significantly greater number of control lymphocytes than untreated control macrophages ($p<0.001$) and the numbers of lymphocytes bound were comparable with those obtained in co-cultures of dusted macrophages and autochthonous lymphocytes or syngeneic control lymphocytes at 1 hr (Fig. 1). The proportion of $NaIO_4$-treated macrophages binding lymphocytes after 1 hr was also similar to that seen with dusted macrophages (Fig. 2). A strong similarity was also noted between the number of control lymphocytes bound at 22 hr by $NaIO_4$-treated and dusted alveolar macrophages, but periodate treatment did not produce the sustained clustering effect at 22 hr, which was detected in co-cultures of autochthonous dusted macrophages and lymphocytes (Fig. 1).

Binding of lymphocytes to dusted macrophages and periodate-treated macrophages pre-treated with L-cysteine. Since similar lymphocyte binding properties were demonstrated by dusted macrophages and $NaIO_4$-treated control alveolar macrophages, L-cysteine, a mild general reducing agent and an antagonist of $NaIO_4$-induced lymphocyte blastogenesis (22) was used in some experiments, in order to establish whether it could abolish the non-specific clustering of lymphocytes around periodate-treated and dusted macrophages. When dusted lymphocytes were incubated with cysteine-treated dusted macrophages for 1 hr, considerably less lymphocytes were bound, compared with those bound to unteated dusted macrophages (Fig. 4). The number of attached lymphocytes now approximated that found in cultures containing control macrophages (Fig. 1). Treatment with L-cysteine produced a similar effect with respect to the percentage of the macrophage population with attached lymphocytes at 1 hr (Fig. 2). As expected, sequential treatment of control macrophages with $NaIO_4$ and L-cysteine reduced the number of control lymphocytes bound at 1 hr to levels noted with untreated control macrophages (Fig. 4).

When comparisons were made between the number of dusted lymphocytes bound at 1 hr and 22 hr to cysteine-treated dusted macrophages, there was no decline in lymphocyte attachment after 22 hr (Figs. 4 & 5), indicating that the prolonged physical interaction between dusted autochthonous lymphocytes and macrophages was not abrogated by cysteine treatment. On the other hand, pretreatment of the dusted macrophages with L-cysteine produced a sharp decline in the number of control lymphocytes bound to these

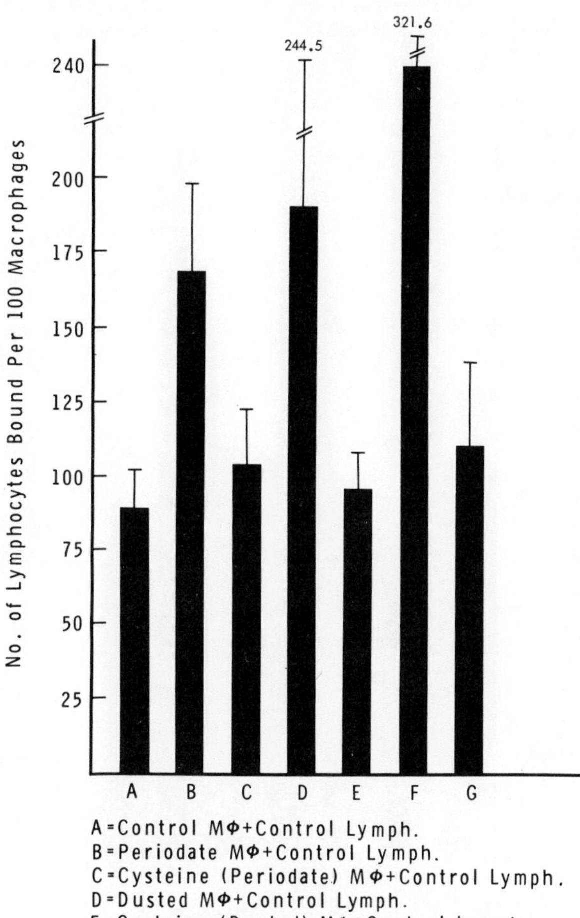

Fig. 4. Effects of L-cysteine treatment on the binding of T cell-enriched spleen suspensions to $NaIO_4$-treated control alveolar macrophages and dusted alveolar macrophages at 1 hr. Each result expressed as mean + S. D. Cysteine (periodate) M = control alveolar macrophage treated sequentially with $NaIO_4$ and L-cysteine.

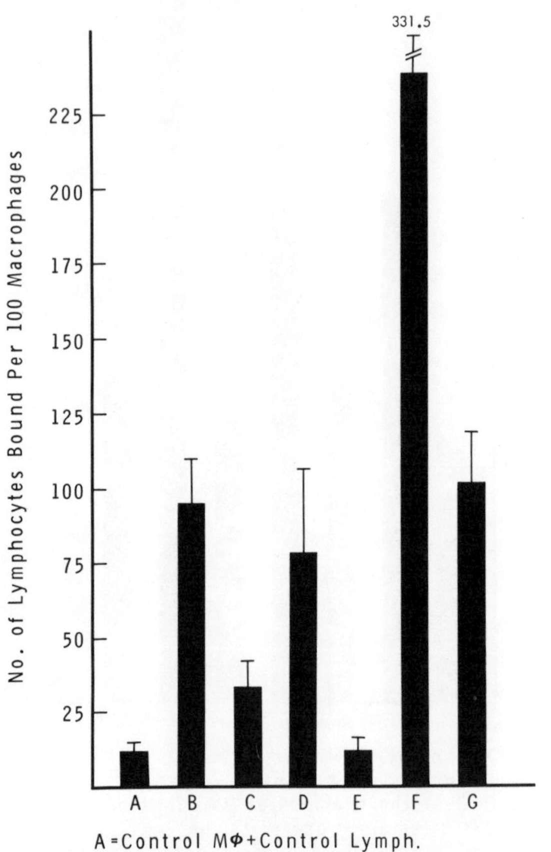

Fig. 5. Effects of L-cysteine treatment on the binding of T cell-enriched spleen suspensions to $NaIO_4$-treated control alveolar macrophages and dusted alveolar macrophages at 22 hr. Each result expressed as mean + S. D. Cysteine (periodate) M = control alveolar macrophage treated sequentially with $NaIO_4$ and L-cysteine.

macrophages after 22 hr (Fig. 5). Similar effects were noted when control macrophages were sequentially treated with $NaIO_4$ and L-cysteine (Figs. 4 & 5).

Effect of histocompatibility differences on lymphocyte binding to macrophages. Studies were also performed, to ascertain whether there was a requirement for histocompatibility restriction between the alveolar macrophages and the T cell-enriched spleen cell population. A number of experiments were performed across allogeneic barriers, using two inbred rat strains which differ at the major histocompatibility complex (MHC). After 1 hr of culture, lymphocytes from both strains of rats were bound to control macrophages, from either strain, in a similar fashion. Dusted macrophages similarly bound both contol and dusted lymphocytes (irrespective of whether the lymphocytes were of allogeneic or syngeneic origin) equally avidly after 1 hr. Distinct MHC-associated differences were, however, apparent at 22 hr (Fig. 6). When syngeneic co-cultures of dusted macrophages and dusted lymphocytes were used, no decrease in lymphocyte binding was observed between 1 hr and 22 hr of incubation. When dusted lymphocytes from one strain were incubated with dusted macrophages from the other strain, however, although a considerable number of lymphocytes was still attached to the macrophage after 22 hr, the number of lymphoid cells bound had decreased by 50-60%, compared with the 1 hr cultures.

Lymphocyte blastogenic assays. The aforementioned morphologic observations were extended, to include parallel lymphocyte proliferative assays, in order to assess whether lymphocyte blastogenesis could be induced by dusted macrophages. Peak uptake of ^{3}H-TdR was noted after incubation of autochthonous dusted macrophages and lymphocytes for 96 hr (11,838 ± 2,515 dpm) and was considerably higher than values obtained for 96 hr autochthonous control cell cultures, (1,851 ± 327 dpm). Dusted macrophages also induced the transformation of control lymphocytes. The peak incorporation of ^{3}H-TdR was observed, in this instance, after only 72 hr (15,440 ± 4,368 dpm), an effect which was abrogated by L-cysteine treatment of the macrophages, as reflected by a decline in ^{3}H-TdR incorporation to 3,168 ± 279 dpm at 72 hr. L-cysteine did not, however, influence the blastogenic affect of dusted macrophages on autochthonous lymphocytes, which still peaked after 96 hr (11,805 ± 1,647 dpm). Treatment of control macrophages with $NaIO_4$ produced a peak uptake of ^{3}H-TdR at 72 hr (35,591 ± 10,298 dpm) and, as expected, this phenomenon was inhibited by the presence of L-cysteine, which decreased the incorporation of ^{3}H-TdR to 8,922 ± 2,530 dpm at 72 hr.

Effect of in vitro crocidolite phagocytosis by control macrophages on lymphocyte binding. The *in vitro* phagocytosis of cro-

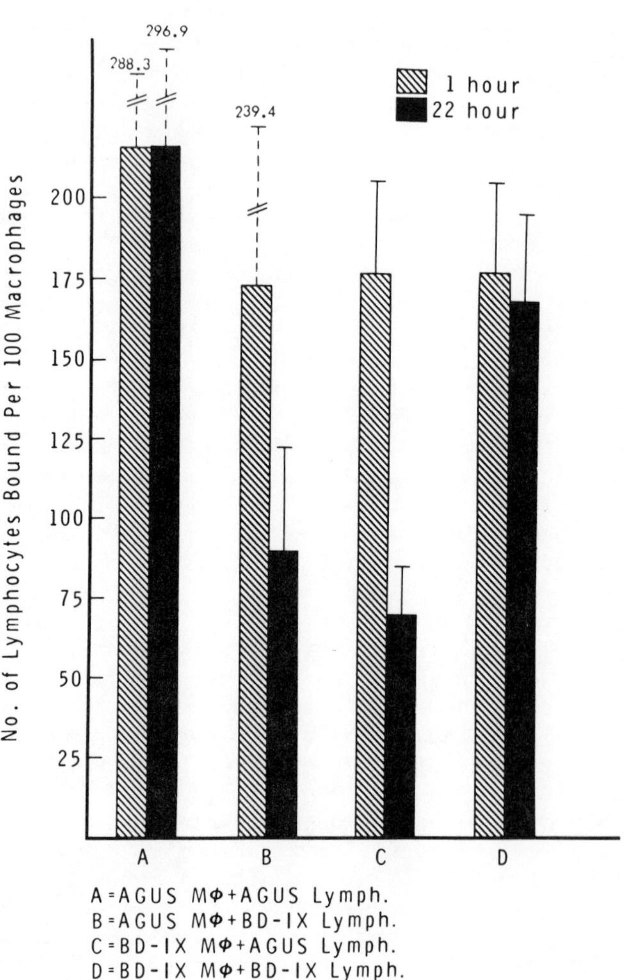

Fig. 6. Effects of histocompatibility differences on the binding of dusted splenic lymphocytes to dusted alveolar macrophages after incubation for 1 hr and 22 hr. Cells were obtained from AGUS and BD-IX inbred rat strains. Each result expressed as mean + S. D.

cidolite by control macrophages induced no obvious morphologic or functional changes in lymphocyte-macrophage interactions, which were analagous to those produced by dusted macrophages.

DISCUSSION

Macrophages are known to play a fundamental role in a number of immunologically-mediated events, including the processing of antigens, the effective presentation of immunogenic moieties to T cells, the optimal expression of _in vitro_ antigen-directed T cell proliferation, T cell-B cell collaboration, lymphokine production and the induction of delayed hypersensitivity reactions (2,23,28). The alveolar macrophage, a primary component of pulmonary defenses, is strategically located to participate in the induction and amplification of local cellular and humoral immunologic processes. This phagocyte is an important constituent of evolving lesions in both clinical and experimental asbestosis (3,17,24) and is known to participate in a variety of cell-mediated immune reactions in the lung, including primary and accelerated granulomatous responses to intravenous injections of BCG (19) and the response to aerosol challenge with _Listeria monocytogenes_ (4).

Rosenthal and co-workers (26-28), using soluble antigens, studied the physical interactions between peritoneal macrophages and T cells in a guinea pig model and identified 2 phases in the attachment of lymphocytes to macrophages. The first step was the reversible binding of lymphocytes, which attained a maximum after incubation for 1 hr. This occurred in the absence of antigen, was temperature dependent and did not require MHC-linked identity between the lymphocytes and the macrophages. The second phase, however, was a sustained, antigen-dependent event, which required the presence of immune lymphocytes, was maximal at 20 hr and needed the presence of histocompatible macrophages and lymphocytes. These findings were extended by other workers, using both peritoneal and alveolar macrophages (13,14,20,25). The avidity of lymphocyte binding can be enhanced by treatment of the cells with mitogenic agents, such as $NaIO_4$ or neuraminidase-galatose oxidase (6), which appear to act through the oxidation and clevage of cell surface glycoproteins, with the generation of surface aldehyde moieties (21). The effects of $NaIO_4$ peroxidation can be antagonised by L-cysteine (22).

The present study has demonstrated 2 separate effects of dusted alveolar macrophages on their interaction with enriched splenic T cell populations, which simulate, in some respects the aformentioned guinea pig model. The first phenomenon, which was analogous to that produced after control alveolar macrophages were pulsed with $NaIO_4$, was observed in co-cultures of dusted macrophages with control lymphocytes. In these cultures maximal lymphocyte clustering occurred at 1 hr, there was no requirement for MHC-linked recognition between the macrophage and the lymphocyte, and a maximal blastogenic response was evident at 72 hr. Since both the asbestos-related and periodate-induced phenomena were abrogated by treatment of the respective macrophages with L-cysteine, it is conceivable that chronic asbestos inhalation may produce an effect akin to alveolar macrophage membrane peroxidation. This asbestos-related phenomenon, through the nonspecific triggering of lymphoproliferation, provides a functional correlate of the adjuvant-like morphologic characteristics described previously in dusted macrophages (15) and may provide a rational explanation for the accentuated humoral immune response noted in asbestosis patients (9,11).

Another asbestos-related effect was illustrated in co-cultures of dusted macrophages and dusted lymphocytes, where sustained clustering was observed after 22 hr, MCH restriction was required between the macrophage and the lymphocyte and a peak lymphocyte proliferative response occurred only after 96 hr. This effect, which was not abolished by L-cysteine, correlates well with previous studies of antigen-induced lymphocyte clustering (20,26-28). The secondary clustering of dusted lymphocytes around primarily dusted macrophage-associated lymphocytes at 22 hr (Fig. 3b) parallels the observations of Nielsen *et al*. (20) with soluble protein antigens. Since splenic lymphocytes were used in the present study, these findings are consistent with systemic immune recognition of an asbestos-related, macrophage-associated antigen. The failure to demonstrate this phenomenon with control macrophages, which had phagocytosed crocidolite *in vitro*, provided further support for this postulate. Such an asbestos-related macrophage neo-antigen, if immunogenic, would explain why dusted rats develop a humoral immune response against autochtonous alveolar macrophages (16) and why patients with asbestosis develop non-organ-specific autoantibodies (1,11,30).

The findings in this study have important implications regarding the pathogenesis of asbestosis. Interest in the fibrogenic effects of asbestos has mainly centered on the structural and aerodynamic properties of asbestos fibers (12,29), but the participation of dusted macrophages in both cell-mediated and humoral immune reactions clearly focuses attention on the equally important role of host factors amplifying mechanically-related events. The induction of cell-mediated immunity in the lung by dusted macrophages could then initiate a chain-reaction, involving the interplay of lymphokines, lysosomal hydrolytic enzymes (1) and macrophage-related chemotactic substances (18), with pulmonary fibrosis as the ultimate end-result.

ACKNOWLEGEMENT

This work was carried out by one of us (K. M.) in partial fulfillment of the requirements for a Ph.D. degree from the University of the Witwaterstrand, Johannesburg.

REFERENCES

1. Allison, A. C. and Davies, P., In: Mononuclear Phagocytes in Immunity, Infection and Pathology (Ed. R. Van Furth), Blackwell, Oxford (1975) 487.
2. Basten, A., and Mitchell, J., In: Immunobiology of the Macrophage (Ed. A. S. Rosenthal), Academic Press, New York (1976) 45.
3. Becklake, M. R., Amer. Rev. Respir. Dis. 114 (1976) 187.
4. Cantey, J. R. and Hand, W. L., J. Clin. Invest., 54 (1974) 1125.
5. Greaves, M. F., Janossy, G. and Curtis, P., In: In Vitro Methods in Cell-Mediated and Tumor Immunity (Ed. B. R. Bloom and J. R. David), Academic Press, New York (1976) 217.
6. Greineder, D. K. and Rosenthal, A. S., J. Immunol. 115 (1975) 932.
7. Haslam, P. L., Lukoszek, A., Merchant, J. A. and Turner-Warwick, M., Clin. Exp. Immunol., 31 (1978) 178.
8. Kagan, E., Solomon, A., Cochrane, J. C., Beissner, E. I., Gluckman, J., Rocks, P. H. and Webster, I., Clin. Exp. Immunol. 28 (1977) 261.
9. Kagan, E., Solomon, A., Cochrane, J. C., Kuba, P., Rocks, P. H. and Webster, I., Clin. Exp. Immunol., 28 (1977) 268.
10. Kang, K. Y., Sera, Y., Okochi, T. and Yamamura, Y., N. Engl. J. Med., 291 (1974) 735.
11. Lange, A., Smolik, R., Zatoński, W. and Szymańska, J., Int. Arch. Arbeitsmed., 32 (1974) 313.
12. Lewinsohn, H. C., J. Soc. Occup. Med., 24 (1974) 2.
13. Lussier, L. M., Chandler, D. K. F., Sybert, A. and Yeager, H., Jr., Physiologist, 20 (1977) 59.
14. Lussier, L. M. and Yeager, H., Jr., Amer. Rev. Respir. Dis., 117, Part 2 (1978) 71.
15. Miller, K. and Kagan, E., J. Reticuloendothel. Soc., 20 (1976) 159.
16. Miller, K. and Kagan, E., Clin. Exp. Immunol., 29 (1977) 152.
17. Miller, K., Webster, I., Handfield, R. I. M. and Skikne, M. I., Pathology, in press.
18. Miller, K., Calverley, A. and Kagan, E., in preparation.
19. Moore, V. L. and Myrvik, Q. N., J. Reticuloendothel. Soc., 21 (1977) 131.
20. Nielsen, M. H., Jensen, H., Braendstrup, O. and Werdelin, O., J. Exp. Med., 140 (1974) 1260.

21. Novogrodsky, A. and Katchalski, E., Proc. Natl. Acad. Sci., 69 (1972) 3207.
22. Novogrodsky, A., In: Immune Recognition (Ed. A. S. Rosenthal), Academic Press, New York (1975) 43.
23. Oppenheim, J. J. and Seeger, R. C., In: Immunobiology of the Macrophage (Ed. D. S. Nelson), Academic Press, New York, (1976) 112.
24. Parkes, W. R., Br. J. Dis. Chest, 67 (1973) 261.
25. Petri, J., Braendstrup, O. and Werdelin, O., Cell Immunol., 35 (1978) 427.
26. Rosenthal, A. S. and Shevach, E. M., J. Exp. Med., 138 (1973) 1194.
27. Rosenthal, A. S., Lipsky, P. E. and Shevach, E. M., In: Mononuclear Phagocytes in Immunity, Infection and Pathology (Ed. R. van Furth) Blackwell, Oxford (1975) 813.
28. Rosenthal, A. S., Blake, J. T., Ellner, J. J., Greineder, D. K. and Lipsky, P. E., In: Immunobiology of the Macrophage (Ed. A. S. Rosenthal), Academic Press, New York (1976) 131.
29. Timbrell, V., In: Biologic Effects of Asbestos (Ed., P. Bogovski, J. C. Gilson, V. Timbrell and J. C. Wagner), World Health Organization, Lyon (1973) 295.
30. Turner-Warwick, M., Proc. Roy. Soc. Med., 66 (1973) 927.

TOBACCO SMOKE AND THE PULMONARY ALVEOLAR MACROPHAGE

D. B. DRATH, P. DAVIES, M. L. KARNOVSKY and G. L. HUBER

Harvard Medical School and Beth Israel Hospital

Boston, Massachusetts (USA)

The pulmonary alveolar macrophage (PAM) has been shown by numerous investigators to be responsible for maintaining sterility of the lower respiratory tract (4, 8). This key host defense cell must interact with and destroy invading microorganisms, as well as inactivate and remove various non-viable particulates to which the lung is exposed. Perhaps the most common particulate in this class is tobacco smoke, a complex chemical aerosol comprised of over 3,000 separate gaseous, liquid and solid components. The lung is the primary target organ affected by tobacco smoke and the first line of resistance to the inhaled smoking products is the alveolar macrophage. Failure on the part of this phagocyte to deal effectively with this environmental inhalant could conceivably lead to an increased susceptibility to microbial infection, as well as an altered pulmonary integrity. We have investigated, therefore, the effects of tobacco smoke on the structure, function, and metabolism of alveolar macrophages harvested by bronchopulmonary lavage from rats previously exposed to carefully quantified dosages of tobacco smoke for periods of 30-180 consecutive days.

MATERIALS AND METHODS

Animals, smoking and exposure schedule. Three groups of male CD rats, weighing approximately 150 g at the onset of exposure regimen, were used. They were divided as follows: (a) those animals exposed to tobacco smoke on a daily basis for 30-180 days; (b) age matched, non-exposed animals serving as shelf controls, and when possible, (c) an age-matched, sham-treated control group.

Rats were placed in individual conical plastic containers with an opening at the narrower end through which the animal's snout projected. Foam plastic stoppers wedged firmly into the container behind each animal prevented retraction of the animal's head. Each container was loaded onto a communal rack, such that an air-tight seal was formed between the container and the channel delivering the freshly generated smoking product. A rack accepted a total of 50 containers and was connected to a multiportal smoking machine programmed to produce a 35 ml puff of fresh whole smoke to 2 sec duration using 2R1 reference research cigarettes from the University of Kentucky (Lexington, Kentucky). The smoke aerosol was diluted immediately with air in a 1:10 ratio before delivery to the animals. The standard exposure utilized 10 cigarettes over a 10 min period and was repeated 3 times over several hr for a daily total of 30 cigarettes. The amount of smoke to which the animals were exposed has been shown by the use of smoke tracers and intrapulmonary deposition curves to correspond to approximately 1-1½ packs of unfiltered cigarettes per day in man (9). On the day following the last smoke exposure, rats were injected intraperitoneally with sodium pentobarbital. The abdominal aorta was severed to exsanguinate the animals, the trachea cannulated, and the intact lung lavaged with physiologic saline as described by LaForce *et al*.(11).

Quantitative morphology. The lavaged cell pellets were resuspended in a fixative solution consisting of a mixture of glutaraldehyde and osmium. Samples of cells from individual animals were collected in the form of a filtered pellicle to ensure a distribution of cells that was unbiased for size (1). After embedding in Epon, the cell pellicles were cut into convenient blocks for microtomy. Sections 1 μm thick were prepared and stained in alkaline toluidine blue for light microscopic morphometry. Measurements were made of PAM profile maximum diameters and the data analyzed by the Schwartz-Saltykov method in order to determine the mean maximum cell diameter, as well as the mean cell volume (19). The same blocks were used to prepare thin sections for ultrastructural analysis. At the electron microscope, randomly selected PAM profiles were photographed onto 35 mm film at as many as 3 levels of magnification. Level I (11,000 x) utilized the whole cell profile; level II (24,000 x), the majority of the cell excluding the nuclear profile; and level III (63,000 x) isolated a randomly selected portion of the cytoplasm. The 35 mm images were projected onto a ground glass screen and analyzed by point and intersection counting to determine the fractional volumes (volume densities) of subcellular compartments and the surface densities of cellular membranes, all relative to a reference compartment which, in this case, was total cytoplasm.

Functional and metabolic studies. Phagocytosis was measured by uptake of viable (^{14}C-labeled Staphylococcus aureus) and non-viable (^{14}C-labeled starch) particles by monolayers of PAM, as previously described by Michell *et al.* (14).

Oxygen consumption was measured polargraphically. Superoxide release was determined by cytochrome C reduction, as previously described (3). Hydrogen peroxide release was measured by the scopoletin technique of Root and co-workers (16) and glucose oxidation was determined by $^{14}CO_2$ production from glucose ^{14}C, as described by Michell *et al.*(14).

RESULTS

Quantitative morphology. After 30, 60 and 90 consecutive days of experimental smoke exposure, there was an increase in mean maximum diameters of PAM over the values of cells from age-matched control animals. The maximum change was exhibited after 60 days exposure, with a mean cell diameter of 14.4 µm, compared with a control value of 11.2 µm. Mean cell volumes for controls were 872 μm^3 at 30 and 60 days, and 623 μm^3 at 90 days. After smoke exposure, the values were 988, 1825 and 1168 μm^3 at 30, 60 and 90 days, respectively.

PAM lavaged from the lungs of control animals were recognized in the electron microscope by their mononuclear profile and heterogeneous collection of lysosomal granules. After experimental smoke exposure for periods of 30 to 90 days, the most distinctive qualitative change was the massively increased presence of lipid inclusions, many of them membrane-bound, within the cytoplasm. These inclusions were oil red O-positive in light microscope preparations. In the electron microscope they exhibited a variable density, presumably as a result of leaching out by lipid solvents. With prolonged osmication, however, their electron density was increased. Lysosomal granules assumed complicated shapes, while tubular structures, similar to those described in PAM by Sorokin (18) were prominent.

The subcellular morphology of PAM from control animals, as defined by stereologic techniques, remained fairly consistent at all periods studied. The nature and direction of the morphologic changes induced by the smoking regimen were also similar from 30 to 90 days of exposure. Figs. 1-5 present the volume densities of subcellular compartments in cells from control and smoke-exposed animals, expressed as a percent value relative to total cytoplasm. The volume density of nucleus in total cytoplasm was significantly less than controls in cells from animals exposed to smoke (Fig. 1). The volume density of mitochondria was slightly increased after 30 to 60 days of smoke exposure. The control value at 90 days was greater and there was no increase in this

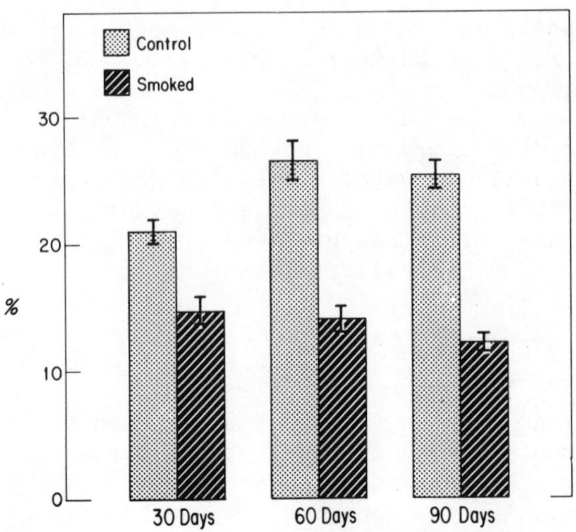

Fig. 1. Volume density of nucleus in total cytoplasm.

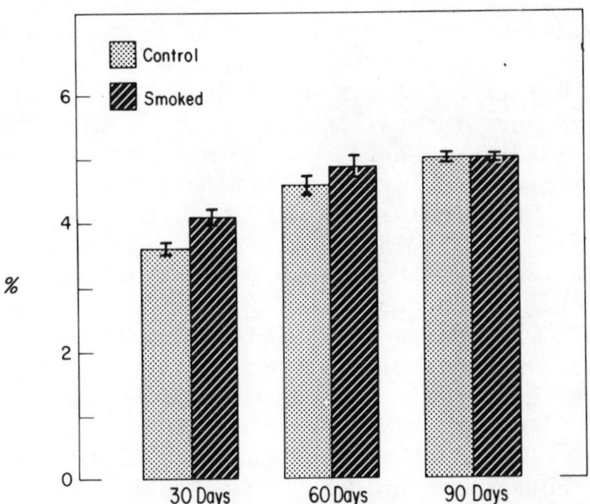

Fig. 2. Volume density of mitochondria in total cytoplasm.

parameter after smoke exposure (Fig. 2). A numerical count of mitochondria also indicated no change after 90 days exposure. The volume density of lipid inclusions was increased 10-fold after 30 days and nearly 20-fold after 90 days of animal smoke exposure (Fig. 3). The volume density of lysosomal granules was consistently less than control values after all periods of exposure (Fig. 4).

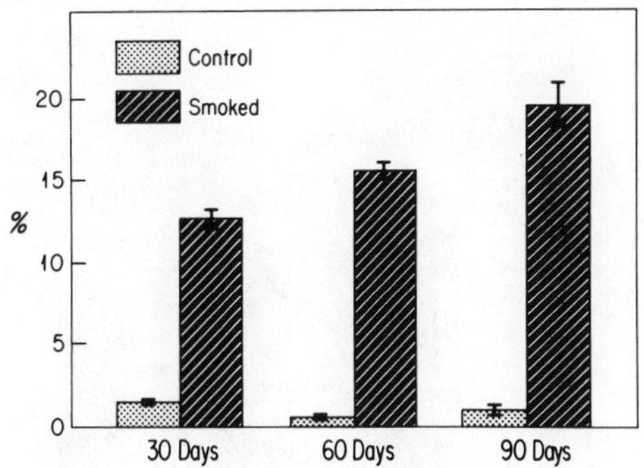

Fig. 3. Volume density of lipid inclusions in total cytoplasm

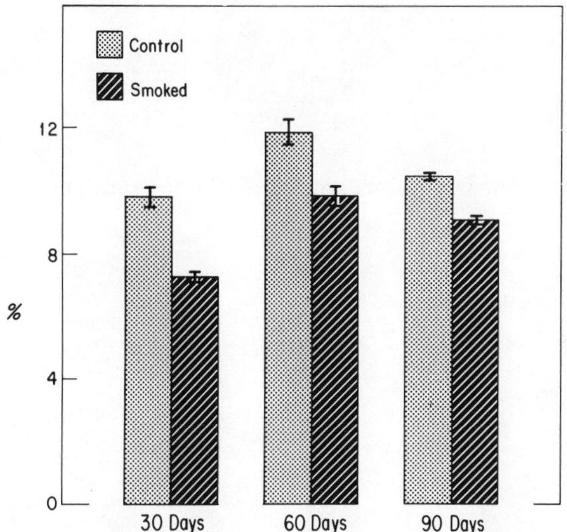

Fig. 4. Volume density of lysosomal granules in total cytoplasm.

Remaining cytoplasm constituted the cytoplasmic matrix, reticular network and golgi complex. The volume density of this compartment was also consistently less than control values in cells from smoke-exposed animals (Fig. 5).

Measurements on the surface densities of subcellular membranes was made only after 90 days of experimental smoke inhalation. The results, expressed in square microns per cubic micron of total cytoplasm, are presented in Fig. 6. The surface density of mitochondrial inner membrane in total cytoplasm was increased, relative

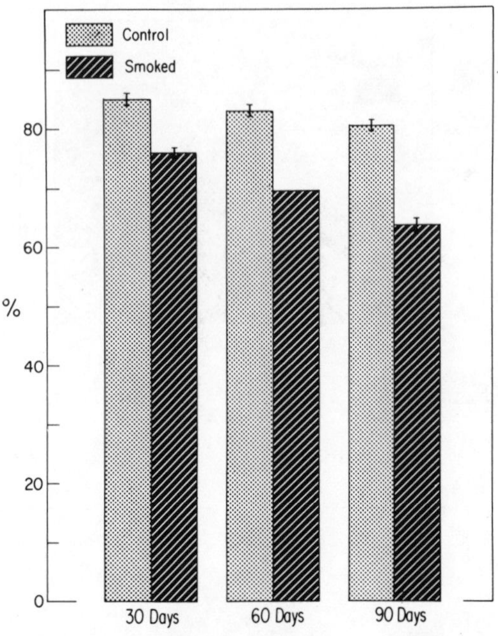

Fig. 5. Volume density of remaining cytoplasm in total cytoplasm.

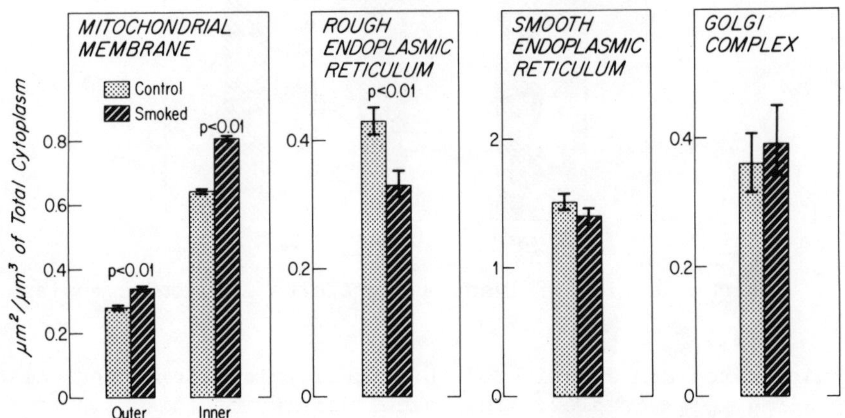

Fig. 6. Surface densities of subcellular membranes in μm^2 per μm^3 of total cytoplasm.

to control values, by a factor of 27%. If the results were expressed per unit volume of mitochondria, the relative changes would be 19% and 9%, respectively. The surface density of rough endoplasmic reticulum was significantly decreased by a factor of 23%. The surface densities of smooth endoplasmic reticulum and golgi membranes, however, exhibited no significant changes at the 5% level.

Functional studies. As an indicator of the functional capability of PAM, we have measured their uptake of viable ^{14}C labeled *Staphylococcus aureus* and inert ^{14}C starch particles when isolated from control, 30 and 180 day smoke-exposed animals. Results are shown in Figs. 7 and 8 and are expressed as the relative uptake or ratio of particles taken up (in micrograms) by smokers over controls (s/c). Values above the dashed line indicate an enhancement of phagocytosis and those below an inhibition. Following 30 days of exposure, an enhancement of phagocytic ability was shown towards the starch particles by cells from the smoke-exposed animals (Fig. 7A). This situation was reversed with the more chronic exposure (180 days) where an inhibition of approximately 35% resulted after 30 min in PAM from smoke-exposed rats (Fig. 7B). *S. aureus* presented a different picture than starch. No effect on uptake of the bacterium was shown following the short term exposure when compared with controls (Fig. 8A). More chronic exposures showed a similar pattern as for starch in that approximately a 40% inhibition in bacterial uptake was evident (Fig. 8B).

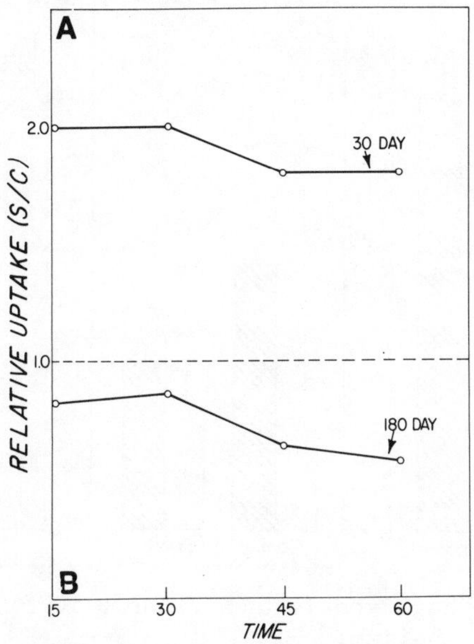

Fig. 7. Relative uptake of ^{14}C-labeled starch particles following 30 and 180 days of tobacco smoke exposure.

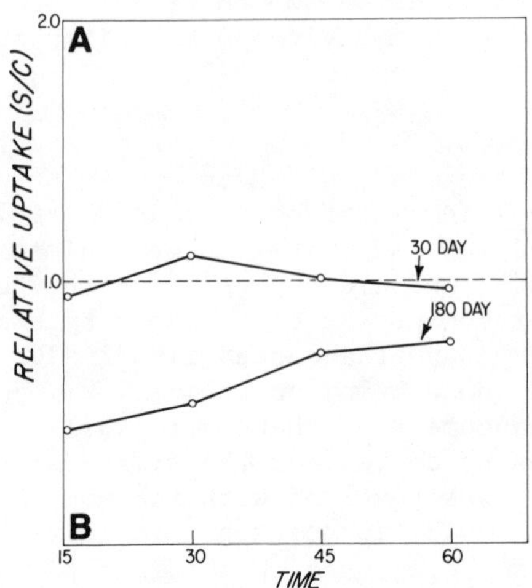

Fig. 8. Relative uptake of ^{14}C-labeled Staphylococcus aureus following 30 and 180 days of tobacco smoke exposure.

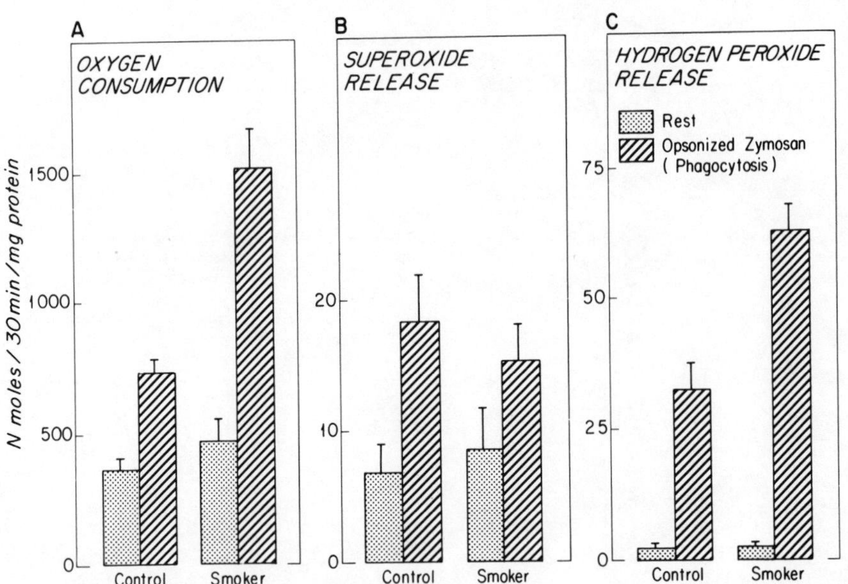

Fig. 9. Effect of phagocytosis and 30 days of tobacco smoke exposure on oxygen metabolism.

Oxygen metabolism. All studies reported herein were performed on PAM from control, 30 and 180 days smoke-exposed rats. Shown in Fig. 9 are the effects of 30 consecutive days of smoke inhalation on oxygen consumption (A), superoxide (B) and hydrogen peroxide release (C). As expected, an increase in oxygen consumption was seen upon phagocytosis of opsonized zymosan. The 2-fold increase observed was further doubled in response to smoke exposure. Superoxide release, while increased as a result of phagocytosis, was surprisingly unaffected by tobacco smoke, whereas hydrogen peroxide was elevated in response to both the phagocytic particle and the smoking regimen. This information may be compared with that of Fig. 10, which illustrates results obtained from animals subjected to a more chronic smoke exposure (180 days). Several observations are immediately apparent. Superoxide release following 180 consecutive days of smoke exposure is markedly elevated over control levels, a situation not observed following 30 day exposures. Control levels of superoxide release, however, are considerably less dramatic than were seen in Fig. 9 (shorter exposure). Oxygen consumption and hydrogen peroxide release are again elevated during phagocytosis and this is further stimulated by smoking, though not as dramatically as was shown for the short term smokers. Of interest was the finding that tobacco smoke of either duration had no effect on the metabolism of resting macrophages.

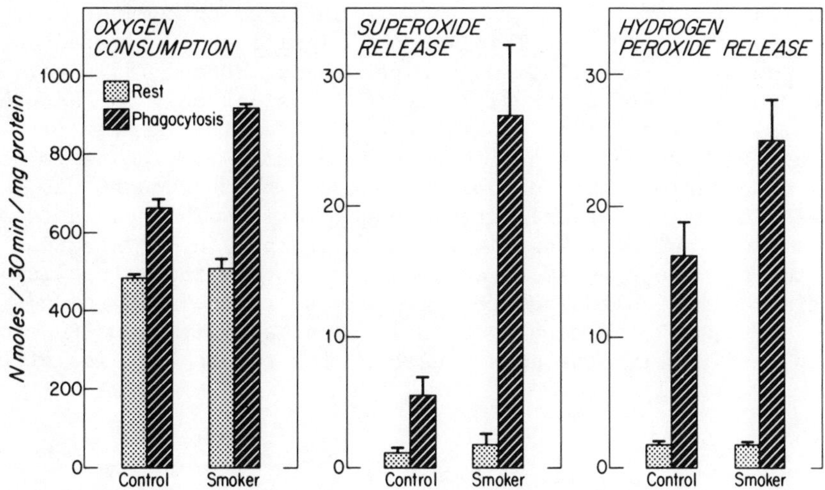

Fig. 10. Effect of phagocytosis and 180 days of tobacco smoke exposure on oxygen metabolism.

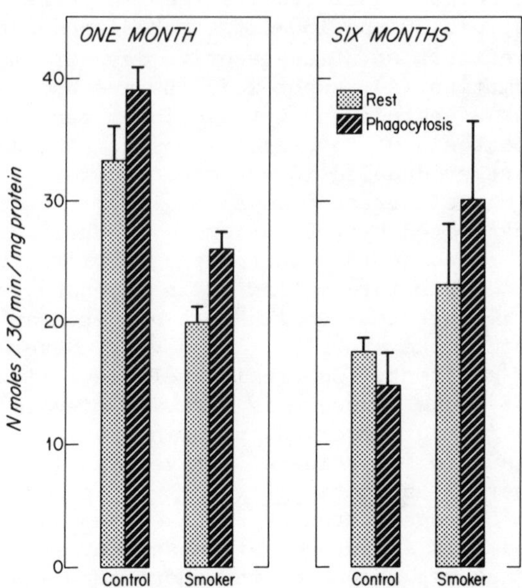

Fig. 11. Hexose monophosphate shunt activity following 30 and 180 days of tobacco smoke exposure.

Glucose metabolism. Oxidation of glucose labeled in the carbon 6 position was completely unremarkable when compared to the situation in other phagocytic cells following particle uptake. Approximately 2 nmoles of glucose were oxidized on a mg of protein basis in 30 min at rest. This was not significantly altered during phagocytosis and following smoke exposures of 30 and 180 days. Hexose monophosphate shunt activity (C-1 oxidation), on the other hand, was affected by the smoking regime. As seen in Fig. 11, shunt activity was not significantly affected by phagocytosis at either time period, but following the short term exposure was depressed both at rest and during phagocytosis. The reason for this remains unclear. This is the sole example in our studies where tobacco smoke exposure caused an effect on the metabolism of a resting cell. Following prolonged exposure, shown in the adjacent panel, an elevation is seen in shunt activity, a situation more in keeping with the data presented for tobacco and its effects on oxygen metabolism.

DISCUSSION

The increase in cell volume after smoke exposure has been shown to be contributed mainly by the total cytoplasm compartment, while the volume of the nucleus remained virtually unchanged (2).

Although the volume density of mitochondria underwent only a small increase or showed no change, the absolute volume and absolute number of mitochondria must have increased in roughly the same proportions as the increase in cell volume. Evidence for mitochondrial replication was not found, however, nor is the mechanism known. Mitochondrial inner membrane is recognized as the site of oxidative phosphorylation. Thus, an increase in the surface density of the membrane indicates a potentially increased level of oxidative phosphorylation in the cells from smoke-exposed animals. Lipid inclusions have been reported as being present in PAM from human smokers (7, 15, 21) and from animals experimentally exposed to tobacco smoke (2, 13) and it has been suggested that they may contain lipid soluble tobacco smoke components (20). They have also been reported to be present in PAM after exposure of animals to inert aerosols (6), so that tobacco smoke exposure may act as a non-specific stimulus to their formation. Several reports have demonstrated cytochemical acid phosphatase activity in association with the lipid inclusions and we can conclude that the lipid accumulates within heterolysosomes. Thus, the decrease in the volume density of lysosomal granules, found at all stages of smoke exposure investigated, was most probably due to a utilization of primary lysosomal granules in the formation of heterolysosomes, many of which contained lipid. The remaining cytoplasm compartment included the cytoplasmic matrix, the site for certain energy-producing pathways, including the glycolytic pathway. The enzymes necessary for the direct oxidation of glucose (the hexose monophosphate shunt) are also present within the cytosol. The decrease found in the volume densities of this compartment after all periods of smoke exposure may, therefore, have serious repercussions in terms of available energy supply of the cell. A reduced level of protein synthesis would be a probable concomitant of the decreased surface density of rough endoplasmic reticulum found after smoke exposure.

Despite the fact that a decrease in the volume density of cytosol occurred and, with it, a potential decrease in production of glycolytic energy, there was no concomitant decrease in phagocytic capability by smokers following 30 days of exposure. In fact, phagocytosis of starch particles was increased following this exposure regimen. Although Green et al.(5) described an inhibition of the glycolytic enzyme, glyceraldehyde 3-phosphate dehydrogenase, following the administration of smoke to macrophages in cell culture, there is no compelling evidence to suggest that glycolysis supplies the energy for phagocytosis in these cells. An equally feasible view is that a cell in such an aerobic environment might rely more heavily on oxidative phosphorylation than on glycolysis for its energy source. The lack of an inhibitory effect on phagocytosis, which we observed, was transient, however, in that with more prolonged exposures of 180 days a definite inhibition in particle uptake occurred, suggesting that the effects of tobacco smoke on the phagocytic machinery were cumulative. Whether particle uptake, shown by us to be inhibited in vitro, is also impaired in the intact host following chronic smoke exposure remains to be seen. If impairment of this key host defense cell were to occur, however, it would undoubtedly lead at the very least to an increased susceptibility on the part of the host to microbial infection.

The metabolism of alveolar macrophages was also affected by tobacco smoke, the final product being a cell which in many respects was similar to phagocytes commonly described as "activated". Short term exposure (30 days) produced more variable effects on metabolism in that oxygen consumption and hydrogen peroxide release were elevated while superoxide release was unchanged and hexose monophosphate shunt activity was depressed. Longer exposures showed a pattern more consistent with activation, with all metabolic parameters elevated. It is important to note that the effects of tobacco smoke on oxygen metabolism only occurred during phagocytosis and did not alter the basal metabolism of the resting cell. Such an occurrence distinguishes this type of activation as a consequence of an immune reaction (12) or nonspecifically by casein or thioglycolate elicitation (10). Our finding may be more consistent with the idea that various receptors which initiate the metabolic phenomena accompanying particle engulfment are uncovered during phagocytosis and are thus more susceptible to stimulation by tobacco smoke.

Of potentially greater importance than the mechanism of activation is the result of such activation. It is known, for example, that in polymorphonuclear leukocytes (PMN) the products of oxygen metabolism, such as hydrogen peroxide and superoxide, are important in microbial killing. It is therefore not unreasonable to postulate that a similar situation exists in alveolar macrophages which are because of their location more accessible to oxygen than PMN. Our results indicate that with longer exposures (180 days) these cells release increased amounts of hydrogen peroxide and superoxide. Under non-smoking conditions these agents may actively participate in microbial killing. During smoking, however, the increased release of these reactive compounds may directly affect the functional capability of the macrophage and/or damage the pulmonary parenchyma. Salin and McCord (17) have shown that PMN exhibit a loss of viability following phagocytosis, which could be prevented by inhibitors of either superoxide, hydrogen peroxide or hydroxyl radical, a potent biological oxidant. In other studies from our laboratory we have shown that PAM produce hydroxyl radicals. Unfortunately, information on the effects of tobacco smoke on radical formation is not presently available. We do know, however, that short term exposures (30 days) cause an approximate 35% inhibition of superoxide dismutase (SOD) activity. This enzyme occupies a key position in the control of hydroxyl radical production through its action on superoxide generation. Smoking may therefore result in an overproduction of hydroxyl and other oxygen radicals through both a direct effect on oxygen metabolism and indirectly via its depressant effect on enzymes (SOD) which control oxygen radical formation. These radicals, once produced, may affect the integrity of the alveolar macrophage, rendering it incapable of meeting a microbial challenge, and/or affect its viability as does occur in PMN. No information is currently available about the relationship of smoking, radical production and viability. If, however, a loss of viability were to occur, the result would be a release of lysosomal enzymes from damaged macrophages, which could conceivably lead to inflammation and destruction of surrounding parenchymal tissue.

SUMMARY

Our results indicate that tobacco smoke exposure of varying duration causes morphological, biochemical and functional alterations in pulmonary alveolar macrophages. The results of these changes is a population of alveolar macrophages made up of larger cells, with a reduced nucleus-cytoplasmic ratio, which are heavily loaded with heterolysosomes containing lipid. Though their fractional complement of mitochondria remains the same, an increase in the inner mitochondrial membrane surface area may be related to an enhanced oxidative metabolism. The cell is biochemically activated particularly following chronic exposure and is functionally impaired with respect to phagocytosis.

REFERENCES

1. Davies, P., Sornberger, G. C. and Huber, G. L. Amer. Rev. Resp. Dis. 116 (1977) 1113.
2. Davies, P., Sornberger, G. C. and Huber, G. L. Lab. Invest. 37 (1977) 297.
3. Drath, D. B. and Karnovsky, M. L. J. Exp. Med. 145 (1975) 257.
4. Green, G. M. Ann. Rev. Med. 19 (1968) 315.
5. Green, G. M., Powell, G. M. and Moriss, T. G. J. Clin. Invest. 50 (1971) 40a.
6. Gross, P. and DeTreville, R. T. P. Arch. Environ. Hlth. 17 (1968) 720.
7. Harris, J. O., Swenson, E. W. and Johnson, J. E. J. Clin. Invest. 49 (1970) 2086.
8. Huber, G. L., Johanson, W. G. and LaForce, F. M. In: Lung biology in health and disease (Ed. C. Lenfant) Vol. 5, Marcel Dekker, Inc. New York (1977) 979.
9. Huber, G. L. , Pochay, V. E., Mahajan, V. K., McCarthy, C. R. Hinds, W. C., Davies, P., Drath, D. B. and Sornberger, G. C. Bull. Eur. Physiopathol. Respir. 13 (1977) 145.

10. Karnovsky, M. L., Lazdins, J. and Simmons, S. In: Mononuclear phagocytes in immunity, infection and pathology (Ed. R. Van Furth), Blackwell Scientific Publications, Oxford, England (1975) 423.
11. LaForce, F. M., Kelly, W. J. and Huber, G. L. Am. Rev. Resp. Dis. 108 (1973) 784.
12. MacKaness, G. B. J. Expt. Med. 120 (1964) 105.
13. Matulionis, D. H. and Traurig, H. H. Lab. Invest. 37 (1977) 314.
14. Michell, R. H., Pancake, S. J., Moseworthy, J. and Karnovsky, M. L. J. Cell. Biol. (1969) 216.
15. Pratt, S. A., Smith, M. H., Ladman, A. J. and Finley, T. N. Lab. Invest. 24 (1971) 331.
16. Root, R. K., Metcalf, J., Oshino, M. and Chance, B. J. Clin. Invest. 55 (1974) 945.
17. Salin, M. L. and McCord, J. M. Clin. Invest. 56 (1975) 1319.
18. Sorokin, S. O. In: Lung biology in health and disease (Ed. C. Lenfant) Vol. 5, Marcel Dekker, Inc., New York (1977) 711.
19. Underwood, E. E. In: Quantitative stereology. Addison-Wesley, Reading, Massachusetts (1970) 119.
20. Vassar, P. S., Culling, C., Saunders, A. M. Arch. Pathol. 70 (1960) 649.
21. Warr, G. A. and Martin, R. R. J. Reticuloendo. Soc. 23 (1978) 53.

EFFECTS OF PESTICIDES ON THE RETICULOENDOTHELIAL SYSTEM

W. S. CEGLOWSKI, C. D. ERCEGROVICH, AND N. S. PEARSON

Department of Microbiology and Cell Biology and Pesticide Research Laboratory, The Pennsylvania State University, University Park, Pennsylvania (USA)

Pesticide is a rather broad, general term utilized to describe a diverse group of compounds which have been widely utilized to control a variety of organisms considered as pests. In the United States, pesticides are described in the Federal Environmental Pesticide Control Act as any substance or mixture of substances intended for preventing, destroying, repelling or mitigating any pest. A pest may be an insect, rodent, nematode, fungus, weed, other forms of terrestrial or aquatic plant or animal life, viruses, bacteria, or other micro-organisms on or inside humans as well as animals, which the Administrator declares to be a pest. Substances which are utilized as plant regulators, defoliants or dessicants are also identified as pesticides. Pesticides discussed in this paper include the following:

Common Name	Chemical Name
Ametryne	2-ehtylamino-4-isopropylamino-6-methylmercapto-s-triazine
Carbaryl	1-naphthyl-N-methylcarbamate
Chlordimeform	N'-(4-chloro-o-toyl)-N,N-dimethylformamidine
DDT	1,1,1-trichloro-2,2-bis(p-chlorophenyl)ethane
Malathion	S-(1,2-dicarbethoxyethyl)-0,0-dimethyldithiophotphate
Mirex	(dodecachlorooctahyro-1,3,4,-metheno-2H-cyclobuta(cd)pentalene)

Common Name	Chemical Name
Parathion	0,0-diethyl-0-p-nitrophenylphosphorothioate

In contrast to many environmental pollutants which are by-products of manufacturing processes and may be inadvertently introduced into the environment, pesticides represent an example of large group of chemicals which are intentionally introduced into the environment in substantial quantities. Pesticides have been widely utilized, particularly since the Second World War. Indeed, it is generally acknowledged that extensive utilization of pesticides has contributed significantly to the increasing production of agricultural products. Estimates suggest that in the United States alone approximately 10 billion pounds of pesticides were utilized in the time period of 1945-1970 (8). Even greater quantities of pesticides have been produced and utilized since that time. For example, it has been estimated (8) that in the year 1971 alone approximately 1 billion pounds of pesticides were produced in the United States. Contributing to this total were 55 million pounds of the insecticide Carbaryl, 45 million pounds of the insecticide DDT, and 30 million pounds of the insecticide Malathion. The recent restrictions in the production and application of certain pesticides have resulted in a significant increase in the utilization of other approved pesticides with no reduction in the total amounts of pesticides utilized.

It has been estimated that approximately 85% of the human pesticide burden can be attributed to the diet (2). Extensive studies (2) have demonstrated that many commonly used pesticides can frequently be detected in randomly sampled fresh foods. Other studies (1) have documented the presence of detectable levels of pesticide residues in human adipose tissue and blood. As might be expected individuals who because of their occupation may be exposed to high concentrations of pesticides can exhibit blood and tissue pesticide levels up to 25 times that of the general population.

Most studies concerned with the effects of pesticides on human health have concentrated attention on their acute toxicity (4, 8). In contrast fewer studies have been concerned with the effects of either acute or chronic exposure to pesticides on functions of the reticuloendothelial system.

Several studies, however, have been performed to assess the effects of a limited number of pesticides on humoral immunity. For example, an early study by Wasserman *et al.* (12) examined the effect of one of the organochlorine pesticides, DDT, on the immune response. These investigators utilized rats as the experimental animal, and DDT in the drinking water at a concentration of 200 ppm as the pesticide. Animals exposed to DDT for 35 days exhibited significantly lower weight spleens and livers than did appropriate control animals. A group of ovalbumin-immunized DDT-treated animals developed levels of antibody such that the mean titer of the treated group was 70% that of the control. In addition the immunized, DDT-treated animals exhibited a rise in the percentage of serum albumin with a decrease in the gamma globulin serum fraction.

In a more recent study Wasserman _et al._ (13) have assessed the effect of DDT on the immune response of rabbits, to either _Salmonella typhi_ or sheep erythrocytes. In these studies, rabbits were exposed to DDT in the drinking water at a concentration of 200 ppm for a total of 38 days. Agglutinin titers were determined at 1 and 7 weeks post-immunization. Salmonella agglutinin titers were significantly lower in the DDT-treated animals at both time intervals post-immunization. In contrast, while agglutinin titers to sheep erythrocytes were reduced, this reduction was not statistically significant. Comparison of the control and DDT-treated animals confirmed the previous observation of reduced gamma globulin concentrations in the serum and revealed that the decrease in total gamma globulin concentration was a consequence of a reduction in the 7S component of this fraction. These investigators also observed that the plasma levels of DDT were significantly higher in the DDT-treated Salmonella-immunized group than the DDT-treated sheep erythrocyte-immunized group. This observation was interpreted as evidence for a bi-directional relationship between the degree of detoxication of DDT and magnitude of the immune response to the antigens tested.

In a related study Kosutzky _et al._ (7) examined the effect of feeding DDT at a concentration of 100 mg DDT/Kg of feed on the immune responsiveness of chickens and ducks to the antigen, human serum albumin. In these studies, animals were fed the DDT-containing feed for 14 days prior to immunization and the immune response was assessed at several time intervals post immunization. While the antibody titers of the DDT-treated birds were reduced, the differences did not achieve statistical significance.

More recently, Janezic _et al._ (5) have studied immune responses to bovine serum albumin in rats following daily oral administration of DDT at a rate of 20 and 40 mg/K body weight for 21 days prior to immunization. Antibody titers were determined at 7, 14, 28 and 35 days post-immunization. In this study, significant elevations in antibody titers were observed in every group except for the 28 day post-immunization group receiving 20 mgm DDT/K.

In a more recent study, Subba Rao and Glick (11) examined the effect of feeding a food containing 100 ppm DDT to newly hatched chicks for the first 40 days of life on their subsequent immune responsiveness to sheep erythrocytes. While they observed no significant subsequent reduction in the agglutinin titers to sheep erythrocytes, assaying for mercaptoethanol sensitive and resistant agglutinins revealed a significant depression in mercaptoethanol resistant antibody and a marked increase in the mercaptoethanol sensitive antibody levels at both 5 and 7 days post-immunization. At no time in this experiment were any differences observed between the treated and control groups in either body weight or bursa, spleen, thymus or liver weights. Similar experiments were performed with newly hatched chicks exposed to a feed containing 100 ppm of the pesticide Mirex. These studies also revealed no change in total agglutinin titers with a depression in mercaptoethanol resistant antibody and an increase in mercaptoethanol sensitive antibody levels.

Recent studies (14) in our laboratory have investigated the effect of a single oral administration of DDT at either 300 mg/K (1 LD_{50}) or 30 mg/K (0.1 LD_{50}) on the subsequent immune response of mice to sheep erythrocytes. The administration of 30 mg/K DDT at either 5 days before, the day of, or 2 days after immunization with sheep erythrocytes did not affect the number of splenic antibody plaque forming cells observed at the peak of the primary immune response. Administration of a single high dose (300 mg DDT/K) at the same time intervals resulted in no significant depression of the splenic antibody plaque forming cell response except in the group receiving DDT 2 days after immunization. Additional groups of mice were administered 30 mgm/K DDT daily for either 8 or 28 days prior to immunization with sheep erythrocytes. There was no significant decrease in the number of splenic antibody forming cells in either group. There was a slight, though not significant, increase in the number of antibody plaque forming cells in the group exposed to DDT for 28 days prior to immunization.

The organophosphorus group of compounds is another widely utilized type of pesticide. The effect of an extensively used representative of this group, Malathion, on immune reactions in rats has been studied by Popeskovic et al. (10). In these studies rats were administered daily doses of 0.61 mg of Malathion per K of body weight from either 15 days prior to immunization or the day of immunization until 30 days post-immunization. All mice were subsequently assayed for humoral immunity at 10, 20 and 30 days post-immunization. Significant reductions in antibody titers were observed in both groups at 10 and 20 days post-immunization. Antibody titers observed at 30 days post-immunization while reduced did not differ significantly from control levels. However,

Arthus reactivity was observed to be significantly suppressed at all three time intervals tested.

In our recent study (14) mice were administered a single dose of the organophosphorus compound, Parathion, orally at either 22.3 (1 LD_{50}) or 2.2 mg/K (0.1 LD_{50}). Immunization with sheep erythrocytes was performed either five days after, the day of, or two days prior to the administration of the pesticide. All animals were assayed for antibody plaque forming cells four days after immunization. Significant reductions in the number of antibody forming cells were observed only in animals receiving the highest (22.3 mg/K) dose 2 days after immunization. Daily administration of the lowest (2.2 mg/K) dose tested for eight days also resulted in a significant reduction in splenic antibody plaque forming cells.

We have performed similar studies with the compounds Ametryne (a herbicide of the S-triazine class), Carbaryl (an insecticide of the carbamate class) and chlordimeform (an insecticide of the formamidine class) (14). A single dose of Ametryne was administered orally at either 879 (1 LD_{50}) or 88 mg/K (0.1 LD_{50}) 5 days before, the day of, or 2 days after immunization with sheep erythrocytes. Upon assay for antibody plaque forming cells four days later, all animals receiving the high dose exhibited significant depressions in splenic plaque forming cell numbers. Animals receiving the low dose either in a single administration or for eight or twenty-eight consecutive days prior to immunization exhibited no significant reduction in antibody plaque forming cell numbers.

Identical studies with Carbaryl at doses of either 153 mg/K (1 LD_{50}) or 15.3 mg/K (0.1 LD_{50}) revealed no significant change in the plaque forming cell numbers in animals receiving the low dose for either 8 or 28 days prior to immunization. Suppression of plaque forming cell numbers was observed only when the single high dose was administered two days after immunization. In additional studies with Carbaryl, mice have received oral doses of either 2.2 mg/K or 0.2 mg/K at weekly intervals for a total of 10 months. Groups of mice were immunized with sheep erythrocytes after 3, 8 and 10 months exposure to the pesticide. None of the experimental groups exhibited antibody plaque forming cell numbers which differed significantly from those of appropriate controls.

Additional studies utilizing the insecticide chlordimeform at 14.8 mg/K (0.1 LD_{50}) revealed no change in plaque forming cell numbers following oral administration for either 8 or 28 consecutive days prior to immunization with sheep erythrocytes. Oral administration of a single dose of 148 mg/K (1 LD_{50}) of chlordimeform at either the time of immunization or two days after immunization also resulted in a significant reduction in plaque forming cell numbers. Intraperitoneal administration of a single dose of chlordimeform at 30.5 mg/K at two days post-immunization also resulted in a significant depression in humoral immunity whereas the same dose administered at either 5 days before or the day of immunization was without any significant suppressive effect.

While a limited number of studies have been performed on humoral immunity even fewer studies have been performed on the effect of pesticides on phagocytic capacity of the RE system. A study by Kaliser (6) examined the effect of daily oral administration of DDT on the ability of rat leukocytes to phagocytose *Staphylococcus epidermidis* in both an *in vivo* and an *in vitro* system. Rats were treated with daily doses of DDT at a rate of 0.2 mg/K for up to 31 days. *In vivo* studies were performed in which rats were treated with DDT for 10, 21 or 31 days prior to the intracardial inoculation of *S. epidermidis*. *In vitro* studies were also performed in which blood collected from rats after 10, 21 or 31 days of exposure to DDT was incubated with *S. epidermidis*. Following 25 min of incubation in the *in vivo* and *in vitro* systems blood smears were prepared and stained and two determinations were made. The first concerned the percentage of polymorphonuclear leukocytes which had engulfed *S. epidermidis* and the second concerned the average number of bacteria present within polymorphonuclear leukocytes which had ingested at least one bacterium. Analysis of the data generated in this study revealed that while statistically significant differences were observed between groups tested on different days, no statistically significant differences between DDT-treated and control groups resulted at any single experimental time point studied.

In a recent study Pipy *et al.*(9) examined the effect of the insecticide Carbaryl on the phagocytic activity of the reticuloendothelial system in the rat. Carbaryl at rates of 3.75, 7.5, 15.0 and 30.0 mg/K was administered 1 hr prior to the intravenous inoculation of colloidal carbon. Calculation of the rate of carbon removal from the circulation revealed a dose-dependent decrease in phagocytic activity as a consequence of Carbaryl treatment.

SUMMARY

The information available concerning the effects of compounds utilized as pesticides on functions of the reticuloendothelial system is quite limited. Review of selected examples of such studies in this and other reports (3) reveals considerable diversity in terms of species of experimental animal, purity and dose of pesticide, length of exposure, and class of pesticide employed. Observations include depression, enhancement, or no significant effect on the selected reticuloendothelial system function studies. With the present available information it is difficult to formulate general conclusions or to predict whether or not any individual pesticide will consistently and significantly alter any specific function of the reticuloendothelial system. At the present time, it is not known if pesticides within a single chemical class act in a similar manner in regard to their ability to influence reticuloendothelial system function. In addition, the relationship, if any, between the toxic, mutagenic, teratogenic, or carcinogenic potential of any pesticide and its ability to alter the reticuloendothelial system is also unknown. More extensive systematic studies in experimental animal models would appear to be required before protocols to effectively evaluate the potential of pesticides to influence reticuloendothelial system functions in man can be developed.

ACKNOWLEDGEMENT

These studies were supported in part by Biomedical Research Support Grant of The Pennsylvania State University.

REFERENCES

1. Davies, J. E. In: Environmental Pollution by Pesticides (Ed. C. A. Williams) p. 313, Plenum Press, London. 1973.
2. Duggan, R. E. and Duggan, M. B. In: Environmental Pollution by Pesticides (Ed. C. A. Williams) p. 334, Plenum Press, London. 1973.
3. Ercegovich, C. D. Fed. Proc. 32 (1973) 2010.
4. Hayes, W. J., Jr. In: Toxicology of Pesticides. Williams and Wiklins, Baltimore. 1975.
5. Janezić, A., Popesković, L., Adamovic, M. and Janković, B. D. Proc. Yugoslav. Immunol. Soc. 3 (1971) 130.
6. Kaliser, L. A. Toxicol. Appl. Pharmacol. 13 (1968) 353.
7. Košutzký, J., Adamec, O., Ledeč, M. and Bobáková, E. In: Environmental Quality and Safety, Suppl. Vol. III. (Ed.: F. Coulston and F. Korte) p. 573, G. Thieme, Stuttgart. 1975.
8. Matasumura, F. Toxicology of Pesticides. Plenum Press, New York. 1975.
9. Pipy, B., Bérand, M. and Gaillard, D. Experientia 34 (1978) 87.
10. Popesković, L., Lukić, M. and Janković, B. D. Proc. Yugoslav. Immunol. Soc. 3 (1974) 124.
11. Subba Rao, D. S. V. and Glick, B. Proc. Soc. Exptl. Biol. Med. 154 (1977) 27.
12. Wasserman, M., Wasserman, D., Gershon, Z. and Zellermayer, L. Ann. N. Y. Acad. Sci. 160 (1969) 393.

13. Wasserman, M., Wasserman, D., Kedar, E. and Djavaherian, M. Bull. Environm. Contam. Toxicol. 6 (1971) 426.
14. Wiltrout, R. W., Ercegovich, C. D. and Ceglowski, W. S. Bull. Environm. Contam. Toxicol., in press.

SUBSTANCES FROM MARINE ORGANISMS INFLUENCING TUMOR GROWTH AND IMMUNE RESPONSES

M. M. SIGEL, W. LICHTER, A. GHAFFAR, L. L. WELLHAM and A. J. WEINHEIMER
University of Miami, Miami, Florida; University of South Carolina, Columbia, South Carolina, and University of Oklahoma, Norman, Oklahoma (USA)

The sea which is a readily accessible receptacle for man-made wastes and pollution of coastal water has become the concern of environmentalists and public health authorities alike. What has escaped their attention is that, in addition to exogenous pollution, the sea can receive conglomerates of substances produced by its inhabitants which can affect its biosphere in a favorable or deleterious way.

Marine organisms produce substances with toxic properties which may serve their defensive needs or which can be turned into offensive weapons. To be of use, these substances would have to be secreted or excreted by the living animals into the environment. In addition, there are substances concerned with inner processes of the animals which are released when the animals die. Not all products of the marine biosphere are toxic; some may function as attractants and others may provide growth promoting or regulatory factors. In the aggregate, they may exert biological effects which shape and modify the ecosystem.

The sporadic outbreaks of red tide are well recognized phenomena traceable to marine dinoflagellates. Periodic fish kills are also being reported and commercial as well as sports fishermen are complaining about a variety of conditions causing malformation and destruction of fish scales, fins and muscles. Infectious agents, as well as chemicals, are suspect in some of these epizootic and endozootic occurrences. It is not surprising to find these problems in estuarine polluted waters. What is surprising are the occurrences of pathological conditions in waters remote from human and industrial pollution. Fig. 1 illustrates papillomas in green turtles caught in the Caribbean--at a site generally regarded as

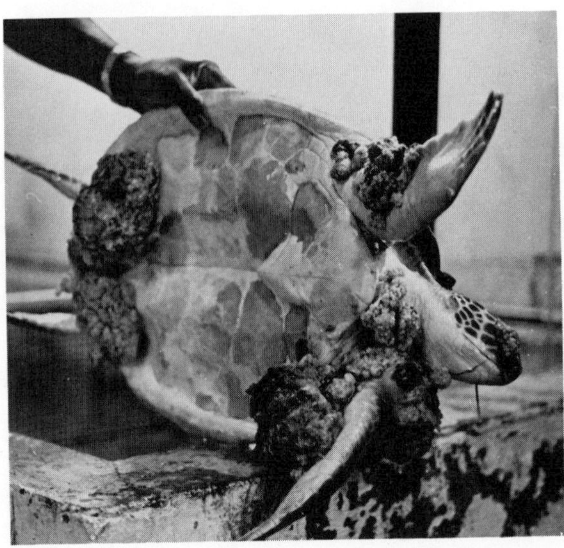

Fig. 1. Generalized papillomas in a green turtle (Animal provided by Mr. Joe Quick, Jr.; photograph courtesy of Dr. Delfin Rippe).

free of man-made pollution. Although Herpesvirus has been incriminated as an agent responsible for severe skin diseases in captive turtles (5), the papillomas found on these turtles caught in the open sea were not caused by this virus (and no other virus could be isolated from them).

Our studies have addressed biologically active substances endogenous in invertebrates inhabiting the reefs in the Caribbean. Figs. 2-4 show species of special interest. The early work was mainly concerned with substances with cytostatic or cytocidal effects (14). Some of these substances were shown to exert _in vitro_ cell growth inhibition or cell destruction, and some have been effective in restraining growth of transplanted tumors in mice. Extracts of _Ecteinascidia turbinata_ (Ete) have been most interesting in this respect because they have not only displayed antitumor activity but have also manifested powerful immunosuppressive action. This will be discussed in more detail below. In the meantime, we would like to recall that prostaglandins have been isolated from gorgonians (16,10,13) and that gorgonians have yielded several terpenoid compounds (1,17) including isoprenoid furans (18. The structures of two of these are shown in Fig. 5. Sterols with hormonal regulatory functions, like ecdyson, have been isolated from marine species (2). At the recent Conference on Food-Drugs from the Sea, Hadfield and Ciereszko (4)

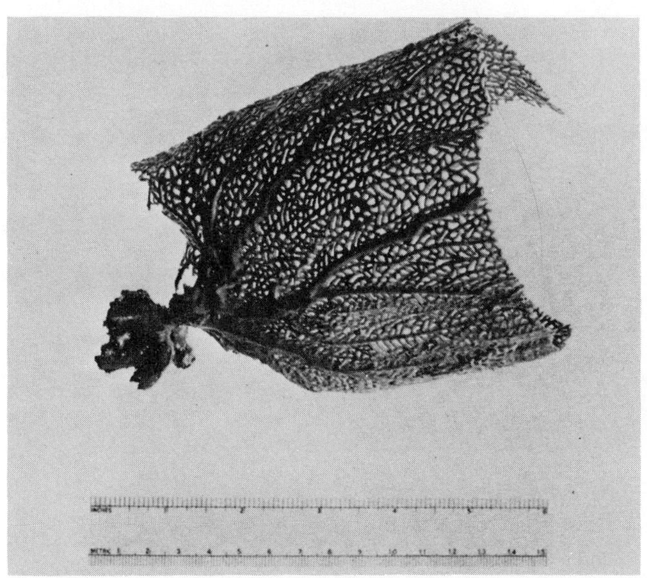

Fig. 2. Gorgonia ventalina (sea fan)

reported that some of the marine diterpenes are gastropod larvae. In the same Conference, much consideration was given to other substances with powerful biological effects on the heart (12), endocrine system (6) and the CNS (7).

Several years ago, we embarked on a study of invertebrates as sources of substances with antitumor activity (14). One hundred thirty two species from 13 phyla, 59 families and 104 genera were collected from the waters surrounding the Florida Keys and the Island of Bimini. Under the auspices of what is now the Division of Cancer Treatment, NCI (Bethesda, MD), we prepared extracts from these animals for tests against tumor cells in vitro and in vivo. Twenty species yielded products with some protective activity against murine leukemia P388; 27 extracts inhibited the growth of KB cells in tissue culture at a concentration of less than or equal to 50 ug/ml; seven of these were inhibitory at a concentration of less than 10 ug/ml. Ete stood out among these extracts because it actually afforded some cures to leukemic mice (Table I).

Subsequent studies demonstrated that Ete had other interesting biologic effects (8). It inhibited antibody production when administered intraperitoneally prior to and after antigen (Table II); diminished graft vs host reactions (Table III); and prolonged the survival of allografts (Table IV). More recently, we demonstrated that Ete was capable of inhibiting (and possibly reversing) blasto-

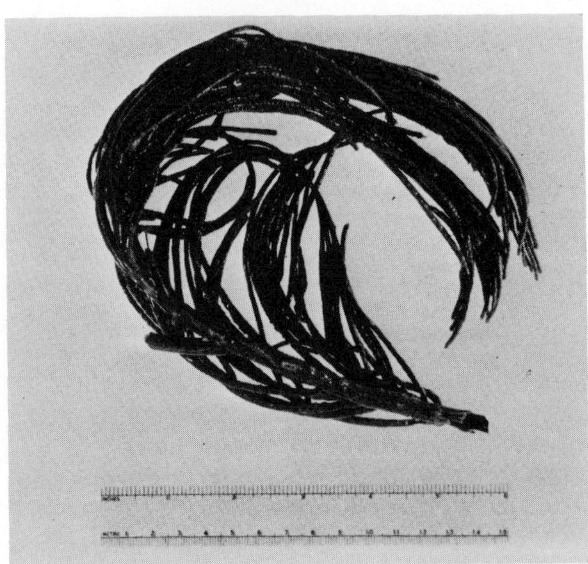

Fig. 3. Pseudopterogorgia americana (gorgonian, sea whip)

TABLE I

Antitumor[a] Effect of Ecteinascidia Turbinata Extract

Test Material	Dose[b] mg/kg	% Survival Time Treated/Controls	Cures
Ete-1[c]	265	140	2/6
Ete-2	265	270	4/6
Ete-4	50[d]	200	
Ete-5	100	181	
Ete-7	100	148	
Ete-8	175	230	1/6
Ete-10	100	167	
Ete-11	300[e]	149	
Ete-12	300[e]	149	

[a]tested in mice with lymphocytic leukemia (P388)

[b]optimal dose

[c]lot number

[d]higher doses were toxic

[e]lower doses were inactive

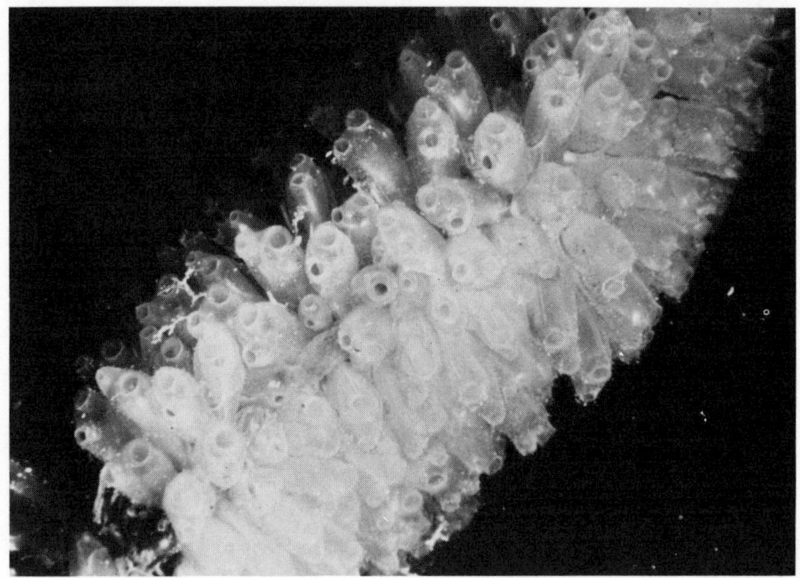

Fig. 4. Ecteinascidia turbinata (tunicate, sea squirt)

genic transformation reactions (9). As shown in Table V, Ete was effective when given to cells as late as 24 hrs after stimulation with PHA.

All experiments measuring humoral and cellular responses have pointed to suppression by Ete. We have recently obtained evidence that suppression is at least in part due to activation of suppressor

Pseudoplexaura porosa *Eunicea mammosa*

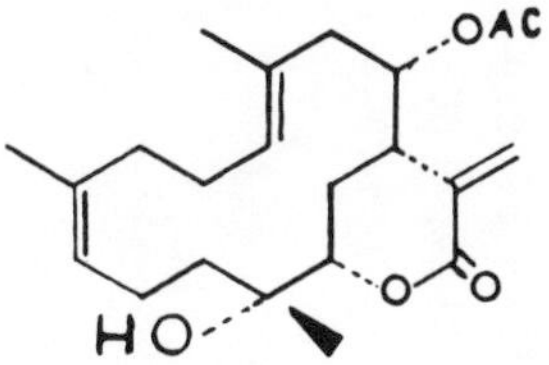

crassin acetate eunicin

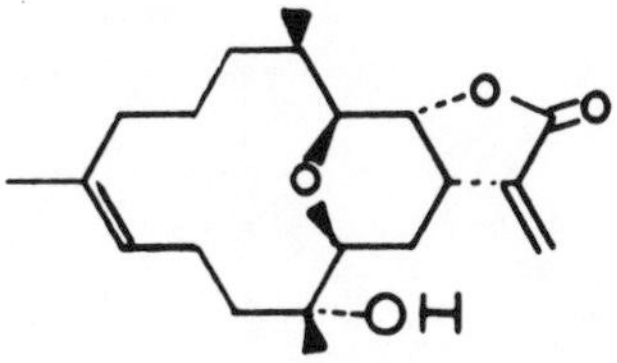

Fig. 5. Structures of two diterpenes isolated from gorgonians.

TABLE II

Immunosuppressive Effect of *Ecteinascidia turbinata* Extract on Humoral Immune Response[a]

Group	Days 1-5	Day 8		Days 9-12	SRBC HA Titer Day 17	% Inhibition of Control Titer
		AM	PM			
1	Ete	Ete	SRBC[b]	Ete	<1:2	>99.0
2	Ete	HBSS[c]	SRBC[b]	HBSS[c]	1:48	87.5
3	HBSS[c]	Ete	SRBC[b]	Ete	1:192	50.0
4	HBSS[c]	HBSS[c]	SRBC[b]	HBSS[c]	1:384	-

[a]Comparison of treatments given prior to and after antigen

[b]SRBC = sheep RBC

[c]HBSS = Hanks balanced salt solution

cells. Cells induced by treatment of mice with Ete were added to lymphocytes of untreated mice and inhibited their response to mitogens. This effect could be abrogated by antibody to Thy 1 antigen plus complement, indicating that the cells were of the T lineage. Suppression was also obtained in adoptive transfer experiments measuring production of plaque-forming cells in response to immunization with SRBC. It has not yet been ascertained whether the cells involved in the *in vivo* suppression are also T cells.

What is of equal importance is that Ete was also capable of activating macrophages. This was demonstrated in three kinds of experiments which are herewith presented as new data.

CLEARANCE OF COLLOIDAL CARBON

C_3H/HeN mice were treated with Ete (250 mg/kg) by the i.p. route and 3 days later injected intravenously with colloidal carbon in the form of a 20% suspension of India ink. Tests of carbon clearance from the blood (measured spectrophotometrically at 800 nm) were performed at intervals of 0, 3, 6, 10, 15 and 20 mins. Results were expressed as K values of phagocytic indices calculated by the standard formula (15). The results are given in Fig. 6. It can be seen that Ete caused a significant increase in the rate of clearance. In fact, the increase was substantially greater than that caused by the better-known macrophage activator, *Corynebacterium parvum*, but this difference may be more apparent than real since the relative concentrations of the relevant components in Ete and *C. parvum* are not known.

TABLE III

Graft Versus Host Reaction

Group	Range of Sp/K[a] Ratio	Mean Sp/K
Ete-treated	0.70 - 1.00	0.87
HBSS	1.07 - 1.62	1.36
Negative control (syngeneic)	0.38 - 0.60	0.46

[a]$Sp/k = \frac{\text{weight of spleen}}{\text{weight of kidney}}$

TABLE IV

Skin Graft Survival

Group	Treatment	Mean of 50% Skin Graft Survival	50% Mice with 10% Skin Graft Survival
1	3 days before graft and 0 days after	11 days	13 days
2	3 days before graft and 3 days after	11 days	13½ days
3	3 days before graft and 5 days after	11 days	12½ days
4	3 days before graft and until rejection	11 days	14½ days
5	0 days before graft and 3 days after	15 days	17½ days
6	0 days before graft and until rejection	17 days	19½ days
7	Control; no treatment	10 days	10 days

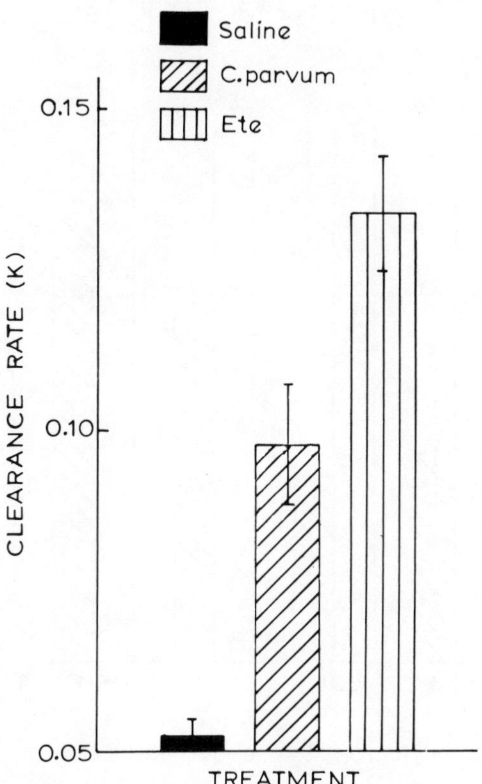

Fig. 6. Enhanced clearance of colloidal carbon by Ete and Corynebacterium parvum.

INHIBITION OF GROWTH OF TUMOR CELLS

Antitumor cell activity of macrophages was measured by exposing P388 leukemic cells to peritoneal exudate cells (PEC). The test depends on nonspecific action of peritoneal macrophages from nonimmunized syngeneic or allogeneic mice. In the procedure employed, the target P388 cells were labelled with ^{3}H-thymidine after exposure to the effector PEC obtained from Balb/c mice treated 4 days earlier with Ete (3). The amount of radioactivity denotes the number of cells surviving the attack by the effectors and the assay measures both cytolysis and cytostasis. The results given in Fig. 7 indicate that at all effector-to-target ratios, PEC from Ete-treated mice were more effective than PEC from untreated mice.

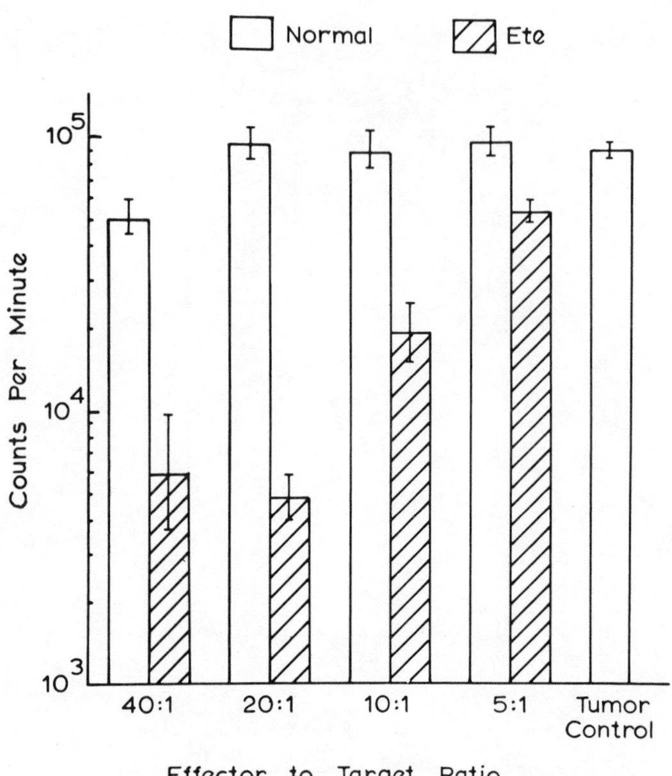

Fig. 7. Activation of peritoneal macrophages by Ete as measured by cytolysis/cytostasis of P388 cells. Counts/min detect viable P388 cells.

The functional changes evoked by treatment with Ete correlated with increases in the size of the liver and spleen. This is shown in Fig. 8. Preliminary studies have disclosed that the increase was associated with higher numbers of T cells and macrophages.

Twenty years ago Ross Nigrelli (11) wrote about the impact of endogenous growth promoting and growth inhibiting substances on marine animals and spoke eloquently about the potential role of these molecules in the life of marine communities. Our studies which were largely inspired by the work of Nigrelli and George Ruggieri have demonstrated that, in addition to controlling growth, some of the substances can influence the reticular system and other compartments of the immune mechanism. The effect on phagocytic activity may be crucial to invertebrates as this is a dominant activity of primitive organisms which constitute much of the marine biosphere.

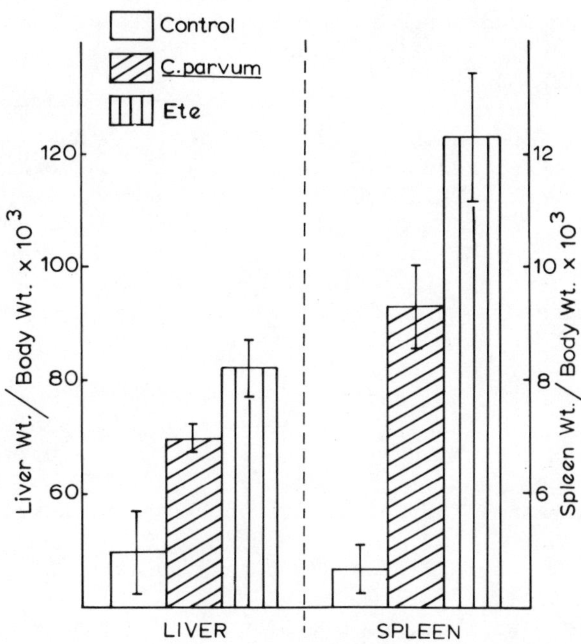

Fig. 8. Splenomegaly and hepatomegaly induced by Corynebacterium parvum and Ete.

ACKNOWLEDGEMENTS

The initial work was supported by USPHS Contract numbers PH43-67-1179, PH43-63-622 and PH43-64-890 and by a Sea Grant awarded to the University of Miami. Recent work was supported in part by USPHS Contract number NO1-CM-57041.

REFERENCES

1. Faulkner, D. J., Stallard, M. O., Fayos, J. and Clardy, J. J. Am. Chem. Soc. 95 (1973) 3413.
2. Galbraith, M. N., Horn, D. H. S., Middleton, E. J. and Hackney, R. J. Chem. Commun. (1968) 83.
3. Ghaffar, A. and Cullen, R. T. J. Reticuloendothel. Soc. 20 (1976) 349.
4. Hadfield, M. G. and Ciereszko, L. S. In: Food and Drugs from the Sea. Myth or Reality? (Eds. P. N. Kaul and C. J. Sindermann) The University of Oklahoma, Norman, Oklahoma (1978) 145.
5. Haines, H. Marine Fisheries Review 40 (1978) 33.

6. Hollenbeak, K. H., Schmitz, F. J., Kaul, P. N. and Kulkarni, S. K. In: Food and Durgs from the Sea. Myth or Reality? (Eds. P. N. Kaul and C. J. Sindermann) The University of Oklahoma, Norman, Oklahoma (1978) 81.
7. Kaul, P. N., Kulkarni, S. K., Schmitz, F. J. and Hollenbeak, K. H. In: Food and Drugs from the Sea. Myth or Reality? (Eds. P. N. Kaul and C. J. Sindermann) The University of Oklahoma, Norman, Oklahoma (1978) 99.
8. Lichter, W., Wellham, L. L., Van der Werf, B. A., Middlebrook, R. E., Sigel, M. M. and Weinheimer, A. J. In: Food-Drugs from the Sea Proceedings 1972 (Ed. L. R. Worthen) Marine Technology Society, Washington, D. C. (1973) 117.
9. Lichter, W., Lopez, D. M., Wellham, L. L. and Sigel, M. M. Proc. Soc. Exp. Med. Biol. 150 (1975) 475.
10. Nakano, J. J. Pharm. Pharmacol. 21 (1969) 782.
11. Nigrelli, R. F. Trans. N. Y. Acad. Sci. 20 (1958) 248.
12. Norton, T. R., Kashiwagi, M. and Shibata, S. In: Food and Drugs from the Sea. Myth or Reality? (Eds. P. N. Kaul and C. J. Sindermann) The University of Oklahoma, Norman, Oklahoma (1978) 37.
13. Schneider, W. P., Hamilton, R. D. and Ruhland, L. E. J. Amer. Chem. Soc. 94 (1972) 2122.
14. Sigel, M. M., Wellham, L. L., Lichter, W., Dudeck, L. E., Gargus, J. L. and Lucas, A. H. In: Food-Drugs from the Sea Proceedings 1969 (Ed. H. W. Youngken, Jr.) Marine Technology Society, Washington, D. C. (1970) 281.
15. Stuart, A. E. In: Handbook of Experimental Immunology (Ed. D. M. Weir) Blackwell Scientific Publishers, Oxford (1968) 1034.
16. Weinheimer, A. J. and Spraggins, R. L. Tetrahedron Lett. 15 (1969) 5185.
17. Weinheimer, A. J., Schmitz, F. J. and Ciereszko, L. S. In: Drugs from the Sea (Ed. H. D. Freudenthal) Marine Tech. Soc., Washington, D. C. (1968) 135.
18. Weinheimer, A. J. and Washecheck, P. H. Tetrahedron Lett. 14 (1969) 3315.

EFFECTS OF UV RADIATION ON THE IMMUNE SYSTEM: CONSEQUENCES FOR UV CARCINOGENESIS

M. L. KRIPKE

Cancer Biology Program
NCI Frederick Cancer Research Center
Frederick, Maryland (USA)

Since the early 1900's, UV light has been suspected of being the causative agent for certain types of human skin cancer (1). Clinical and epidemiological data, as well as animal experiments, have provided strong evidence in support of this hypothesis (2). However, recent evidence from animal studies suggests that UV light can, in addition, affect immunologic functions, and that these immunologic perturbations may be important in the pathogenesis of UV light-induced skin cancer.

Influence of UV Radiation on the Immune Response to UV-Induced Tumors

The experiments leading to the latter conclusion were based on the observation that the skin tumors in C3Hf mice by UV radiation are highly antigenic. In fact, most of these fibrosarcomas and squamous carcinomas are immunologically rejected upon transplantation to normal syngeneic recipients (8). Therefore, the primary tumors must have some means of escaping immunologic destruction, because if left undisturbed, the tumors will grow progressively and eventually kill the animals in which they arose. In investigating how these highly antigenic tumors were able to avoid immunologic rejection in the primary host, we discovered that the UV irradiation, itself, rendered the mice anergic to challenge with syngeneic or autochthonous UV-induced fibrosarcomas (12). Long before primary tumors could be detected on UV-irradiated mice, these animals were unable to resist the growth of UV-induced tumors transplanted subcutaneously to unirradiated sites.

The immunologic nature of this inability to reject UV-induced tumors was established in a series of cell transfer experiments (4). Lethally X-irradiated mice were reconstituted by an intravenous injection of lymphoid cells from syngeneic UV-irradiated or untreated donors and challenged with a tumor implant. Cells from the UV-treated animals failed to restore tumor resistance in the recipients, whereas lymphoid cells from normal donors conferred resistance against challenge with a syngeneic UV-induced tumor. This indicated that the inability of UV-irradiated mice to reject the tumor implants was due to an alteration in the lymphoid cells. To determine whether this alteration represented the absence of reactive cells or the presence of suppressor cells, lymphoid cells from normal and UV-irradiated donors were mixed and used to reconstitute lethally X-irradiated recipients. These recipients were unable to resist challenge with UV-induced tumors, suggesting that the UV-irradiated animal had contributed suppressor lymphoid cells to the mixture. Additional studies have shown that the spleens and lymph nodes of UV-irradiated mice contain T lymphocytes that suppress the induction of a tumor rejection response (5).

Effects of UV Radiation on Other Immune Responses

The specificity of the immunologic unresponsiveness in UV-irradiated mice has been studied in some detail. With few exceptions, UV-irradiated mice are indistinguishable from untreated, age-matched animals in their responses to exogenous antigens (13, 14). Furthermore, in the tests performed thus far, UV-treated mice do not appear to be impaired in their reactivity against most syngeneic tumors that are not etiologically related to UV radiation (11).

However, there is an early, transient depression of two immunologic reactions that can be detected in UV-irradiated C3H mice. One reaction is delayed hypersensitivity to dinitrochlorobenzene (DNCB), measured by footpad swelling; the other is the host component of the graft-versus-host reaction, measured by the popliteal lymph node weight gain assay in UV-irradiated F_1 hybrid recipients (13). Both of these reactions are depressed early in the course of UV irradiation, but return to normal levels at about the time the animals reach maximum susceptibility to challenge with UV-induced tumors. This suggests that the mechanism of the transient depression of these reactions differs from that causing the failure of tumor rejection. Nonetheless, these transiently depressed reactions may reflect physiologic or immunologic changes that are related indirectly to the subsequent anergy to UV-induced tumor antigens. For this reason, we have examined in more detail the basis for the early, transient depression of DNCB reactivity in UV-irradiated mice.

Mechanisms of Energy to DNCB

The mechanism of this depressed reactivity to DNCB has been investigated in BALB/c mice (7). This albino strain is more sensitive to the carcinogenic effects of UV radiation than C3H (agouti) mice (10); in addition, susceptibility to the growth of transplanted UV-induced fibrosarcomas also occurs earlier in this strain. In these experiments, BALB/c mice were shaved dorsally with electric clippers once per week and exposed to a bank of 6 Westinghouse FS40 sunlamps for 1 hr, 3 times per week (Mon., Wed., Fri.). The mice were housed 5 per cage on a shelf 20 cm below the light source. The average dose rate of the irradiator within the wavelength range between 280 and 340 nm was 2.8 $J/m^2/sec$. Approximately 80% of the energy from the light source is emitted within this wavelength range. For tumor challenge, a 1 mm^3 tumor fragment was implanted in each recipient subcutaneously with a trocar. The tumor tissue was maintained by serial passage in immunosuppressed mice (adult thymectomy + 450R whole-body X-irradiation), and was used in the fourth to the sixth transplant generations. Reactivity to DNCB was measured using the method described in (6). Mice were sensitized by injecting 2 mg DNCB in 0.1 ml dimethylsulfoxide (DMSO) subcutaneously into the flank. For challenge, the mice were injected subcutaneously 10 days later with 0.05 mg DNCB in 0.05 ml of 50% DMSO (in 0.15 M NaCl) into the hind footpad. The percent footpad swelling was determined 24 hr later by measuring both hind footpads with a micrometer, where:

$$\% \text{ footpad swelling} = \left(\frac{\text{thickness of injected footpad} - \text{thickness of uninjected footpad}}{\text{thickness of uninjected footpad}} \right) \times 100$$

The % footpad swelling was compared to that observed in a group of animals treated in an identical manner, except that the DNCB was omitted from the sensitizing injection.

Table I shows that mice treated with UV light for 1 or more months are susceptible to challenge with a syngeneic UV-induced fibrosarcoma (#2C16), whereas unirradiated mice are resistant to challenge. The reactivity of these mice to DNCB is also impaired for the first 2 months of UV irradiation, but this activity returns to a normal level by the third month of treatment. The mechanisms of these phenomena were analyzed by means of lymphoid cell transfer experiments.

The lack of tumor rejection in UV-irradiated mice could be transferred with spleen cells to lethally X-irradiated (800R) syngeneic recipients. Five x 10^7 spleen cells from normal or UV-treated mice were injected intravenously into lethally X-irradiated

TABLE I

Reactivity of UV-irradiated BALB/c Mice to a Syngeneic UV-induced Fibrosarcoma and to Sensitization with DNCB

Treatment	Susceptibility to Tumor Challenge[a]	Reactivity to DNCB (% Specific Footpad Swelling)[b]
1 month UV[c]	9/10	4
Control	0/10	30[d]
2 months UV[c]	7/10	8
Control	1/10	24[e]
3 months UV[c]	10/10	22[e]
Control	0/10	26[e]

[a]Number of progressively growing tumors/number of mice challenged with a syngeneic UV-induced fibrosarcoma (#2C16)
[b]7-10 Mice per group. Percent footpad swelling of sensitized mice minus % swelling in unsensitized controls
[c]Mice were shaved weekly and exposed to UV radiation for 1 hr 3 times per week until used for testing. Controls are age- and sex-matched animals
[d]$P < 0.01$ versus unsensitized control mice (Student's t-test)
[e]$P < 0.001$ versus unsensitized control mice

BALB/c mice, and these recipients were challenged with implants of fibrosarcoma #2C16. Table II shows that when normal spleen cells were used to reconstitute the recipients, these animals were capable of rejecting the tumor challenge (group 3). In constrast, mice reconstituted with spleen cells from UV-irradiated donors were susceptible to tumor growth (group 4). We conclude that the lymphoid cells from UV-irradiated mice are unable to respond to UV-induced tumor antigens, even when they are removed from the UV-irradiated host.

The inability of mice to respond to challenge with DNCB during the first 2 months of UV irradiation could have been due to the failure of sensitization (afferent block), or to the failure of an effector mechanism (efferent block), or both. A series of cell transfer experiments were performed to distinguish among these possibilities; these are summarized in Table III. In experiment 1, 1 x 10^7 spleen cells from DNCB-sensitized donors

TABLE II

Growth of UV-induced Fibrosarcoma in Lethally X-irradiated BALB/c Mice Reconstituted with Spleen Cells from Normal or UV-irradiated Donors

Group	Donor Spleen Cells[a]	Recipients[b]	Tumor Incidence[c]
1	None	Normal	0/10
2	None	UV-irradiated	10/10
3	Normal	800R	1/9
4	UV	800R	7/7

[a]5×10^7 spleen cells from normal or UV-irradiated BALB/c mice were injected intravenously 24 hr after X-irradiation
[b]Recipients were challenged subcutaneously with fragments of tumor #2C16 24 hr after reconstitution
[c]Number of progressively growing tumors/number of mice challenged

TABLE III

Studies on Adoptive Transfer of Reactivity to DNCB[a]

Exp	Treatment of Spleen Cell Donor	Treatment of Recipient	% Specific Footpad Swelling in Recipient[b]
1	DNCB	None	21 ($P < 0.01$)
	DNCB	UV 1 month	16 ($P < 0.01$)
2	1 month UV, DNCB	None	0
	DNCB	None	12 ($P < 0.05$)
3	1 month UV	800R, DNCB	19 ($P < 0.01$)
	None	800R, DNCB	26 ($P < 0.001$)

[a]See text for experimental details
[b]5-10 mice per group. Percent footpad swelling of sensitized mice minus percent swelling in unsensitized control mice. P = probability of no difference from unsensitized control group by Student's t-test

were injected intraperitoneally into normal or UV-irradiated recipients. The recipients were challenged with 0.05 mg DNCB in the footpad immediately after the cell transfer, and the footpad swelling was measured 24 hr later. Both normal and UV-irradiated recipients reacted against the DNCB challenge, indicating that there was no impairment in the effector portion of the reaction in UV-irradiated mice. In experiment 2, 1 x 10^7 spleen cells from DNCB-sensitized unirradiated or UV-irradiated donors were injected intraperitoneally into untreated recipients to adoptively transfer reactivity. The reactivity to DNCB was detected in the same way as described for experiment 1. Table III shows that no reactivity was transferred with spleen cells from UV-irradiated DNCB-sensitized donors (experiment 2), indicating that the UV-irradiated mice had not become sensitized to the DNCB (afferent block). To determine whether this afferent block was due to a deficiency in antigen-reactive lymphoid cells, we tested the ability of spleen cells from UV-irradiated mice to become sensitized to DNCB following their transfer into mice that had been lethally X-irradiated. Twenty-four hr after X-irradiation (800R), BALB/c mice were reconstituted with an intravenous injection of 5 x 10^7 spleen cells from normal or UV-irradiated donors. One day later, the recipients were sensitized by injecting 2 mg of DNCB subcutaneously, and they were footpad tested for reactivity 10 days later. As indicated in Table III, experiment 3, spleen cells from UV-irradiated donors were as effective as normal spleen cells in reconstituting the recipients for reactivity to DNCB. This result demonstrates that spleen cells from mice UV-irradiated for 1 month are capable of recognizing DNCB and responding to it when they are removed from the UV-irradiated mouse. This suggests that the temporary inability of UV-irradiated mice to respond to DNCB sensitization is due to a block in antigen processing or antigen presentation, since the lymphocytes from these animals can be sensitized to DNCB if they are transferred to a different host.

From these experiments we conclude that the two immunologic dysfunctions in UV-irradiated mice are mediated by different mechanisms, even though both are induced by UV radiation. The inability of UV-treated mice to reject UV-induced tumors is due to an inability of the lymphoid cells to respond to these tumor antigens, probably because of the presence of specific suppressor T-lymphocytes (4, 5, 7). In contrast, the temporary inability of UV-treated mice to respond to DNCB seems to be due to a block in antigen processing or presentation, perhaps at the level of the macrophage or the Langerhans cell. Since this block selectively affects DNCB reactivity and does not seem to influence the immune response to other types of antigens (13, 14), this suggests that the early steps in the induction of this particular type of immune response may differ from those of other immune responses. This could perhaps occur through the involvement of Langerhans cells, which reside in the epidermis and collect certain antigens for presentation to lymphocytes (15).

Whether this impairment of antigen processing activity is related to the subsequent inability of UV-irradiated mice to reject UV-induced tumors is not known. However, this may be another example of the pathway proposed by Feldmann in *in vitro* studies of the antibody response (3). He found that when antigen was taken up by macrophages and then combined with lymphocytes, antibody formation occurred. In contrast, when antigen was added directly to lymphocytes, immunologic tolerance resulted. By analogy, we could speculate that the temporary impairment of antigen processing by UV radiation permits a UV-induced antigenic photoproduct to act directly on lymphocytes, thereby inducing suppressor activity, rather than effector activity.

Evidence for a UV-induced Photoproduct

Whether or not this accurately represents the sequence of events involved in the induction of suppressor cells by UV light, it seems likely that a UV-induced photoproduct is involved. We know from previous experiments that the lack of tumor rejection in UV-irradiated mice is induced by the light that falls on the skin (9). Since this immunologic unresponsiveness is relatively specific for tumors induced by UV radiation (11, 13, 14), this suggests that the light does not act directly on the immune system in a nonspecific manner. Therefore, something produced in the skin by UV irradiation must serve as the intermediate between the UV light and the immune system. Further, this "something" must bear some antigenic relationship to the tumors induced by UV light, since the resulting anergy is directed toward UV-induced tumors.

Preliminary experiments performed by Edmund Palaszynski in this laboratory provide evidence that supports the existence of a UV-induced skin photoproduct. In these experiments, large, circumferential skin grafts are prepared from UV-irradiated donors, and grafted onto normal, syngeneic recipients. These grafts cover the dorsal and ventral surfaces of the recipients in the area between the hind- and fore-limbs. After a six-week healing period, these recipients and mice grafted with unirradiated skin are challenged subcutaneously with a UV-induced fibrosarcoma. It should be noted that the challenge tumors are implanted under the intact skin of the recipient, and not under the skin graft. The results of two such experiments are depicted in Table IV. More of the challenge tumors grew progressively in mice grafted with UV-irradiated skin than in those grafted with normal skin (12/16 versus 5/17; $P < 0.01$, Chi square test). In addition, mice that received grafts of normal skin exhibited a slight increase in

TABLE IV

Transfer of Susceptibility to Tumor Challenge with Skin Grafts from UV-irradiated Donors

Treatment of Tumor Recipient	Tumor:	Final Tumor Incidence #1316	#1591	Totals
Graft of UV-irradiated skin[a]		6/8	6/8	12/16 (75%)
Graft of normal skin		1/8	4/9	5/17 (29%)
None		0/10	0/5	0/15 (0%)
Immunosuppression (adult thymectomy + 450R)		4/5	5/5	9/10 (90%)

[a]Mice were grafted with large areas of skin from syngeneic mice in UV-irradiated for 3 months and challenged with tumor fragments 6 weeks later

susceptibility to tumor challenge compared to untreated animals (5/17 versus 0/15; $P < 0.05$, Chi square test). It is not clear at present whether this represents nonspecific suppression due to trauma associated with the grafting procedure, or whether this is a specific phenomenon that results from the release of a substance present in normal skin whose concentration is elevated following UV irradiation. However, this experiment shows that grafts of UV-irradiated skin can increase the susceptibility of mice to challenge with UV-induced tumors, relative to that of mice grafted with normal skin (Palaszynski and Kripke, unpublished data). Studies are underway to determine whether this increased susceptiblity to tumor challenge is due to the induction of suppressor cells in the graft recipients. Thus far, however, these experiments are consistent with our hypothesis that there is a photoproduct (or an elevated level of a normal skin component) in UV-irradiated skin that provides the link between UV light and the immune system.

SUMMARY

UV radiation has a profound effect on the immune response to skin tumors induced by UV light. Although many of these antigenic tumors are rejected by normal syngeneic recipients, they grow progressively in UV-irradiated animals. The amount of exposure required for the induction of this effect differs for different challenge tumors and with different mouse strains. However, regardless of the test system employed, susceptibility to tumor challenge precedes the development of primary UV-induced skin tumors.

The mechanism by which UV irradiation prevents immunologic rejection of UV-induced tumors is not entirely clear. However, several steps in this process have been identified. First, UV light impinges upon the skin causing cellular damage, cellular proliferation, the release of pharmacologically active substances, and at some point, neoplastic transformation. At least one of these processes results in the production of an antigen in skin that serves as the intermediate between the immune system and UV light. Second, UV radiation produces a transient depression in the ability of mice to effectively process certain types of antigens introduced via the skin. This may be the reason why suppressor cells, rather than effector cells, are induced in response to the photoproduct. In any event, suppressor T lymphocytes appear in the lymphoid tissue of UV-irradiated mice. These cells act to prevent the induction of an immune response against transplanted UV-induced tumors. It seems likely that these cells also are responsible for the development and progressive growth of the primary tumors induced by UV light, and experiments are currently underway to test this hypothesis directly. If this is the case, it would suggest that a surveillance system against this type of skin cancer not only exists, but plays an important role in tumor induction. It is possible that the long induction period required for the development of these tumors represents a period during which there is immunologic elimination of newly transformed cells. Eventually, however, this surveillance system is depressed, either specifically by UV irradiation, or nonspecifically by aging or immunosuppression, and primary tumors begin to grow unchecked. Whether this process can be prevented or reversed by some form of immunologic intervention remains to be explored.

ACKNOWLEDGEMENTS

Research sponsored by the National Cancer Institute under Contract No. N01-CO-75380 with Litton Bionetics, Inc. (USA).

REFERENCES

1. Dubreuilh, W. Annal. Dermat. Syph. viii (1907) 387.
2. Emmet, E. A. Crit. Rev. Toxicol. 2 (1973) 211.
3. Feldmann, M. Nature New Biol. 242 (1973) 82.
4. Fisher, M. S. and Kripke, M. L. Proc. Natl. Acad. Sci., USA, 74 (1977) 1688.
5. Fisher, M. S. and Kripke, M. L. Immunol., in press.
6. Jessup, J. M., Cohen, M. H., Tomaschewski, M. M. and Felix, E. L. J. Natl. Cancer Inst. 57 (1976) 1077.
7. Jessup, J. M., Hanna, N., Palaszynski, E. and Kripke, M. L.

Cell. Immunol. 38 (1978) 105.
8. Kripke, M. L. J. Natl. Cancer Inst. 53 (1974) 1333.
9. Kripke, M. L. Photochem. Photobiol. 24 (1976) 599.
10. Kripke, M. L. Cancer Res. 37 (1977) 1395.
11. Kripke, M. L. J. Reticuloendothel. Soc. 22 (1976) 599.
12. Kripke, M. L. and Fisher, M. S. J. Natl. Cancer Inst. 57 (1976) 211.
13. Kripke, M. L., Lofgreen, J. S., Beard, J., Jessup, J. M. and Fisher, M. S. J. Natl. Cancer Inst. 59 (1977) 1227.
14. Norbury, K. C., Kripke, M. L. and Budmen, M. B. J. Natl. Cancer Inst. 59 (1977) 1231.
15. Stingl, G., Katz, S. I., Shevach, E. M., Schreiner, E. and Green, I. J. Immunol. 120 (1978) 570.

IN VITRO AND *IN VIVO* PARAMETERS OF HUMORAL AND CELLULAR IMMUNITY IN AN ANIMAL MODEL FOR PROTEIN-CALORIE MALNUTRITION

M. A. TAYLOR, B. A. ISRAEL, M. R. ESCOBAR and D. BERLINERMAN

Medical College of Virginia, Virginia Commonwealth University, Richmond, Virginia (USA)

As a result of recent advances in immunology innumerable reports have emerged in the literature on the general field of nutrition-immunocompetence-disease interactions (2). Originally, questions arising from human observations led to animal experimentation much of which yielded often conflicting findings. Although nutritional modulation of the immune response may be an important factor influencing morbidity and mortality associated with a variety of human disease processes, including cancer, the data generated from a large number of pertinent studies in humans and animals have to be interpreted with caution. That is, many components of the immune system have been studied frequently in isolation from other parameters and apparently out of context with other critical environmental and genetic variables which influence the clinical onset and course of many pathologic conditions.

Some of the reasons for this problem are based on differences among the laboratory animals used. These differences relate to: (a) the genetic background and health state of the parents; (b) age of the animal at the point of nutritional stress (postnatal); (c) length and degree of food deprivation; (d) defined qualitative and quantitative characteristics of the diet; (e) the dosage, purity and biological nature of the infectious agent or tumor cells employed to test the immunocompetence of the host; and (f) the control and monitoring of a broad spectrum of environmental factors to which the laboratory animals are subjected. It is difficult to learn from clinical studies the true nature of the interrelationships among nutrition, immunity and disease since susceptibility to the latter is multifactorial. Therefore, the present investigation was undertaken in an effort to use a "holistic" approach to test certain *in vitro* and *in vivo* parameters of humoral and cell-mediated immune responses in an inbred guinea pig model.

MATERIALS AND METHODS

Animals. Pregnant Hartley strain guinea pigs (Camm Research Laboratories, Wayne, N. J.) and Seawell-Wright, strain 2, guinea pigs (NCI, Frederick Cancer Research Center, Frederick, MD) were employed throughout these studies. Newborn guinea pigs remained with their mother until 24-48 hr post-partum and were housed in groups of not more than 8 animals per cage.

Diet regimens. The newborn animals were divided into two categories, control and experimental. The control animals included: (a) those designated "W" (weanling) which remained with their mother until age 28 days; (b) those designated "N" (normal) which were fed *ad libitum* after separation from their mother at age 24-48 hr. The experimental group consisted of animals designated: (a) "STM" (short-term malnourished) which were fed enough food for 10 days after separation from their mother at age 24-48 hr to maintain them within ± 10% of their birth weight; (b) "LTM" (long-term malnourished) which were fed enough food for 15 days after separation from their mother at age 24-48 hr to maintain them to within ± 15% of their birth weight. An additional group included animals that were fed barely enough food for 19 days after separation from their mother at age 24-48 hr to maintain them to within ± 20% of their birth weight but were not studied further due to the mortality incidence of virtually 100%, Purina Guinea Pig Chow (Ralston Purina Co., St. Louis, MO) and water (Animals in each of the above groups were allowed unlimited access to water) supplemented with VI-Daylen multiple vitamins (Ross Laboratories, Columbus, OH) at a concentration of 6 cc/480 cc of water daily. All animals were weighed daily and they were isolated from their respective group only if more than ± 2.5% deviation from the mean gain of the group was observed. All animals were individually numbered at 24 hr with aluminum ear tags (Scientific Products, McGaw Park, Ill).

Total serum protein and albumin. These tests were carried our essentially as manual analogs of the SMA 12/60 method, (Technicon, Tarrytown, N. Y.). The results obtained were expressed as grams/dL of serum.

Single radial immunodiffusion for immunoglobulin quantitation. Quantitative determination of guinea pig serum immunoglobulins was done according to Mancini (8) by the limit diffusion method using rabbit anti-guinea pig IgG, IgA and IgM (Behring Diagnostics, Somerville, N. J.).

Assays for complement level. Guinea pig sera were tested for hemolytic complement activity by hemolytic radial diffusion after a modification of the Mancini procedure (8) and by the LBCF Complement Fixation Microtiter Method (Center for Disease Control, Atlanta

Ga). The C3 complement component was immunochemically quantitated by the single radial immunodiffusion technique similar to the one described above for immunoglobulin determinations employing goat anti-guinea pig C3 (Cappel Laboratories, Inc., Cochranville, PA).

Assay for plasma cortisol. Total plasma cortisol was determined with a commercial Cortisol Radioassay kit (The Schwarz-Mann, Orangeburg, N. Y.) by competitive protein binding using tritiated cortisol as tracer and transcortin as the binding reagent.

Dinitrochlorobenzene (DNCB) sensitization. The sensitizing dose was given at 4 weeks of age and consisted of 0.02 ml of a 10% solution of DNCB (Eastman Chemicals, Rochester, N. Y.) in acetone. Fourteen days later, two test doses on different sites were administered consisting of 0.03 ml of 0.1% and 0.05% solutions of DNCB respectively. Acetone, 0.03 ml, was used on a separate site as a control.

Lymphocyte transformation. This assay was performed with purified lymphocytes obtained from the anterior cervical lymph nodes which were placed in microculture and stimulated with PHA (Burroughs-Wellcome Co., Triangle Park, N. C.) at dilutions of 1:1, 1:2, 1:5, 1:10, 1:20 and 1:40 in triplicate. After 48 hr incubation in 5% CO_2 in air, 2 μCi of ^{3}H-thymidine (Schwarz-Mann Co., Orangeburg, N. Y.) were added to each microculture. Cultures were harvested 16 hr later using an automated multiple harvester (Otto-Hilar Co., Madison, Wisconsin) onto glass filter paper (Whatman #GF-81). Radioactivity was measured with a Beckman LS-330 Liquid Scintillation System.

Spontaneous E rosette assay. This test was performed with lymphocytes from thymus and cervical lymph nodes purified as described earlier at a concentration of 5 x 10^5 cells/ml. A 0.75% suspension of rabbit erythrocytes containing 0.1% BSA was prepared and 0.5 ml of this suspension was gently mixed with 0.5 ml of the lymphocyte suspension; mixtures prepared in duplicate were then centrifuged at low speed for 5 minutes at 25 C and incubated at 4 C for 1 hr. Each pellet was gently resuspended and a drop of methylene blue dye added to the suspension before counting 200 lymphocytes per sample.

Tumor cells. A hepatocellular carcinoma induced in a strain 2 male guinea pig by oral administration of diethylnitrosamine and adapted to intradermal growth and designated line 10 as described by Rapp *et al*. (10) was used in this study as the source of tumor cells. Fresh viable tumor cells were obtained via intraperitoneal inoculation of 1 - 10 x 10^6 cryo-preserved tumor cells in adult guinea pigs. Intradermal inoculations of tumor cells were made at doses of 1 x 10^4, 1 x 10^5 and 1 x 10^6.

Bacillus Calmette-Guerin (BCG) preparation. The BCG preparation was obtained from the Trudeau Institute (Saranac Lake, N. Y., mycobacterial culture collection, TMC#1032, Lot #3). It was stored in 1 cc aliquots containing 2.0 x 10^8 organisms/cc at -70 C.

Animal inoculation with tumor cells and BCG.. Some animals received BCG and tumor cells at a 100:1 ratio and others received tumor cells alone. Each animal was weighed and the tumor size was recorded at regular intervals after the 5th day post-inoculation. The approximate area was determined by measuring with calipers the longest axis of the tumor and the width of the perpendicular axis. This was possible since the tumor had characteristic growth away from the surface of the body to approximately 1 cm in height at which point the tumor became necrotic and spread laterally.

Statistical measurements. These were performed as indicated below with respect to each parameter tested.

RESULTS

Total serum protein and albumin. Serum values of total protein determined on control (W and N) and STM animals at 10 days of age were 3.8 g/dL and 4.0g/dL, respectively. At 42 days of age total protein levels were 4.2-4.5g/dL for both groups. Albumin levels at 10 days of age were 2.8g/dL and 3.1g/dL for control and STM animals, respectively. At 42 days of age albumin levels were similar for both groups: 3.0 ± 0.3g/dL in control animals and 2.9 ± 0.3g/dL for the STM group. There was no significant difference for total serum protein among the W, N and STM groups based on the Student's t test at the 5% of 1% confidence levels. Similarly, there was no statistically significant difference among these 3 groups for albumin at the 1% confidence level. However, there was a significant difference for albumin between the W and STM groups at the 5% confidence level.

Plasma cortisol level. The total plasma control was not significantly elevated in the STM group when compared to the W and N groups, probably indicating that malnutrition was not severe enough.

Serum immunoglobulins and complement levels. There were no statistically significant differences according to the Student's t test at the 1% and 5% confidence levels for IgG, IgA and IgM or for complement levels by all assays among the W, N and STM groups.

Dinitrochlorobenzene sensitization. The ability to respond to DNCB at 42 days of age was significantly depressed in the STM group when compared to the animals in the control groups as can be seen in Table I.

Lymphocyte transformation. Peak stimulation of lymphocytes by PHA occurred at 1:2 dilution in 75% of animals in the N group and 80% of those in the STM group. The lymphocytes of the other animals in each of these groups, however, responded to a PHA dilution of 1:5. When stimulation ratios of counts/min in stimulated cultures to counts/min in unstimulated cultures were averaged for all the animals within one group, the mean peak stimulation ratio for the N animals was 102.2 ± 163.1, and for the STM animals of 84.0 ± 81.8. The difference is not significant by the Student's t test.

TABLE I

Response to DNCB in 42 Day Old Guinea Pigs

Group	No. of Animals	Percent Positive in 48 hr	
		0.1% DNCB	0.05% DNCB
W and N	17	94.1%	41.2%
STM	21	38.0%	4.7%

Spontaneous E rosette assay. There was no statistically significant difference in the percentage of spontaneous rosette forming cells (RFC) in the thymus of STM (83.6% ± 5.6) as compared to N animals (85.0% ± 4.7) lymph node cells from the anterior cervical nodes were examined in 5 N and 6 STM animals and were found to contain an average of 57.8% ± 11.9 RFC and 48.3% ± 19.6 RFC respectively. This difference is not significant by the Student's t test.

In vivo response to challenge with tumor cells. Inoculation of tumor cells produced a palpable bleb. By the fifth day this swelling was usually undetectable. No erythematous reaction was noted at the inoculation site. Tumor growth was shown by the formation of a nodule which progressed to a large size and metastisized to the axillary and occasionally to the inguinal lymph nodes. Following metastasis there was frequently a rapid further increase in tumor size, which was usually associated with a marked elevation in body weight to 30-50% weight increase within 10 days.

It was found that a high dose of tumor cells alone (1×10^6) produced metastatic tumors in all animals of the 4 groups tested (W, N, STM, and LTM). However, at the lower tumor cell dose (1×10^4) the STM and LTM groups had more rapid tumor growth than the W and N animals.

When induced regression of tumors was attempted via the concomitant inoculation of tumor cells and BCG at the same site, the STM and LTM animals had significantly shorter regression times than either the W or N group.

No correlation was found between tumor growth and lack of response to DNCB, although induced tumor regression and DNCB reactivity appeared to be related.

DISCUSSION

Although Kramer and Good (4) state that the immune system of the guinea pig reacts in a way similar to that of the mouse and the rat, there are several practical and biological advantages for using the guinea pig as a model. These include: (a) its relative biological independence soon after birth so that weaning can be started within hours because they are able to eat solid food by themselves; (b) the larger size at birth which permits the collection of more sample material for testing; (c) the ontogeny of its immune response is similar to that of the human, according to physiologic age equivalence formulas devised by Solomon (6,11).

In contrast to other studies (5,7,9), the period of malnutrition in this study was started soon after birth during their normal sucking period which is more in accord with the actual circumstances surrounding infantile marasmus. In fact, even 24-48 hr after birth is not early enough for malnutrition to modulate the ontogeny of the immune response which is more susceptible to irreversible changes during early fetal life. In addition, the *in utero* environmental factor and the endogenous effects of a malnourished mother, with all its complications on the developing embryo, are aspects that need to be considered if one is going to extrapolate from animals to humans. The external environmental factors must also be emphasized as certainly their role may vary from study to study. For example, as shown elsewhere in this section (La Via, *et al*.) the disinfectants used in cleaning animal hardware were discovered accidentally to have effects on the immune response of mice. The degree of contamination of the environment in which the animals are kept as well as the interaction of immunity and malnutrition with subclinical or clinical infections in the animals under study are also important.

In considering the incidence of spontaneous tumors in children or young adults who have a long history of malnutrition, going back several generations, one must ponder on: (a) the role of infection and population genetics or immunogenetics as additional factors and (b) the provoking studies reported by several investigators and reviewed by Cohen (3) dealing with immunologic effects of corticosteroids, personality and stress and their relationship to the incidence of cancer.

The major purpose in presenting the data generated by our group during the last several years is: (a) to demonstrate that conflicting results are not uncommon and are undoubtedly due to the basic differences among the models and experimental protocols used by various investigators in the field as well as to the environmental and technical limitations prevailing in this type of scientific research. Most critical are the qualitative and quantitative characteristics of the diet regimen as well as the severity of malnutrition as regards its impact depending on the age of the animal and the length of deprivation. It must be reiterated that a suitable model is lacking in which malnutrition could be instituted during the early gestational period including a familial background of deficiency as is actually the case in human situations.

As stated by Good _et al_. (4) chronic moderate protein restriction may result in enhancement of cell-mediated responses but more severe dietary protein deprivation can actually produce the opposite effect. With the recent knowledge that several subpopulations of T and B lymphocytes and of macrophages exist the interpretation of immunologic results becomes much more difficult and even misleading unless those tests have acceptable degrees of sensitivity and specificity.

In summary, we decided to publish this report mainly to emphasize on the basis of our own data that much work still remains to be done in the general field of nutrition-immunocompetence-disease interactions. In this connection, studies concerning the effects of obesity or overnutrition and the role of aging in each of the facets outlined in this presentation should also prove fruitful.

REFERENCES

1. American Society for Experimental Pathology. Symposium: The Role of Nutrition in the Pathogenesis of Disease (organized by H. Sidransky), Am. J. Path. 84 (1976) 597.
2. Chandra, R. K. and Newberne, P. M., Nutrition, Immunity and Infection: Mechanisms of Interactions, Plenum Press, New York (1977).
3. Cohen, J. J., Symposium on Pharmacology of The Reticuloendothelial System. XV National Meeting of the RE Society, Charleston, S. C. (1978).
4. Good, R.A., Fernandes, E. J., and Yunis, _et al_., Am. J. Path. 84 (1976) 599.
5. Jose, D. G. and Good, R. A., Nature 241 (1973) 57.
6. Leslie, R. G. Q. and Cohen, S., The Biochem. J. 120 (1970) 787.

7. Lopez, V., Davis, S. D. and Smith, N., Pediat. Res. 6 (1972) 779.
8. Mancini, G., Carbonara, A. O. and Heremans, J. F., Immunochem. 2 (1965) 235.
9. McAnulty, P. A. and Dickerson, J. W. T., Pediat. Res. 7 (1973) 778.
10. Rapp, H. J., Churchill, W. H., Jr., Kronman, B. S., *et al.*, J. Nat. Cancer Instit. 41 (1968) 1.
11. Solomon, J. B., Foetal and Neonatal Immunology. Amsterdam Elsevier Publ. Co., Amsterdam, The Netherlands (1971).

PARTICIPANTS

ABRAMOFF, P.
Marquette University
Milwaukee, Wisconsin

ADES, E.
Comprehensive Cancer Center
University of Alabama
Birmingham, Alabama

ADLER, A.
Hadassah Medical School
Hebrew University
Jerusalem, Israel

AKSAMIT, R.
National Cancer Institute, NIH
Bethesda, Maryland

ARONSON, M.
Sackler School of Medicine
Tel Aviv University
Tel Aviv, Israel

BABNIK, J.
J. Stefan Institute
Ljubljana, Yugoslavia

BAR-ELI, M.
Hadassah Medical School
Hebrew University
Jerusalem, Israel

BARTH, R. F.
Mount Sinai Medical Center
Milwaukee, Wisconsin

BASIC, I
Faculty of National Sciences
and Mathematics and Central
Institute for Tumors and Allied
Health Diseases
Zagreb, Yugoslavia

BATTISTO, J. R.
Cleveland Clinic Foundation
Cleveland, Ohio

BENDINELLI, M.
University of Pisa
Pisa, Italy

BENNEDSEN, J.
Statens Seruminstitut
DK-2300, Copenhagen S, Denmark

BERTOK, L.
National Research Institute
for Radiobiology and
Radiohygiene
Budapest, Hungary

BERTOLI, F.
Via Donzelle No 1
Bologna, Italia

BLIZNAKOV, E. G.
New England Institute
Ridgefield, Connecticut

BOEHME, D. H.
Veterans Administration Hospital
East Orange, New Jersey

BOLTZ-NITULESCU, G.
Institute of General and
Experimental Pathology
University of Vienna
Vienna, Austria

BONAVIDA, B.
University of California at
Los Angeles
Los Angeles, California

CASS, I. M.
79 Old Forest Hill Road
Toronto, Canada

CEGLOWSKI, W. S.
Pennsylvania State University
University Park, Pennsylvania

CHAUVET, G.
Centre de Physiologie
et d' Immunologie Cellulaires
Inserm U. 104
CNRS et Ass. Cl. Bernard
Hospital St-Antoine
Paris Cedex 12
France

CLOUGH, J. D.
Cleveland Clinic Foundation
Cleveland, Ohio

COHN, D. A.
York College
City University of New York
Jamica, New York

COOPER, D. A.
Department of Immunology
St. Vincent's Hospital
Sydney, Australia

DAMAIS, C.
Immunotherapie Experimentale
Institut Pasteur
Paris, France

DAVIES, W. A.
Prince of Wales Children's Hosp.
Randwick, N. S. W.
Australia

DE HALLEAUX, F.
Brocades Belga
Blvd. General Jacques, 26
Brussels, Belgium

DELVILLE, J.
School of Public Health
Universite Catholique de Louvain
1200 Brussels, Belgium

DI LUZIO, N. R.
Tulane University School of
Medicine
New Orleans, Louisiana

DIXON, J.
University of Southern California
School of Medicine
Los Angeles, California

DRATH, D.
Harvard Medical School
Boston, Massachusetts

DUBROFF, L. M.
Hahnemann Medical College
Philadelphia, Pennsylvania

EISENSTEIN, T. K.
Temple University School of
Medicine
Philadelphia, Pennsylvania

ESCOBAR, M. R.
Medical College of Virginia
Richmond, Virginia

FABIAN, I.
Sackler School of Medicine
Tel Aviv University
Tel Aviv, Israel

FIDLER, I. J.
Frederick Cancer Center
Frederick, Maryland

FILKINS, J. P.
Loyola University Medical Center
Maywood, Illinois

FRANK, M.
National Institutes of Health
Bethesda, Maryland

FLEMMING, K. B. P.
University of Freiburg
Freiburg, Germany

FORD, P. M.
Queen's University
Kingston, Ontario
Canada

FORSTER, O.
Institute of General and
Experimental Pathology
University of Vienna
Vienna, Austria

FRIEDMAN, H.
University of South Florida
College of Medicine
Tampa, Florida

GABIZON, A.
The Weizmann Institute of
Science
Rehovot, Israel

GHAFFAR, A.
Department of Microbiology and
Immunology
University of South Carolina
Columbia, South Carolina

GILLET, J.
School of Public Health
Universite Catholique de Louvain
1200-Brussels, Belgium

GINSBURG, H.
Technicon University
School of Medicine
Haifa, Israel

GINSBURG, I.
Hadassah School of
Dental Medicine
Hebrew University
Jerusalem, Israel

GLOBERSON, A.
Hadassah Medical School
Hebrew University
Jerusalem, Israel

GOLDBLUM, N.
Hadassah Medical School
Hebrew University
Jerusalem, Israel

GOLDMAN, R.
Weizmann Institute
Rehovot, Israel

GOLUB, S. H.
Department of Surgery
University of California
at Los Angeles
Los Angeles School of Medicine
Los Angeles, California

GORCZYNSKI, R. M.
Ontario Cancer Institute
Toronto, Ontario Canada

GORELICK, E.
Hadassah Medical School
Hebrew University
Jerusalem, Israel

GREENBLATT, C.
Hebrew University
Jerusalem, Israel

HALL, J. M.
Proctor Foundation
University of California
San Francisco, California

HAMBURGER, J.
Hadassah Medical School
Hebrew University
Jerusalem, Israel

HANNA, M. G., Jr.
Frederick Cancer Center
Frederick, Maryland

HARAN, Ghera, J.
Tel Aviv University
Tel Aviv, Israel

HARRIS, S.
The Children's Hospital of
Philadelphia and School
of Medicine
University of Pennsylvania
Philadelphia, Pennsylvania

HARRIS, T. N.
University of Pennsylvania
Children's Hospital
Philadelphia, Pennsylvania

HAYASHI, T.
Fukushima Medical College
Fukushima, Japan

HELLMAN, A.
National Cancer Institute
Bethesda, Maryland

HEMSTREET, G. P.
University of Alabama at
Birmingham
Birmingham, Alabama

HENSEN, E.
Department of Immunohematology
University Hospital
Leiden, The Netherlands

HERBERMAN, R. B.
National Cancer Institute
Bethesda, Maryland

HERMAN, F.
School of Public Health
Universite Catholique de Louvain
1200-Brussels
Belgium

HERSCOWITZ, H. B.
Georgetown University
Medical Center
Washington, D. C.

HIBBS, J. B., Jr.
Veterans Administration Hospital
and University of Utah
Medical College
Salt Lake City, Utah

HOFFMAN, M. K.
Memorial Sloan-Kettering
Cancer Center
New York, New York

HOLDEN, H. T.
Laboratory of Immunodiagnosis
National Cancer Institute
Bethesda, Maryland

HOLY, H. W.
Technicon International
Division S. A.
12-14 Chemin Rieu
1208 Geneva
Switzerland

HOOGHE, R.
Weizmann Institute of Science
Rehovot, Israel

ISAKOV, N.
Department of Cell Biology
Weizmann Institute of Science
Rehovot, Israel

JACQUES, P. J.
Catholic University of Louvain
Brussels, Belgium

JAKAB, G.
Department of Environmental
Health Sciences
Johns Hopkins University
Baltimore, Maryland

JANICKI, B. W.
National Institutes of Health
Bethesda, Maryland

KAGAN, E.
Department of Pathology
Georgetown University
Medical Center
Washington, D. C.

KALTER, S. S.
Southwest Foundation for
Research and Education
San Antonio, Texas

KAMPSCHMIDT, R. F.
S. R. NObel Foundation
Ardmore, Oklahoma

KAPLAN, A. M.
Medical College of Virginia
Richmond, Virginia

KAPLOW, L. S.
Veterans Administration Hospital
West Haven, Connecticut

KIESSLING, R.
Karolinska Institute
Stockholm, Sweden

KFIR, S.
Hebrew University of Jerusalem
Jerusalem, Israel

KLEIN, M.
Temple University Medical School
Philadelphia, Pennsylvania

KODITSCHEK, L. K.
409 Highland Avenue
Upper Montclair, New Jersey

KOJIMA, M.
Fukushima Medical College
Fukushima, Japan

KOPITAR, M.
J. Stefan Institute
Ljubljana, Yugoslavia

KOREN, H. S.
Division of Immunology and
Department of Pathology
Duke University
Durham, North Carolina

KRAKAUER, R. S.
Departments of Dermatology
and Immunology
Cleveland Clinic Foundation
Cleveland, Ohio

KRIPE, M.
Frederick Cancer Center
Frederick Maryland

LA VIA, M.
Medical University of
South Carolina
Charleston, South Carolina

LEFLER, A. M.
Jefferson Medical College of
Thomas Jefferson University
Philadelphia, Pennsylvania

JEJEUNE, F. J.
Institut Jules Bordet
Universite Libre de Bruxelles
Brussels, Belgium

LEONARD, E. J.
National Institutes of Health
Bethesda, Maryland

LESPINATS, G.
Institute for Cancer Research
Villejuif, France

LICHTER, W.
University of Miami School of
Medicine
Miami, Florida

LINNA, T. J.
Temple University School of
Medicine
Philadelphia, Pennsylvania

LONAI, P.
Weizmann Institute
Rehovot, Israel

LOOSE, L. D.
Institute of Comparative
and Human Toxicology
Albany Medical College
Albany, New York

LOWELL, G. H.
Walter Reed Army Institute
Washington, D. C.

LOWY, I.
Immunotherapie Experimentale
Institut Pasteur
75015 Paris, France

LUCAS, D. O.
Department of Microbiology
University of Arizona
Tucson, Arizona

LUMB, J. R.
Atlanta University
Atlanta, Georgia

MADDISON, S. E.
Parasitology and
Pathology Divisions
Center for Disease Control
Atlanta, Georgia

MARSHALL, N. B.
Department of Hypersensitivity
Diseases
The Upjohn Company
Kalamazoo, Michigan

MEKORI-FELSTEINER, T.
Rambam Medical Center
Haifa, Israel

MELTZER, M. S.
National Cancer Institute
Bethesda, Maryland

MOORE, M.
Paterson Laboratories
Christie Hospital and
Hold Radium Institute
Manchester M20 9BX
England

MORRELL, R. M.
Neurology Service
Veterans Administration Hospital
Allen Park, Michigan

MYRVIK, Q. N.
Bowman Gray School of Medicine
Winston-Salem, North Carolina

NACHTIGAL, D.
Weizmann Institute
Rehovot, Israel

NAJJAR, V. A.
Tufts University
Boston, Massachusetts

NELSON, D. S.
Kolling Institute of
Medical Research
Sydney, Australia

NELSON, M.
Kolling Institute of
Medical Research
Royal North Shore Hospital
Sydney, Australia

NGUYEN, B. T.
Service Microbiologie
Clinique Universitaire Saint Luc
Universite de Louvain
Brussels 1200
Belgium

NORMANN, S. J.
University of Florida
Gainesville, Florida

NOWOTNY, A.
Temple University Medical School
Philadelphia, Pennsylvania

OMURA, Y.
Fukushima Medical College
Fukushima, Japan

OPPENHEIM, J. J.
National Institute of
Dental Research
Bethesda, Maryland

PARANT, M.
Immunotherapie Experimentale
Institut Pasteur
Paris, France

PATRIARCA, P.
University of Trieste
Trieste, Italy

PELED, A.
Department of Chemical
Immunology
Weizmann Institute of Science
Rehovot, Israel

PENNY, R.
St. Vincent's Hospital
Sydney, Australia

PITT, J.
Columbia University College of
Physicians and Surgeons
New York, New York

PLUZNIK, D. H.
Bar-Ilan University
Ramat-Gan, Israel

POLAKOW
Hadassah Medical School
Hebrew University
Jerusalem, Israel

POUPON, M.
Institute for Cancer Research
Villejuif, France

PRIBNOW, J. F.
Proctor Foundation
University of California
San Francisco, California

PRESANT, C.
Jewish Hospital
of St. Louis
St. Louis, Missouri

QUASTEL, M.
Soroka Medical Center
Beer-Sheba, Israel

RABINOWITZ, R.
Hadassah Medical School
Hebrew University
Jerusalem, Israel

RACHMILEWITZ, M.
Hebrew University
Hadassah Medical School
Jerusalem, Israel

REGELSON, W.
Department of Medicine
Medical College of Virginia
Virginia Commonwealth University
Richmond, Virginia

REICHARD, S. M.
Medical College of Georgia
Augusta, Georgia

ROMEO, D.
University of Trieste
Trieste, Italy

ROOS, D.
Netherlands Red Cross Blood
Transfusion Service
The Netherlands

ROSENBERG, R.
Accurate Chemical Scientific Corp
New York, N. Y.

ROSENBERG, S. A.
National Cancer Institute
National Institutes of Health
Bethesda, Maryland

ROSENSTEIN, M. M.
Department of Zoology
and Physiology
Rutgers University
Newark, New Jersey

ROSENTAHL, A. S.
National Institute of Allergy
and Infectious Diseases
Bethesda, Maryland

ROSSI, F.
University of Trieste
Trieste, Italy

RUPOLD, H.
Heitzinger Hauptstr. 18 A 16
Vienna, Austria

RUN, R.
Hadassah Medical School
Hebrew University
Jerusalem, Israel

RUTTER, V.
Weizmann Institute of Science
Rehovot, Israel

SALEM, H.
Cannon Lab, Inc.
Reading, Pennsylvania

SAMAK, R.
Chemotherapy Unit
University of Paris
XIII. CHU Bobigny
93000 France

SAUDER, D. N.
Department of Dermatology
and Immunology
Cleveland Clinic Foundation
Cleveland, Ohio

SCHECHTER, G.
Veterans Administration
Hospital and George Washington
University Medical Center
Washington, D. C.

SCHILDT, B. E.
University of Linkoping
Regional Hospital
S-581 85 Linkoping
Sweden

SCHIRRMACHER, V.
Institute of Immunology and
Genetics
Deutsches Krebsforschungszentrum
Heidelberg, Federal Republic
of Germany

SCHLESINGER, M.
Hebrew University
Jerusalem, Israel

SCOTT, M. T.
The Wellcome Research
Laboratories
Beckenham, Kent
England

SEGAL, S.
The Weizmann Institute of
Science
Department of Cell Biology
Rehovot, Israel

SIECK, R. K.
University of Heidelburg
Heidelburg, Germany

SIEDHI, B.
Hadassah Medical School
Hebrew University
Jerusalem, Israel

SIEGEL, B. V.
University of Oregon
Medical School
Portland, Oregon

SIEGEL, J. I. M.
University of Oregon Health
Sciences Center
Portland, Oregon

SIGEL, M. M.
University of South Carolina
School of Medicine
Columbia, South Carolina

SILKWORTH, J.
Institute of Comparative
and Human Toxicology
Albany Medical College
Albany, New York

SILVERSTEIN, E.
State University of New York
Downstate Medical Center
Brooklyn, New York

SOROUDI, M.
5360 Rural Ridge
Anaheim, Canada

SYNDERMAN, R.
Duke University
Durham, North Carolina

SOLOMON, J. B.
University of Aberdeen
Aberdeen, Scotland

STERN, K.
Bar-Ilan University
Tel Aviv, Israel

STIFFEL, C.
Curie Foundation
Institute of Radium
Paris, France

STINNETT, J. D.
University of Cincinnati
Medical Center
Cincinnati, Ohio

STRAUSS, R. R.
Albert Einstein Medical Center
Philadelphia, Pennsylvania

STRAUSSER, J. L.
National Cancer Institute
National Institutes of Health
Bethesda, Maryland

STUART, A. E.
University of Edenburgh
Eidenburgh, Scotland

SULITZEANU, D.
Dept. of Immunology
Hadassah Medical School
Hebrew University of Jerusalem
Jerusalem, Israel

TAL, C.
Hadassah Medical School
Hebrew University
Jerusalem, Israel

TAUB, R. N.
Medical College of Virginia
Richmond, Virginia

TIMAR, M.
Chemical-Pharmaceutical
Research Institute
Vitan 112 Bucuresti 4
Romania

TRAININ, N.
Weizmann Institute
Rehovot, Israel

UETSUKA, A.
Laboratory of Medical Mycology
Department of Infectious Diseases
Institute of Medical Science
University of Tokyo, Japan

URBASCHEK, R.
Institute of Hygiene and
Medical Microbiology
University of Heidelberg
Heidelberg, Germany

VERCAMMEN-GRANDJEAN, A.
Institut Jules Bordet
Centre des Tumeurs
de l'Universite
libre de Bruxelles
Brussels, Belgium

WARD, H. A.
Department of Pathology
and Immunology
Monash Medical School
Victoria, Australia

WEEKS, B. A.
University of South Carolina
Columbia, South Carolina

WERTHEIM, G.
Hebrew University of Jerusalem
Jerusalem, Israel

WHEELOCK, E. F.
Thomas Jefferson University
Philadelphia, Pennsylvania

YOFFEY, J.
Hadassah Medical School
Hebrew University of Jerusalem
Jerusalem, Israel

ZIEGLER, J.
Prince of Wales Hospital
Randwick, Australia

ZLOTNIK
Hadassah Medical School
Hebrew University
Jerusalem, Israel

INDEX

ACE, see Angiotensin converting enzyme
Acid β-glycerophosphatase, in liver, 229-230
Acid deoxyribonuclease, 226
Acid-fast bacteria, glucan in treatment of infection from, 246-251
Acid μ-glycerophosphatase, 226
Adenocarcinoma, glucan inhibitory effect on, 276
Adenosine triphosphatase activity, see ATPase activity
Adenosine triphosphate
  antimycin A effect on, 33-34
  enzymatic splitting of, 43
Adherent cells, 487, see also Spleen cells
  in antigen binding to T cells, 451-458
  in antigen processing, 455
  depletion of, in PFC response, 465
AFB, see Acid-fast bacteria
Aged mice, see also Mouse
  energy metabolism reduction in, 367
  immunologic responsiveness vs. coenzyme Q deficiency in, 361-368
  organ weight change in, 363
AKR lymphocytic leukemia, glucan modification of, 277
  see also Lymphocytic leukemia
AKR mice, see also Mouse
  glucose-induced enhancement in survival of, 296
  spontaneous leukemia in, 279
Albumin, amino terminal sequences of, 170
Alveolar macrophages, see also Macrophages
  binding of lymphocytes to, 542-551
  calcium uptake and secretion of granule enzymes, 44
  exocytosis of granules from, 47
  lysates and plasma membrane fraction of in rabbit, 40-44
  PFC response and, 470, 473
  plasma membrane of, 38
  preparation of, 54
  pulmonary, see Pulmonary alveolar macrophages
  of rat, see Rat alveolar macrophages
  respiratory burst in, 53-70
  splenic lymphocyte interaction with, following asbestos inhalation in rat, 539-552
AM, see Alveolar macrophages
Ametryne, 569, 573
Amyloidosis
  defined, 167
  murine, 167-168
Amyloid proteins, 167
Angiotensin I, as decapeptide, 149

Angiotensin II
  histidyl-leucine release and, 143
  tuftsin and, 143
Angiotensin-converting enzyme, 149-155
  cAMP and, 152
  dexamethasone and, 153
  human monocyte level of, 154
  in lymphocytes, 155
  in mouse peritoneal macrophages, 151
  in rabbit alveolar macrophages, 153
  synthesis of in mononuclear phagocytes, 150
Anionic polyelectrolysis, inhibition of bacteriolysis by, 123-128
Anopheles stephensi, 308
Antibody formation, immunopharmacology and, 224
Antibody-forming cells, suppression of by rat spleen macrophages, 485-494
Antibody-mediated immunity, modification of by environmental chemicals, 499
  see also Immune response; Immune system
Antibody response
  of FLV-infected splenocytes, 317
  lipopolysaccharides in, 315-321
Anticoagulant studies, 216
Antigen binding
  _H-2_ restriction in, 451-458
  kinetics of, 454
  temperature dependence in, 453
Antigen processing, adherent cells in, 455
Antileukocyte antibodies, 53
Anti (LNPI) serum
  analysis of, 86
  immunoelectrophoresis of, 86-89
Antimycin, 44
Antimycin A, 31-33
Arachidonic acid, phagocytosis and, 415
Asbestos inhalation, alveolar-macrophage-splenic lymphocyte interactions following, 539-552
Asbestosis, pathogenesis of, 552
ATPase activity
  calcium-dependent, 31-42, 44
  calcium-induced, 41
  lysates and rabbit alveolar macrophages in, 42
  magnesium-dependent, 43-44
ATP splitting enzymes, 39
Azur granules, endogenous peroxidase activity in, 204
  see also Granule enzymes; Granules

Bacillus Calmette-Guerin, 269, 602
  mouse leukemia and, 286-287
Bacterial clearing, tuftsin and, 138
Bacteriolysis, _see also_ Bacterial clearing
  inhibition of by anionic polyelectrodes, 123-128
BCG, _see_ Bacillus Calmette-Guerin
N-Benzoyl-DL-argenine-2-naphthylamide, 76
Beta adrenergic blockers, 101
Blood cells, peroxidase staining of, 214-220
  see also Sheep red blood cells
Blood glucose level, carbon clearance half-times and, 393-394
Blood granulocytes, stimulation of phagocyte activity in by tuftsin, 133-134
Blood samples
  cytograf scattergrams of, 213
  histograms of, 215

B lymphocytes, in generation of LPS-induced cerebrospinal fluid, 438-443
Bone marrow reticular cells
  cytological characteristics of, 195-208
  as major cell constituent of reticular meshworks, 206
  ultrastructural morphology of, 197-198

Calcium buffering systems
  intracellular, see Intracellular calcium buffering systems
  properties of, 37-50
Calcium concentration
  in biological fluids, 37-38
  in polymorphonuclear leukocytes and macrophages, 37
Calcium-dependent ATPase activity, 38-42 see also ATPase activity
cAMP level
  angiotensin converting enzyme and, 152
  PHA and, 501
Cancer cells, destruction of with tuftsin as activator, 140, 144
  see also Lung carcinoma; Mammary carcinoma
Candida tropicalis, 265
Carbaryl, 569, 573
Carbon clearance, glucocorticoids and, 107
Carbon clearance half-times, blood glucose level and, 393-394
Carcinogenesis, ultraviolet, 589-597
  see also Cancer cells
Cat, asbestos inhalation in, 539-552
Catalase, inhibition of in neutrophil respiration, 30
Cathepsin B, 76
  alpha-1-antitrypsin and, 85
  inhibition of, 77, 80
Cathepsin D
  molecular weight inhibitors of, 78-79
  effect on LNPI-1 and 2, 76-81
  glucocorticoids and, 103-106
CB, see Cytochalasin B
Cell-mediated immune response
  developmental phases of, 503
  and dietary administration of contaminants, 516-521
  effector stage of, 502
  environmental chemical-induced modification of, 499-521
  mixed lymphocyte culture in, 504
Cell-mediated lymphocytotoxicity, 504
Cellular metabolism, immune response and, 14-17
Cerebrospinal fluid generation
  from macrophage-T-lymphocyte interaction, 435-438
  streptococcal enterotoxin B in, 437, 444-445
Cetyltrimethylammonium bromide, 94-95
Chemoluminescence, phagocytosis and, 3
Chicken polymorphonuclear leukocytes, 54, 111-120
Chicken red blood cells, phagocytosis of, 352-357
China black ink, pinocytosis of, 261
Chlordimeform, 569
Chloroleukemia, allogenic Shay, 291
Cholera toxin treatment
  modulation of T cells and macrophages by, 343-349
  sheep red blood cells and, 343
Choline, in calcium-dependent ATPase activity, 43
Chymotripsin-like neutral proteinase, inhibition of, 77-79, 82
δ-Chymotripsin treatment, 160-161
Circulatory shock, glucocorticoids in, 103-106

CML, see Cell-mediated lymphocytotoxicity
Coenzyme Q, defined, 361
Coenzyme Q Bioavailability, in immunological senescence, 367
Coenzyme Q deficiency, in aged mice, 361-368
Colloidal carbon clearance
  endotoxin and, 392
  in marine biology, 583-585
Colloidal iron, phagocytic impairment and, 494
Complement, chemotactic fragments of, 53
Complement-coated giant cells, phagocytosis of, 327
Complement receptor, phagocytosis mediation by, 324-327
Concanavalin A, 53
  cytochalasin B and, 69
  in DNA synthesis suppression, 459
Contaminants, manmade, 523-524
Copper metabolism, RES role in, 403-409
Coriolus versicolor extract, 256
  pinocytosis and, 260, 265-266
Corticosteone, 151, see also Glucocorticoids
Cortisone, 151
Corynebacteria, 224
Corynebacterium parvum, 255, 269, 307, 324, 328, 583, 585, 587
  activation of pleural macrophages by, 333-341
  mice mammary carcinomas and, 335
  systemic effects of injection of, 336
Corynebacterium parvum-activated pleural macrophages, *in vitro* destructive effects of, 339
Corynebacterium parvum-induced antitumor resistance, 333
CP, see *Corynebacterium parvum*
CRBC, see Chicken red blood cells
Crocidolite, phagocytosis of, 552
CSF, see Cerebrospinal fluid
CT, see Cholera toxin treatment
CTAB, see Cetyltrimethylammonium bromide
Cycloheximide, in degradation of Fc-receptor activity, 160-164
Cyclophosphamide
  glucan and, 295, 300-301
  immunosuppressive doses of, 384-387
  priming and, 382
  in rabbit secondary ocular immune response, 381-388
  secondary response and, 382-387
Cytochalasin B, in oxygen and hydrogen peroxide production during phagocytosis, 66
Cytograf oscilloscope displays, 219
Cytograf scattergrams, of blood samples, 213
Cytotoxicity, enhancement of by tuftsin, 140-141
Cytoxan, see Cyclophosphamide

DDT, immune response and, 569-575
Delayed hypersensitivity, to dinitrochlorobenzene, 590-595
Deoxycholate, 41
11-Deoxycorticosterone, 152
2-Deoxyglucose
  glucose addition and, 7
  intraperitoneal injection of, 5-6
  and mouse PFC response to sheep red blood cells, 6
  time as factor in mouse PFC response to, 6
Dexamethasone, 104, 151
  angiotensin converting enzyme and, 153

o-Dianisidine, 97-98
Diethylnitrosamine, tumor cells and, 601
Digitonin treatment, in plasma membrane purification, 188-191
Dinitrochlorobenzene
  delayed hypersensitivity to, 590-595
  protein-calorie malnutrition and, 601
  sensitization to, 601
  tumor regression and, 604
Dinoflagellates, red tide and, 577
DNA synthesis, suppression of, 459-460
DNCB, see Dinitrochlorobenzene
DOG, see 2-Deoxyglucose
DPFC, see IgM plaque-forming cells

Ecteinascidia turbinata, 578-579, 581-583, 585-587
EDTA (ethylenediaminetetra-acetate), as anticoagulant, 216
EGTA-ATPase activity, 40
Elastase
  enzyme activity of, 76
  inhibition of, 78
Endogenous peroxidase activity
  localization of, 204
  ultracytochemical localization of, 208
Endotoxin-induced SAA protein elevation, in mouse, 167-172
Endotoxins
  colloidal carbon clearance and, 392
  in murine amyloidosis induction, 167-168
  phagocytes and, 53
  plasma glucose levels and, 392
Endotoxin shock
  hypoglycemia and, 24
  lead salt sensitization to, 21-27
Environmental contaminants, damaging effect of, 523-524
Enzyme stains, in leukocyte enzyme assays using flow cytophotometry, 212-217
Eosinophil peroxidase
  biochemical properties of, 91-98
  defined, 91
E rosette assay, 601-603
Escherichia coli, 168, 438
  blood clearing of, 137
  tryptan blue dose-response effects on, 15
  tuftsin chemotactic effect on, 134
Escherichia coli endotoxin, 4
Ete, see Ecteinascidia turbinata
Ethylenediaminetetraacetate, as anticoagulant, 216

Fc-receptors
  cycloheximide and, 160, 162-164
  of macrophages, 157
Fish kills, marine organisms and, 577-578
Flavonoids, in PMNL respiration, 372-375
Flow cytophotometers, defined, 211
Flow cytophotometry, leukocyte enzyme assays using, 211-221
Flow systems, blood cell examination, 219-220
FLV, see Friend leukemia virus
Foreign substances, intraperitoneal injection of, 323
Formylmethionyl peptides, polymorphonuclear leukocytes and, 37
Friend leukemia virus, 315

Gallic acid, in mouse spleen cultures, 534-537
Glucagon, 101

Glucan, see also *Coriolus versicolor* extract; Lentinan
  administration route of in malaria prophylaxis, 310
  antitumor activity of, 273-274, 284
  bactericidal effect of, 250
  and cyclophosphamide-treated mice, 295-298
  effect of in leukemic mice, 294-295
  immunopotentiating effect of, 287
  as immunoprophylactic agent, 286
  induction of *Staphylococcus aureus* infection by, 291-304
  inhibiting effect on adenocarcinoma BW 15091A, 276
  inhibiting influence on melanoma B16[a], 273
  intralesional administration of, 295
  as *in vivo* mitogen, 242
  lowered efficacy of in malaria treatment, 311
  lysosomes and, 225-236
  as macrophage activator, 242
  modification of lymphocytic leukemia by, 277
  mononuclear phagocyte response to, 237, 241
  mortality reduction through, 298-299
  in mouse lymphocytic leukemia, 303-304
  in mouse malaria prophylaxis, 307-312
  in *Mycobacterium leprae* infection, 245-251
  nonantigenic nature of, 270
  as protection against staphylococcal disease, 302
  renal tubule dilatation and, 299
Glucan (cont'd)
  in resistance to bacterial sepsis, 304
  as reticuloendothelial system stimulator in leprosy, 245-251
  serum lysozyme and, 287
  suppressor cell induction and reticuloendothelial cell activation produced by, 235-243
  in syngeneic tumor models, 284-285
  tumor growth and, 269-288
  water-soluble polysaccharides and, 233
Glucocorticoids (glucocorticosteroids)
  ACE synthesis and, 150-151
  carbon clearance of, 107
  cathepsin D and, 103-106
  in circulatory shock, 101
  and lysosomal integrity of control, 104
Gluconeogenesis, lead acetate and, 22-25
Glucoregulation, RES role in, 21-27
Glucose homeostasis, RES function in, 391-401
Glucose metabolism, tobacco smoke and, 564
Glucose oxidation
  lead acetate and, 22, 26
  in respiratory burst, 56
Glucose-stimulated immunoreactive insulin, RES depression and, 401
Glucose tolerance
  lead acetate and, 21-23
  RES depression and, 396
Glucose utilization, phagocytosis and, 3
Glutathione disulfide, 14
Glutathione peroxidase, 14, 57
Glycemia-stimulated serum insulin levels, lead acetate and, 24
Gorgonia ventalina, 579

Graft-versus-host response, 502-503
diet and, 510, 518-519
reduction in, 509
spleen index and, 505
Gram-negative rods, 224
Granule enzymes, calcium uptake and secretion of, 44, 46
Granules, exocytosis of from rabbit alveolar macrophages, 47
Granulocytes
in host resistance and inflammation, 433-434
neutrophilic, *see* Neutrophils
Granulopoesis, macrophages as regulators of, 433-447
Granulopoietic system, lipopolysaccharides and, 434
Guinea pig peritoneal macrophages
biochemical analysis of, 184
purification of plasma membranes from 183-192
GVHR, *see* Graft-versus-host response

HCB, *see* Hexachlorobenzene
Heparin
anticoagulant effect of, 175
desulphation of by macrophages, 179-181
metabolic fate of, 175-179, 181
polyornithine and, 177
uptake of by macrophages, 177-179
Hepatic gluconeogenesis, RES function depression and, 396-399
Hepatic phagocytosis, glucocorticoid protection of, in hypoxia, 101-108
Hexachlorobenzene, 500
cell-mediated immune function impairment by, 518-520
Hexose monophosphate pathway, of rabbit polymorphonuclear leukocytes and alveolar macrophages, 64
Hippuryl-L-histidyl-L-leucine, 149
Histidyl-leucine, angiotensin II and, 143
Histiocytes, tissue macrophages of, 207
Homovanillic acid, 116
Horseradish peroxidase, 116, 119
Host resistance, chemical-induced alteration of, 499-520
H-2 restriction, in antigen binding to T cells, 451-458
Humans, immunodepressive effects in, 524-525
Hydrocortisone, 151
Hydrogen peroxide
accumulation of by rabbit polymorphonuclear leukocytes and alveolar macrophages, 65
concanavalin A in production of, 70
fluorometric assay of, 112
increased accumulation of, 63
in vitro immunosuppression in presence of, 16
measurement of in respiratory burst, 56
and mouse in vitro PFC production, 7
from phagocytosing chicken polymorphonuclear leukocytes, 111-120
production of in alveolar macrophage respiratory burst, 53-70
production of during NADPH oxidation, 61
production of by neutrophils and monocytes, 30
release of from phagocytosing rabbit polymorphonuclear leukocytes and alveolar macrophages, 68
17-α-Hydroxyprogesterone, 152
Hyperchlorinated water, macrophage-mediated cytoxicity following intake of, 526

Hyperinsulinemia, RES depression and, 401
Hypoglycemia
  depression of RES phagocytosis in, 391-393
  in endotoxin shock, 24
Hypoxia, hepatic phagocytosis protection in, 101-108

IgG immunoglobulin, macrophage receptors for, 157
IgM immunoglobulin, as sheep red blood cell coating, 324
IgM plaque forming cells, number of, 530
Immune response, see also PFC response
  alveolar macrophage in suppression of, 459-483
  cell-mediated, see Cell-mediated immune response
  DDT and, 571-575
  factors in development of, 501
  leukocyte metabolic activities and, 3-18
  macrophage participation in, 459
  marine organism substances and, 577-587
Immune system
  environmental chemical toxicity and, 500-501
  ultraviolet radiation and, 589-597
Immunodepressive effects, in humans, 524-525
Immunological killing, lysosomes in, 226
Immunological responsiveness, supression of in aged mice, 361-368
Immunomodulation, protein-calorie malnutrition and, 498
Immunopharmacology, 224
Immunosuppressed mice, glucan and, 296
Immunosuppression
  lysosomal enzymes and, 17
Immunosuppression (cont'd)
  macrophage-mediated, 461-483
Inflammatory exudates, inhibition of bacteriolysis by, 123-128
Insulin hypoglycemia, RES depression and, 395
Insulin lethality
  lead acetate and, 21-22
  RES depression and, 395
Insulin levels, RES function and, 399-401
Insulin sensitivity, RES function and, 393-396
Intracellular calcium buffering system
  mechanism of, 38
  role of, 37-50
Intracellular leukocyte proteinase inhibitor, 75
  immunological studies of, 85-90
Iron metabolism, RES role in, 403-409

Kallikrein, polymorphonuclear leukocytes and, 37
N-Ketoprogesterone, 152
Krebs Ringer phosphate buffer, 55
Kuppfer cells, 226, 232

Lactate production, by human neutrophils and monocytes, 36
Lactic dehydrogenase activity, following liver perfusion, 103
Lead acetate
  gluconeogenesis and, 22-25
  glucose oxidation and, 22-23
  glucose tolerance and, 21-23
  insulin lethality and, 21-22
  serum insulin levels and, 24-26
Lead salt sensitization, to endotoxin shock, 21-27
LEM, see Leukocytic endogenous mediator

Lentinan, spreading effect of on macrophage monolayers, 256-257, 265-266
Leprosy, glucan as reticuloendothelial system stimulator in treatment of, 245-251
Leukemic mice, experimental _Staphylococcus aureus_ infection in, 291-304, _see also_ Mouse
Leukemic splenocytes, restoration of depressed antibody responses of, 315-321
Leukocyte activity, immune response and, 3-18
Leukocyte enzyme assays, flow cytophotometry in, 211-221
Leukocyte extracts, lysis of staphylococci by, 123-128
Leukocyte inhibitors, Lewis lung carcinoma and, 81
Leukocyte intracellular inhibitors, of proteinases, 75-83
Leukocyte migration, tuftsin and, 139
Leukocyte neutral proteinase inhibitors, 76-78
  tumor growth and, 81-82
Leukocyte proteinases
  biochemical and biological properties of, 75-83
  defined, 75
Leukocytes
  peroxidase activity of, 95-96
  polymorphonuclear, _see_ Polymorphonuclear leukocytes
  scattergram and histogram of, 216
  sub-populations of, 211, 216
Leukocytic endogenous mediator, as RES adjunct in body metabolism, 403-409
Leukokinin, enzymes in release of tuftsin from, 132-133
Leukokininase, phagocytic activity of, 132-133
Lewis lung carcinoma, 81
Lipopolysaccharides
  activation of mouse B cells by, 461
  antibody responses and, 315-321
  B lymphocytes in generation of CSF induced by, 438-443
  combination of with MDP, 318
  dose response for stimulation by, 318
  granulopoietic system and, 434
  immunostimulatory effects of supernatants from, 319
  macrophage supernatants and, 441-442
  from _Salmonella typhimurium_, 353
Listeria monocytogenes, 136-137, 460, 551
Liver, hydrolytic capacity of, vs. parasitic disease control by, 232
LNPI-1 and 2 (leukocyte neutral proteinase inhibitors), 76-78
  see also Molecular weight inhibitors
LPS, _see_ Lipopolysaccharides; _see also_ _Escherichia coli_ endotoxin
LTN, _see_ Lentinan
Lung carcinoma, leukocyte inhibitors and, 81
Lymphocyte activation, lymphocyte clones and, 501
Lymphocytes
  angiotensin converting enzyme activity in, 155
  CSF generation by, 440
  micogen-stimulated, 462
  purified splenic, _see_ Purified splenic lymphocytes

Lymphocytic leukemia, glycan modification of, 277, 303-304
Lysates, marker enzyme activities in, 40
Lysosomal deoxyribonuclease, concentration of in liver, 229-230
Lysosomal marker enzymes in immunosuppression, 17, 226-227
Lysosomes
  glucan and, 225-226
  immunological killing and, 226

Macrophage activities, regulation of, 37-50
Macrophage bactericidal activity, tuftsin augmentation of, 135
Macrophage depleted spleen cells, 486, 494
Macrophage immunogenic function, tuftsin and, 138
Macrophage-mediated cytotoxicity, following hyperchlorinated water intake, 526
Macrophage monolayers
  lentinan spreading effect on, 257
  PSK spreading effect on, 257
Macrophage plasma membrane ATPases, activities of, 41, 45
Macrophage population
  acid phosphatase and 5'-nucleotidase activity in, 325
  activation in, 327-328
  sheep red blood cells and, 326
  stimulated, see Stimulated macrophage populations
Macrophage prostaglandins, functions of in phagocytes, 413-416
Macrophage receptors, proteinase sensitivity and, 157
Macrophages
  activated, 327-328
  alveolar, see Alveolar macrophages
  antitumor activity of, 327-331, 585
  calcium concentration in, 37
  EA-rosetting reaction in, 158
  endocytosis of, 256
  enzyme treatment of, 158
  Fc-receptors of, 157-158
  function of, 3
  in granulopoiesis regulation, 433-437
  guinea pig peritoneal, see Guinea pig peritoneal macrophages
  hemopoiesis and, 419-420
  heparin desulphation by, 179
  in immune response, 459
  modulation of by cholera toxin treatment, 343-349
  peritoneal, see Peritoneal macrophages
  pleural, see Pleural macrophages
  suppressive effects of, 459-460
  tissue, see Tissue macrophages
  transcobalamin secretion by, 428
  tuftsin and immunogenic function of, 137-139
  tuftsin augmentation of in destruction of cancer cells, 140-141, 144
Magnesium-dependent ATPase activity, 43
Major histocompatibility complex, PFC response and, 479
Malaria, host defense in, 307
Malathion, 569
Mammary carcinoma, pleural macrophages and, 338
Manmade contaminants, damaging effect of, 523-524
Marine organism substances, in tumor growth and immune responses, 577-587

Marker enzymes, activity of in lysates and plasma membrane fractions of macrophages, 40
Mastocytoma target cells, growth inhibition of, 352-354
MDP, see Muramyl dipeptide
Melanoma tumors, glucan inhibitory effect on, 273-274, 283, 287
Metabolism, RES role in, 403-409
Methylprednisolone, 101
MF, see Peritoneal adherent cells
Mice, see Mouse
Mirex, 569
Mitochondria
  coenzyme Q in, 367
  in human neutrophils and monocytes, 31
Mitogen, Nocardia water-soluble, see Nocardia water-soluble mitogen
Mixed lymphocyte culture
  in cell-mediated immune reaction, 504
  stimulation index and, 509, 511-515
Mixed lymphocyte response, inhibition or stimulation of, 506
Mixed spleen cells, PFC response and, 489-493
Molecular weight inhibitors, leukocyte inhibitors and, 76
Monocyte cells
  cytological characteristics of, 195-208
  tissue culture of, 201
Monocyte macrophage, in host defense, 419-420
Monocytes
  angiotensin-converting enzyme in, 149-155
  function of, 3
  lactate production by, 36
  metabolic comparison of with neutrophils, 29-36
  mitochondria in, 31
Mononuclear phagocyte system, hemopoiesis and, 419-429
Mouse (mice), see also Murine (adj.)
  aged, see Aged mice
  angiotensin-converting enzyme in macrophage of, 150
  cholera toxin in immune response of, 348
  delayed hypersensitivity to dinitrochlorobenzene in, 590-595
  glucan effects in, 235-243
  glucan in susceptibility to systemic S. aureus infection in, 293-294
  hemolytic PFC response of to sheep red blood cells, 5
  human leprosy bacilli injections in, 246-251
  immunological senescence in, 363-364
  Mycobacterium leprae infections in, 245-251
  reticuloendothelial cell activation in, 235-243
  splenoperoxidase activity of, following heterologous or syngeneic erythrocytes, 8
  spontaneous leukemia in, 279-281
  suppressor cell induction in, 235-243
Mouse hemolytic plaque formation, trypan blue injection and, 13-14
Mouse malaria, glucan in casual prophylaxis of, 307-312
Mouse peritoneal cells, cytochemistry of, 236
Mouse spleen cells
  antibody response to, 345
  peroxidase activity in, 8-10
  response of to sheep red blood cells, 5-6
  and trypan blue/phytohemagglutinin stimulation of ^{3}H-thymidine uptake by, 15

MP, _see_ Methylprednisolone
Muramyl dipeptide, 224, 316
Murine amyloidosis, endotoxin in induction of, 167
Murine leukemia virus, tuftsin and, 135
  see also Mouse
Murine peritoneal macrophages, _in vivo_ activation of by _Nocardia_ water-soluble mitogen, 351-358
Murine tumors
  glucan-induced inhibition of, 269-288
  syngeneic and spontaneous models of, 271
Mycobacteria, 224
Mycobacterium leprae infections, glucan in treatment of, 245-251
Mycobacterium tuberculosis, 307
Myeloperoxidase, 16
  biochemical properties of, 91-98
  defined, 91
  inhibition of, 30
  in staphylococci lysis, 123-128
Myeloperoxidase-deficient subjects, 92-93

NADPH (reduced nicotinamide adenine dinucleotide phosphate) oxidase activity, 113-114
  inhibition of, 373
  and _in vitro_ immunosuppression in presence of hydrogen peroxide, 16-17
  phagocytosis and, 3
NADPH oxidation
  chicken PMN granules in, 117-118, 120
  hydrogen peroxide production in, 60-61
NAP activity, _see_ Neutrophil alkaline phosphatase activity
Napthol AS-D chloroacetate asterase activity, 218
Neutrophil alkaline phosphate activity, 213
  flow-cytophotometric interpretations of, 215
Neutrophilic granulocytes, 29
Neutrophils
  ATP level in, 33-35
  function of, 3
  lactate production by, 36
  metabolic comparison with monocytes, 29-36
  respiration of, 30
Nocardia water-soluble mitogen, 351-358
5'-Nucleotidase distribution, in plasma membrane purification, 187
NWSM, _see_ _Nocardia_ water-soluble mitogen

Octapeptide, angiotensin II as, 149
Oleic acid, in phagocytosis, 415
Oligomycin, 44
OPP, _see_ Orthophenylphenol
Orthophenylphenol, toxicity of, 526-530, 533-537
Oxidative metabolism, stimulation of, 53-72
Oxygen consumption
  measurement of in respiratory burst, 56
  metabolic pathway in, 59
  in phagocytosing PMNL, 65, 68
  phagocytosis and, 3
  reactions involved in, 57-58
Oxygen metabolism tobacco smoke and, 563
Oxygen production, during respiratory burst in alveolar macrophages, 53-72
Oxygen uptake, by phagocytosing chicken polymorphonuclear leukocytes, 115-116

PAM, _see_ Pulmonary alveolar macrophage

Papillomas, in turtles,
577-578
Parathion, 570
PCB, see Polychlorinated biphenyl
Peritoneal adherent cells, in
in antigen binding to
T cells, 451-458
Peritoneal exudate cells, 585
Peritoneal macrophages
acid phosphatase activity in,
241
activation of by Ete, 586
antigen-treated, 355
Corynebacterium parvum and,
337
glucan interaction with, 284
growth inhibition of
mastocytoma cells by,
354
murine, see Murine peritoneal
macrophages
PHA and LPS inhibition by, 238
similarity and diversity of,
323-331
suppression of immune response
by addition of,
492-493
Peptidyl dipeptidase, 149
Peroxidase activity
in blood cell staining, 214-217
in mouse spleen cells, 8-10
phagocytosis and, 3
Peroxidase production, 3,
see also Hydrogen
peroxide
Pesticides
in food, 570
in human adipose tissue and
blood, 570
reticuloendothelial system and,
569-575
PFC response, see Plaque-forming
cell response
Phagocytes
hydrogen peroxide production
and degradation in, 59
"respiratory burst" in, 53-70
Phagocyte system, mononuclear,
see Mononuclear phagocyte
system
Phagocytic cells
physiological activities of,
37
types of, 29
Phagocytosing chicken
polymorphonuclear
leukocytes, hydrogen
peroxide and, 111-120
Phagocytosis
arachidonic acid in, 415
of bone marrow reticular cells,
198
of C3b-coated yeast cells,
327
of chicken red blood cells,
352
cytochalasin B and, 66
defined, 3
glucose utilization and, 3
hepatic, see Hepatic
phagocytosis
inhibition of by spleen
macrophages, 414
mediation of by complement
receptor, 324-327
mitochondrial oxygen
consumption in, 30
oleic acid and, 415
oxidative phosphorylation in,
31
by polymorphonuclear
leukocytes, 15
polysaccharide effect in,
259-260
prostaglandin role in,
413-416
"respiratory burst" in, 53-70
tobacco smoke exposure and,
563-564
PHA-P, see Phytohemagglutinin-P
Phenol derivatives,
immunodepressive effect
of, 523-528
Phenols, 498
Phorbol myristate acetate, 53
Phosphodiesterase I, as plasma
membrane marker enzyme,
39
Phospholipase C,
53

Phytohemagglutinin, 4
  in DNA synthesis suppression, 459
  RNA synthesis and, 501
Phytohemagglutinin response, of spleen cells, 500
Phytohemagglutinin stimulation, trypan blue effect on, 15
Pig peripheral leukocytes, disrupted, 76
Pinocytosis, PSK effect on, 260
Plaque-forming cell response
  alveolar macrophages and, 470, 477-478
  hydrogen peroxide and, 7
  Jerne hemolytic plaque assay for, 486
  in leukocyte-immune response studies, 4-5
  of macrophage-depleted lymphoid cells, 460, 465, 468
  RES suppression and, 489
  suppression of, 482
Plasma membranes
  digitonin in purification of, 188-191
  purification of from guinea pig peritoneal macrophages, 183-192
  ultrastructure analysis of, 186, 188
Plasma proteinase inhibitors, purification and properties of, 85-87
Plasmadium berghei, 307-308, 500, 524
Pleural cavity, nucleated cells in, 334-338
Pleural macrophages
  activation of by Corynebacterium parvum, 333-334
  antitumor activity of, 335
  mammary carcinoma and, 338
  tumor growth and, 335, 340
PMNL, see Polymorphonuclear leukocytes
Polycations, differential effect of on uptake and desulphation of heparin, 175-181
Polychlorinated biphenyl, 499
Polymorphonuclear leukocytes
  binding of peptides and compounds to, 371
  calcium concentration in, 37
  compared with monocytes in "respiratory burst," 57-58
  flavonoids in respiratory stimulation of, 372-373
  migration of, 377
  oxygen metabolism products in, 566
  phagocytosing chicken type, 111-120
  phagocytosis by, 15
  preparation of, 54-55
  regulation of by quercetin, 371-378
Polyornithine, in heparin uptake, 177-180
Polyphenolic disinfectant
  composition of, 527
  immunodepressive effect of, 531-532
Polysaccharides
  antitoxoplasmic effect of, 257
  HeLa cell monolayers and, 258
  mouse peritoneal macrophages and, 258
  particulate vs. water-soluble, 255-266
  phagocytic activity of macrophages treated with, 256-257
  phagocytosis and, 259-260
  toxoplasma infection and, 263
Prednisone, 152
Pronase treatment, 160, 163
Prostaglandins, in phagocytosis, 413-416
Proteinases
  chymotrypsin-like, 76
  leukocyte, see Leukocyte proteinases

Proteinases (cont'd)
  leukocyte intracellular inhibitors of, 75-83
  in rat macrophage binding receptors, 157-165
Protein-calorie malnutrition
  animal model of, 599-605
  humoral and cellular immunity in, 599-605
  immunomodulation and, 498
Pseudopterogorgia americana, 580
PSK, see Coriolus versicolor extract
Pulmonary alveolar macrophage, see also Alveolar macrophage
  sub-cellular morphology of, 557
  tobacco smoke and, 555-567
Purified splenic lymphocytes, SSF generation in, 441
Purulent exudates, of staphylococci, 126-127

Quercetin
  and Con-A-induced glycogen aggregation, 374
  as inhibitor of PMNL respiratory stimulation, 372-373
  in PMNL regulation and motility, 371-378
Rabbit alveolar macrophages
  angiotensin-converting enzyme and, 149-155
  BCG-induced, 39
  degradation of oxygen and hydrogen peroxide in, 59-60
  enzyme activity and, 44-50, 54, 62
Rabbits
  angiotensin-converting enzyme in macrophages of, 149-155
  "respiratory burst" in, 53-72
  secondary ocular immune response in, 381, 388
Rat alveolar macrophages, proteinase effect on binding receptors of, 157-165
Rat liver, increased hydrolytic capacity of, 232
Rat liver lysosomes, glucan and, 225-236
Rat peritoneal macrophages, proteinase effect on binding receptors of, 157-165
Rats
  angiotensin-converting enzyme in macrophages of, 150
  multiple LEM injections in, 408
Rat spleen macrophages, suppression of antibody-forming cells by, 485-494
Red tide, dinoflagellates and, 577-578
RES, see Reticuloendothelial system
Resorcinol, inhibition of leukocyte peroxidase activity by, 95
"Respiratory burst"
  in alveolar macrophages, 53-70
  concanavalin A and, 69
  hydrogen peroxide production and, 63
  oxygen consumption in, 56
Reticular cells
  of bone marrow, see Bone marrow reticular cells
  phagocytosis in, 198
  tissue culture and, 201
Reticuloendothelial cell activation, by glucan, 235-243
Reticuloendothelial clearance techniques, 103
Reticuloendothelial system
  altered insulin sensitivity and, 393-396
  in amyloidosis, 167
  blocking agents for, 486

Reticuloendothelial system (cont'd)
  of bone marrow, 195
  Corynebacterium parvum and, 333
  depression of, see Reticuloendothelial system depression
  factors incluencing function of, 390
  flow-cytophotometric studies of, 220-221
  glucose homeostasis and, 391-401
  lead acetate depression of, 23-25
  metabolism and, 403-409
  pesticides and, 569-575
  role of in lead salt sensitization to endotoxin shock, 21-27
  shock stimuli and, 101
  suppression of, 489-490
Reticuloendothelial system depression
  glucose tolerance and, 395-396
  hepatic gluconeogenesis and 396-399
  insulin lethality and, 395
  serum insulin levels and, 399-401
RNA synthesis, phytohemagglutinin and, 501

SAA protein, 167-172
  endotoxin-induced, 171
  enzyme inhibitors of, 171
  generation of by amloidogenic and nonamyloidogenic substances, 169
  purification of, 168
Saccharomyces cerevisiae, 225-234, 245, 269, 272, 288, 291, 304, 324-325
Salmonella bern, 499
Salmonella enterides, 391-392
Salmonella typhimurium, 137, 353, 409
Schizophyllan micro, 256
SEB, see Staphylococcal enterotoxin B
Serratia marcescens, 315, 321
Sheep erythrocytes, see Sheep red blood cells
Sheep red blood cells
  aged mice and, 364
  cholera toxin in antibody response to, 348-349
  IgM coating for, 324-326
  mouse hemolytic PFC response to, 5
  and mouse spleen cell peroxidase activity, 5-6, 8
  orthophenylphenol toxicity and, 532-533
  pooled rabbit antisera against, 158
  in PFC response, 469-480, 488, 491-493
  in phagocytosis studies, 2
Skin grafts
  marine organism substances and, 584
  ultraviolet-irradiated, 596
Smoking, see Tobacco smoke
SOD, see Superoxide dismutase
Spleen cells, see also Spleen macrophages
  co-cultivation with cells for CT-treated mice, 345-346
  in generation of CSF, 441-442
  mitogenic index of, 240
  phagocytosis inhibition by, 416, 532
Spleen weight, lymphocyte proliferation and, 239
Splenic lymphocytes
  binding of to alveolar macrophages, 542-551
  interaction with alveolar macrophages following asbestos inhalation, in rat, 539-552
Splenoperoxidase activity
  in mouse, 8-10
  redistribution and increase in, 17

Splenoperoxidase activity (cont'd)
  sub-cellular distribution of, 11
SPO, see Splenoperoxidase activity
SRBC, see Sheep red blood cells
Staphylococcal disease, glucan protection against, 302
Staphylococcal enterotoxin B, in CSF generation, 434-437, 444-445
Staphylococci, purulent exudates of, 127
Staphylococcus aureus, 134, 137, 287, 303, 434, 561-562
  experimental infection with, 291-304
  glucan-induced modification of, in mice, 291-304
  lysis of, 123-127
  mouse susceptibility to, 293-294
Staphylococcus epidermidis, 574
Stimulated macrophage populations, lysosomal enzyme level in, 324
Staphylococcus faecalis, lysis of, 123-127, 302
Superoxide anion
  for phagocytosing chicken polymorphonuclear leukocytes, 111-120
  phagocytosis and, 3
  production of, 113-114
Superoxide dismutase
  cytochrome c2 reduction and, 56-57
  as catalyst, 57
  cytochrome C reduction and, 113
  inhibition of, 566
Suppressor cell
  glucan and, 235-253
  properties of, 469
Syngeneic tumor models, glucan activity in, 284-285

TDCC, see 2,3,7,8-Tetrachloro-dibenzo-p-dioxin
T cells
  antigen binding to, 451-458
  modulation of by cholera toxin treatment, 343-349
2,3,7,8-Tetrachlorodibenzo-p-dioxin, 499-500
Tetrapeptide, see Tuftsin
^{3}H-Thymidine
  incorporation studies for, 4
  uptake of, 328-329
Tissue macrophages, see also Macrophages
  cytological characteristics of, 195-208
  endogenous peroxidase activity of, 198-202
  as "histiocytes," 207
  ultrastructural morphology of, 197
  in cerebrospinal fluid generation, 435-438
Tobacco smoke
  glucose metabolism and, 564
  oxygen metabolism and, 563
  phagocytosis and, 563
  pulmonary alveolar macrophage and, 555-567
Toxoplasma gondii, 255, 264
Toxoplasma infection
  cell-mediated immunity in, 255
  polysaccharides and, 263
Transcobalamin
  assay of, 422-423
  bleeding and, 425
  in bone marrow, 425-426
  concentration of, 425
  in peritoneal exudate cells, 425-427
  production of *in vitro*, 424
  serum concentrates of in health and disease, 421
  synthesis site for, 420
Triton X-100, 41
Trypan blue
  effect of on LPS-mediated mitogenesis by mouse spleen cells, 16

Trypan blue (cont'd)
  and immune response to sheep red blood cells in mice, 12-13
Trypsin treatment, on EA (IgG)-binding of rat macrophages, 159-160
Tuftsin
  activity of in free tetrapeptide state, 143
  analogs of, 142
  angiotensin II system and, 143
  assay of, 131-132
  in augmentation of macrophage activity to destroy cancer cells, 140-141
  bactericidal activity of, 136-138
  biological activity of, 137, 144
  biological and biochemical characteristics of, 131-145
  defined, 131
  enzymes in release of from leukokinin, 132-133
  and macrophage bactericidal activity, 135
  in phagocytosis stimulation, 144
  Rauscher murine leukemia virus and, 135
Tuftsin deficiency, acquired or congenital, 142
Tuftsin endocarboxypeptidase, 132
Tuftsin reception sites, 139
Tumor growth
  glucan-induced inhibition of, 269-288
Tumor growth (cont'd)
  LNPI effect in, 81-82
  marine organism substances and, 577-587
Tumor regression, DNCB and, 604
Tumors, ultraviolet radiation induction of, 589-597
Turtles, skin diseases of, 578

Ubiquinone, 361-368, see also Coenzyme Q deficiency
Ultraviolet-induced photoproduct, 595-596
Ultraviolet radiation
  carcinogenesis and, 589-597
  and delayed hypersensitivity to dinitrochlorobenzene, 590-595
  immune system and, 589-597

Vibrio cholerae, 343
Vitamin B_{12} binding proteins, 419-420
  see also Transcobalamin

White blood cells, residual myeloperoxidase activity of, 94
  see also Leukocytes

Yeast glucan, see Glucan

Zinc metabolism, RES role in, 403-409
Zymosan-stimulated cells
  metabolic inhibitors of oxygen consumption in, 32
  oxygen metabolism of, 30

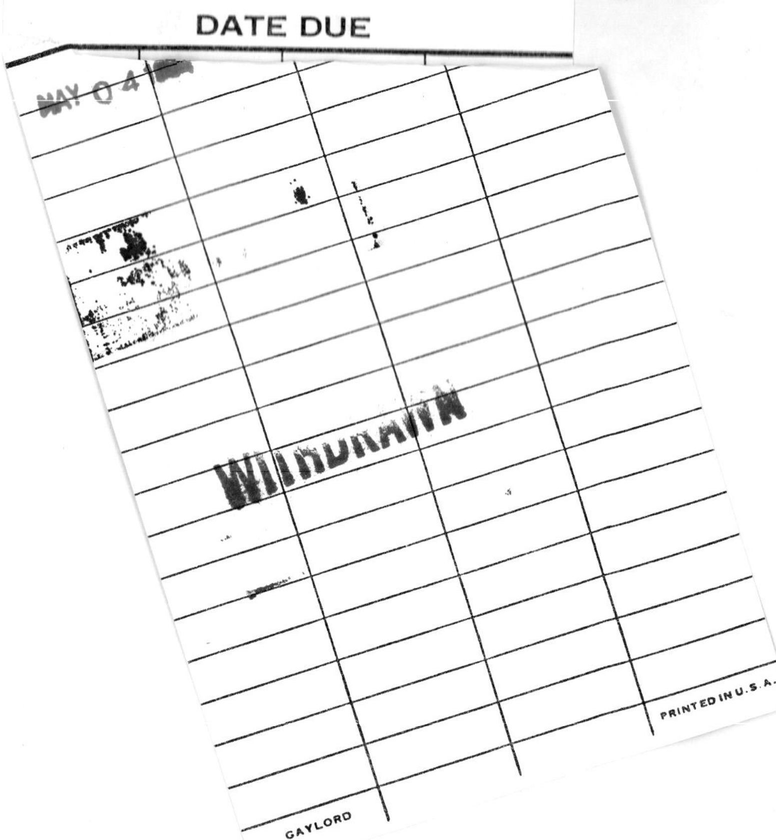
DATE DUE

MAY 0 4

WITHDRAWN

GAYLORD

PRINTED IN U.S.A.